MEDICAL ASSISTING
REVIEW

Passing the CMA, RMA, and Other Exams
Third Edition

Jahangir Moini, M.D., M.P.H.
Professor and Former Director of Allied Health Sciences
including Medical Assisting Program
Everest University, Melbourne, Florida

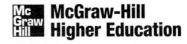

McGraw-Hill
Higher Education

Boston   Burr Ridge, IL   Dubuque, IA   New York   San Francisco   St. Louis
Bangkok   Bogotá   Caracas   Kuala Lumpur   Lisbon   London   Madrid   Mexico City
Milan   Montreal   New Delhi   Santiago   Seoul   Singapore   Sydney   Taipei   Toronto

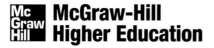
**McGraw-Hill
Higher Education**

MEDICAL ASSISTING REVIEW: PASSING THE CMA, RMA, AND OTHER EXAMS
Published by McGraw-Hill, a business unit of The McGraw-Hill Companies, Inc., 1221 Avenue of the Americas, New York, NY, 10020. Copyright © 2009 by The McGraw-Hill Companies, Inc. All rights reserved. Previous editions © 2001 and 2005. No part of this publication may be reproduced or distributed in any form or by any means, or stored in a database or retrieval system, without the prior written consent of The McGraw-Hill Companies, Inc., including, but not limited to, in any network or other electronic storage or transmission, or broadcast for distance learning.

Some ancillaries, including electronic and print components, may not be available to customers outside the United States.

This book is printed on acid-free paper.

3 4 5 6 7 8 9 0 DOW/DOW 0 9

ISBN 978-0-07-352087-2
MHID 0-07-352087-X

Vice President/Editor in Chief: *Elizabeth Haefele*
Vice President/Director of Marketing: *John E. Biernat*
Senior sponsoring editor: *Debbie Fitzgerald*
Managing developmental editor: *Patricia Hesse*
Freelance developmental editor: *Becky Barnhart, S4Carlisle Publishing Services*
Editorial assistant: *Shelle Mills*
Executive marketing manager: *Roxan Kinsey*
Lead media producer: *Damian Moshak*
Media producer: *Marc Mattson*
Director, Editing/Design/Production: *Jess Ann Kosic*
Lead project manager: *Susan Trentacosti*
Senior production supervisor: *Janean A. Utley*
Designer: *Srdjan Savanovic*
Senior photo research coordinator: *Lori Hancock*
Media project manager: *Mark A. S. Dierker*
Typeface: *10/12 Giovanni Book*
Compositor: *ICC Macmillan Inc.*
Printer: *R. R. Donnelley*
Cover credits: *Computer, blood draw, applying lead wires: Kathryn Booth, Total Care Programming, Inc.; DAQbilling® Practice Management Software screen shots were provided by Antek HealthWare, LLC. www.antekhealthware.com; blood pressure image: John Lund/Tiffany Schoepp, ©Gettyimages; background: David Gould, ©Gettyimages*
Credits: The credits section for this book begins on page 581 and is considered an extension of the copyright page.

Library of Congress Cataloging-in-Publication Data
Moini, Jahangir, 1942-
    Medical assisting review : passing the CMA, RMA, and other exams / Jahangir
Moini. -- 3rd ed.
        p. ; cm.
    Includes index.
    ISBN-13: 978-0-07-352087-2 (alk. paper)
    ISBN-10: 0-07-352087-X (alk. paper)
    1. Medical assistants--Examinations, questions, etc. 2. Physicians' assistants--
Examinations, questions, etc. I. Title.
    [DNLM: 1. Allied Health Personnel--Examination Questions. 2. Clinical Medicine--
methods--Examination Questions. W 18.2 M712m 2009]
R728.8.M653 2009
610.73'7069076--dc22

                                    2007052535

WARNING NOTICE: The clinical procedures, medicines, dosages, and other matters described in this publication are based upon research of current literature and consultation with knowledgeable persons in the field. The procedures and matters described in this text reflect currently accepted clinical practice. However, this information cannot and should not be relied upon as necessarily applicable to a given individual's case. Accordingly, each person must be separately diagnosed to discern the patient's unique circumstances. Likewise, the manufacturer's package insert for current drug product information should be consulted before administering any drug. Publisher disclaims all liability for any inaccuracies, omissions, misuse, or misunderstanding of the information contained in this publication. Publisher cautions that this publication is not intended as a substitute for the professional judgment of trained medical personnel.

The Internet addresses listed in the text were accurate at the time of publication. The inclusion of a Web site does not indicate an endorsement by the authors or McGraw-Hill, and McGraw-Hill does not guarantee the accuracy of the information presented at these sites.

www.mhhe.com

This book is fondly dedicated to:
The living memory of my father and my sister Pari
My loving mother and caring family:
My wife, Hengameh, and my daughters Mahkameh
and Morvarid
My colleagues, staff, past and present students at
Everest University
This book is dedicated to all medical assistants across the
United States.

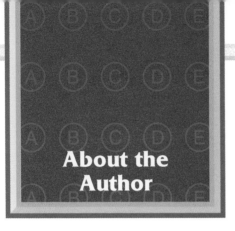

About the Author

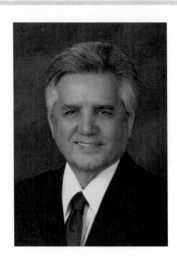

Dr. Moini was assistant professor at Tehran University School of Medicine for 9 years, teaching medical and allied health students. The author is a professor and former director (for 15 years) of allied health programs at Everest University (formerly Florida Metropolitan University). Dr. Moini re-established the Medical Assisting Program in 1990 at Everest University's Melbourne campus. He also established several other new allied health programs for Everest University.

Dr. Moini has been physician liaison of the Florida Society of Medical Assistants since 2000. He has been a marketing strategy team member of the National AAMA and president of the Brevard County chapter of the AAMA. He has been a published author of various allied health books since 1999.

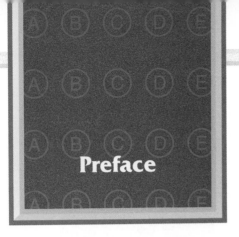

Preface

Medical Assisting Review: Passing the CMA, RMA, and Other Exams, third edition, is a comprehensive approach to reviewing the key competencies of a medical assisting program for the student preparing to take the CMA or RMA Medical Assistant certification exams. The book is divided into three parts: *Theory Review*, *Self-Evaluation*, and *Answers and Rationales*.

Theory Review

The first part, *Theory Review*, provides easy-to-read essential material summaries, which highlight key areas of a Medical Assistant's program. The chapters are organized into three sections that cover general, administrative, and clinical medical assisting knowledge. Chapters 1 through 8 cover General Medical Assisting, Chapters 9 through 14 cover Administrative Medical Assisting, and Chapters 15 through 24 cover Clinical Medical Assisting.

COMPETENCY CORRELATIONS

Each chapter correlates to the AAMA Role Delineation Competencies and RMA (AMT) Certification Exam Topics.

AT A GLANCE TABLES

At a Glance tables throughout the chapters summarize key information for quick review.

STRATEGIES TO SUCCESS

We have collected a number of tips that will help students study for and pass the certification exams. We call these tips *Strategies to Success*. There are two *Strategies to Success* features placed in every chapter, one at the beginning and one at the end of the chapter. In each chapter, the first tip will provide material to help improve a student's study skills and the second tip will enhance a student's test-taking skills. These skills are as essential as the material covered in this book.

CHAPTER REVIEW

At the end of each chapter, there are 20 to 40 multiple choice review questions that correlate with actual CMA and RMA-style questions. Each chapter review is followed by an answer key, so the book can be easily used for self-study.

Self-Evaluations with Answers and Rationales

This book contains three self-evaluations—General, Administrative, and Clinical—which correspond not only to the chapter divisions but also to the actual parts of the certification exams. The test for general medical assisting knowledge contains 250 questions, and it covers material contained in the first 8 chapters of the book, as well as some communication and professionalism content covered in Chapter 10. The test for administrative medical assisting knowledge contains 250 questions, and it covers material reviewed in Chapters 9 through 14. The last test covers the clinical medical assisting part of the book in 250 questions. Similar to the quizzes at the end of each chapter, these questions also follow both the CMA and RMA style. We recommend students answer as many of the questions as possible to familiarize themselves with the content covered on the exams. Practicing answering exam-style questions will increase the student's understanding of the material and raise confidence and test-taking abilities.

After students have taken a self-evaluation exam, they can find the correct answer and rationale for each question in the last section of the book. These rationales are not intended to be a complete review of the material; however, they can be used to refresh a student's memory about a specific topic and help him or her focus on areas that need improvement through further study and review.

HOW TO USE THIS BOOK

This book is intended for use in a Medical Assistant review course or for self-study before taking either the CMA or RMA exam. There are a number of ways to use this book.

In a classroom, it might be best to teach the *Theory Review* chapter by chapter and, at the end of the course, allow students to take the exams contained in the *Self-Evaluation* section to assess their knowledge. Instructors can tear out the perforated sheets and give students timed exams in the classroom or ask students to answer questions at home and check their own answers. Students can then come back to class with questions, and the class can review the material together.

A student using this book for self-study might find it more useful to begin with the *Self-Evaluations,* which can pinpoint strengths and weaknesses. If the answers and rationales are not sufficient in answering the student's questions, the student can consult the *Theory Review* section to refresh his or her memory about a specific topic.

STUDENT TUTORIAL AND TEST PREP CD-ROM SYSTEM REQUIREMENTS

To get the optimal results with the CD, your computer should have:

System Requirements

Windows

- Microsoft® Windows® 2000/XP/Vista™
- Minimum 256 MB main memory
- Internet browser

Macintosh

- OS X 10.2, OS X 10.3, or OS X 10.4
- Minimum 256 MB main memory
- Internet browser

RUNNING THE CD-ROM

If the CD-ROM does not start automatically, follow the instructions below:

Windows

1. Insert the CD-ROM into your CD-ROM drive.
2. Click on the Start button and select Run.
3. Type D:\Start_Here.exe and click OK (where D is your CD-ROM drive).

Macintosh

1. Insert the CD-ROM into your CD-ROM drive.
2. Double-click on the CD-ROM icon on the desktop.
3. Double-click the icon labeled Start_Here.

ABOUT THE CD-ROM

The software contains more than 1300 questions, which are a combination of questions taken from the text and new questions. Students will be able to take multiple chapter quizzes as well as comprehensive RMA- or CMA-style practice exams. We recommend that after reading each chapter, the student take the quiz for the chapter. After completing all the chapters in the *Theory Review* section, the student can start taking practice exams. If the student's scores are below 60% on these practice exams, the student should return to the appropriate chapters in the book to review the material. Please consult the help files on the CD-ROM for more information.

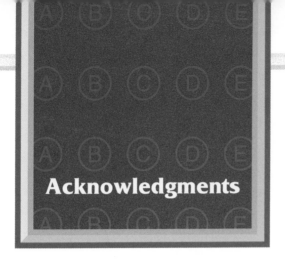

Acknowledgments

Sincere thanks go to the following McGraw-Hill staff for their considerable efforts, invaluable assistance, and vital guidance during the development of this book: Roxan Kinsey, Marketing Manager; Patricia Hesse, Developmental Editor; and the production team. The author would also like to thank Leesa Whicker, whose contribution made this text a more valuable tool in exam preparation.

Additionally, I would like to express my appreciation to McGraw-Hill for providing the artwork that helped illustrate this book.

REVIEWERS

Mary Barko, MAEd/AEDL
Ohio Institute of Health Careers
Elyria, OH

Barbara C. Berger, BSN, RN, MS, CMA
Northwestern Connecticut Community College
Winsted, CT

Mary Ellen Brown, CMA, PBT(ASCP)
Stone Academy, Medical Assisting Department
Hamden, CT

Diana Brumm
Professional Health Training Academy
Ocala, FL

Stephanie M. Denney, CMA, MS
Bryant & Stratton College
Syracuse, NY

David Drumm
CLN
Mechanicsburg, PA

Marianne Durling
Vance-Granville Community College
Henderson, NC

Brenda K. Frerichs
Colorado Technical University
Sioux Falls, SD

Dana L. Garrett, CMA
National American University–
    Albuquerque Campus
Albuquerque, NM

Tamra Greco
Davenport University
Kalamazoo, MI

Marsha Perkins Hemby
Pitt Community College
Winterville, NC

Dolly R. Horton, CMA, BS, M.Ed.
Mayland Community College
Spruce Pine, NC

Peggy Hughes
Allegany College of MD
Cumberland, MD

Nina Huntington, RN BSN, BA
Andover College
Portland, ME

Sheila Lambert
FastTrain
Clearwater, FL

Brian E. Lessard
American Commercial College
Wichita Falls, TX

Sandra Lessard, RN, CMA
Sawyer School
Hamden, CT

Dr. Conrado Martinez, MD
Health Occupations Dept. Cerritos College
Norwalk, CA

Angela N Mathews, NRCMA, NCET, NCPT
MedVance Institute of Ft. Lauderdale
Plantation, FL

Maureen M Mattia
Quinnipiac University, 1987–Stone Academy
Hamden, CT

Jean McGillvary, RN, BAAS
American Commercial College
Wichita Falls, TX

Monica M. Mitzenmacher, CPC
FastTrain
Miami, FL

Darlene Nelson
Gibbs College RI
Cranston, RI

Peggy Populo, BS, CMA
Duff's Business Institute
Pittsburgh, PA

Patricia E. Rondini, MALS, RRT
Branford Hall Career Institute
Southington, CT

Lynn G. Slack, CMA
ICM School of Business & Medical Careers
Pittsburgh, PA

Margie F. Smith
Ivy Tech Community College of Indiana
Greencastle, IN

Danielle Schortzmann Wilken
Goodwin College
East Hartford, CT

Victoria Wise
Owens Community College
Findlay, OH

Previous Reviewers

Second Edition:

Janet Roberts-Andersen, BS, MS, MT
Director of the Medical Assistant Program
Hamilton College
Urbandale, IA

Niccole Ostroff-Bologna, BS, CMA
Adjunct Professor and Academic Advisor
Florida Metropolitan University
Melbourne, FL

Susan Boulden, BSN, RN, CMA
Medical Assisting Program Director/Instructor
Mt. Hood Community College
Gresham, OR

Michael L. Decker, BS, MA
Instructor
Omaha College of Health Careers
Omaha, NE

Beulah A. Hofmann, RN, MSN, CMA
Ivy Tech State College
Terre Haute, IN

Deborah E. Holmes, RN, CMA, MLT
Medical Assistant Program Coordinator
Nebraska Methodist College
Omaha, NE

Charlotte A. Jensen, BS, MPS/HAS, CMA
Director of Medical Assistant Department
Cabrillo College
Aptos, CA

Barbara Lato, BSN, CMA
Program Director of the Medical Assistant Program
Mid-State Technical College
Marshfield, WI

Pat Gallagher Moeck, BA, MBA, CMA
Director of the Medical Assisting Program
El Centro College/Mountain View College
Dallas, TX

Susan Perreira, BS, CMA, RMA
Assistant Professor
Capital Community College
Hartford, CT

Teri A. Provenzano, CMA
VP, Owner, and Program Coordinator of the
Medical Assistant Program
Medical Careers Training Center
Somerville, NJ

Dyiane Saban, CMA
Medical Program Director
Bryman College
Gardena, CA

Beatrice Salada, BAS, CMA
Davenport University
Lansing, MI

Susan Schilling, BS, AA, CMA
Dean of Instruction
Bryant & Stratton
Syracuse, NY

Janet Sesser, BS, CMA, RMA
Corporate Director of Education, Allied Health
    Programs
Hightech Institute
Phoenix, AZ

Lynn G. Slack, CMA
Director, Medical Program
ICM School of Business and Medical Careers
Pittsburgh, PA

Janice Vermigilo-Smith, RN, MS, PhD
Central Arizona College
Apache Junction, AZ

Dana Stidham, BS, MS, TC
Medical Assisting Program Chair
Ivy Tech State College
Columbus, IN

Sylvia Taylor, AS, BS
Assistant Professor/MOA Director
Cleveland State Community College
Cleveland, TN

Barbara Ulto
Branford Hall Career Institute
Branford, CT

Fred Valdes, MD
City College
Ft. Lauderdale, FL

Bennita W. Vaughans, BA, MS
Medical Assisting Technology Program Director
H. Council Trenholm State Technical College
Montgomery, AL

Brenda Vetere, BS, MT
Externship Coordinator/Adjunct Faculty
Capital Community College
Hartford, CT

Leesa G. Whicker, BA, CMA
Program Chair, Medical Assisting
Central Piedmont Community College
Charlotte, NC

First Edition:

Janet Roberts-Andersen, BS, MS, MT
Director of the Medical Assistant Program
Hamilton College
Urbandale, IA

Susan Boulden, BSN, RN, CMA
Medical Assisting Program Director/Instructor
Mt. Hood Community College
Gresham, OR

Michael L. Decker, BS, MA
Instructor
Omaha College of Health Careers
Omaha, NE

Deborah E. Holmes, RN, CMA, MLT
Medical Assistant Program Coordinator
Nebraska Methodist College
Omaha, NE

Charlotte A. Jensen, BS, MPS/HAS, CMA
Director of the Medical Assistant Program
Cabrillo College
Aptos, CA

Barbara Lato, BSN, CMA
Program Director of the Medical Assistant
    Program
Mid-State Technical College
Marshfield, WI

Pat Gallagher Moeck, BA, MBA, CMA
Director of the Medical Assisting Program
El Centro College/Mountain View College
Dallas, TX

Susan Perreira, BS, CMA, RMA
Assistant Professor
Capitol Community College
Hartford, CT

Teri A. Provenzano, CMA
VP, Owner, and Program Coordinator of the
    Medical Assistant Program
Medical Careers Training Center
Somerville, NJ

Dyiane Saban, CMA
Medical Program Director
Bryman College
Gardena, CA

Susan Schilling, BS, AA, CMA
Dean of Instruction
Bryant & Stratton
Syracuse, NY

Janet Sesser, BS, CMA, RMA
Corporate Director of Education, Allied Health
    Programs
Hightech Institute
Phoenix, AZ

Lynn G. Slack, CMA
Director, Medical Programs
ICM School of Business and Medical Careers
Pittsburgh, PA

Dana Stidham, BS, MS, TC
Medical Assisting Program Chair
Ivy Tech State College
Columbus, IN

Sylvia Taylor, AS, BS
Assistant Professor/MOA Director
Cleveland State Community College
Cleveland, TN

Barbara Ulto
Branford Hall Career Institute
Branford, CT

Bennita W. Vaughans, BA, MS
Medical Assisting Technology Program Director
H. Council Trenholm State Technical College
Montgomery, AL

Brenda Vetere, BS, MT
Externship Coordinator/Adjunct Faculty
Capitol Community College
Hartford, CT

AAMA Role Delineation Study Areas of Competence (2003) Correlation Chart

Areas of Competence	Chapters
I. ADMINISTRATIVE	
A. Administrative Procedures	
1. Perform basic administrative medical assisting functions.	9, 10, 11
2. Schedule, coordinate, and monitor appointments.	9
3. Schedule inpatient/outpatient admissions and procedures.	9
4. Understand and apply third-party guidelines.	13, 14
5. Obtain reimbursement through accurate claims submissions.	13, 14
6. Monitor third-party reimbursement.	13
7. Understand and adhere to managed care policies and procedures.	13
* *Negotiate managed care contracts.*	
B. Practice Finance	
1. Perform procedural and diagnostic coding.	14
2. Apply bookkeeping principles.	12
3. Manage accounts receivable.	12
* *Manage accounts payable.*	12
* *Process payroll.*	12
* *Document and maintain accounting and banking records.*	12
* *Develop and maintain fee schedules.*	
* *Manage renewals of business and professional insurance policies.*	
* *Manage personnel benefits and maintain records.*	12
* *Perform marketing, financial, and strategic planning.*	
II. CLINICAL	
A. Fundamental Principles	
1. Apply principles of aseptic technique and infection control.	5, 15, 16, 17, 24
2. Comply with quality assurance practices.	16, 17, 24
3. Screen and follow up patient test results.	15, 16, 17, 20, 21, 22, 24
B. Diagnostic Orders	
1. Collect and process specimens.	16, 24
2. Perform diagnostic tests.	16, 17, 20, 21, 24
C. Patient Care	
1. Adhere to established patient screening procedures.	20, 23
2. Obtain patient history and vital signs.	20, 23, 24
3. Prepare and maintain examination and treatment areas.	16
4. Prepare patient for examinations, procedures, and treatments.	16, 20, 21, 22

Areas of Competence	Chapters
5. Assist with examinations, procedures, and treatments.	16, 20, 21, 22
6. Prepare and administer medications and immunizations.	19
7. Maintain medication and immunization records.	18, 19
8. Recognize and respond to emergencies.	20, 23, 24
9. Coordinate patient care information with other health-care providers.	13, 23
10. Initiate IV and administer IV medications with appropriate training and as permitted by state law.	19
III. GENERAL	
A. Professionalism	
1. Display a professional manner and image.	1, 8, 9, 10, 17
2. Demonstrate initiative and responsibility.	1, 9
3. Work as a member of the health-care team.	1, 9, 10, 17, 20, 21, 22
4. Prioritize and perform multiple tasks.	1, 9, 23
5. Adapt to change.	9
6. Promote the CMA credential.	1, 8
7. Enhance skills through continuing education.	1, 8
8. Treat all patients with compassion and empathy.	15, 16, 17, 20
9. Promote the practice through positive public relations.	1
B. Communication Skills	
1. Recognize and respect cultural diversity.	7, 8, 9, 10, 16, 17, 20
2. Adapt communications to individual's ability to understand.	7, 9, 10, 16, 17, 20, 24
3. Use professional telephone technique.	8, 9, 10
4. Recognize and respond effectively to verbal, nonverbal, and written communications.	9, 10, 16, 17, 20
5. Use medical terminology appropriately.	2, 3, 4, 5, 6, 7, 9, 10
6. Utilize electronic technology to receive, organize, prioritize, and transmit information.	8, 9, 11, 13
7. Serve as liaison.	9, 10
C. Legal Concepts	
1. Perform within legal and ethical boundaries.	1, 8, 9, 15, 16, 17, 20
2. Prepare and maintain medical records.	8, 9, 16, 22
3. Document accurately.	8, 9, 15, 16, 17, 20, 24
4. Follow employer's established policies dealing with the health-care contract.	8, 9, 13

Areas of Competence	Chapters
5. Implement and maintain federal and state health-care legislation and regulations.	8, 13, 15, 16, 18, 24
6. Comply with established risk management and safety procedures.	15, 17, 18, 20, 24
7. Recognize professional credentialing criteria.	1, 8, 24
* Develop and maintain personnel, policy, and procedure manuals.	8, 9, 20
D. Instruction	
1. Instruct individuals according to their needs.	6, 7, 9, 10, 15, 16, 21, 22
2. Explain office policies and procedures.	9, 16
3. Teach methods of health promotion and disease prevention.	7, 15, 16, 17
4. Locate community resources and disseminate information.	9, 15, 23
* Develop educational materials.	17
* Conduct continuing education activities.	
E. Operational Functions	
1. Perform inventory of office supplies and equipment.	23
2. Perform routine maintenance of administrative and clinical equipment.	
3. Apply computer techniques to support office operations.	11
* Perform personnel management functions.	
* Negotiate leases and prices for equipment and supply contracts.	
* Advanced skill	

AMT Registered Medical Assistant (RMA) Certified Exam Topics Correlation Chart

Exam Topics	Chapters
I. GENERAL MEDICAL ASSISTING KNOWLEDGE	
A. Orientation	
1. Introduction and review of program	1
2. Employment outlook	1
3. General responsibilities	1
B. Anatomy and Physiology	
1. Anatomy and physiology	3, 4
2. Diet and nutrition	7
3. Study of diseases and etiology	4, 5, 15
4. All body systems	3, 4
5. Diagnostic/treatment modalities	20, 21, 24
C. Medical Terminology	
1. Basic structure of medical words (roots, prefixes, suffixes, spelling, and definitions)	2
2. Combining word elements to form medical words	2
3. Medical specialties and short forms	2
4. Medical abbreviations	2
D. Medical Law and Ethics	
1. Ethical decisions, medical jurisprudence, and confidentiality	8
2. Legal terminology pertaining to office practice	8
3. Medical/ethical issues in today's society	8
4. Risk management	8
E. Psychology of Human Relations	
1. Dealing with difficult patients with normal/abnormal behavior	10
2. Caring for patients with special and specific needs	7, 10, 15, 16
3. Caring for cancer and terminally ill patients	10, 15
4. Emotional crisis/patients and/or family	10, 21
5. Various treatment protocols	15, 16
6. Basic principles	9, 10, 16
7. Developmental stages of the life cycle	
8. Hereditary, cultural, and environmental influences on behavior standards	7, 10

Exam Topics	Chapters
F. Career Development	
1. Instruction regarding internship rules and regulations	1
2. Job search, professional development, and success	1
3. Goal setting, time management, and employment opportunities	
4. Resume writing, interviewing techniques, and follow-up	
5. Dressing for success	1
6. Professionalism	1
II. ADMINISTRATIVE MEDICAL ASSISTING	
A. Medical Office Business Procedures/Management	
1. Manual and computerized records management	8, 9
(1) Patient case histories (confidentiality)	8, 9
(2) Filing	9
(3) Appointments and scheduling	9
(4) Inventory/control	
2. Financial Management	
(1) Basic bookkeeping	12
(2) Billing and collections	12
(3) Purchasing	12
(4) Banking and payroll	12
3. Insurance (including HMOs, PPOs, co-pays, CPT coding, etc.)	13, 14
4. Equipment and supplies (including ordering/maintaining/ storage/inventory)	
5. Reception, public, and interpersonal relations	10
(1) Telephone techniques	9
(2) Professional conduct and appearance	9, 10
(3) Professional office environment and safety	9
6. Office safety and security	
B. Basic Keyboarding	
1. Office machines, transcriptions, computerized systems/medical data processing	11
2. Transcribing medical correspondence and medical reports	11
3. Medical terminology review	11
III. CLINICAL MEDICAL ASSISTING	
A. Medical Office Clinical Procedures	
1. Basic clinical skills (e.g., vital signs)	16

Exam Topics	Chapters
2. Basic skills and procedures used in medical emergencies	23
3. Patient examination	16
(1) Patient histories	16, 23, 24
(2) Patient preparation	16
(3) Physical exam	16, 20, 21, 22
(4) Instruments	16
(5) Assisting the physician	16, 20, 21, 22
(6) Housekeeping	16
4. Medical Equipment	
(1) Electrocardiogram, centrifuge, etc.	16, 20
(2) Physical therapy	22
(3) Radiology	
(a) Safety	21
(b) Patient preparation	21
(c) Radiography of chest and extremities	21
(4) Medical asepsis/sterilization and minor office surgery	5
(5) Specialties	16
(6) First Aid, CPR	20, 22, 23, 24
(7) Injections (dosage calculations)	19
(a) IM	19
(b) Subq	19
(c) ID	19
(8) Universal precautions in the medical office	5, 15, 16, 17, 20, 24
B. Medical Laboratory Procedures	
1. Orientation	
(1) Laboratory equipment and maintenance	24
(2) Safety	24
(3) Storage of chemicals and supplies	24
(4) Fire safety	24
(5) Care of microscope (introduction)	24
2. Urinalysis	
(1) Specimen collection	24
(2) Physical exam	24

Exam Topics	Chapters
(3) Chemical analysis	24
(4) Microscopic exam	24
3. Hematology	
(1) Personal protection equipment	24
(2) Specimen collection	24
(a) Venipuncture	24
(b) Finger puncture	24
(3) Hemoglobin	24
(4) Hematocrit	24
(5) WBC	24
(6) RBC	24
(7) Slide preps	24
(8) Serology	24
(a) Blood typing	24
(b) Blood morphology	24
(9) Quality control	24
4. Basic blood chemistries	24
5. HIV/AIDS and blood-borne pathogens	15, 24
6. OSHA compliance rules and regulations	15, 17, 24
C. Pharmacology	
1. Occupational math and metric conversions (drug calculations)	18, 19
2. Use of PDRs and medication books	18, 19
3. Common abbreviations used in prescription writing	18, 19
4. Legal aspects of writing prescriptions	18, 19
5. PDA and state laws	18, 19
6. Medications prescribed for the treatment of illness and disease based on a systems method	18, 19

Brief Table of Contents

Part 3	**Self-Evaluation Answers and Rationales**	

Table of Contents

Theory Review

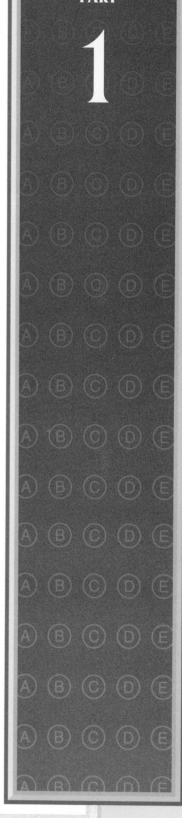

PART

1

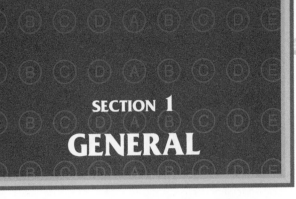

SECTION 1
GENERAL

MEDICAL ASSISTING KNOWLEDGE

Theory Review

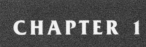

CHAPTER 1

The Profession of Medical Assisting

CHAPTER OUTLINE

The Profession of Medical Assisting

The Duties of a Medical Assistant
Specialization

Membership in a Medical Assisting Association

Certification and Registration

Medical Assisting Credentials

State and Federal Regulations
CMA Certification
RMA Registration

CMA and RMA Examination Topics

Externships

References and Portfolios

Preparing for Employment

Personal Attributes

MEDICAL ASSISTING COMPETENCIES

COMPETENCY	CMA	RMA
General/Legal/Professional		
Respond to and initiate written communications by using correct grammar, spelling, and formatting techniques	X	X
Recognize and respond to verbal and nonverbal communications by being attentive and adapting communication to the recipient's level of understanding	X	X

MEDICAL ASSISTING COMPETENCIES (concl.)

COMPETENCY	CMA	RMA
General/Legal/Professional		
Be aware of and perform within legal and ethical boundaries	X	X
Demonstrate knowledge of and monitor current federal and state health-care legislation and regulations; maintain licenses and accreditation	X	X
Exercise efficient time management		X
Project a positive attitude		X
Be a "team player"		X
Exhibit initiative		X
Adapt to change		X
Evidence a responsible attitude		X
Be courteous and diplomatic		X
Conduct work within scope of education, training, and ability		X
Be impartial and show empathy when dealing with patients		X
Understand allied health professions and credentialing		X

The Profession of Medical Assisting

Medical assisting is one of the most versatile health-care professions. Men and women can be equally successful as medical assistants. They are able to work in a variety of administrative and clinical positions within health care. According to the U.S. Department of Labor's *Occupational Outlook Handbook,* medical assisting is one of the 10 fastest growing occupations through the year 2008.

The Duties of a Medical Assistant

Medical assistants are skilled health-care professionals who work primarily in ambulatory settings such as medical offices and clinics. The duties a medical assistant may perform include administrative and clinical duties.

Administrative duties: Administrative medical assisting duties include the following:

- Greeting patients
- Handling correspondence
- Scheduling appointments
- Answering telephones
- Using computers, facsimile (fax) machines, and other automated office equipment

- Communicating with patients, families, and coworkers
- Creating and maintaining patient medical records
- Handling billing, bookkeeping, and insurance claim form processing
- Performing medical transcription
- Arranging for hospital admissions and testing procedures
- Organizing and managing office supplies
- Educating patients

Clinical duties: Medical assistants' clinical duties vary according to state law. They may include the following:

- Asepsis and infection control
- Preparing the examination and treatment areas
- Interviewing patients and documenting patients' vital signs and medical histories
- Preparing patients for examinations and explaining treatment procedures to patients
- Assisting the physician during examinations
- Disposing of contaminated (soiled or stained) supplies
- Performing diagnostic tests, such as electrocardiograms (ECGs)

- Giving injections (where allowed by local or state law)
- Performing first aid and cardiopulmonary resuscitation (CPR)
- Preparing and administering medications as directed by the physician, and following state laws for invasive procedures
- Removing sutures or changing the dressings on wounds
- Sterilizing medical instruments
- Assisting patients from diverse cultural backgrounds, as well as assisting patients with hearing or vision impairments, or physical or mental disabilities
- Educating patients

Medical assistants' clinical duties may also include processing various laboratory tests. Medical assistants may prepare the patient for the test, collect the sample, complete the test, report the results to the physician, and report information about the test from the physician to the patient. Specific laboratory duties may include:

- Performing tests, such as a urine pregnancy test, in the physician's office laboratory (POL)
- Collecting, preparing, and transmitting laboratory specimens, including blood and urine specimens
- Teaching patients to collect specific specimens properly
- Arranging laboratory services
- Meeting safety standards and fire protection mandates
- Performing as an Occupational Safety & Health Administration (OSHA) compliance officer

Specialization

A medical assistant may work with a wide variety of allied health professionals. In addition, medical assistants may choose to specialize in a specific field of health care, either in an administrative or clinical area. For example, ophthalmic medical assistants help ophthalmologists (physicians who provide eye care) by administering diagnostic tests, measuring and recording vision, testing the functioning of a patient's eyes and eye muscles, and performing other duties.

Administrative specialty areas include the following:

- Ward secretary
- Medical office administrator
- Dental office administrator
- Medical transcriptionist
- Medical record technologist
- Coding, billing, and insurance specialist

Clinical specialty areas include the following:

- Histologic technician
- Surgical technologist
- Physical therapy assistant
- CPR instructor
- Medical laboratory assistant
- Phlebotomist

Membership in a Medical Assisting Association

Certification and Registration

Certification or registration is not required to practice as a medical assistant. You may practice with a high school diploma or the equivalent. However, you will have more career options if you graduate from an accredited school and become certified or registered.

A solid medical assisting program provides the following:

- Facilities and equipment that are up to date
- Job placement services
- A cooperative education program and opportunities for continuing education

Medical Assisting Credentials

Professional associations set high standards for quality and performance in a profession. They define the tasks and functions of an occupation. They also provide members with the opportunity to communicate and network with one another.

State and Federal Regulations

Certain provisions of the Occupational Safety and Health Act (OSHA) and the Clinical Laboratory Improvements Act of 1988 (CLIA '88) are making mandatory credentialing for medical assistants a logical step in the hiring process. Currently, OSHA and CLIA '88 do not require that medical assistants be credentialed. However, various components of these statutes and their regulations can be met by demonstrating that medical assistants in a clinical setting are certified.

One of the CLIA regulatory categories based on their potential risk to public health is waived tests. Waived tests are: "Laboratory examination and procedures that have been approved by the Food and Drug Administration for home use or that, as determined by the secretary, are simple laboratory examinations and procedures that have an insignificant risk of an erroneous result."

CMA Certification

The Certified Medical Assistant (CMA) credential is awarded by the Certifying Board of the American Association of Medical Assistants (AAMA). The AAMA works to raise the standards of medical assisting to a more professional level. It is the only professional association devoted exclusively to the medical assisting profession. Figure 1-1 shows the pin worn by medical assistants who are certified by the AAMA.

The idea for a national association of medical assistants, which eventually became the AAMA, began at the 1955 annual state convention of the Kansas Medical Assistants Society. The next year, at an American Medical Association (AMA) meeting, the AAMA was officially created. In 1978, the U.S. Department of Health, Education, and Welfare declared medical assisting an allied health profession. The AAMA's website address is www.aama-ntl.org.

The AAMA Role Delineation Study: In 1996, the AAMA formed a committee. Its goal was to revise and update the standards it used for the accreditation of medical assisting programs. The committee's findings were published in 1997 under the title of the "AAMA Role Delineation Study: Occupational Analysis of the Medical Assisting Profession." Included in the publication was a new Role Delineation Chart that outlined the areas of competence entry-level medical assistants must master. The Role Delineation Chart was further updated in 2003. The AAMA's certification examination evaluates the mastery of medical assisting competencies on the basis of the 2003 Role Delineation Study. The National Board of Medical Examiners (NBME) also provides technical assistance in developing the tests. Its website address is www.nbme.org.

The areas of competence listed in the AAMA Role Delineation Study must be mastered by all students enrolled in accredited medical assisting programs. Each of the three areas of competence—administrative, clinical, and general (or transdisciplinary)—contains a list of statements that describe the medical assistant's role.

According to the AAMA, the Role Delineation Chart may be used to:

- Describe the field of medical assisting to other health-care professionals
- Identify entry-level competency areas for medical assistants
- Help practitioners assess their own current competence in the field
- Aid in the development of continuing education programs
- Prepare appropriate types of materials for home study

Professional support for CMAs: When you become a member of the AAMA, you will have a large support group of active medical assistants. Membership benefits include:

- Professional publications, such as *CMA Today*
- A large variety of educational opportunities
- Legal counsel
- Group insurance

RMA Registration

The Registered Medical Assistant (RMA) credential is given by the American Medical Technologists (AMT), an organization founded in 1939. RMA credentialing by the AMT ensures that you have taken and passed the AMT certification examination for the Registered Medical Assistant. RMA is a generic term used by the American Registry of Medical Assistants since 1950 and by the AMT since 1984. Figure 1-2 shows the pin worn by medical assistants who are certified by the AMT. The AMT's website address is www.amt1.com.

Professional support for RMAs: The AMT offers many benefits for RMAs. These include:

- Membership in the AMT Institute for Education
- Group insurance programs, including liability, health, and life
- State chapter activities
- Legal representation in health legislative matters
- Annual meeting and educational seminars

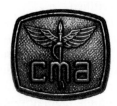

Figure 1-1 *This pin is worn by members of the American Association of Medical Assistants.*

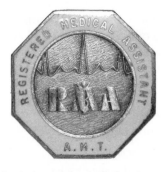

Figure 1-2 *This pin is worn by medical assistants registered by the American Medical Technologists.*

CMA and RMA Examination Topics

The CMA and RMA qualifying examinations are rigorous. Participation in an accredited program, however, will help you learn what you need to know. The examinations cover several distinct areas of knowledge. These include:

- Administrative knowledge, including medical records management, collections, insurance processing, and HIPAA (Health Insurance Portability and Accountability Act)
- Clinical knowledge, including examination room techniques; the preparation, calculation, and administration of medications; performing ECGs; and specimen collection
- General medical knowledge, including terminology, behavioral science, and medical law and ethics

Externships

An externship offers you work experience while you complete a medical assisting program. You will practice skills learned in the classroom in an actual medical office environment. The term "externship" is interchangeable with "internship"; these two words have the same meaning. A medical assisting extern must be able to accept constructive criticism, be flexible, and also be willing to learn. In an externship, you may be exposed to some procedures that are not performed exactly as you were taught. It is not professional to argue with the externship preceptor—there is usually more than one way to get the desired result in patient care.

References and Portfolios

In addition to enhancing medical assisting skills, an externship offers an opportunity to acquire a good reference. A medical assistant's reference is usually written by a supervisor. This reference will describe the student's performance, strengths, and skills. A reference is one part of the medical assistant's portfolio. In addition to a letter of reference, a portfolio typically contains a list of references, the student's resume, any certifications acquired (for example, CPR certification), and other documents of interest that detail volunteer service in a health-related field.

Preparing for Employment

The next phase of beginning a new career is seeking a position as a medical assistant. Most accredited schools have a Career Services department whose primary focus is job placement after graduation. Career Services employees will assist you with your resume, interviewing skills, and learning about positions in your field. Medical assistants can also learn about available positions by using classified ads, Internet sites, and employment services and by networking with colleagues, relatives, and friends.

Personal Attributes

Medical assistants can be more effective and productive if they have the personal qualifications of professionalism, empathy, flexibility, self-motivation, integrity, and honesty. A neat and professional appearance is also essential.

Professionalism: A medical assistant should demonstrate courtesy, conscientiousness, and a generally businesslike manner at all times. It is essential for medical assistants to act professionally with patients, doctors, and coworkers. You represent the physician's practice and should treat all patients with dignity and kindness. It is important to begin acting like a professional even while you are in the classroom studying to become a medical assistant. Present a neat appearance, and show courtesy and respect for peers and instructors.

Professionalism is also displayed in your attitude. The medical assistant is a skilled professional on whom many people, including coworkers and patients, depend. Your attitude can make or break your career. A professional always projects a positive, caring attitude. In the workplace environment, a professional medical assistant is pleasant and courteous and conducts herself in a businesslike and professional manner.

Empathy: Empathy is the ability to put yourself in someone else's situation—to identify with and understand another person's feelings. Patients who are sick, frustrated, or frightened appreciate empathetic medical personnel.

Flexibility: An attitude of flexibility will allow you to adapt to and to handle situations with professionalism. For example, when a physician's schedule changes to include evening and weekend hours, the staff may also be asked to change their schedules. Therefore, you must be flexible and meet the employer's needs.

Self-motivation: You must be self-motivated and offer assistance with work that needs to be done, even if it is not your assigned job. For example, if a coworker is on sick leave or vacation, offer to pitch in and work extra time to keep the office running smoothly.

Integrity and honesty: A medical assistant with integrity holds himself to high standards. Every task must be performed with the goal of excellence. Individuals with integrity have great pride in everything they do. Integrity may be characterized by honesty, dependability, and reliability. The most important elements in providing superior customer service to patients are integrity and honesty. If you make an error, be honest about it. In order to have integrity, you must be dependable and reliable. Everyone in the office must be able to trust you and the decisions you make.

Neat appearance: Medical facilities expect externs and their staff to appear as medical professionals. Most require a uniform that consists of a scrub top and bottom and a lab jacket. Your scrubs should be clean, pressed, and well fitting. Shoes should be clean, white, and in good repair. Your name tag or badge should always be worn and visible to patients. Nails should be clean and trimmed. Facial and tongue piercings are not acceptable when working with patients, and visible tattoos must be covered. Your hair should be a natural color and pulled back from your face and off the collar. If you wear makeup, it should be conservative and in good taste. Perfumes and colognes should be avoided because patients with respiratory conditions or allergies may not be able to tolerate them.

CHAPTER 1 REVIEW

D1122306

Instructions:

Answer the following questions. Check your answers in the *Answer Key* that follows this section.

1. Which of the following words best describes a medical assistant who works effectively as a team member in the medical office?

   A. Passive
   B. Obtrusive
   C. Argumentative
   D. Accountable
   E. Aggressive

2. Accreditation may be defined as

   A. A contract that specifies an agreement
   B. Permission to engage in a profession
   C. Permission to be licensed
   D. An assessment of an individual's performance
   E. A process in which recognition is granted to an education program

3. Which one of the following organizations declared medical assisting an allied health profession?

   A. U.S. Department of Justice
   B. U.S. Department of Health, Education, and Welfare
   C. U.S. Department of Health and Human Services
   D. Occupational Safety and Health Administration
   E. American Association of Medical Assistants

4. Which of the following organizations offers the Registered Medical Assistant credential?

   A. AMA
   B. AAMA
   C. AMT
   D. CDC
   E. NBME

5. The CMA and RMA examinations cover all of the following distinct areas of knowledge except

   A. Calculations for preparing medications
   B. HIPAA
   C. Criminal justice
   D. Medical records
   E. Behavioral science

6. Which of the following organizations publishes the journal *Professional Medical Assistants?*

   A. Centers for Disease Control and Prevention
   B. AMT
   C. AMA
   D. AAMA
   E. The Medical Labor Union

7. Which of the following professional attributes indicates the ability to understand someone else's situation?

   A. Empathy
   B. Professionalism
   C. Self-motivation
   D. Integrity
   E. Flexibility

8. The goal of the 1996 AAMA Role Delineation Study was to

   A. Revise and update the CMA exam questions
   B. Revise and update the standards used for the accreditation of medical assisting programs
   C. Create a new role and policy of practicing medicine
   D. Establish a new organization that would combine the AAMA and AMT into one organization
   E. Publish all materials needed for medical assisting programs

9. The initials CMA listed after a medical assistant's name indicate
   A. A professional person
   B. Registration
   C. A multiskilled person
   D. Compliance
   E. Credentials

10. After you become a certified medical assistant, how often is recertification required?
    A. Every year
    B. Every 2 years
    C. Every 3 years
    D. Every 5 years
    E. Every 7 years

11. Which of the following terms refers to legal, mental, or moral responsibility?
    A. Knowledge
    B. Trust
    C. Accountability
    D. Reputation
    E. Concern

12. Which of the following is allowed as long as the medical assisting credential remains current?
    A. Registration
    B. Reciprocity
    C. Accreditation
    E. Endorsement
    F. Recertification

13. Which of the following behaviors might be displayed by a medical assistant who is behaving unprofessionally?
    A. Knocking on the door before entering the examination room
    B. Using a term of endearment when talking to a patient
    C. Explaining long delays to patients waiting in the reception area
    D. Being calm while dealing with an angry patient
    E. Thanking a patient for paying for services

14. Which of the following terms describes behaving courteously, conscientiously, and in a generally businesslike manner?
    A. Self-motivation
    B. Professionalism
    C. Job description
    D. Ethics
    E. Morals

ANSWER KEY

1.	D	8.	B
2.	E	9.	E
3.	B	10.	D
4.	C	11.	C
5.	C	12.	E
6.	D	13.	B
7.	A	14.	B

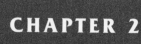

CHAPTER 2

Medical Terminology

MEDICAL ASSISTING COMPETENCIES

COMPETENCY	CMA	RMA
General/Legal/Professional		
Use appropriate medical terminology		X

▶ *Study Skills*

Organize and manage!

Organize your notes after class. Doing so will not only help you review material but also make it easier to understand your notes when you go back to them to study for an exam. Organizing your notes right away will also give you plenty of time to ask your instructor to clarify something you didn't understand.

Word Building

Root: The main part of a word that gives the word its central meaning. The root is the basic foundation of a word that can be made more complex through the addition of other word parts.

Prefix: A structure at the beginning of a word that modifies the meaning of the root. Not all medical words have a prefix. An example of a prefix can be found in the word *hypolipemia. Hypo-* is the prefix, *lip* is the root, and *-emia* is the suffix. For a list of common prefixes, see Table 2-1.

Suffix: A word ending that modifies the meaning of the root. Not all words have a suffix. An example of a suffix can be found in the word *ganglionectomy. Ganglion* is the root and *-ectomy* is the suffix. For a list of common suffixes, see Table 2-2.

Combining vowels: When a medical term is formed from many different word parts, these parts are often joined by a vowel. This vowel is usually an *o* and occasionally an *i*. For example, *o* serves as a combining vowel in the word *hyperlipoproteinemia (hyper / lip / o / protein / emia)*. The vowel *o* is the most common combining vowel. The combining vowel is used to ease

AT A GLANCE	Common General Prefixes		
Prefix	**Meaning**	**Example**	**Definition**
a-	Without	Aphonia	Inability to produce sound
ab-	From, away from	Abduct	To move away from the midline of the body
ad-, ac-, af-, ag-, al-, ap-, ar-, as-, at-	Toward, increasing	Adduct	To move toward the midline of the body
alb-	White	Albinism	Whiteness of skin, hair, and eyes caused by the absence of pigment
ambi-	Both	Ambidextrous	Able to use both hands effectively
ana-	Up, upward, toward	Anaphylactic	Characterized by an exaggerated reaction to an antigen or toxin
ante-	Before	Antepartum	Before childbirth
anti-	Against	Antibiotic	Acting against microorganisms

Table 2-1

Prefix	Meaning	Example	Definition
auto-	Self	Autodermic	Of the patient's own skin (said of skin grafts)
bi-	Two, both	Bilateral	Pertaining to both sides
bio-	Life	Biology	Study of life
circum-	Around	Circumcision	Removal of the skin around the tip of the penis
con-, col-, com-, cor-	Together, with	Congenital	Accompanying birth, present at birth
contra-	Against	Contraceptive	Preventing conception
de-	Away from, down, not	Decalcify	To decrease or remove calcium
dia-	Through	Diagnosis	Knowledge through testing
dis-	Apart, separate	Dislocation	Removal of any part of the body from its normal position
dys-	Bad, difficult, painful, poor	Dysuria	Painful urination
ec-	Out, away	Ectopic	Pertaining to something outside its normal location
ecto-	Outside	Ectoplasm	Outermost layer of cell protoplasm
en-, em-	In	Endemic	Occurring continuously in a population
		Empyema	Pus in a body cavity
endo-	Within	Endoscope	Instrument to examine something from within
epi-	Upon, over	Epidermal	Upon the skin
eu-	Good	Eupnea	Normal, good breathing
ex-, e-	Out, away	Exhale	To breathe out
		Emanation	Something given off
hemi-	Half	Hemicardia	Half of the heart
hyper-	Excessive, beyond	Hyperlipemia	Condition of excessive fat in the blood

Table 2-1, continued

Prefix	Meaning	Example	Definition
hypo-	Below, under	Hypoglycemia	Low blood sugar
in-, il-, im-, ir-	Not	Impotence	Inability to achieve erection
infra-	Below, under, beneath	Inframammary	Below the breast
inter-	Between	Intercellular	Between cells
intra-	Within	Intravenous	Within a vein
iso-	Equal	Isometric	Of equal dimension
juxta-	Near, beside	Juxtaarticular	Near a joint
mal-	Bad	Malaise	Discomfort
mega-, megal- / o	Large	Megacephaly	Abnormal enlargement of the head
mes- / o	Middle	Mesoderm	Middle layer of the skin
meta-	Beyond, after	Metastasis	Spread of disease from one part of the body to another
micro-	Small	Microscope	Instrument used to view small organisms
milli-	One-thousandth	Milliliter	One-thousandth of a liter
mono-	One, single	Mononuclear	Having only one nucleus
multi-	Many	Multidisciplinary	Pertaining to many areas of study
neo-	New, recent	Neonatal	Pertaining to the period after birth
non-	Not	Noninvasive	Not invading the body through any organ, cavity, or skin (said of a diagnostic or therapeutic technique)
para-	Near, beside, beyond, opposite, abnormal	Paramedic	Person who provides emergency medical care (alongside other medical personnel)
per-	Through	Percutaneous	Through the skin
peri-	Around, surrounding	Perianal	Around the anus
poly-	Many	Polyarthritis	Inflammation of many joints

Table 2-1, continued

Prefix	Meaning	Example	Definition
post-	After	Postmortem	After death
pre-	Before	Premature	Before maturation
primi-	First	Primiparous	Having given birth for the first time
re-	Again, back	Reactivate	To make active again
retro-	Back, backward, behind	Retrograde	Going backward
rube-	Red	Rubella	Viral disease characterized by red rashes, among other things
semi-	Half	Semiconscious	Half conscious
sub-	Under, below	Sublingual	Under the tongue
super-	Above, excessive	Superficial	Near or above the surface
supra-	Above, over	Suprapubic	Above the pubic area
syn-, sym-	Together	Symbiosis	Mutual interdependence
tri-	Three	Triceps	Muscle with three heads
uni-	One	Unicellular	One-celled
ultra-	Beyond, excessive	Ultrasound	Sound with a very high frequency, used to obtain medical images

Table 2-1, concluded

Suffix	Meaning	Example	Definition
-ac	Pertaining to	Cardiac	Pertaining to the heart
-ad	Toward	Cephalad	Toward the head
-al	Pertaining to	Thermal	Pertaining to the production of heat
-ar	Pertaining to	Articular	Pertaining to a joint
-desis	Binding	Arthrodesis	Surgical binding or fusing of a joint

Table 2-2

Suffix	Meaning	Example	Definition
-e	Noun marker	Dermatome	Instrument used to cut the skin
-ectomy	Excision, removal	Hysterectomy	Removal of the entire uterus
-emesis	Vomit	Hyperemesis	Excessive vomiting
-form	Resembling, like	Vermiform	Shaped like a worm
-genic	Beginning, originating, producing	Toxigenic	Producing toxins
-genetic	Beginning, originating, producing	Virogenetic	Caused by a virus, having a viral origin
-gram	Record	Electrocardiogram	Record of the variations in electrical potential caused by the heart muscle
-graph	Instrument for recording	Electrocardiograph	Instrument for making electrocardiograms
-graphy	Process of recording	Electrocystography	Process of recording the changes of electric potential in the urinary bladder
-iasis	Condition, formation	Lithiasis	Formation or presence of stones
-iatric	Pertaining to medical treatment	Pediatric	Pertaining to the treatment of children
-iatry	Study or field of medicine	Psychiatry	Study of the human psyche
-ic	Pertaining to	Thoracic	Pertaining to the thorax
-ical	Pertaining to	Neurological	Pertaining to nerves
-ism	Condition	Cryptorchidism	Condition of undescended testes
-ist	Specialist	Gynecologist	Physician who specializes in the female reproductive system
-itis	Inflammation	Appendicitis	Inflammation of the appendix
-logist	Specialist in the study of	Microbiologist	Biologist who specializes in the study of microorganisms
-logy	Study of	Microbiology	Study of microorganisms
-lysis	Destruction, breaking down	Hemolysis	Breaking down of blood

Table 2-2, continued

Suffix	Meaning	Example	Definition
-megaly	Enlargement	Cardiomegaly	Enlargement of the heart
-meter	Instrument used to measure	Scoliosometer	Instrument for measuring the curves of the spine
-oma	Tumor	Carcinoma	Cancerous, malignant tumor
-ory	Pertaining to	Auditory	Pertaining to hearing
-osis	Condition, disease	Leukocytosis	Condition of increased leukocytes in the blood
-pathy	Disease	Hemopathy	Disease of the blood
-penia	Abnormal reduction	Leukocytopenia	Decrease in the number of white blood cells
-philia	Attraction	Necrophilia	Attraction to dead bodies
-phobia	Abnormal fear	Photophobia	Fear of light
-plasia	Development	Dysplasia	Faulty formation
-plasty	Molding, surgical repair	Rhinoplasty	Surgical repair of the nose
-ptosis	Drooping, prolapse, falling	Mastoptosis	Drooping of the breast
-rrhage, -rrhagia	Excessive flow, discharge	Hemorrhage	Bursting forth of blood
-rrhea	Discharge, flow	Amenorrhea	Absence of menstrual flow
-rrhexis	Rupture	Cardiorrhexis	Rupture of the heart
-scope	Instrument used to view	Oscilloscope	Instrument that displays visual representation of electrical variations
-scopy	Process of viewing with a scope	Opthalmoscopy	Process of examining the interior of the eye by using an opthalmoscope
-stasis	A standing still, control, stoppage	Hemostasis	A stopping of the flow of blood
-stomy	Surgical creation of a new opening	Colostomy	Creation of an opening between the colon and the surface of the body
-tomy	Incision, cutting	Phlebotomy	Incision into a vein

Table 2-2, concluded

Abbreviation	Meaning	Abbreviation	Definition
Ht	Height	R	Right
Hx	History	R/O	Rule out
I & D	Incision and drainage	re✓	Recheck
inj	Injection	ref	Referral
IV	Intravenous	ROS/SR	Review of systems/systems review
L	Left	Rx	Prescription
L & W	Living and well	s.c./subq.	Subcutaneously
lab	Laboratory studies	sig	Sigmoidoscopy
MM	Mucous membrane	S/R	Suture removal
N & V	Nausea and vomiting	SOB	Shortness of breath
NP	New patient	stat	Immediately
NYD	Not yet diagnosed	STD	Sexually transmitted disease
P	Pulse	surg	Surgery
P &P	Pap smear (Papanicolaou smear) and pelvic examination	T	Temperature
Pap	Pap smear	TPR	Temperature, pulse, respirations
PE	Physical examination	Tx	Treatment
pH	Hydrogen concentration (acidity/alkalinity)	UCHD	Usual childhood diseases
PI	Present illness	US	Ultrasound
PMH	Past medical history	VS	Vital signs
PMS	Premenstrual syndrome	WDWN	Well-developed and well-nourished
pt	Patient	WNL	Within normal limits
PT	Physical therapy	Wt	Weight
Px	Physical examination	y.o.	Year old

Table 2-4, concluded

Abbreviation	Meaning	Abbreviation	Meaning
cc	Cubic centimeter (1 cc = 1 mL)	deca-	× 10
cm	Centimeter (2.5 cm = 1 inch)	hect-	× 100
km	Kilometer	kilo-	× 1000
mm	Millimeter	deci-	÷ 10
g, gm	Gram	centi	÷ 100
kg	Kilogram (1 kg = 1000 gm = 2.2 pounds)	milli-	÷ 1000
L or l	Liter = 1000 ml (1 gallon = 4 quarts = 8 pints = 3.785 L; 1 pint = 473.16 ml)	micro-	÷ 1,000,000

Table 2-5

Abbreviation	Meaning	Abbreviation	Meaning
a	Before	IM	Intramuscular
a.c.	Before meals	IV	Intravenous
ad lib.	As desired	noc., n.	Night
AM, a.m.	Morning	NPO	Nothing by mouth
amt	Amount	oint., ung.	Ointment
aq	Water	$\bar{p}$	After
b.i.d., BID	Twice a day	p.c.	After meals
buc	Buccal	per	By, through
$\bar{c}$	With	PM, p.m.	After noon
cap	Capsule	p.o., PO	By mouth
d	Day	PR	Through the rectum
Fl.	Fluid	p.r.n., PRN	As needed
h, hr	Hour	PV, vag.	Through the vagina
h.s.	At bedtime, at the hour of sleep	q)	Every
ID	Intradermal	qh	Every hour

Table 2-6

AT A GLANCE — Integumentary System—Suffixes

Suffix	Meaning	Example	Definition
-malacia	Softening	Onychomalacia	Softening of the nails
-phagia	Eating, swallowing	Onychophagia	Nail-biting

Table 2-9

AT A GLANCE — Integumentary System—Abbreviations

Abbreviation	Meaning
Bx	Biopsy
Derm	Dermatology
SC, sub-Q, SQ, subcu, subq	Subcutaneous

Table 2-10

Musculoskeletal System

AT A GLANCE — Musculoskeletal System—Common Combining Forms

Combining Form	Meaning	Example	Definition
ankyl / o	Stiff	Ankylosis	Complete loss of movement in a joint
arthr / o	Joint	Arthralgia	Pain in the joint
bucc / o	Cheek	Buccinator	Cheek muscle
burs / o	Bursa	Bursolith	Stone in a bursa
calc / o	Calcium	Hypercalcemia	Excessive amount of calcium in the blood
carp / o	Wrist	Carpal	Pertaining to the wrist
cervic / o	Neck	Cervical	Pertaining to the neck
chondr / o	Cartilage	Osteachondroma	Benign bone tumor
cost / o	Rib	Intercostal	Between the ribs
crani / o	Cranium (skull)	Cranial	Pertaining to the skull
dors / o	Back	Dorsal	Pertaining to the back

Table 2-11

Combining Form	Meaning	Example	Definition
fasci / o	Band of fibrous tissue	Fasciotomy	Operation to relieve pressure on the muscles by making an incision into the fascia
fibr / o	Fiber	Fibroma	Benign tumor of the connective tissues
kyph / o	Hump	Kyphosis	Excessive curvature of the spine, "humpback"
lamin / o	Lamina	Laminectomy	Surgical removal of the lamina
lei / o	Smooth muscle	Leiomyoma	Benign tumor of smooth muscle
lord / o	Curve	Lordosis	Inward curvature of the spine
my / o	Muscle	Myalgia	Muscle pain
myos / o	Muscle	Myositis	Inflammation of muscle tissue
oste / o	Bone	Osteoporosis	Condition in which bones become porous and fragile
pector / o	Chest	Pectoral	Pertaining to the chest
rhabd / o	Striated, skeletal muscle	Rhabdomyolysis	Destruction of muscle tissue accompanied by the release of myoglobin
spondyl / o	Vertebra	Spondylitis	Inflammation of the joints between the vertebrae in the spine
synov / i	Synovia	Synovial membrane	Membrane lining the capsule of a joint
ten / o, tend / o, tendin / o	Tendon	Tendinitis	Inflammation of the tendons

Table 2-11, concluded

Suffix	Meaning	Example	Definition
-asthenia	Weakness	Myasthenia gravis	Disorder of neuromuscular transmission marked by weakness

Table 2-12

AT A GLANCE **Musculoskeletal System—Suffixes**

Suffix	Meaning	Example	Definition
-clasia	Breaking	Arthroclasia	Artificial breaking of adhesions of an ankylosed joint
-desis	Binding	Arthrodesis	Surgical binding or fusing of a joint
-physis	Growth	Metaphysis	The growing portion of a long bone
-schisis	Splitting	Rachischisis	Failure of vertebral arches and neural tube to fuse
-trophy	Development	Hypertrophy	Excessive development

Table 2-12, concluded

AT A GLANCE **Musculoskeletal System—Abbreviations**

Abbreviation	Meaning
C1, C2, . . . C7	Individual cervical vertebrae (first through seventh)
Ca	Calcium
CTS	Carpal tunnel syndrome
EMG	Electromyography
fx	Fracture
ortho	Orthopedics
ROM	Range of motion
SLE	Systemic lupus erythematosus

Table 2-13

AT A GLANCE **Actions of Muscles**

Motion	Meaning
Abduction	Movement away from the midline
Adduction	Movement toward the midline
Circumduction	Movement in a circular motion

Table 2-14

Actions of Muscles

Motion	Meaning
Depression	Act of lowering a body part from a joint
Dorsiflexion	Act of pointing the foot upward
Elevation	Act of raising a body part from a joint
Eversion	Act of turning outward
Extension	Increase in the angle of a joint
Flexion	Decrease in the angle of a joint
Hyperextension	Increase in the angle of a joint beyond what is normal
Inversion	Act of turning inward
Plantar flexion	Act of pointing the foot downward
Pronation	Act of turning downward or inward
Protraction	Movement of a body part anteriorly
Retraction	Movement of a body part posteriorly
Rotation	Act or process of turning on an axis
Supination	Act of turning upward or outward

Table 2-14, concluded

Nervous System

Nervous System—Common Combining Forms

Combining Form	Meaning	Example	Definition
cerebell / o	Cerebellum	Cerebellar	Pertaining to the cerebellum
cerebr / o	Cerebrum	Cerebral cortex	Outer layer of the cerebrum
dur / o	Dura mater	Subdural hematoma	Bleeding between the dural and arachnoidal membranes
encephal / o	Brain	Encephalitis	Inflammation of the brain
mening / o	Membrane	Meningomyelocele	Protrusion of the spinal cord through a defect in the vertebral column

Table 2-15

Nervous System—Common Combining Forms

Combining Form	Meaning	Example	Definition
myel / o	Spinal cord, bone marrow	Myelogram	Radiographic study of the spinal subarachnoid space
neur / o	Nerve	Neuralgia	Pain in a nerve
poli / o	Gray matter	Poliodystrophy	Wasting of gray matter
psych / o	Mind	Psychosomatic	Pertaining to the influence of the mind on the body

Table 2-15, concluded

Nervous System—Prefixes

Prefix	Meaning	Example	Definition
hemi-	Half	Hemihypesthesia	Diminished sensation in one side of the body
tetra-	Four	Tetraparesis	Weakness of all four extremities

Table 2-16

Nervous System—Suffixes

Suffix	Meaning	Example	Definition
-algesia	Excessive sensitivity to pain	Analgesia	Without a sense of pain
-algia	Pain	Neuralgia	Nerve pain
-esthesia	Feeling sensation	Anesthesia	Loss of sensation
-kinesia	Movement	Bradykinesia	Decrease in spontaneity and movement
-kinesis	Movement	Hyperkinesis	Excessive muscular activity
-lepsy	Seizure	Epilepsy	Chronic brain disorder, often characterized by seizures
-paresis	Slight paralysis	Hemiparesis	Weakness on one side of the body
-phasia	Speech	Aphasia	Impairment of language ability
-plegia	Paralysis	Hemiplegia	Paralysis of one side of the body
-praxia	Action	Apraxia	Impairment of purposeful movement

Table 2-17

Abbreviation	Meaning
ALS	Amyotrophic lateral sclerosis
CAT	Computed axial tomography
CNS	Central nervous system
CP	Cerebral palsy
CSF	Cerebrospinal fluid
CT	Computed tomography
CVA	Cerebrovascular accident
EEG	Electroencephalogram
LP	Lumbar puncture
MRI	Magnetic resonance imaging
MS	Multiple sclerosis
TIA	Transient ischemic attack

Table 2-18

Cardiovascular System

Combining Form	Meaning	Example	Definition
angi / o	Vessel	Angiogram	X-ray image of a blood vessel
aort / o	Aorta	Aortic stenosis	Narrowing of the aorta
arter / o, arteri / o	Artery	Arteriosclerosis	Thickening of arterial walls
atri / o	Atrium	Atrial	Pertaining to an atrium
bas / o	Base	Basophil	Cell with granules that stain specifically with basic (alkaline) dyes
cardi / o	Heart	Cardiomegaly	Enlargement of the heart
coagul / o	Clotting	Anticoagulant	Drug that prevents clotting of the blood

Table 2-19

AT A GLANCE | Respiratory System—Common Combining Forms

Combining Form	Meaning	Example	Definition
adenoid / o	Adenoid	Adenoidectomy	Operation to remove adenoid growths
alveol / o	Air sac	Alveolar	Pertaining to a small cell or cavity
bronch / i, bronch / o	Bronchus	Bronchitis	Inflammation of the mucous membrane of the bronchial tubes
capn / o	Carbon dioxide	Hypercapnia	Excessive carbon dioxide in the blood
coni / o	Dust	Pneumoconiosis	Pulmonary disease caused by prolonged inhalation of fine dust
cyan / o	Blue	Cyanosis	Bluish discoloration of the skin caused by a deficiency of oxygen in the blood
laryng / o	Larynx	Laryngitis	Inflammation of the mucous membrane in the larynx
lob / o	Lobe of the lung	Lobectomy	Excision of a lobe
nas / o	Nose	Paranasal sinuses	Accessory sinuses in the bones of the face that open into the nasal cavities
ox / o, ox / i	Oxygen	Hypoxia	Deficiency of oxygen in tissue cells
phon / o	Voice	Dysphonia	Hoarseness
phren / o	Diaphragm	Phrenohepatic	Pertaining to the diaphragm and liver
pneum / o, pneum / a, pneumat / o	Breath	Pneumatosis	Abnormal presence of air or other gas
pneum / o, pneumon / o	Lung	Pneumonia	Inflammation of the lung parenchyma
pulmon / o	Lung	Pulmonary	Pertaining to the lungs

Table 2-22

Respiratory System—Common Combining Forms

Combining Form	Meaning	Example	Definition
rhin / o	Nose	Rhinorrhea	A watery discharge from the nose
spir / o	Breathing	Spirometer	Gasometer used to measure respiration
tonsill / o	Tonsil	Tonsillectomy	Removal of the tonsil

Table 2-22, concluded

Respiratory System—Suffixes

Suffix	Meaning	Example	Definition
-ema	Condition	Empyema	Condition of having pus in a body cavity as a result of a lung infection
-oxia	Oxygen	Anoxia	Absence of oxygen from blood or tissues
-pnea	Breathing	Apnea	Inability to breathe
-ptysis	Spitting	Hemoptysis	Coughing up and spitting out blood
-sphyxia	Pulse	Asphyxia	Impairment of oxygen intake
-thorax	Chest	Hemothorax	Blood in the pleural cavity

Table 2-23

Respiratory System—Abbreviations

Abbreviation	Meaning
ARDS	Acute respiratory distress syndrome
COPD	Chronic obstructive pulmonary disease
CPR	Cardiopulmonary resuscitation
CXR	Chest X-ray
PFT	Pulmonary function test
TB	Tuberculosis
URI	Upper respiratory infection

Table 2-24

Combining Form	Meaning	Example	Definition
calc / i	Calcium	Hypercalcemia	Elevated concentration of calcium in the blood
cortic / o	Cortex, outer region	Corticosteroid	Steroid produced by the adrenal cortex
crin / o	Secretion	Endocrinologist	Physician who specializes in endocrinology
dips / o	Thirst	Polydipsia	Prolonged excessive thirst
epinephr / o	Adrenal gland	Epinephritis	Inflammation of an adrenal gland
glyc / o	Sugar	Hyperglycemia	High blood sugar
gonad / o	Sex gland	Gonadotropin	Hormone that promotes gonadal growth
home / o	Like, similar	Homeostasis	State of bodily equilibrium
hormon / o	Hormone	Hormonal	Pertaining to hormones
kal / i	Potassium	Hypokalemia	Lack of potassium in the blood as a result of dehydration, excessive vomiting, and diarrhea
lact / o	Milk	Prolactin	Hormone that stimulates milk production during pregnancy
natr / i	Sodium	Hyponatremia	Low concentration of sodium in the blood
parathyroid / o	Parathyroid gland	Parathyroidectomy	Excision of the parathyroid gland
somat / o	Body	Somatotropic	Having a stimulating effect on body growth
ster / o	Solid structure	Steroid	Pertaining to the steroids, some of which increase muscle mass
thyr / o	Thyroid gland	Thyrotropin hormone	Hormone that stimulates growth of the thyroid gland
thyroid / o	Thyroid gland	Thyroiditis	Inflammation of the thyroid gland

Table 2-28, concluded

AT A GLANCE — Endocrine System—Prefixes

Prefix	Meaning	Example	Definition
oxy-	Rapid, sharp	Oxytocin	Hormone that influences contractions of the uterus
pan-	All	Panhypopituita-rism	State of inadequate or absent secretion of pituitary hormones
tri-	Three	Triiodothyronine	Hormone secreted by the thyroid gland that regulates metabolism

Table 2-29

AT A GLANCE — Endocrine System—Suffixes

Suffix	Meaning	Example	Definition
-agon	Assemblage, a gathering together	Glucagon	Hormone produced by the pancreas that causes an increase in blood sugar
-in, -ine	A substance	Epinephrine	Stress hormone secreted by the adrenal gland
-uria	Urine condition	Glycosuria	Urinary excretion of sugar

Table 2-30

AT A GLANCE — Endocrine System—Abbreviations

Abbreviation	Meaning
ACTH	Adrenocorticotropic hormone
BMR	Basal metabolic rate
Ca	Calcium
DI	Diabetes insipidus
DM	Diabetes mellitus
FBS	Fasting blood sugar
FSH	Follicle-stimulating hormone
GH	Growth hormone

Table 2-31

Endocrine System—Abbreviations

Abbreviation	Meaning
GTT	Glucose tolerance test
IDDM	Insulin-dependent diabetes mellitus
K	Potassium
Na	Sodium
NIDDM	Non-insulin-dependent diabetes mellitus
PRL	Prolactin
TFT	Thyroid function test

Table 2-31, concluded

Sensory System

The Eye

The Eye—Common Combining Forms

Combining Form	Meaning	Example	Definition
aque / o	Water	Aqueous	Containing, or like water
blephar / o	Eyelid	Blepharitis	Inflammation of the eyelids
conjunctiv / o	Conjunctiva	Conjunctivitis	Inflammation of the conjunctiva, pinkeye
cor / o, core / o	Pupil	Corepraxy	Procedure to widen a small pupil
dacry / o	Tear, tear duct	Dacryoadenitis	Inflammation of the lacrimal gland
dipl / o	Double	Diplopia	Condition in which one object is perceived as two objects
glauc / o	Gray	Glaucoma	Eye disease that may result in blindness
ir / o	Iris	Iritis	Inflammation of the iris
lacrim / o	Tear	Lacrimal	Pertaining to tears
mi / o	Smaller, less	Miosis	Contraction of the pupil
nyct / o, noct / o	Night	Nyctalopia	Poor night vision

Table 2-32

The Eye—Common Combining Forms

Combining Form	Meaning	Example	Definition
ocul / o	Eye	Intraocular	Inside the eye
opt / o	Vision	Optometer	Instrument for determining refraction of the eye
ophthalm / o	Eye	Ophthalmologist	Physician who specializes in treating eyes
palpebr / o	Eyelid	Palpebral	Pertaining to the eyelid
phot / o	Light	Photophobia	Fear and avoidance of light
presby / o	Old age	Presbyopia	Loss of accommodation in the eye resulting from aging
pupill / o	Pupil	Pupillary	Pertaining to the pupil
retin / o	Retina	Retinitis	Inflammation of the retina
scot / o	Darkness	Scotoma	Blind spot in which vision is absent or depressed
uve / o	Vascular layer of the eye	Uveitis	Inflammation of the uveal tract
vitre / o	Glassy	Vitreous humor	Fluid component of the transparent vitreous body

Table 2-32, concluded

The Eye—Suffixes

Suffix	Meaning	Example	Definition
-opia	Vision	Hyperopia	Farsightedness
-tropia	A turning	Esotropia	Inward turning of the eye, toward the nose

Table 2-33

The Eye—Abbreviations

Abbreviation	Meaning
ast	Astigmatism
IOP	Intraocular pressure

Table 2-34

The Eye—Abbreviations

Abbreviation	Meaning
OD	Right eye
OS	Left eye
OU	Each eye, both eyes
PERRLA	Pupils equal, round, reactive to light and accommodation
REM	Rapid eye movement
VA	Visual acuity
VF	Visual field

Table 2-34, concluded

The Ear

AT A GLANCE The Ear—Common Combining Forms

Combining Form	Meaning	Example	Definition
acou, acous / o	Hearing	Acoustic	Pertaining to hearing
audi / o	Hearing	Audiometer	Instrument for measuring hearing
audit / o	Hearing	Auditory	Pertaining to the sense or organs of hearing
aur / i	Ear	Aural	Pertaining to the ear
cochle / o	Cochlea	Cochlear	Pertaining to the cochlea
mastoid / o	Mastoid process	Mastoiditis	Inflammation of the mastoid process
ot / o	Ear	Otic	Pertaining to the ear
tympan / o	Eardrum	Tympanoplasty	Operation on a damaged middle ear

Table 2-35

The Ear—Suffixes

Suffix	Meaning	Example	Definition
-cusis, -acousia	Hearing	Presbycusis, presbyacousia	Nerve deafness caused by aging
-otia	Ear condition	Macrotia	Enlarged ears

Table 2-36

AT A GLANCE The Ear—Abbreviations

Abbreviation	Meaning
AD	Right ear
AS	Left ear
AU	Both ears
EENT	Eyes, ears, nose, and throat
oto	Otology

Table 2-37

Urinary System

AT A GLANCE Urinary System—Common Combining Forms

Combining Form	Meaning	Example	Definition
albumin / o	Protein	Albuminuria	Protein in the urine
bacteri / o	Bacterium, bacteria	Bacteriuria	Bacteria in the urine
cali / o	Calix (calyx)	Caliectasis	Dilation of the calices
cyst / o	Urinary bladder	Cystitis	Inflammation of the urinary bladder
ket / o	Ketone bodies	Ketosis	Enhanced production of ketone bodies
lith / o	Stone	Nephrolithiasis	Presence of a renal stone or stones
meat / o	Opening, passageway	Meatoscope	Speculum for examining the urinary meatus

Table 2-38

Urinary System—Common Combining Forms

Combining Form	Meaning	Example	Definition
nephr / o	Kidney	Nephropathy	Disease of the kidney
olig / o	Scanty, few	Oliguria	Scanty urine production
pyel / o	Renal pelvis	Pyelolithotomy	Operation to remove a stone from the kidney
ren / i, ren / o	Kidney	Renography	Radiography of the kidney
ur / o, urin / o	Urine, urinary tract	Urodynia	Pain on urination
vesic / o	Urinary bladder	Perivesical	Surrounding the urinary bladder

Table 2-38, concluded

Urinary System—Suffixes

Suffix	Meaning	Example	Definition
-tripsy	Crushing	Lithotripsy	Crushing of a stone in the renal pelvis, ureter, or bladder
-uria	Urination	Dysuria	Difficulty or pain in urinating

Table 2-39

Urinary System—Abbreviations

Abbreviation	Meaning
ADH	Antidiuretic hormone; vasopressin
ARF	Acute renal failure
BUN	Blood urea nitrogen
Cath	Catheter
CFR	Chronic renal failure
ESRD	End-stage renal disease
HD	Hemodialysis
IVP	Intravenous pyelogram
KUB	Kidney, ureter, and bladder

Table 2-40

Abbreviation	Meaning
PKU	Phenylketonuria
UA	Urinalysis
UTI	Urinary tract infection

Table 2-40, concluded

Reproductive System

Combining Form	Meaning	Example	Definition
amni / o	Amnion	Amniocentesis	Aspiration of amniotic fluid for diagnosis
balan / o	Glans penis	Balanitis	Inflammation of the glans penis
cervic / o	Cervix, neck	Endocervicitis	Inflammation of the mucous membrane of the cervix
colp / o	Vagina	Colporrhaphy	Repair of a rupture in the vagina
culd / o	Cul-de-sac	Culdocentesis	Aspiration of fluid from the cul-de-sac
crypt / o	Hidden	Cryptorchism	Failure of one or both testes to descend
epididym / o	Epididymis	Epididymitis	Inflammation of the epididymis
galact / o	Milk	Galactorrhea	Abnormal, persistent discharge of milk
gon / o	Generation, genitals	Gonorrhea	Contagious inflammation of the genital mucous membrane
gynec / o	Female	Gynecomastia	Excessive development of the mammary glands in a male
hyster / o	Uterus	Hysterectomy	Removal of the uterus
lact / i, lact / o	Milk	Lactation	Production of milk
mamm / o	Breast	Mammogram	Breast X-ray
mast / o	Breast	Mastectomy	Excision of the breast

Table 2-41

Combining Form	Meaning	Example	Definition
men / o	Menses	Amenorrhea	Absence or abnormal cessation of menses
metr / o	Uterus	Metrorrhagia	Irregular bleeding from the uterus between periods
nat / i	Birth	Neonatal	Pertaining to the first month of life
orchi / o, orchid / o	Testis, testicle	Orchiectomy	Removal of one or both testes
ov / o	Egg	Ovum	Female sex cell, or egg
prostat / o	Prostate gland	Prostatitis	Inflammation of the prostate
terat / o	Monster	Teratoma	Neoplasm composed of tissues not normally found in the organ
test / o	Testis, testicle	Testicular	Pertaining to the testes
vagin / o	Vagina	Vaginitis	Inflammation of the vagina
vas / o	Vessel, duct	Vasectomy	Removal of a section of the vas deferens
vert / i, vers / i	A turning	Cephalic version	Turning of the fetus so that the head is correctly positioned for delivery

Table 2-41, concluded

Suffix	Meaning	Example	Definition
-arche	Beginning	Menarche	Time of the first menstrual period
-gravida	Pregnant	Primigravida	Woman in her first pregnancy
-one	Hormone	Testosterone	Hormone related to masculinization and reproduction
-pause	Cessation	Menopause	The cessation of menses

Table 2-42

AT A GLANCE — Reproductive System—Suffixes

Suffix	Meaning	Example	Definition
-pexy	Fixation, fastening	Orchiopexy	Surgical treatment of an undescended testicle
-stomy	(New) opening	Vasostomy	Surgical procedure of making a new opening into the vas deferens
-tocia	Labor, birth	Dystocia	Difficult childbirth

Table 2-42, concluded

AT A GLANCE — Reproductive System—Abbreviations

Abbreviation	Meaning
AB	Abortion
AIDS	Acquired immunodeficiency syndrome
BPH	Benign prostatic hyperplasia
CS, C-section	Cesarean section
CX	Cervix
D & C	Dilation and curettage
ECC	Endocervical curettage
EMB	Endometrial biopsy
FHT	Fetal heart tones
FSH	Follicle-stimulating hormone
GYN	Gynecology
HCG	Human chorionic gonadotropin
HIV	Human immunodeficiency virus
HSV	Herpes simplex virus
LH	Luteinizing hormone
Multip	Multipara
Pap smear	Papanicolaou smear (test for cervical or vaginal cancer)

Table 2-43

Abbreviation	Meaning
PMS	Premenstrual syndrome
PSA	Prostate-specific antigen
STD	Sexually transmitted disease

Table 2-43, concluded

STRATEGIES TO SUCCESS

▶ *Test-Taking Skills*

Think success!

Approach the exam with confidence. It's unlikely that you will get all the questions right. Don't panic or become stressed when you can't answer a question. Relax, and imagine yourself doing wonderfully. A positive attitude will help you stay in control and allow you to focus on all the questions that you do know.

Instructions:

Answer the following questions. Check your answers in the *Answer Key* that follows this section.

1. A prefix is
   A. The first part of a word
   B. A word structure at the end of a term that modifies the root
   C. A word structure at the beginning of a term that modifies the root
   D. Found on all medical terms
   E. The last part of a word that gives the word its root meaning

2. Which of the following suffixes means "inflammation"?
   A. -iasis
   B. -trophy
   C. -itis
   D. -osis
   E. -desis

3. The abbreviation for the word *diagnosis* is
   A. Diag
   B. DG
   C. dgs
   D. D
   E. Dx

4. Which of the following prefixes is matched correctly with the meaning?
   A. hypo / above
   B. peri / around
   C. antero / back
   D. endo / over
   E. micro / large

5. The prefix *ab-* means
   A. Without
   B. Toward
   C. Against
   D. Away from
   E. Previous or before

6. The combining form is the
   A. Word root
   B. Word root with the combining vowel attached (written with a separating vertical slash)
   C. Word root with the prefix and suffix attached (written with a separating vertical slash)
   D. Word root with the prefix and suffix attached (written without a slash)
   E. Combining vowel

7. Which of the following suffixes means "lack of strength"?
   A. -algia
   B. -tomy
   C. -asthenia
   D. -trophy
   E. -phasia

8. Which of the following words is misspelled?
   A. Abscess
   B. Homostasis
   C. Venous
   D. Prostate
   E. Integumentary

9. When the combining form *cyan / o* is used, it means that
   A. The skin is involved
   B. The object is blue
   C. The object is oily
   D. The muscles are involved
   E. Something is poisonous

10. The combining form *oste / o* means
    A. Tendon
    B. Vertebra
    C. Muscle
    D. Calcium
    E. Bone

11. Which of the following abbreviations means "every day"?

 A. b.i.d.
 B. q.e.d.
 C. t.i.d.
 D. q.i.d.
 E. q.d.

12. The prefix *intra-* means

 A. Between
 B. Below
 C. Within
 D. Beside
 E. Above

13. The abbreviation *stat* means

 A. Immediately
 B. Do not change
 C. Stay on alert
 D. Daily
 E. Statistics

14. The suffix *-stasis* means

 A. Condition
 B. Control
 C. Destruction
 D. Discharge
 E. Unchanged

15. The suffix *-pathy* means

 A. Disease
 B. Spasm
 C. Treatment
 D. Tumor
 E. Excision

16. Which of the following combining forms refers to the brain?

 A. myel / o
 B. encephal / o
 C. cortic / o
 D. alveol / o
 E. psych / o

17. The combining form *audi / o* means

 A. Speaking
 B. Hearing
 C. Seeing
 D. Learning through personal experience
 E. Learning from reported experience, or "book-learning"

18. The prefix *epi-* means

 A. Good
 B. Out
 C. Off
 D. Within
 E. Upon

19. *Nephr / o* and *ren / o* both refer to which of the following?

 A. The lungs
 B. The heart
 C. The bladder
 D. The kidney
 E. The rectum

20. The suffix *-gravida* refers to

 A. A pregnancy
 B. The condition of aging
 C. A serious condition
 D. A stomach ache
 E. A malignancy

21. The prefix *peri-* means

 A. Behind
 B. Underneath
 C. Inside
 D. Half
 E. Surrounding

22. The underlined portions of the words *pneumo-coniosis* and *pneumonoconiosis* represent which of the following word parts?

 A. Prefix
 B. Root
 C. Suffix
 D. Combining form
 E. None of the above

23. Which of the following contains the central meaning of a word?
    A. Prefix
    B. Suffix
    C. Root
    D. Combining form
    E. Both C and D

24. The abbreviation *q.o.d.*, as used in prescriptions, means
    A. Every hour
    B. Every two hours
    C. Twice a day
    D. Four times a day
    E. Every other day

25. The prefix *retro-* means
    A. Behind
    B. Around
    C. Below
    D. Before
    E. Above

26. The underlined portion of the word *hypolipemia* represents which of the following word parts?
    A. Prefix
    B. Root
    C. Suffix
    D. Combining form
    E. None of the above

27. Which of the following words is misspelled?
    A. Peritoneum
    B. Dissect
    C. Homerous
    D. Metastasis
    E. None of the above

28. Which of the following words is misspelled?
    A. Vacsine
    B. Sphincter
    C. Parietal
    D. Osseous
    E. Asthma

29. Which of the following prefixes means "bad, difficult, painful"?
    A. ex-
    B. dis-
    C. dys-
    D. dia-
    E. meta-

30. The suffix *-kinesia* means
    A. Mind
    B. Muscle
    C. Pain
    D. Touch
    E. Movement

31. The combining form *cheil / o* means
    A. Cheek
    B. Lip
    C. Gum
    D. Tongue
    E. Mouth

32. The prefix *rube-* means
    A. Rotation
    B. Small
    C. Spots
    D. Abnormal
    E. Red

33. Which of the following words is misspelled?
    A. Neruon
    B. Malaise
    C. Humerus
    D. Desiccation
    E. Glaucoma

34. The prefix *milli-* means
    A. One-thousandth
    B. Many
    C. One
    D. One-hundredth
    E. One-tenth

35. Which of the following suffixes means "beginning, origin, production"?

    A. -iasis
    B. -genic
    C. -genetic
    D. Both B and C
    E. Both A and B

36. The suffix -*scope* means an instrument for

    A. Measuring
    B. Viewing
    C. Creating a new opening
    D. Recording
    E. Illuminating

37. The combining form *xer / o* refers to something

    A. Dry
    B. Yellow
    C. Multiple
    D. Pertaining to hair
    E. Pertaining to x-rays

38. The combining form *ot / o* means

    A. Hearing
    B. Seeing
    C. Light
    D. Eye
    E. Ear

39. The plural of *diverticulum* is

    A. Diverticulums
    B. Diverticuli
    C. Diverticulae
    D. Diverticulumes
    E. Diverticula

40. The plural of *calculus* is

    A. Calculus'
    B. Calcula
    C. Calculi
    D. Calculuses
    E. Calculus

ANSWER KEY

1.	C		21.	E
2.	C		22.	D
3.	E		23.	E
4.	B		24.	E
5.	D		25.	A
6.	B		26.	A
7.	C		27.	C
8.	B		28.	A
9.	B		29.	C
10.	E		30.	E
11.	E		31.	B
12.	C		32.	E
13.	A		33.	A
14.	B		34.	A
15.	A		35.	D
16.	B		36.	B
17.	B		37.	A
18.	E		38.	E
19.	D		39.	E
20.	A		40.	C

CHAPTER 3

Anatomy and Physiology

CHAPTER OUTLINE

Levels of Organization

Cell Structure

Organelles
Cell Division
Movement of Substances Across the Cell Membrane

Chemistry

Tissues of the Body

Body Membranes

Division Planes and Body Cavities

Division Planes
Body Cavities

Integumentary System

Musculoskeletal System

Skeletal System
Muscular System

Nervous System

Nerve Cells and Neurotransmitters
Central Nervous System
Peripheral Nervous System

Sensory System

Smell
Taste
Sight
Hearing

Cardiovascular System

The Blood
Blood Cell Types
The Heart and Blood Vessels
Lymphatic System

Respiratory System

Digestive System

Additional Organs and Processes Involved with Digestion

Endocrine System

Control of Hormonal Secretions

Urinary System

Body Fluids
Organs and Function of the Urinary System

Reproductive System

Male Reproductive System
Female Reproductive System

MEDICAL ASSISTING COMPETENCIES

COMPETENCY	CMA	RMA
General/Legal/Professional		
Conduct work within scope of education, training, and ability		X
Use appropriate medical terminology		X

STRATEGIES TO SUCCESS

▶ Study Skills

Find a good place to study!
Think about what atmosphere you study best in. Are you distracted by the slightest noise? Do you like a certain level of noise to keep you going and focused? Do you like studying alone or in groups? Also consider how comfortable you want to be. Do you find yourself drifting off when you study on your bed or in a comfortable chair? Is studying at a desk too uncomfortable? There's no right place or way to study. Some people pace the halls whereas others find a secluded place in their house where their family and friends can't bother them. We do suggest that you find a place that is well lighted. Unnecessary eye strain could cause you to become tired too soon. Whatever place you pick, make sure it's right for you and make it a habit to study there regularly.

Levels of Organization

The human body is composed of atoms that join together to form molecules at the chemical level. The other levels of organization of the body are shown in Figure 3-1.

Cell Structure

Cell: The basic structural unit of all organisms. Cells have three main parts: the cell membrane, the cytoplasm, and the nucleus. See Figure 3-2.
1. Cell membrane: A bilayer of phospholipid and protein molecules that controls the passage of materials in and out of the cell.
2. Cytoplasm: The medium for chemical reactions in the cell. It contains water, dissolved ions, nutrients, and different organelles. The cytoplasm surrounds the nucleus and is encircled by the cell membrane.

3. Nucleus: The largest and innermost organelle in the cell. It is a roughly spherical body near the center of the cell, and it contains DNA, which regulates the cell's activities.
DNA: Deoxyribonucleic acid. DNA consists of long chains of chemical bases along a sugar-phosphate backbone; the chains are joined in pairs by bonds between complementary bases and twist around each other in a double helix. This pattern of bases carries genetic information that directs all cell activities.
Chromatin: The genetic material contained in the nucleus of a nondividing cell. It consists primarily of chromosomes, made of DNA bound in clumps to proteins.
Nucleolus: A dense body within the nucleus, also known as the little nucleus, composed of DNA, RNA, and protein molecules. It is the site for synthesis of ribosomal RNA (rRNA).
RNA: Ribonucleic acid. RNA consists of long, single chains of chemical bases along a sugar-phosphate backbone.

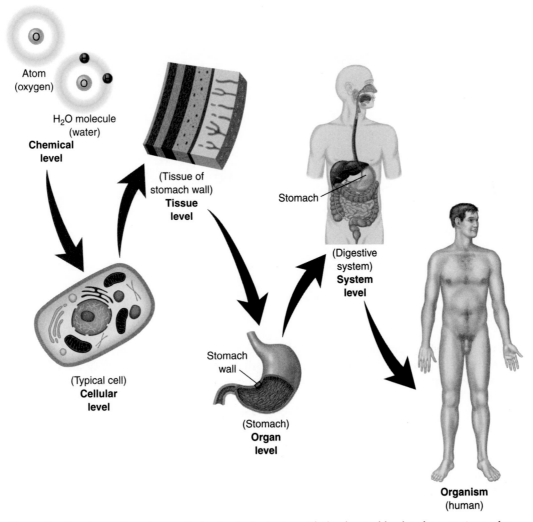

Figure 3-1 *The human body is organized in levels, beginning with the chemical level and progressing to the cellular, tissue, organ, system, and organism (whole body) levels.*

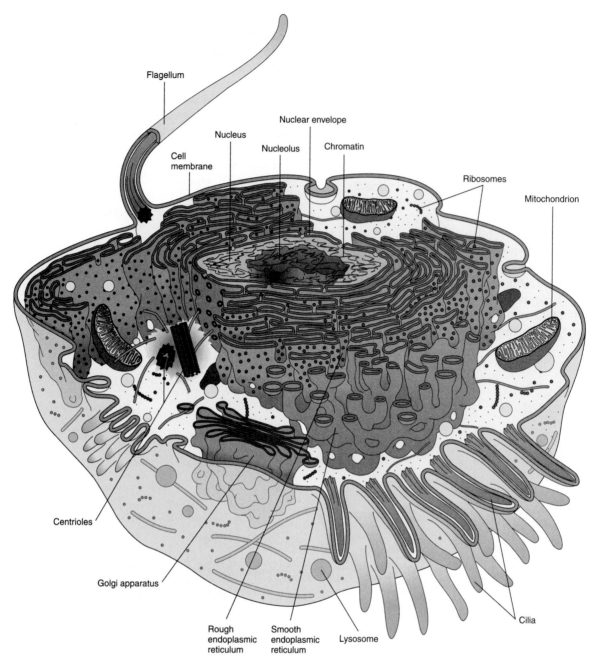

Flagellum

Cell
membrane

Nucleus

Nuclear envelope

Nucleolus

Chromatin

Ribosomes

Mitochondrion

Centrioles

Golgi apparatus

Rough
endoplasmic
reticulum

Smooth
endoplasmic
reticulum

Lysosome

Cilia

Figure 3-2 *A composite cell. Organelles are not drawn to scale.*

RNA molecules are transported from the nucleus into the cytoplasm, where they direct the formation of proteins.
Organelle: A specialized part of a cell that performs a particular function.

Organelles

Ribosome: A granular cytoplasmic organelle composed of RNA. Ribosomes provide enzymes that link amino acids for protein synthesis.
Mitochondrion: A small, rod-shaped organelle that serves as the power plant of the cell because it provides energy.

Lysosomes: Cytoplasmic particles that digest material that comes into the cell. They are often referred to as the garbage disposals of the cells because they break down nutrient molecules and foreign particles.
Endoplasmic reticulum: A network of tubules that transports material through the cytoplasm and aids in the synthesis of proteins and lipids.
Golgi apparatus: A small membranous structure found in most cells that forms the carbohydrate side chains of glycoproteins. The Golgi apparatus consists of a stave of about six flattened membranous sacs that refine and alter glycoproteins. It is also called the Golgi body or Golgi complex.

Cytoskeleton: The cytoplasmic elements that coordinate the movement of organelles.

Centriole: An intracellular, rod-shaped body involved with cell division and organizing mitotic spindles.

Cilium: One of numerous small, hairlike extensions that move substances across the surface of a cell.

Flagellum: A long, whiplike extension from a cell that aids in movement. The only human cell with a tail (flagellum) is sperm. Otherwise, flagellum is usually associated with a parasite.

Cell Division

Mitosis: The division of a somatic cell to form two new cells, each identical to the parent cell.

Meiosis: A type of nuclear division in which the number of chromosomes is reduced to one half the number found in a normal body cell. It results in the formation of an egg or sperm.

Cytokinesis: Separation of the cytoplasm into two cells after nuclear division has occurred.

Movement of Substances Across the Cell Membrane

Diffusion: The movement of molecules from a region of higher concentration to a region of lower concentration, a concentration gradient.

Osmosis: The diffusion of water through a selectively permeable membrane in response to the concentration gradient.

Facilitated diffusion: Diffusion through a membrane by means of proteins acting as carrier molecules.

Filtration: The movement of fluid through a membrane in response to hydrostatic pressure.

Active transport: The movement of substances against a concentration gradient, from a region of lower concentration to a region of higher concentration. It requires a carrier molecule and uses energy.

Endocytosis: The formation of vesicles in the cell membrane to transfer particles and droplets from the outside into the cell. Phagocytosis (ingestion of solids) and pinocytosis (ingestion of liquids) are two such processes.

Exocytosis: The discharge from a cell of particles too large to pass through the cell membrane by diffusion.

Isotonic solution: A solution that has the same concentration (osmotic pressure) as the fluids within a cell.

Hypertonic solution: A solution that has a higher concentration (osmotic pressure) than the fluids within a cell.

Hypotonic solution: A solution that has a lower concentration (osmotic pressure) than the fluids within a cell.

Chemistry

Element: The simplest form of matter with unique chemical properties. Oxygen, iron, gold, and other elements cannot be broken down into different substances by ordinary chemical means. All matter, living and nonliving, is composed of elements.

Atom: The smallest particle of an element, consisting of electrons surrounding a nucleus composed of protons, neutrons, and other entities.

Atomic number: The number of protons in the nucleus of the atom. The hydrogen atom, for example, has one proton and its atomic number is 1. Carbon has six protons and its atomic number is 6.

Atomic weight: The relative weight of an atom, determined by the number of protons and neutrons together and compared with the standard carbon atom (which has a mass of 12 and an atomic weight of 12).

Ionic bond: A relatively weak attraction formed when one or more electrons are transferred from one atom to another. It is easily disrupted in water.

Covalent bond: The chemical bond formed when two atoms share a pair of electrons. It is the strongest type of chemical bond.

Ion: An atom that has acquired a charge through the gain or loss of one or more electrons.

Anion: A negatively charged ion.

Cation: A positively charged ion.

Compound: A molecule composed of two or more different elements, such as carbon dioxide (CO_2).

Mixture: A combination of substances that are not chemically combined and can be separated by physical means.

Suspension: A mixture in which a solid is distributed but not dissolved. It will separate unless it is shaken.

Electrolyte: A substance that permits the transfer of electrons in solution. Common electrolytes include acids, bases, and salts.

pH: The number used to indicate the exact strength of an acid or base.

pH scale: A scale, ranging from 0 to 14, that measures the hydrogen ion concentration of a solution. See Figure 3-3.

Acid: A substance with a pH less than 7.0 that ionizes in water to release hydrogen ions. Because a hydrogen ion consists of a proton, an acid is referred to as a *hydrogen ion donor* or a *proton donor*.

Base: A substance with a pH greater than 7.0. It is referred to as a *hydrogen ion acceptor* or a *proton acceptor*. Bases contain higher concentrations of hydroxyl ions (OH^-), whereas acids contain higher concentrations of hydrogen ions (H^+).

Buffer: A substance that prevents or reduces changes in pH and counterbalances the addition of an acid or base.

Buffer system: A system that uses chemical reactions occurring in body fluids to maintain a particular pH. The acid-base balance is regulated by two buffer systems in the body: the lungs and the kidneys.

ATP: The abbreviation for adenosine triphosphate. ATP is the primary provider of energy for a cell.

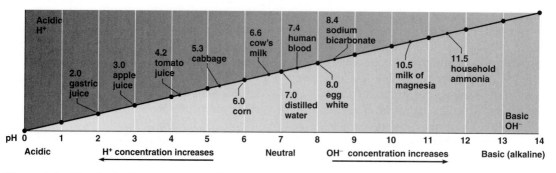

Figure 3-3 *pH scale. As the concentration of hydrogen ions (H^+) increases, a solution becomes more acidic and the pH decreases. As the concentration of hydroxyl ions (OH^-) increases, a solution becomes more basic and the pH increases.*

Tissues of the Body

Histology: The microscopic study of tissues.

Tissue: A collection of similar cells acting together to perform a particular function. Types include epithelial (see Table 3-1), connective, muscular, and nervous.

Gland: An organ that contains special cells that secrete substances. Some glands lubricate; others produce hormones (see Table 3-2 on p. 57).

Unicellular glands: Glands that consist of only one cell.

Multicellular glands: Glands that may be classified on the basis of structure (simple or compound), type of secretion (mucous, serous, or mixed), presence or absence of ducts (exocrine or endocrine), characteristics of secreting units (alveolar or acinar), and manner of secretion (merocrine, apocrine, or holocrine).

Goblet cell: The only unicellular exocrine gland. Goblet cells produce mucus in digestive, respiratory, urinary, and reproductive tracts.

Connective tissue: Tissue that connects, protects, supports, and forms a framework for all body structures. Connective tissue includes loose fibrous tissue, adipose tissue, dense fibrous tissue, cartilage, bone, and blood.

Loose fibrous tissue: Tissue that fills spaces in the body and binds structures together.

Adipose tissue: A specialized form of loose fibrous tissue that provides insulation; it is commonly called fat.

Dense fibrous tissue: Connective tissue that forms tendons and ligaments.

Cartilage: A hard, dense connective tissue consisting of cells embedded in a matrix that can withstand considerable pressure and tension. It provides support, a framework, and attachment; protects underlying tissues; and forms structural models for many developing bones. It is bluish-white or gray and semi-opaque. Cartilage does not contain any nerves or blood supply. There are three types of cartilage: hyaline, fibrous, and elastic.

Bone: A hard, connective tissue consisting of specialized cells embedded in a matrix of hardened mineral salts. It is the most rigid connective tissue.

AT A GLANCE	Types of Epithelial Tissue	
Type	**Description**	**Location**
Simple squamous	Single layer of thin, flat cells	Alveoli of lungs, capillary walls
Simple cuboidal	Single layer of cube-shaped cells	Ovary, thyroid gland
Simple columnar	Single layer of tall cells	Intestines, stomach
Stratified squamous	Several layers of cells with flat cells at the free surface	Skin, vagina, anus
Transitional	Tissue specialized to change in response to increased tension; cells become thinner when distended	Urinary bladder

Table 3-1

Secretion Mode	Meaning	Examples
Merocrine	Pertaining to a secretory cell that remains intact during secretion	Salivary glands, certain sweat glands, pancreatic glands
Apocrine	Pertaining to a secretory cell that contributes part of its protoplasm to the secretion	Mammary glands and certain sweat glands
Holocrine	Pertaining to a secretory cell that produces secretions consisting of altered cells of the same gland	Sebaceous glands

Table 3-2

Blood: The only type of connective tissue that is liquid, composed of cells suspended in a fluid matrix called plasma.

Nervous tissue: Tissue found in the brain, spinal cord, and nerves.

Muscle tissue: Tissue that provides movement, maintains posture, and produces heat. Muscle tissue is composed of elongated muscle fibers that can contract and thereby move body parts. There are three types of muscle tissue: skeletal, smooth, and cardiac. Skeletal muscles attach to bones and are controlled voluntarily. Smooth muscles, which lack the striations of skeletal muscles, line the walls of hollow internal organs. Cardiac muscles, which are striated, are found only in the heart. Both smooth and cardiac muscles are controlled involuntarily.

Sarcoma: A malignant tumor that forms in connective tissue.

Body Membranes

Membrane: A layer of tissue that lines body cavities, covers organs, or separates structures.

Cutaneous membrane: The membrane that covers the body. It is also known as the skin.

Epithelial membranes: Mucous and serous membranes.

Serous membranes: The pleura, pericardium, and peritoneum.

Connective tissue membranes: Synovial membranes and the meninges.

Meninx: One of three connective tissue coverings, or meninges, around the brain and spinal cord. The three layers, from the outermost to the innermost, are the dura mater, arachnoid, and pia mater.

Adenoma: A benign tumor of glandular epithelial cells.

Adenocarcinoma: A malignant tumor originating in glandular epithelium.

Division Planes and Body Cavities

Division Planes

Division plane: One of three imaginary planes (frontal, sagittal, and transverse) used as references in describing positions of the body or of parts of the body. See Figure 3-4.

Frontal plane: A plane that divides the body into front and back halves. This plane is also referred to as the coronal plane.

Sagittal plane: A plane that divides the body into left and right halves. This plane is also referred to as the lateral plane.

Midsagittal plane: A plane that passes along the midline and divides the body into left and right halves. This plane is also referred to as the median plane.

Transverse plane: A plane that divides the body into upper and lower halves. This plane is also referred to as the horizontal plane.

Body Cavities

Body cavity: Either of two main cavities in the body, the dorsal and the ventral. See Figure 3-5.

Dorsal cavity: The main body cavity consisting of the cranial cavity, which contains the brain, and the spinal cavity, which contains the spinal cord.

Ventral cavity: The main body cavity consisting of the thoracic, the abdominal, and the pelvic cavities. It is much larger than the dorsal cavity.

The division of the abdominal area: The two most common ways to subdivide the abdominal area are into either nine regions or four quadrants. See Figure 3-6.

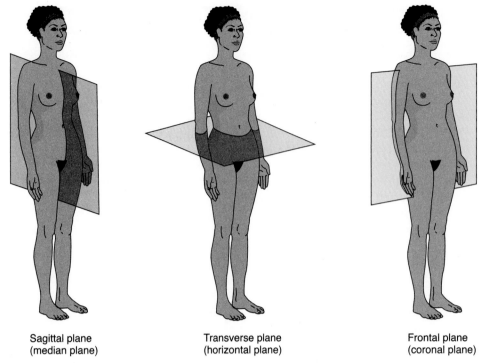

Sagittal plane
(median plane)

Transverse plane
(horizontal plane)

Frontal plane
(coronal plane)

Figure 3-4 *Sectioning the body along various planes.*

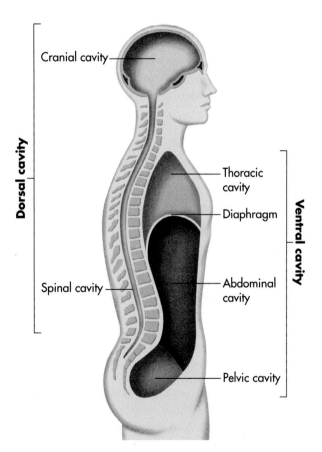

Cranial cavity

Dorsal cavity

Thoracic cavity

Diaphragm

Ventral cavity

Spinal cavity

Abdominal cavity

Pelvic cavity

Figure 3-5 *The two main body cavities are dorsal and ventral.*

Integumentary System

Integumentary system: The skin and its derivatives. Functions of the skin include protection, the regulation of body temperature, sensory reception, and the synthesis of vitamin D.

Cutaneous membrane: The medical term for skin. It consists of three layers: the epidermis, the dermis, and subcutaneous tissue. See Figure 3-7.

Epidermis: The outermost layer of the skin. It contains no blood vessels, but it does contain melanin, which gives skin its characteristic color, and keratin, which is a waterproof barrier against pathogens and chemicals. Specialized cells in the epidermis called melanocytes produce melanin. The more melanin in skin, the darker its color. The epidermis consists of five layers, or strata. They are, from outermost to innermost, the stratum corneum, the stratum lucidum, the stratum granulosum, the stratum spinosum, and the stratum germinativum.

Dermis: The layer of skin containing hair follicles, nails, glands (that secrete oil or sebum), fibers, sense receptors, and blood vessels. It is also called true skin.

Subcutaneous tissue: The bottom layer of the cutaneous membrane, beneath the true skin.

Stratum lucidum: A translucent band that is seen best in thick, glabrous skin.

Stratum corneum: Dead, keratinized cells located on the outer surface of the epidermis.

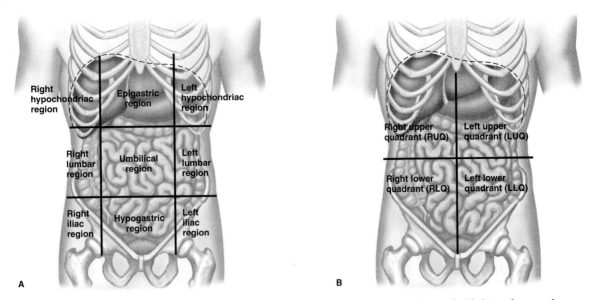

Figure 3-6 *(A) The abdominal area divided into nine regions and (B) the abdominal area divided into four quadrants.*

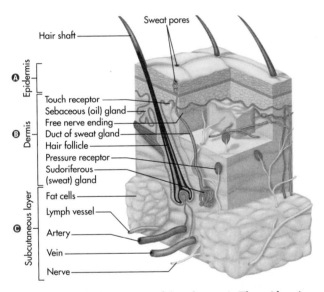

Figure 3-7 *The skin consists of three layers. A. The epidermis (outer layer) is made entirely of epithelial cells. B. The dermis (middle layer) contains connective tissue, nerve endings, hair follicles, and the sweat and oil glands. C. The subcutaneous (innermost) layer contains fat cells, loose connective tissue, and blood and lymph vessels.*

Keratinization: A process by which epithelial cells lose their moisture, which is replaced by keratin (protein).

Sebaceous gland: An oil gland, associated with hair follicles. Sebaceous glands secrete sebum and are abundant in the scalp, external ear, face, nose, mouth, and anus.

Sweat gland: A gland that secretes sweat, either directly to the skin's surface (eccrine type) or indirectly through hair follicles (apocrine type). Also called sudoriferous glands, sweat glands are widely distributed over the body, except for the lips, nipples, and parts of the external genitalia.

Musculoskeletal System

Skeletal System

Bone: An individual unit of osseous tissue, part of the body's supporting framework. Although they appear hard and lifeless because of the calcium contained in them, bones are living tissue. Bones also produce blood cells, act as a storage area for calcium, and protect delicate organs of the body.

Types: There are two types of bone tissue: compact and spongy bone tissue. The three types of cells in bone are osteoblasts, osteoclasts, and osteocytes.

Classification: Bones are classified into four types according to their shape: long, short, flat, and irregular. The femur, radius, and humerus are long bones. The carpals and tarsals are short bones. The ribs, scapula, skull, and sternum are flat bones. The vertebrae, sacrum, and mandible are irregular bones. The adult human skeleton is made up of 206 named bones. See Figure 3-8 and Table 3-3.

Diaphysis: The shaft of a long bone, located between the epiphyses.

Epiphysis: Spongy bone tissue, located at the ends of a long bone.

Endochondral ossification: During development, most bones originate as hyaline cartilages. Each cartilage is a miniature model of the bone that will occupy that particular position in the adult skeleton. These cartilage model are gradually converted to bone through the process of **endochondral ossification.**

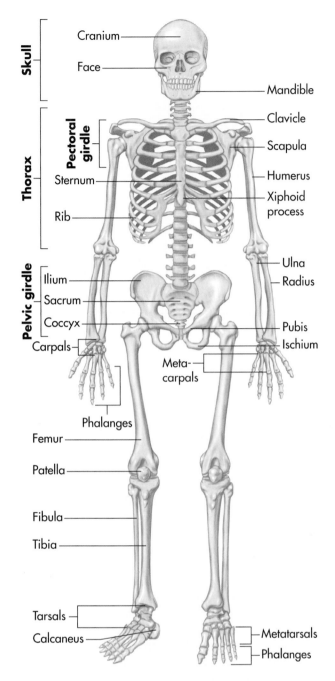

Skull
Thorax
Pelvic girdle
Pectoral girdle

Cranium
Face
Mandible
Clavicle
Scapula
Humerus
Xiphoid process
Sternum
Rib
Ulna
Radius
Ilium
Sacrum
Coccyx
Pubis
Ischium
Carpals
Meta-carpals
Phalanges
Femur
Patella
Fibula
Tibia
Tarsals
Calcaneus
Metatarsals
Phalanges

Figure 3-8 *The skeletal system is composed of bones, joints, and related connective tissue.*

Articulation, or **joint:** A place of junction between two or more bones of the skeleton. There are three types of articulation: immovable (synarthrosis), slightly movable (amphiarthrosis), and freely movable (diarthrosis). Diarthrosis joints are the most common type in the human body.

Classification of synovial joints: Synovial joints are classified according to the shapes of their parts and the movements they permit:

- Ball-and-socket joint
- Condyloid joint
- Gliding joint

Axial skeleton	80 bones

Skull, consisting of:	28 bones, as follows:
a. Cranial bones	8
b. Facial bones	14
c. Auditory ossicles	6

Thoracic cage	25 bones

Appendicular skeleton:	126 bones, as follows:
a. Upper extremity	60
b. Lower extremity	60
c. Pelvic girdle	2
d. Pectoral girdle	4

Table 3-3

- Hinge joint
- Pivot joint
- Saddle joint

Table 3-4 summarizes these types of joints.

Hyoid bone: A U-shaped bone in the neck that supports the tongue. This bone does not articulate directly with any other bone.

Vertebral column, or **spinal column:** The portion of the skeleton consisting of vertebrae (26 in the human adult) and intervertebral disks. There are four curvatures: cervical curve, thoracic curve, lumbar curve, and sacral curve.

Atlas: The first cervical vertebra. It articulates with the occipital bone and the axis.

Axis: The second cervical vertebra, with which the atlas bone articulates. This articulation allows the head to be turned (rotated), extended, and flexed.

Coccyx: The last bone at the base of the vertebral column. The coccyx, also called the tailbone, attaches to the end of the sacrum.

Sternum: The bone that forms the anterior portion of the thoracic cage. It consists of the manubrium, the body (or gladiolus), and the xiphoid process. It supports the clavicles and articulates directly with the first seven pairs of the ribs.

True ribs: Seven pairs of ribs, which attach to the sternum directly by their individual costal cartilages.

False ribs: Ribs in pairs 8 through 10, which attach to the sternum indirectly.

Floating ribs: Ribs in pairs 11 and 12, which do not attach to the sternum.

Pectoral girdle: The skeletal structure consisting of the two clavicles, or collarbones, and the two scapulae, or shoulder blades.

Type of Joint	Description	Possible Movements	Example
Fibrous	Articulating bones are fastened together by a thin layer of dense connective tissue.	None	Suture between bones of skull, joint between the distal ends of tibia and fibula
Cartilaginous	Articulating bones are connected by hyaline cartilage or fibrocartilage.	Limited movement, as when back is bent or twisted	Joints between the bodies of vertebrae, symphysis pubis
Synovial	Articulating bones are surrounded by a joint capsule of ligaments and synovial membranes; ends of articulating bones are covered by hyaline cartilage and separated by synovial fluid.	Allow free movement (see the following list)	
1. Ball-and-socket	Ball-shaped head of one bone articulates with cup-shaped cavity of another.	Movements in all planes and rotation	Shoulder, hip
2. Condyloid	Oval-shaped condyle of one bone articulates with elliptical cavity of another.	Variety of movements in different planes, but no rotation	Joints between the metacarpals and phalanges
3. Gliding	Articulating surfaces are nearly flat or slightly curved.	Sliding or twisting	Joints between various bones of wrist and ankle, sacroiliac joints, joints between ribs 2-7 and sternum
4. Hinge	Convex surface of one bone articulates with concave surface of another.	Flexion and extension	Elbow, joints of phalanges
5. Pivot	Cylindrical surface of one bone articulates with ring of bone and ligament.	Rotation around a central axis	Joint between the proximal ends of radius and ulna
6. Saddle	Articulating surfaces have both concave and convex regions; the surface of one bone fits the complementary surface of another.	Variety of movements	Joint between the carpal and metacarpal of thumb

Table 3-4

Clavicle: One of the pair of long bones that form the anterior part of the pectoral girdle. It is commonly called the collarbone.

Scapula: One of the pair of large, flat, triangular bones that form the dorsal part of the pectoral girdle. It is commonly called the shoulder blade.

Olecranon process: A projection on the ulna that forms the bony point of the elbow.

Styloid process: A projection on the temporal bone.

Pelvic girdle: The skeletal structure consisting of the ilium, the sacrum, and the coccyx.

Acetabulum: The deep depression on the lateral surface of the hipbone, on which the ball-shaped head of the femur articulates.

Obturator foramen: A large opening on each side of the lower part of the hipbone.

Patella: A flat, triangular bone at the front of the knee joint. It is also called the kneecap.

Muscular System

Muscle: Connective tissue made up of contractile cells or fibers that produce movement. There are three types of muscle: skeletal, or voluntary; smooth, also called visceral, or involuntary; and cardiac. There are two types of proteins in muscle tissue: actin and myosin. For a list of some of the main muscles of the human body, see Figure 3-9.

Skeletal muscle: A muscle composed of cylindrical, multinucleated, and striated fibers that works together with bones to enable movement. Skeletal muscles are characterized by contractility, elasticity, excitability, and extensibility. There are more than 600 skeletal muscles in the human body. See Table 3-5 for examples of

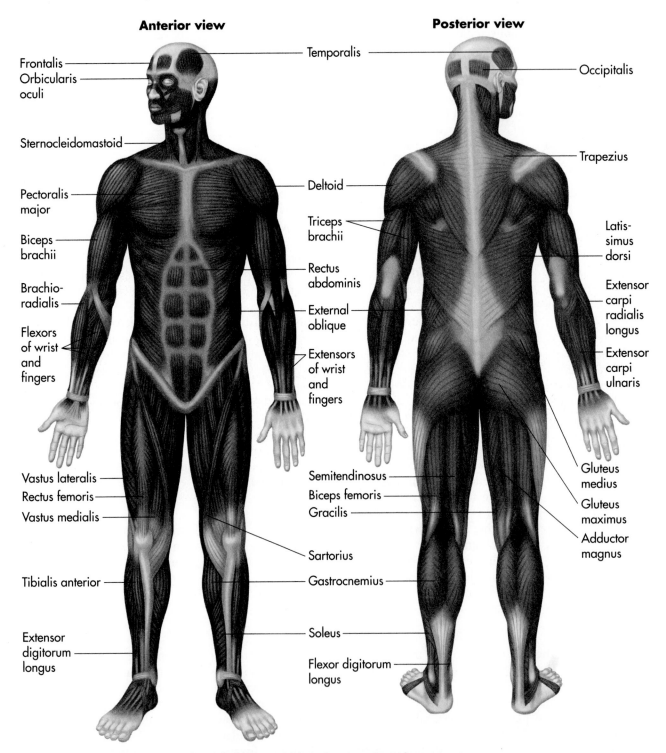

Anterior view

Frontalis
Orbicularis oculi
Sternocleidomastoid
Pectoralis major
Biceps brachii
Brachio-radialis
Flexors of wrist and fingers
Vastus lateralis
Rectus femoris
Vastus medialis
Tibialis anterior
Extensor digitorum longus

Temporalis
Deltoid
Triceps brachii
Rectus abdominis
External oblique
Extensors of wrist and fingers
Semitendinosus
Biceps femoris
Gracilis
Sartorius
Gastrocnemius
Soleus
Flexor digitorum longus

Posterior view

Occipitalis
Trapezius
Latissimus dorsi
Extensor carpi radialis longus
Extensor carpi ulnaris
Gluteus medius
Gluteus maximus
Adductor magnus

Figure 3-9 *Many of the large muscles in the body are visible in these anterior and posterior views.*

Skeletal Muscle	Action
Masseter	Closes the jaw
Temporalis	Closes the jaw
Sternocleidomastoid	Flexes and rotates the head
Trapezius	Extends the head and moves the scapula
Pectoralis major	Adducts and flexes the arm
Deltoid	Abducts the arm
Biceps	Flexes and supinates the forearm
Triceps	Extends the forearm
Brachioradialis	Flexes the forearm
Brachialis	Flexes the forearm
Gluteus maximus	Extends the thigh
Gluteus medius	Abducts and rotates the thigh
Quadriceps femoris	Extends the leg
Sartorius	Flexes the thigh; flexes and rotates the leg
Hamstring	Flexes the leg and extends the thigh
Gastrocnemius	Flexes the foot

Table 3-5

skeletal muscles and their actions. Skeletal muscles are also called striated or voluntary muscles.

Smooth muscle: A spindle-shaped muscle that causes the contraction of blood vessels and viscera such as the intestines and the stomach.

Cardiac muscle: A special striated muscle of the myocardium that pumps blood through the heart and blood vessels. Its contraction is not under voluntary control.

Muscle fiber: Any individual muscle cell.

Myofibril, or myofibrilla: A slender, striated strand of contractile fiber within skeletal and cardiac muscle cells.

Epimysium: The fibrous sheath that surrounds muscle tissue. It may also fuse with a fascia that attaches a muscle to a bone.

Endomysium: The fibrous sheath that surrounds each individual muscle cell.

Fascia: A sheet of fibrous connective tissue that covers, separates, or supports muscle.

Tendon: A band of dense fibrous connective tissue, generally white in color, that attaches muscle to bone.

Ligament: A band or sheet of fibrous tissue that connects two or more bones, cartilages, or other structures.

Sarcoplasm: The cytoplasm of muscle fiber.

Sarcolemma: The cell membrane of a muscle fiber.

Sarcomere: The smallest functional unit of a myofibril.

Neuromuscular junction: The region of contact between the ends of an axon and a skeletal muscle fiber.

Excitability: The ability of muscle tissue to react and respond to stimulation.

Contractility: The ability of muscle tissue to shorten, or contract, in response to a stimulus.

Elasticity: The capacity of tissues to return to their original shape and length after contraction or extension.

Contraction: A shortening or tightening of a muscle. Skeletal muscles need actin, myosin, calcium, ATP, and neurotransmitters to contract. All other muscles need only ATP and calcium.

Actin: A protein that forms the thin fibrils in muscle fibers.

Myosin: A skeletal and cardiac muscle protein that interacts with actin to cause muscle contraction.

Muscle tone: The continual state of slight contraction present in muscles. It is also called tonus.

Flexion: A bending that decreases the angle between two bones of a joint.

Extension: A straightening that increases the angle between two bones of a joint.

Nervous System

Nervous system: One of the body's regulatory systems. It controls all body activities by responding to internal and external stimuli and sending out signals

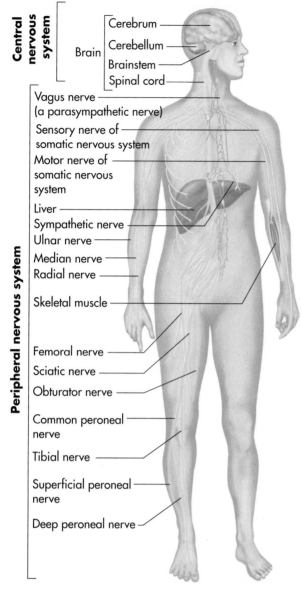

Central nervous system
Brain
- Cerebrum
- Cerebellum
- Brainstem
- Spinal cord

Peripheral nervous system
- Vagus nerve (a parasympathetic nerve)
- Sensory nerve of somatic nervous system
- Motor nerve of somatic nervous system
- Liver
- Sympathetic nerve
- Ulnar nerve
- Median nerve
- Radial nerve
- Skeletal muscle
- Femoral nerve
- Sciatic nerve
- Obturator nerve
- Common peroneal nerve
- Tibial nerve
- Superficial peroneal nerve
- Deep peroneal nerve

Figure 3-10 *The main organs of the nervous system are the brain, the spinal cord, and the nerves. The spinal nerves originate in the spinal cord, whereas the cranial nerves (for example, the vagus nerve) originate in the brain.*

or impulses to other nerves and various body organs. The brain, the spinal cord, and the nerves make up the nervous system, which is divided into two groups: the central nervous system and the peripheral nervous system. See Figure 3-10.

Nerve Cells and Neurotransmitters

Neuron: A nerve cell, the basic unit of the nervous system. It consists of a cell body, one or more dendrites, and a single axon. The two forms of neurons are sensory and motor.

Cell body of a neuron: The main part of the neuron. It is also called the soma.

Dendrite: A nerve cell process that conducts impulses to the cell body.

Axon: A nerve cell process that conducts impulses away from the cell body.

Sensory neuron: A neuron that carries impulses to the spinal cord and the brain. It is also known as an afferent neuron.

Motor neuron: A neuron that carries impulses from the central nervous system out to muscles and glands. It stimulates a muscle to contract or a gland to secrete. It is also known as an efferent neuron.

Myelin: A white, fatty substance, largely composed of phospholipids and protein, that surrounds many nerve fibers.

Synapse: The junction between two neurons.

Neuroglia cell: A type of nerve cell that supports, protects, and nourishes the neuron. There are four kinds: astrocytes, microglia, ependymal cells, and oligodendrocytes.

Astrocyte: A large, star-shaped cell that provides nutrition.

Microglion: One of many small interstitial cells in the brain and spinal cord that serve as phagocytic cells and respond to inflammation.

Ependymal cell: A columnar cell located in the brain that produces cerebrospinal fluid.

Oligodendrocyte: A type of neuroglial cell that produces myelin, the white matter of the nervous system.

Nerve impulse: The electrochemical process involved in neural transmission.

Action potential: The sudden electrical charge transmitted across the cell membrane of a nerve fiber.

Neurotransmitter: A chemical substance that is released from synaptic knobs into synaptic clefts. Neurotransmitters include acetylcholine, dopamine, norepinephrine, epinephrine, serotonin, histamine, and gamma-aminobutyric acid (GABA).

Central Nervous System

Central nervous system: The part of the nervous system consisting of the brain and the spinal cord.

The Brain

Brain: The part of the central nervous system contained within the cranium. The brain consists of four major parts: the cerebrum, the cerebellum, the diencephalon, and the brainstem. See Figure 3-11.

Cerebrum: The largest and uppermost portion of the brain. The cerebrum is divided into two hemispheres, right and left, and five lobes: frontal, parietal, occipital, temporal, and insular.

Right hemisphere: The portion of the brain responsible for controlling the left side of the body. It also controls hearing and tactile and spatial perception.

Left hemisphere: The portion of the brain responsible for controlling the right side of the body. It is also responsible for verbal, analytical, and computational skills.

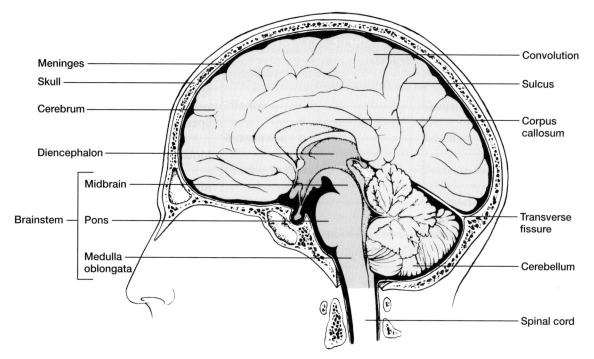

Figure 3-11 *The major portions of the brain include the cerebrum, the cerebellum, and the brainstem.*

Frontal lobe: The part of the brain responsible for complex concentration, planning, and problem solving. It also contains the olfactory cortex, which interprets smells.

Parietal lobe: The part of the brain responsible for the interpretation of sensory input other than sight, sound, and smell. It contains the gustatory area responsible for taste.

Occipital lobe: The part of the brain responsible for visual recognition.

Temporal lobe: The part of the brain responsible for the interpretation of sensory experiences such as hearing and smell. It is also said to be the center for emotion, memory, and personality.

Insular lobe, or **central lobe:** The part of the brain responsible for visceral or primitive emotions, drives, and reactions.

Broca's area: The part of the brain responsible for motor speech and for controlling the muscular actions of the mouth, tongue, and larynx.

Wernicke's area: The part of the brain responsible for language comprehension.

Corpus callosum: A large and transverse band of myelinated nerve fibers that connect the cerebral hemispheres. It is the largest commissure of the brain.

Basal ganglion: One of four islands of gray matter located in the white matter of the cerebrum: the lentiform nucleus, the caudate nucleus, the amygdaloid nucleus, and the claustrum. One function of the basal ganglia is to initiate and regulate muscular activity.

Diencephalon: The centrally located portion of the brain surrounded by the cerebrum that contains the thalamus and hypothalamus.

Thalamus: The subdivision of the diencephalon that sorts sensory impulses and directs them to the appropriate areas in the brain. It is basically a relay station for sensory impulses.

Hypothalamus: The subdivision of the diencephalon that assists in controlling body temperature, water balance, sleep, appetite, emotions of fear and pleasure, and involuntary functions.

Brainstem: The portion of the brain, located between the diencephalon and the spinal cord, that controls vital visceral activities. It consists of the midbrain, the pons, and the medulla oblongata.

Midbrain: The section of the brainstem that controls visual and auditory reflexes, such as turning to listen to a loud noise.

Pons: The section of the brainstem that relays sensory impulses and regulates the rate and depth of breathing in coordination with the medulla oblongata.

Medulla oblongata: The section of the brainstem that contains the cardiac center (which controls heart rate), the vasomotor center (which controls blood pressure), and the respiratory center (which controls the rate, rhythm, and depth of breathing).

Cerebellum: The second largest portion of the brain, located below the occipital lobes of the cerebrum. The cerebellum coordinates skeletal muscle activity. Damage to this area can result in tremors, loss of muscle tone, and loss of equilibrium.

Ventricle: One of four small interconnected cavities within the brain filled with cerebrospinal fluid.

The Spinal Cord

Spinal cord: A part of the central nervous system that conducts sensory and motor impulses, through nerves to the trunk and limbs, and serves as a center for reflex

Granulocyte, or granular leukocyte: A leukocyte that has large granules in its cytoplasm, which stain in different colors under a microscope. Granular leukocytes include neutrophils, basophils, and eosinophils.

Neutrophil: The most frequently occurring leukocyte (55% to 70% of all WBCs). Neutrophils are phagocytic in acute inflammatory response.

Basophil: A granulocyte that mediates allergic reactions. In the tissues, a basophil is called a mast cell. These cells produce heparin and histamine.

Eosinophil: A granulocyte that functions as defense against helminthic and protozoan infections and also participates in allergic reactions.

Phagocyte: A cell that ingests bacteria, foreign particles, and other cells.

Phagocytosis: The process by which special cells engulf and destroy cellular debris and microorganisms. It is also called cell eating.

Pinocytosis: The process by which extracellular fluid is taken into a cell. It is also known as cell drinking.

Agranulocyte: A leukocyte that lacks granules. Nongranular leukocytes include lymphocytes and monocytes.

Lymphocyte: The smallest WBC. These cells travel from the blood to the lymph and lymph nodes and back into circulation. They are the main means of providing the body with immunity. They recognize antigens, produce antibodies, prevent excess tissue damage, and become memory cells. Type B lymphocytes produce antibodies. Type T lymphocytes regulate type B lymphocytes and macrophages.

Monocyte: The largest of the WBCs. Monocytes and neutrophils are largely phagocytic.

Macrophage: A monocyte that has left circulation and settled in tissue. Along with neutrophils, macrophages are the major phagocytic cells of the immune system. They recognize and digest all antigens and also process and present these antigens to T cells, activating the specific immune response.

Thrombocyte: A cell fragment and the smallest formed element of blood. It is also called a platelet. Thrombocytes are essential in blood coagulation.

The Heart and Blood Vessels

Heart: A muscular organ, about the size of a closed fist, that acts as the pump of the circulatory system. It is made up of three layers: the epicardium, the myocardium, and the endocardium. See Figure 3-16.

Endocardium: The innermost layer of the heart.

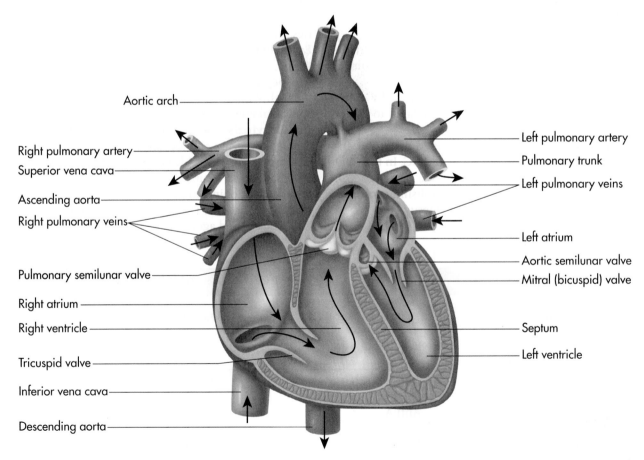

Figure 3-16 *The heart has four main chambers: left and right atria and left and right ventricles. This figure shows the pathway of blood through the heart.*

Myocardium: The middle layer of the heart and the most important structure of the heart. It contains the heart muscles that can regulate cardiac output.

Epicardium: The outermost layer of the heart.

Atrium: A thin-walled chamber that receives blood from the veins. There are two atria in the heart, the right and the left.

Right atrium: The chamber that receives deoxygenated blood from systemic veins.

Left atrium: The chamber that receives oxygenated blood from the pulmonary veins.

Ventricle: A thick-walled chamber that pumps blood out of the heart. There are two ventricles in the heart, the right and the left.

Right ventricle: The chamber that pumps blood to the lungs.

Left ventricle: The chamber that pumps blood to the tissues of the whole body. It is the largest and the most powerful of the four chambers.

Valve: A membranous structure that temporarily closes to permit the flow of fluid through a passage in only one direction. The four valves in the heart are the bicuspid (or mitral) valve, the tricuspid valve, the aortic valve, and the pulmonary valve.

Cardiac cycle: The contraction and relaxation of the ventricles, known as systole and diastole. At a normal heart rate, one cardiac cycle lasts 0.8 seconds.

Systole: The contraction phase.

Diastole: The relaxation phase.

Cardiac center: The control center of the heart located in the medulla oblongata. It has both sympathetic and parasympathetic components.

Cardiac conduction system: A system consisting of specialized cardiac muscle cells. Its components are the sinoatrial (SA) node, the atrioventricular (A-V) node, the A-V bundle (bundle of His), the bundle branches, and the Purkinje fibers.

Cardiac output: The volume of blood pumped per minute by the heart, which increases during exercise.

Stroke volume: The amount of blood that the ventricle discharges with each heartbeat.

Pulse pressure: The pressure exerted by the circulating volume of blood on the walls of the blood vessels. It is proportional to stroke volume.

Myocardial oxygen demand: The demand for oxygen by the heart muscle. It is raised by increases in diastolic blood pressure, contractility, heart rate, and heart size.

Contractility: The force of left ventricular ejection.

Diastolic blood pressure: The blood pressure during diastole, the period of least pressure in the arterial vascular system.

Heart sound: A normal noise produced during the cardiac cycle by the closure of the mitral and tricuspid valves and of the aortic and pulmonic valves.

Murmur: Abnormal heart sound. The three types of murmurs are systolic, diastolic, and continuous murmurs.

Artery: A vessel that carries blood away from the heart.

Capillary: One of many very small vessels that connect arteries and veins.

Vein: A vessel that sends blood toward the heart. Its walls are thinner than those of arteries, and it contains valves, which prevent the backflow of blood.

Systemic artery: An artery that carries oxygenated blood.

Pulmonary artery: An artery that transfers low-oxygen blood to the lungs.

Aorta: The largest artery in the body. It consists of the ascending aorta, the aortic arch, and the descending aorta. The descending aorta consists of the thoracic aorta and the abdominal aorta.

Coronary artery: One of a pair of vessels that supply blood to the myocardium. The coronary arteries are the only vessels that branch from the ascending aorta.

Aortic arch: A part of the aorta from which three vessels branch: the brachiocephalic trunk (or innominate artery), the left common carotid artery, and the left subclavian artery.

External iliac artery: An artery that provides the blood supply for the lower extremities.

Internal iliac artery: An artery that supplies blood to the pelvic organs.

Internal carotid artery: One of the primary vessels that provide blood to the brain.

Vertebral artery: One of the primary vessels that provide blood to the brain.

Internal jugular vein: One of the primary vessels that drain blood from the brain.

Vertebral vein: One of the primary vessels that drain blood from the brain.

Azygous vein: One of the seven veins in the thorax. It drains blood from the thoracic and abdominal walls and empties into the superior vena cava.

Saphenous vein: A superficial vein of the lower extremity. It is the longest vein in the body.

Umbilical cord: The attachment connecting a fetus with the placenta. First formed during the fifth week of pregnancy, it contains two arteries and one vein.

Ductus venosus: The vascular channel in the fetus that is a continuation of the umbilical vein to the inferior vena cava. It becomes the ligamentum venosum of the liver.

Ductus arteriosus: A vascular channel in the fetus located between the pulmonary artery and the aorta. It becomes the ligamentum arteriosum.

Fetal circulation: The pathway of blood circulation in the fetus. Oxygenated blood from the placenta is carried through the umbilical vein to the fetal heart.

Lymphatic System

Lymphatic system: The body system that returns excess interstitial fluid to the blood and protects the body against disease.

Lymph: A thin, watery fluid in the lymphatic vessels that is filtered by the lymph nodes and contains chyle, RBCs, and WBCs, most of which are lymphocytes.

Chyle: A milklike alkaline fluid consisting of digestive products and absorbed fats.

Lymphatic vessel: A vessel that carries lymph. Lymphatic vessels resemble veins, but they have more valves, thinner walls, and lymph nodes, and they carry excess fluid away from the tissues.

Right lymphatic duct: The lymphatic vessel that drains lymph from the upper right quadrant of the body.

Thoracic duct: The lymphatic vessel that drains all the lymph not drained by the right lymphatic duct.

Lymph node: A small, oval structure that filters the lymph and fights infection. Lymph nodes are located along lymphatic vessels except in the nervous system. Superficial nodes are found in the neck, axilla, and groin.

Spleen: The lymph organ that filters and also serves as a reservoir for blood.

Thymus: A gland essential to the maturation and development of the immune system. T-lymphocytes mature in this gland.

Respiratory System

Respiratory system: The body system that provides oxygen to cells and removes carbon dioxide from them. The organs of the respiratory system include the nose, the pharynx, the larynx, the trachea, the bronchi, and the lungs. The nose, pharynx, larynx, and upper trachea are collectively known as the upper respiratory tract. The lower respiratory tract consists of the lower trachea, the bronchi, and the lungs. See Figure 3-17.

Respiratory center: A group of nerve cells in the medulla oblongata and pons of the brain that control the rhythm of breathing in response to changes in oxygen and carbon dioxide levels in the blood and cerebrospinal fluid.

Nose: The projection that serves as the entrance to the nasal cavities. Hairs and cilia in the nose help trap dust, bacteria, and other particles and keep them from entering the body. The nose also warms and moistens the air, and it is involved with the sense of smell.

Larynx: The organ at the upper end of the trachea that contains the vocal cords, which vibrate to make speech.

Trachea: The tube that extends from the larynx and branches into two bronchi that lead to the lungs. It is also called the windpipe.

Lung: A spongy organ in the thorax used for breathing. The two highly elastic lungs are the main component of the respiratory system. The left lung is divided into two lobes, and the right lung is divided into three lobes.

Alveolus: One of many clusters of air sacs at the end of the bronchioles in the lungs. The exchange of gases occurs in the alveoli.

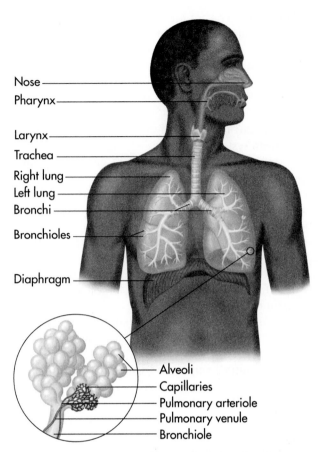

Figure 3-17 *The exchange of oxygen for carbon dioxide between the air and blood occurs within the lungs, where the alveoli and the capillaries are in intimate contact.*

Inspiration: The process of letting air into the lungs, also known as inhalation. The major muscle of inspiration is the diaphragm, the contraction of which creates a negative pressure in the chest.

Expiration: Breathing out, the process of letting air out of the lungs, which is normally a passive process. It is also called exhalation.

External respiration: The exchange of oxygen and carbon dioxide between the air in the lungs and the blood in the surrounding capillaries.

Internal respiration: The exchange of gases between the tissue cells and the blood in the tissue capillaries.

Carbon dioxide transport: A process that moves carbon dioxide from the tissues to the lungs in three forms: as bicarbonate, bound to hemoglobin, as carbaminohemoglobin, and as dissolved carbon dioxide.

Oxygen transport: The transfer of oxygen in the blood. Approximately 3% of oxygen is transported as a dissolved gas in the plasma; 97% is carried by hemoglobin molecules.

Surfactant: Any of certain lipoproteins that are produced by the lungs and that reduce the surface tension within the alveoli, keeping them inflated. Artificial surfactants are administered to premature infants to help prevent their lungs from collapsing.

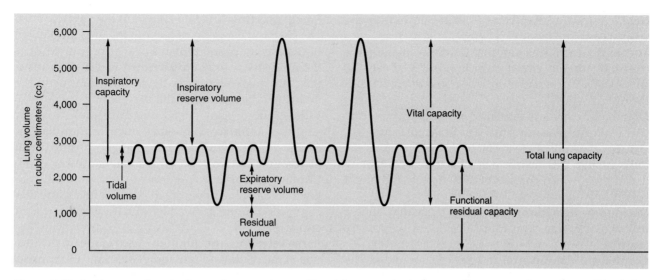

Figure 3-18 *A spirogram showing lung volumes and capacities.* A lung capacity is the sum of two or more lung volumes. The vital capacity, for example, is the sum of the tidal volume, the inspiratory reserve volume, and the expiratory reserve volume. Note that residual volume cannot be measured with a spirometer because it is air that cannot be exhaled. Therefore, the total lung capacity (the sum of the vital capacity and the residual volume) also cannot be measured with a spirometer.

Spirometer: An instrument that measures and records the volume of air that moves in and out of the lungs.
Spirogram: A chart with recorded volumetric information. See Figure 3-18.
Pulmonary function test: The assessment that provides information about airflow, lung volumes, and the diffusion of gas.

Digestive System

Digestive system: The group of organs that change food so that it can be used by the body. The organs of the digestive system include the mouth, the pharynx, the esophagus, the stomach, and the small and large intestines. See Figure 3-19.
Digestive tract, or **alimentary canal:** The digestive tube, running from the mouth to the anus. The wall consists of four layers, or tunics: the mucosa, the submucosa, the muscular layer, and the serous layer, or serosa.
Serosa: The outermost layer of the digestive tract. It is composed of connective tissue. Above the diaphragm, it is known as the adventitia.
Mouth: The cavity where food is chewed into small pieces and is mixed with saliva to form a moist, soft lump called a bolus.
Saliva: A fluid that moistens food and begins the chemical breakdown of carbohydrates. It is produced by the salivary glands located along the upper and lower jaws and under the tongue.
Salivary gland: A gland that secretes saliva. There are three pairs of glands secreting into the mouth: the parotid glands, the sublingual glands, and the submandibular glands.

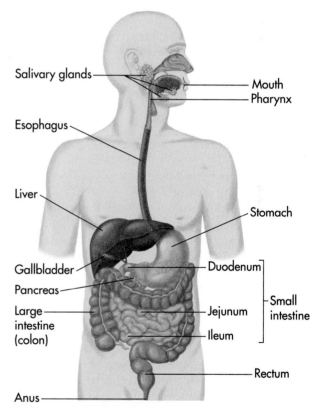

Figure 3-19 *The main organs and accessory organs of the digestive system change food into a form the body can use.*

Parotid gland: The largest salivary gland, which secretes serous fluid.
Sublingual gland: The smallest salivary gland, which secretes mucus.
Submandibular gland: A salivary gland located in the floor of the mouth. It secretes both mucus and serous fluid.

Uvula: A structure of soft tissue hanging down from the soft palate in the mouth.

Tooth: A dental structure that develops in the jaws, consisting of the crown (which projects above the gum), the neck (between the crown and the root), and the root.

Enamel: The hardest substance in the body, covering the crown and consisting mainly of calcium salts.

Dentin: The bulk of the tooth.

Pulp cavity: The interior part of a tooth, containing dental pulp, which consists of cells, nerves, and blood vessels or lymph vessels.

Deciduous dentition: The set of teeth that appear in the mouth first, also called deciduous or primary teeth.

Esophageal sphincter: The sphincter located in the lower portion of the esophagus. It is also called the cardiac sphincter.

Peristalsis: Rhythmic contractions that move food. This action occurs throughout the digestive tract.

Stomach: A muscular J-shaped organ that stores, churns, and further digests food. The stomach produces strong acids and enzymes that, combined with the churning action, begin the chemical breakdown of food.

Gastric gland: One of the glands in the stomach mucosa that secrete hydrochloric acid, mucin, and pepsinogen. Four different types of cells make up the gastric glands: mucous cells (goblet cells), parietal cells, chief cells, and endocrine cells.

Parietal cell: A gastric cell that secretes hydrochloric acid and intrinsic factor, which aids in the absorption of vitamin B_{12}.

Chief cell: A gastric cell that secretes pepsinogen, an active form of the enzyme pepsin.

Endocrine cell: A gastric cell that secretes the hormone gastrin, which regulates gastric activity. See Table 3-9.

Chyme: A mixture of partially digested food, water, and digestive juices that forms in the stomach and passes through the pylorus into the duodenum.

Intestine: One of two long, tubular organs distinguished by the difference in their diameters.

AT A GLANCE	Hormones of the Digestive System

Secretion	Source
Gastrin	Stomach
Secretin	Small intestine
Cholecystokinin	Small intestine

Table 3-9

Small intestine: The longest part of the digestive tract. The chemical digestion of fats and the final breakdown of carbohydrates and proteins take place here. Most of the nutrients in food are absorbed in the small intestine. The small intestine is divided into three parts: the duodenum, the jejunum, and the ileum.

Villus: One of many small, fingerlike projections, or villi, on the surface of the membrane in the small intestine through which digested food is absorbed. Villi increase the surface area of the small intestine.

Cholecystokinin: A hormone that is secreted from the mucosa of the upper small intestine and stimulates contraction of the gallbladder to release bile and pancreatic enzymes.

Large intestine: The intestine joined to the small intestine at the ileum and extending to the anus. It consists of the cecum, the colon, the rectum, and the anal canal. It is divided into ascending, transverse, descending, and sigmoid portions. The large intestine is responsible for making Vitamin K and some B vitamins, absorbing water and electrolytes, and storing and eliminating undigested waste.

Anal canal: The final portion of the digestive tract, between the rectum and the anus. Material that the body cannot use is excreted through the anus as feces. The internal anal sphincter is under involuntary control. The external anal sphincter can be controlled voluntarily.

Additional Organs and Processes Involved with Digestion

Kupffer cell: A cell in the liver responsible for cleansing the blood.

Hepatocyte: A liver cell responsible for storage, synthesis of bile salts, detoxification, synthesis of plasma proteins, and metabolism of carbohydrates, proteins, and lipids.

Liver: An organ of the digestive system whose main role is to produce bile.

Bile: The fluid responsible for excreting bile pigments and cholesterol from the breakdown of hemoglobin. Bile helps the body digest and absorb fat.

Pancreas: An organ that produces enzymes that digest fats, proteins, and carbohydrates. Pancreatic substances also neutralize the acids produced by the stomach.

Metabolism: The physical and chemical processes that take place in a living organism, resulting in growth, production of energy, elimination of wastes, and other body functions. The fundamental metabolic processes are anabolism and catabolism.

Basal metabolism: The minimal energy that is necessary to maintain the body's functions at a low level.

Anabolism: The conversion of simple compounds into more complex substances needed by the body and living matter.

Catabolism: The breakdown of substances into simple compounds that liberates energy for use in work and heat production. It produces carbon dioxide, water, and energy.

Thermogenesis: The production of heat needed to utilize food, especially within the human body.

Core temperature: The temperature around the internal organs.

Shell temperature: The temperature near the body surface.

Endocrine System

Endocrine system: A system of glands whose secretions coordinate many body functions. Its response to change is slower and more prolonged than that of the nervous system. See Figure 3-20.

Endocrine gland: A ductless gland that secretes hormones directly into the bloodstream. See Table 3-10.

Hormone: A protein or steroid carried through the blood to a target organ. Secretion is regulated by other hormones, through a negative feedback system, or by neurotransmitters.

Steroid hormone: A hormone derived from cholesterol. Steroid hormones include the adrenal cortex hormones, androgens, and estrogens.

Control of Hormonal Secretions

Hormone secretion is precisely regulated by the hypothalamus, the anterior pituitary gland, and other groups of glands that respond to the hypothalamus and pituitary glands. See Figure 3-21.

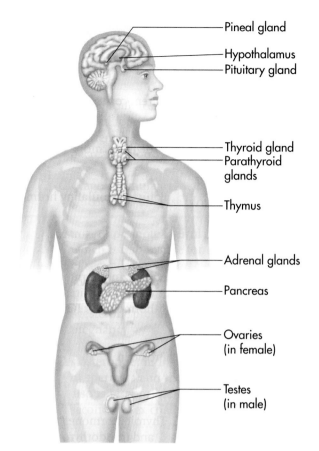

Figure 3-20 *The endocrine system produces hormones that affect activities such as growth, metabolism, and reproduction.*

AT A GLANCE	Endocrine Glands and Their Functions	
Gland	**Hormones**	**Major Functions**
Hypothalamus	Releasing and inhibiting hormones (TRH—Thyrotropin-releasing hormone, CRH—Corticotropin-releasing hormone, GnRH—Gonadotropin-releasing hormone, GHRH—Growth hormone-releasing hormone)	These hormones control the release of anterior pituitary hormones.
Posterior pituitary (hormone storage site)	Vasopressin (antidiuretic hormone)	Vasopressin increases reabsorption of water in kidney tubules and stimulates smooth muscle tissue in blood vessels to constrict.
	Oxytocin	Oxytocin increases the contractility of the uterus and causes milk ejection.
Anterior pituitary	Thyroid-stimulating hormone (TSH)	TSH stimulates the thyroid gland to produce thyroid hormones (T_3 and T_4 secretion).

Table 3-10

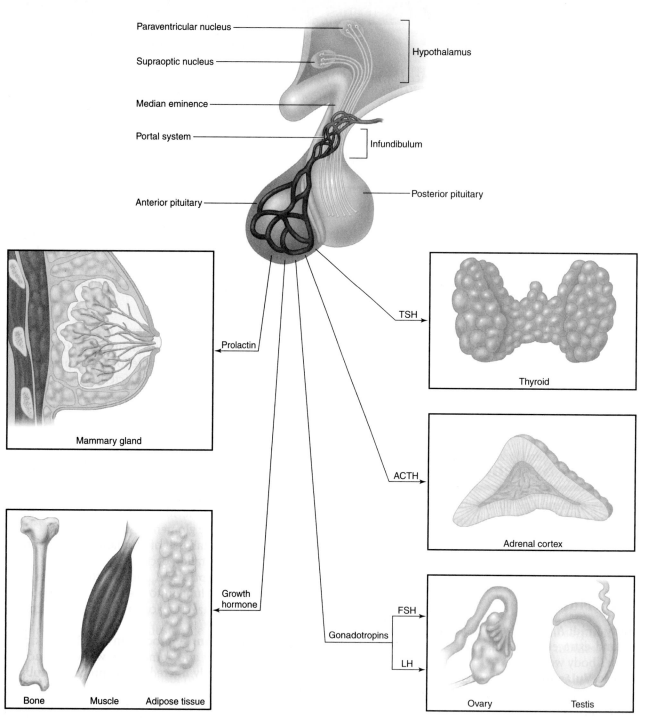

Figure 3-21 *Hormones secreted by the anterior pituitary and their target organs. Notice that the anterior pituitary controls some (but by no means all) of the other endocrine glands.*

and includes multiple actions that conserve sodium and water, resulting in an increased blood volume.

Ureter: One of two long, slender tubes that extend from the kidneys to the urinary bladder.

Urinary bladder: The expandable organ that temporarily stores urine. Stretch receptors in the bladder create the urge to urinate. Urination is also called voiding urine or micturition.

Ruga: A ridge, wrinkle, or fold, as in a mucous membrane. Rugae line the urinary bladder and the stomach.

Detrusor muscle: The smooth muscle of the urinary bladder wall.

Fallopian
(uterine) tube

Uterus

Urinary bladde

Clitoris

Labium minus
(plural, labia n

Labium majus
(plural, labia n

Figure 3-24 *T*
develop.

Progesteror
endometriun
implantation
Corpus albi
face of the o
conception c
Broad ligan
supports the
latum uteri.
Mons pubi:
pubic symph
with pubic h
Menstrual c
in the endon
the endome
ates. The ute
phase, the s
See Figure 3

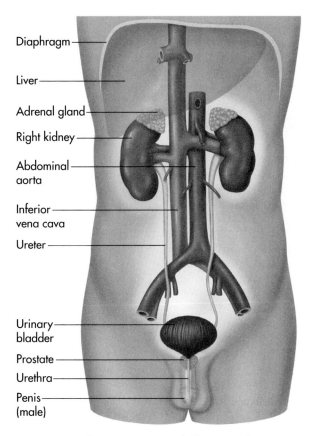

Diaphragm

Liver

Adrenal gland

Right kidney

Abdominal
aorta

Inferior
vena cava

Ureter

Urinary
bladder

Prostate

Urethra

Penis
(male)

Figure 3-22 *The urinary system, also known as the excretory system, removes waste products from the body and maintains the proper balance of body fluids and their chemistry.*

Trigone: A triangular area on the internal floor of the bladder between the opening of the two ureters and the internal urethral orifice.

Urethra: The tube through which urine leaves the body.

Buffer system: A physical or physiological system that tends to maintain constancy. For example, the kidneys act as a buffer system to help regulate blood pH.

Reproductive System

Genitalia: The reproductive organs of males and females.

Gonad: One of the two types of primary reproductive organ, the ovary and the testis, or testicle. Ovaries and testes produce gametes and hormones.

Follicle-stimulating hormone (FSH): The hormone produced by the anterior pituitary that stimulates development of ova in the ovary and spermatozoa in the testes.

Male Reproductive System (Figure 3-23)

Testis: The male gonad. There are two testes, normally situated in the scrotum, which produce sperm cells and male sex hormones.

Lobule: One of two layers that surround each testis: an outer mesothelial layer (tunica vaginalis) and an inner white capsule (tunica albuginea).

Spermatogonium: A male germ cell that gives rise to spermatocyte early in spermatogenesis.

Spermatocyte: A male germ cell, or gamete, that arises from a spermatogonium.

Spermatozoon: A mature male gamete that develops in the seminiferous tubules of the testes, consisting of a head, a midpiece, and a tail.

Acrosome: A caplike structure over the head of the spermatozoon that helps the sperm to penetrate the ovum during fertilization. It is also called the acrosomal cap.

Ejaculatory duct: The passage formed by the junction of the duct of the seminal vesicles and ductus deferens through which semen enters the urethra.

Seminal vesicle: One of a pair of saclike accessory glands located posterior to the urinary bladder in the male that provide nourishment for sperm.

Prostate: A gland, located below the neck of the bladder in males, that surrounds the proximal portion of the urethra. It is a firm structure composed of muscular and glandular tissue that secretes alkaline phosphatase.

AT A GLANCE	Hormonal Effects on the Kidneys
Hormone	**Stimulus**
Vasopressin (ADH)	Increases plasma osmolarity and increases blood volume.
Aldosterone	Increases blood volume via angiotensin II and decreases plasma potassium ions.
Angiotensin II	Increases blood volume via renin.
Parathyroid hormone	Increases plasma calcium ions.

Table 3-11

Ureter (from kidn

Urinary bladder –
Prostate gland —
Spermatic cord–
Penis–
Epididymis–
Testis –
Urethral orifice–
Scrotum–

Figure 3-23 *The
fertilize an egg.*

**Cowper's glan
base of the per
bourethral glan
Semen, or **sem
the male repro
thra on ejaculat
Epididymis: O
bules along the
and carry sperm
Glans penis: T
Prepuce, or **fo
the glans penis.
Emission: A di
the urethra.
**Tunica albugir
testis in the ma
Phimosis: A ti
on the penis th
skin over the g
and is usually
by infection.
Impotence: Th
to ejaculate afte
Circumcision:
puce of the pe
boys.
Vasectomy: Su
of the ductus (

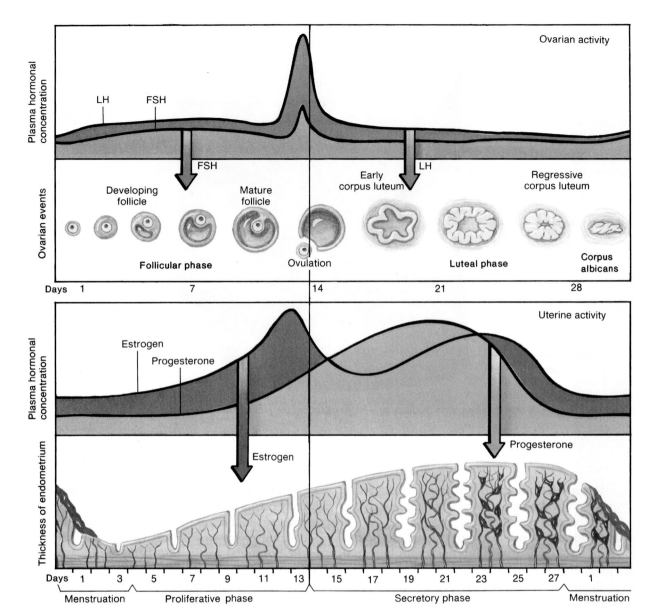

Figure 3-25 *Major events in the ovarian and menstrual cycles.*

Instructions:

Answer the following questions. Check your answers in the *Answer Key* that follows this section.

1. The first period of menstrual bleeding is called
   - A. Menses
   - B. Menopause
   - C. Menstruation
   - D. Menarche
   - E. Mendacious

2. The energy that is necessary to keep the body functioning at a minimal level is known as
   - A. Thermogenesis
   - B. Catabolism
   - C. Metabolite
   - D. Metabolic reaction
   - E. Basal metabolism

3. The portion of the brain that coordinates skeletal muscle activity is the
   - A. Cerebellum
   - B. Pons
   - C. Medulla oblongata
   - D. Thalamus
   - E. Hypothalamus

4. The strands of DNA in the nucleus are called
   - A. Chromatin
   - B. Nucleolus
   - C. Network
   - D. Granules of RNA
   - E. Guanine

5. The part of the nervous system that governs conscious activities is the
   - A. Central
   - B. Autonomic
   - C. Somatic
   - D. Ventral
   - E. Myelin

6. A translucent band that is present in thick skin is called
   - A. Stratum corneum
   - B. Stratum granulosum
   - C. Stratum germinativum
   - D. Stratum spongiosum
   - E. Stratum lucidum

7. Which of the following endocrine glands releases glucagon?
   - A. Adrenal cortex
   - B. Thyroid gland
   - C. Pancreas
   - D. Hypothalamus
   - E. Anterior pituitary

8. Which of the following arteries carries deoxygenated blood from the heart to the lungs?
   - A. Femoral
   - B. Renal
   - C. Pulmonary
   - D. Brachial
   - E. Coronary

28. Which of the following is <u>not</u> a type of muscle tissue?

    A. Striated
    B. Visceral
    C. Skeletal
    D. Smooth
    E. Patella

29. The production of heat needed to utilize food is called

    A. Catabolism
    B. Thermogenesis
    C. Anabolism
    D. Metabolism
    E. Both A and D

30. Pulmonary arteries

    A. Send blood toward the heart
    B. Transfer oxygenated blood away from the heart
    C. Transfer low-oxygen blood away from the heart
    D. Are very small vessels that connect with veins
    E. Transfer blood to the brain

31. The three bones in the middle ear that amplify vibrations are called

    A. Auditory ossicles
    B. Cochlea
    C. Organs of Corti
    D. Vestibule
    E. Malleus

32. The part of the brain responsible for visual recognition is

    A. Occipital lobe
    B. Temporal lobe
    C. Parietal lobe
    D. Broca's area
    E. Pons

33. Which of the following is a type of hormone?

    A. Chyme
    B. Globulin
    C. Bile
    D. Secretin
    E. Agglutinin

34. The thalamus

    A. Controls body temperature
    B. Acts as a relay station for sensory impulses
    C. Is the center of the brain for memory and visual recognition
    D. Connects the two hemispheres of the brain
    E. Has no known function

35. Bitter taste receptors are located on what part of the tongue?

    A. Tip
    B. Right side
    C. Left side
    D. Middle
    E. Back

36. The white and outermost layer of the eye is called the

    A. Retina
    B. Iris
    C. Ciliary body
    D. Vitreous humor
    E. Sclera

37. The hormone epinephrine is produced by the

    A. Ovaries
    B. Adrenal medulla
    C. Thyroid
    D. Anterior pituitary
    E. Testes

38. Secretion of hormones is regulated by

    A. Other hormones
    B. Neurotransmitters
    C. Negative feedback system
    D. All of the above
    E. None of the above

39. All but which of the following are characteristics of the endocrine system?

    A. It is responsible for many conscious and unconscious activities.
    B. Its response is slow and prolonged when compared with that of the nervous system.
    C. Endocrine glands are ductless and release hormones into the bloodstream.
    D. It controls many body functions, such as blood pressure, heart rate, and sexual characteristics.
    E. The endocrine system produces hormones that affect activities such as growth, metabolism, and reproduction.

40. Type A blood has

    A. A antigen on the red blood cells and A antibodies in plasma
    B. B antigen on the red blood cells and A antibodies in plasma
    C. A antigen on the red blood cells and B antibodies in plasma
    D. Both A and B antigens on red blood cells and no antibodies in plasma
    E. No antigens on red blood cells and both A and B antibodies in plasma

41. The sympathetic action of the pupil of the eye is

    A. Constriction
    B. Dilation
    C. Stimulation
    D. Maintaining a constant size
    E. None of the above

42. A synapse is

    A. The junction between two neurons
    B. The junction between two bones
    C. The main part of the neuron
    D. A type of nerve cell that supports, protects, and nourishes the neuron
    E. A type of bone cell that supports, protects, and nourishes the bone

43. Which of the following is the correct spelling for the term describing an area of ossification of bone?

    A. Epifyseal
    B. Epifeseal
    C. Ephyseal
    D. Epiphyseal
    E. Epiphyceal

ANSWER KEY

1.	D		23.	B
2.	E		24.	C
3.	A		25.	A
4.	A		26.	A
5.	C		27.	D
6.	E		28.	E
7.	C		29.	B
8.	C		30.	C
9.	C		31.	A
10.	B		32.	A
11.	D		33.	D
12.	B		34.	B
13.	B		35.	E
14.	E		36.	E
15.	C		37.	B
16.	A		38.	D
17.	E		39.	A
18.	C		40.	C
19.	A		41.	B
20.	E		42.	A
21.	C		43.	D
22.	B			

CHAPTER 4

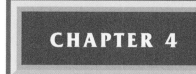

Pathophysiology

CHAPTER OUTLINE

Mechanisms of Disease

Immunology

Nonspecific Defense Mechanism
Specific Immune Response
Organs and Tissues of the Immune System

Hereditary and Congenital Diseases and Conditions

Hereditary Diseases and Conditions
Congenital Conditions

Neoplasia

Common Infectious Diseases

Major Diseases and Disorders

Diseases and Disorders of the Integumentary System
Diseases and Disorders of the Musculoskeletal System
Diseases and Disorders of the Nervous System
Diseases and Disorders of the Cardiovascular System
Diseases and Disorders of the Respiratory System
Diseases and Disorders of the Digestive System
Diseases and Disorders of the Endocrine System
Diseases and Disorders of the Sensory System
Diseases and Disorders of the Urinary System
Diseases and Disorders of the Reproductive System
Diseases and Disorders Specific to Children

COMPETENCY	CMA	RMA
General/Legal/Professional		
Provide patients with methods of health promotion and disease prevention	X	X
Use appropriate medical terminology		X

STRATEGIES TO SUCCESS

▶ *Study Skills*

Don't procrastinate!
   Don't cram for the exam. Leave yourself enough time to review your texts and the material summarized for you in this book, study class notes, and practice answering questions by using the CD-ROM that accompanies this text or by going through the self-evaluation section. Never leave studying to the night before the exam.

Mechanisms of Disease

Pathology: The study of the characteristics, causes, and effects of disease. Also, a condition produced by disease.
Etiology: The study of all factors that cause a disease. Also, the cause of a disease.
Nosocomial: Pertaining to an infection acquired in a hospital or other medical care facility at least 72 hours after admission.
Acute: Characterized by sudden onset and short duration, with marked intensity or sharpness.
Chronic: Developing gradually and persisting for a long period, often for the remainder of a person's lifetime.
Aplastic: Lacking new development, or pertaining to the failure of a tissue to produce normal cell division.
Hypertrophy: An increase in the size of individual cells or an organ, resulting in an enlarged tissue mass. The cells of the heart, kidney, and prostate are particularly prone to hypertrophy.
Ischemia: Inadequate oxygenated blood supply to an organ or tissue, often marked by pain and organ dysfunction.
Infarction: An area of dead cells that results from a lack of oxygen.

Gangrene: An area of necrotic or dead tissue caused by an invasion of bacteria or loss of blood supply (ischemia). The extremities are most often affected, but it can occur in the intestines or gallbladder.

Immunology

Immunity: The quality of being resistant to a disease, often because of the presence of antibodies. Immunity can be acquired in a variety of different ways. See Table 4-1.
Immune system: Includes two major components: nonspecific immune mechanisms and specific immune mechanisms.
Antigen: A marker on the surface of a cell that identifies the cell as self or non-self. A non-self (foreign) antigen stimulates an immune response.
Immunodeficiency disorders: Health conditions caused by a deficiency of the immune system in which individuals are more susceptible to infections and chronic diseases. These diseases may be congenital or acquired, or they may result from therapeutic intervention for transplants.

Nonspecific Defense Mechanism

Nonspecific defense mechanism: The body's initial response to any threat, whether it be trauma, organisms, or chemicals. It is also known as inflammation. It is characterized by heat, redness, swelling, and pain.
Phagocyte: A cell that has the ability to ingest and destroy pathogens such as bacteria and protozoa, as well as cells, cell debris, and dust particles.
Macrophages: The main phagocytic cells of the immune system. They have the ability to recognize and ingest all foreign antigens. These antigens are then destroyed by lysosomes. Macrophages also serve a vital role in processing antigens and presenting them to T cells, thereby activating a specific immune response. Macrophages are present in the lymph nodes, liver, spleen, lungs, bone marrow, and connective tissue and in the blood as monocytes.
Kupffer cells: The fixed macrophages of the liver.

| Ways of Acquiring Immunity

Active Immunity	Passive Immunity
The body produces its own antibodies. Provides long-term immunity.	Antibodies produced outside the body are introduced into the body. Provides temporary immunity.
Natural Active Immunity	**Natural Passive Immunity**
Results from exposure to disease-causing organism.	Results when antibodies from the mother cross the placenta to the fetus.
Artificial Active Immunity	**Artificial Passive Immunity**
Results from the administration of a vaccine with killed or weakened organisms.	Results from immunization with antibodies to a disease-causing organism.

Table 4-1

Neutrophil: A granular leukocyte that is responsible for much of the body's protection against infection. Neutrophils destroy antigens by phagocytosis, and they play a vital role in inflammation and the nonspecific immune response.

Interferons: Antiviral, soluble glycoproteins produced by cells infected with viruses, chlamydiae, rickettsiae, and protozoa (e.g., malaria). They inhibit virus production within the cells and mark infected cells to be destroyed by T cells.

Specific Immune Response

Specific immune mechanisms: Mechanisms required if the nonspecific immune response cannot cope with the invasion or injury to the body. These defenses are directed and controlled by T cells and B cells. They are highly changed after exposure to a pathogen. They can "remember" pathogens such that the next time they invade the body, the specific immune response is quicker and specifically directed at the pathogen.

Cell-mediated immune response: An immune response involving the production of lymphocytes by the thymus (T cells) in response to antigen exposure. This response is important in the rejection of transplants, malignant growths, hypersensitivity, and some infections.

Humoral immune response: An immune response involving the production of plasma lymphocytes (B cells), leading to subsequent antibody formation. This response can produce immunity and hypersensitivity.

Antibody: An immunoglobulin produced by the lymphocytes in response to foreign antigens, such as those on bacteria and viruses.

Autoantibody: An antibody produced in response to a self-antigen. An autoantibody attacks the body's own cells. Autoantibodies are the basis for autoimmune diseases such as rheumatoid arthritis.

Hypersensitivity: An abnormal condition characterized by an exaggerated response of the immune system to an antigen. The four types of hypersensitivity are shown in Table 4-2.

| Types of Hypersensitivity

Type	Example
I	Hay fever, anaphylaxis, asthma, and eczema
II	Transfusion reactions, drug reactions, erythroblastosis fetalis, autoimmune disorders, glomerulonephritis
III	Serum sickness
IV	Tuberculin reaction, contact dermatitis, transplant rejection

Table 4-2

Organs and Tissues of the Immune System

Thymus: The gland located in the mediastinum. It is the site of the maturation and proliferation of the T lymphocytes.

Lymphatic tissue: Tissue containing many lymphocytes that remove foreign matter.

Bone marrow: Soft material that fills the cavity of the bones. Bone marrow is the source of stem cells and lymphocytes, and it is the site where B lymphocytes mature.

Hereditary and Congenital Diseases and Conditions

Hereditary diseases: Diseases caused by an error in the individual's genetic or chromosomal makeup. These diseases may or may not be apparent at birth. Hereditary diseases require a gene from one or both parents, depending on whether the gene is dominant or recessive.

Congenital anomaly: Any abnormality present at birth, which may be inherited or acquired during gestation. It is also called a birth defect.

Hereditary Diseases and Conditions

Albinism: A genetic condition that results in the lack of melanin pigment in the body, increasing the chance of sunburn and skin cancer.

Classic hemophilia: A hereditary bleeding disorder caused by a deficiency of clotting factors. Hemophilia is an X-linked genetic disorder in males.

Color blindness: The hereditary inability to distinguish between certain colors, generally red and green. Color blindness is more common in males.

Galactosemia: An inherited disorder in which the patient lacks the enzyme that converts galactose to glucose. Galactose accumulates in the blood and interferes with development of the brain, liver, and eyes and can lead to anorexia, vomiting, diarrhea, and even death if it goes untreated. This condition is usually present at birth, so it is also congenital. The diagnosis is confirmed by testing the newborn's urine.

Phenylketonuria (PKU): A hereditary congenital disease in which the newborn child is unable to oxidize an amino acid because of a defective enzyme. If not treated early, this condition results in brain damage and severe mental retardation. Some states require that newborns be tested for this disease.

Sickle cell anemia: An inherited disorder that primarily affects Africans and African Americans. Red blood cells become crescent-shaped, rigid, sticky, and fragile and cause chronic anemia, tissue hypoxia, weakness, and fatigue.

Tay-Sachs disease: A fatal hereditary congenital disease that primarily affects people of Ashkenazic (Eastern European) Jewish origin. This enzyme deficiency causes abnormal lipid metabolism in the brain, which leads to mental and physical retardation. Individuals affected with Tay-Sachs disease die at a very young age.

Congenital Conditions

Achondroplasia: Defective cartilage formation in the fetus. As a result, the long bones of the arm and legs are short, the trunk of the body is normal in size, and the head is large.

Down syndrome: A congenital condition caused by trisomy 21 (the presence of an extra autosomal chromosome 21). It results in varying degrees of mental retardation and distinctive physical features.

Klinefelter's syndrome: A congenital endocrine condition caused by the presence of an extra X chromosome, in which the individual appears to be male but has small testes and enlarged breasts.

Polydactyly: A congenital anomaly characterized by the presence of extra fingers or toes.

Turner's syndrome: A congenital endocrine disorder caused by the lack of a second X chromosome in females. The individual appears to be female, but the ovaries do not develop.

Ventricular septal defect: The most common congenital cardiac disease, in which a defect in the septum allows blood to be shunted between the left and right ventricles.

Coarctation of the aorta: Narrowing of the aortic arch, which creates increased left ventricular pressure and decreased blood pressure distal to the narrowing. Signs include left ventricular failure with pulmonary edema, dyspnea, and tachycardia.

Patent ductus arteriosus (PDA): A defect in which the ductus arteriosus, a fetal blood vessel, fails to close after birth. This condition often results in heart failure.

Tetralogy of Fallot: The most common cyanotic cardiac defect, of which there are four symptoms: ventricular septal defect, dextroposition of the aorta, pulmonary stenosis, and right ventricular hypertrophy.

Cyanosis: A bluish or grayish discoloration of the skin due to decreased amounts of hemoglobin in the blood.

Cerebral palsy: The name given to a group of motor impairment syndromes caused by lesions or anomalies in the brain in the early stages of development. Motor impairment generally occurs with secondary defects such as mental retardation or epilepsy. There are three major types: spastic (the most common), athetoid, and ataxic.

Spina bifida: The incomplete closure of the vertebral column. In cases that are not severe, surgery may be performed to close the defect and thus prevent damage to the spinal cord.

Myelomeningocele: Also known as spina bifida cystica, a congenital defect in the walls of the spinal canal that allows the membranes of the spinal cord to push through and form a tumor. It usually occurs within the first 24 hours after birth, and surgical correction is necessary.

Hydrocephalus: A condition in which there is excessive fluid in or around the brain, an abnormal enlargement of the head, and abnormal muscle tone of the legs.

Muscular dystrophy: A progressive degeneration and weakening of the skeletal muscles.

Duchenne's muscular dystrophy: The most common type of muscular dystrophy, mostly affecting males and involving the muscles of the shoulders, hips, and thighs.

Phimosis: A narrowing of the opening of the foreskin.

Congenital pyloric stenosis: A narrowing of the pyloric sphincter at the exit of the stomach. A symptom of this disease is projectile vomiting after feeding that starts at 2 to 3 weeks of age.

Hirschsprung's disease: Also called congenital aganglionic megacolon, an impairment of intestinal motility that causes obstruction of the distal colon. The newborn fails to pass meconium (first feces) within 48 hours after birth.

Congenital myxedema: A condition characterized by severe hypothyroidism and often associated with other endocrine abnormalities. Typical signs of myxedema include lack of growth, mental deficiency, puffy facial features, dry skin, and a large tongue. The condition is also referred to as cretinism.

Neoplasia

Neoplasia: The new and abnormal growth of cells, which may be benign or malignant.

Neoplasm: Literally, a new growth, commonly called a tumor.

Hyperplasia: An increase in the number of cells in a body part that results from an increased rate of cellular division that can cause the formation of a tumor.

Malignant: Invasive and capable of metastasis.

Benign: Not recurrent or progressive; nonmalignant.

Metastasis: Development of a tumor away from the site of origin. It occurs when tumor cells spread to distant parts of the body through lymphatic circulation or the bloodstream and implant in lymph nodes or other organs.

Common Causes of Death in the United States
1. Heart disease
2. Cancer
3. Cerebrovascular diseases
4. Pulmonary diseases and conditions

Table 4-3

Cancer: A neoplasm characterized by the uncontrolled growth of abnormal cells that invade surrounding tissue and metastasize to distant body sites. As shown in Table 4-3, cancer is second only to heart disease as a cause of mortality in the United States. Possible causes of cancer include smoking; viruses; hormones; radiation; genetic predisposition; chemicals used in industry, food, cosmetics, and plastic; and air and water pollution. See Table 4-4 for the most common types of cancer in men, women, and children. See Table 4-5 for the most common types of cancer that result in death for men and women.

Carcinogen: A substance or agent that causes cancer or increases the incidence of cancer.

Carcinogenesis: The process by which normal cells are transformed into cancer cells.

Carcinoma: A malignant tumor of the epithelial cells. This neoplasm tends to infiltrate and metastasize through the lymphatic system or the bloodstream. It develops most often in the skin, large intestine, lungs, stomach, prostate, cervix, or breast.

Sarcoma: A malignant neoplasm of the connective tissues, such as bone or muscle. This type of cancer might affect the bones, bladder, kidneys, liver, lungs, or spleen.

Epidermoid carcinoma: A malignant tumor of epidermal cells of the skin.

Adenocarcinoma: A cancer of glandular epithelial cells.

Teratoma: A congenital tumor composed of different kinds of tissue, none of which normally occur together

Most Common Cancers		
Men	**Women**	**Children**
Prostate	Breast	Leukemia
Lung	Lung	Brain and other nervous system
Colon	Colon	

Table 4-4

Most Common Lethal Cancers	
Male	**Female**
Lung	Lung
Prostate	Breast
Colon and rectum	Colon and rectum
Pancreas	Ovary

Table 4-5

or at the site of the tumor. It is most common in the ovaries or testes.

Dermoid cyst: A cyst containing elements of hair, teeth, or skin that commonly occurs in the ovaries or testes.

Leukemia: A primary cancer of the bone marrow with proliferating leukocyte precursors. Its cause is generally unknown, but environmental risk factors include exposure to radiation and to certain chemicals.

Lymphoma: A cancer of the lymph nodes and lymphoid tissue that usually responds to treatment. The two main kinds are Hodgkin's disease and non-Hodgkin's lymphoma.

Renal carcinoma: A cancer of the kidneys, also called hypernephroma. Painless hematuria is common with this condition. Metastasis to the lungs, liver, bones, and brain is possible.

Prostate cancer: A slowly progressive adenocarcinoma of the prostate that affects males after the age of 50. It is the second leading cause of cancer death among men in the United States. The cause is unknown, but it is believed to be hormone related.

Bladder cancer: The most common cancer of the urinary tract, it occurs more often in men than in women. The risk of bladder cancer increases with cigarette smoking and exposure to aniline dyes and to materials used in the petroleum, paint, plastics, and timber industries.

Cancer of the mouth: A malignancy that may develop in the gums, cheeks, or on the roof of the mouth. In men, it is common to see a cancer of the lower lip, which may be related to pipe smoking.

Stomach cancer: A malignancy of the stomach that is declining in incidence in North America but is common in Japan. It often spreads to the liver.

Colorectal cancer: A malignancy of the large intestine, characterized by a change in bowel habits and the passing of blood. This cancer usually occurs in people older than 50. The risk of colorectal cancer is increased in patients with chronic ulcerative colitis, Crohn's disease, villous adenomas, and familial adenomatous polyposis of the colon.

Laryngeal cancer: A cancer of the larynx that occurs most frequently in those between 50 and 70 years of age. Persistent hoarseness or dysphonia are usually the only symptoms.

Lung cancer: A pulmonary malignancy attributable in the majority of cases to cigarette smoking. Other predisposing factors are exposure to arsenic, asbestos, coal products, ionizing radiation, mustard gas, and petroleum. It is the leading cause of cancer death in the United States. Metastasis is to the brain, bone, and skin.

Cervical cancer: A malignancy of the uterine cervix that can be detected in the early, curable stage by the Papanicolaou (Pap) test. Risk factors include coitus at an early age, relations with many sexual partners, genital herpes virus infections, multiparity, and poor obstetric and gynecological care.

Endometrial cancer: An adenocarcinoma of the endometrium of the uterus. It is the most prevalent malignancy of the female reproductive system, most often occurring in the fifth or sixth decade of life. Some of the risk factors include infertility; anovulation; late menopause; administration of exogenous estrogen; and a combination of diabetes, hypertension, and obesity.

Ovarian carcinoma: A malignant neoplasm of the ovaries rarely detected in the early stage. It occurs commonly in the fifth decade of life. Risk factors include infertility, nulliparity or low parity, delayed childbearing, repeated spontaneous abortion, endometriosis, and group A blood type.

Choriocarcinoma: An epithelial malignancy of fetal origin. The primary tumor usually appears in the uterus and may metastasize to the lungs, liver, and brain. This cancer is more common in older women.

Adenocarcinoma of the vagina: A small percentage of women whose mothers were given the synthetic hormone diethylstilbestrol (DES), used to prevent spontaneous abortion, have developed this form of cancer. Most cases are in women whose mothers did not take the hormone.

Breast cancer: The most common cancer in North American women and the leading cause of death in females 35 to 54 years of age. This adenocarcinoma commonly metastasizes to the lungs, liver, brain, and bone.

Testicular cancer: A malignant neoplastic disease of the testis occurring most frequently in men between 20 and 35 years of age. Patients with early testicular cancer are often asymptomatic, and metastases may be present in lymph nodes, the lungs, and the liver.

Common Infectious Diseases

Common cold: Acute viral inflammation of any or all parts of the respiratory tract, marked by congestion of the nasal mucosa, sneezing, and malaise, among other symptoms. The contagious period begins before the onset of symptoms, and the incubation period is from 12 to 72 hours.

Age Group	Most Common Infective Causes
Neonates	*Streptococcus, Escherichia coli*
Infants	*Haemophilus influenzae*
Adults	*Neisseria meningitidis*
Elderly individuals	*Streptococcus pneumonia*
Overall	*Haemophilus influenzae*

Table 4-6

Influenza: Also known as the flu or grippe, an acute respiratory infection characterized by the sudden onset of fever, chills, headache, and muscle pain or tenderness. Inflammation of the nasal mucous membrane, cough, and sore throat are common. The incubation period is from 1 to 3 days.

Mumps (parotitis): The inflammation of one or both parotid glands caused by viral infection, with an incubation period of 2 to 3 weeks. Complications may include meningoencephalitis, pericarditis, deafness, arthritis, nephritis, and sterility in men.

Chickenpox (varicella): A highly contagious, acute viral infection characterized by spots and an elevated temperature. The incubation period is 2 to 3 weeks. Complications may include encephalitis, meningitis, Reye's syndrome, pneumonia, and conjunctival ulcer. The virus may reemerge later as shingles. Chickenpox can be severely damaging to a fetus.

Measles (rubeola): An acute, highly contagious viral disease. The incubation period is 7 to 14 days. The condition is characterized by spots and a rash. Complications may include otitis media, pneumonia, and encephalitis.

German measles (rubella): Also called 3-day measles, a highly communicable viral disease that has an incubation period of 14 to 21 days. It is characterized by spots. Rubella poses great danger to the fetus.

Meningitis: Any infection or inflammation of the membranes covering the brain and spinal cord. The most common causes for different age groups are summarized in Table 4-6. Aseptic meningitis may be caused by nonbacterial agents such as chemical irritants, viruses, or neoplasms.

Infectious mononucleosis: An acute infectious disease that causes changes in the leukocytes. It is also called glandular fever and the "kissing disease." Mononucleosis is caused by the Epstein-Barr virus and is usually transmitted by direct oral contact. It is rare in those older than 35 years of age.

Epiglottitis: An inflammation of the epiglottis that commonly occurs in children between 3 and 7 years of age. The most common cause is *Haemophilus influenzae* type B bacteria.

Genital lesion: A symptom that usually accompanies a sexually transmitted disease such as herpes or syphilis. It is found in the genital region of either males or females.

Botulism: A severe form of food poisoning from botulinus toxins produced by the *Clostridium botulinum* bacterium.

Gastroenteritis: Stomach and intestinal inflammation caused by a food- or waterborne virus.

Tetanus: An infection of the central nervous system caused by the tetanus bacillus, *Clostridium tetani*. The symptoms include sudden, extremely painful muscle contractions and stiffness of certain muscles such as the neck and the jaw. It is commonly called lockjaw.

Tapeworm: A species of parasitic worm that can infect the intestines when ingested with uncooked meat containing the larvae. Symptoms are often absent, but too many tapeworms can cause intestinal obstruction.

Malaria: An acute and sometimes chronic infection of red blood cells, transmitted by the bite of an infected female mosquito. Symptoms include chills, shaking, discomfort, fatigue, fevers, and headaches.

Yellow fever: An acute infectious viral infection transmitted by mosquitoes. Symptoms include jaundice, abdominal tenderness, vomiting, and fevers.

Major Diseases and Disorders

Diseases and Disorders of the Integumentary System

Viral infections of the skin: Infections that include chickenpox and shingles (varicella), measles (rubeola), German measles (rubella), and warts (condyloma acuminata).

Bacterial infections of the skin: Infections that include scarlet fever (erysipelas), impetigo (a type

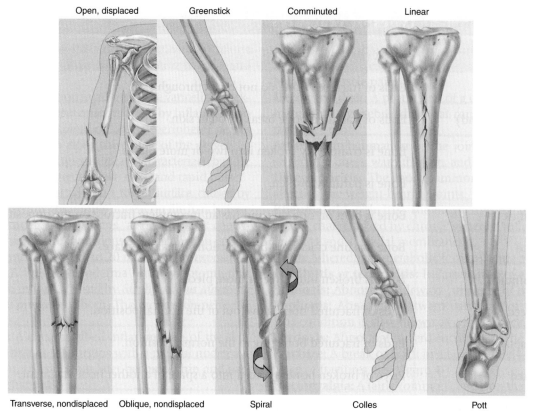

Open, displaced   Greenstick   Comminuted   Linear

Transverse, nondisplaced   Oblique, nondisplaced   Spiral   Colles   Pott

Figure 4-1 *Some types of bone fractures.*

Parkinson's disease: A brain degeneration that appears gradually and progresses slowly. It is also known as shaking palsy. Signs of Parkinson's disease include slowness of movement, resting tremor, and rigidity. The degeneration occurs in the basal ganglia. There is dopamine depletion.

Cerebral hemorrhage: Hemorrhage in epidural, subdural, or subarachnoid spaces in the meninges. The major cause of this condition is hypertension.

Concussion: An immediate loss of consciousness caused by a violent blow to the head or neck. It may last from a few seconds to several minutes.

Contusion: Bruising of the brain, a more serious head injury than a concussion. Permanent damage to the brain may result. It is commonly associated with skull fracture.

Paraplegia: Paralysis of motor or sensory abilities of the lower trunk and lower extremities. The individual may lose bowel and bladder control, and sexual dysfunction is common.

Quadriplegia: Paralysis of the lower and upper extremities (the arms, legs, and trunk) that results from injury to the spinal cord at the fifth, sixth, or seventh cervical vertebra. A major cause of death is respiratory failure.

Hemiplegia: Paralysis on one side of the body.

Epilepsy: A chronic brain disorder characterized by sudden and recurrent episodes of convulsive seizures. There are two major types of seizure: partial seizures and generalized. A simple partial seizure was originally called jacksonian epilepsy. Generalized seizures include absence (petit mal) and tonic–clonic (grand mal).

Bell's palsy: A paralysis of the facial nerve that results from trauma to the nerve, compression of the nerve by a tumor, or an unknown infection. It commonly occurs between 20 and 60 years of age. It is usually self-limiting (temporary paralysis).

Trigeminal neuralgia: Also called tic douloureux, a condition that involves pain in the fifth cranial nerve. Paroxysmal episodes of the pain may last for hours.

Migraine: A type of periodic headache, which may or may not be accompanied by aura or neurological dysfunction. Pain is usually confined to one side, but it can be bilateral.

Diseases and Disorders of the Cardiovascular System

Arteriosclerosis: A disease of the arterial vessels characterized by thickening, hardening, and loss of elasticity in the arteries.

Atherosclerosis: The most common form of arteriosclerosis, marked by cholesterol, lipid, and calcium deposits in arterial linings.

Angina pectoris: A paroxysmal chest pain caused by a temporary oxygen insufficiency as a result of atherosclerosis, spasms of the coronary arteries, or thrombosis.

Myocardial infarction: Necrosis of the myocardium, often resulting from the occlusion of a coronary artery by atherosclerotic plaque, myocardium spasm, or thrombus.

Congestive heart failure: A slowly developing condition in which the heart weakens over time. In time, the heart is no longer able to pump enough blood to meet the body's needs.

Coronary thrombosis: A blood clot in a coronary artery, the most common cause of myocardial infarction.

Myocarditis: Inflammation of the myocardium. It is commonly caused by viruses, bacteria, fungi, or protozoa.

Endocarditis: Inflammation of the lining and valves of the heart due to an invasion of microorganisms or an abnormal immunological reaction. There are several types of endocarditis.

Acute endocarditis: Inflammation of the lining and valves of the heart caused by *Staphylococcus aureus* and group A beta-hemolytic streptococci.

Subacute endocarditis: Inflammation of the lining and valves of the heart commonly caused by *Escherichia coli* or *Streptococcus viridans*.

Pericarditis: Inflammation of the pericardium. It may be caused by myocardial infarction, viral uremia, bacteria, fungi, parasites, or rheumatic fever. There are three types: fibrinous, serous, and suppurative.

Rheumatic fever: A systemic, inflammatory autoimmune disease involving the heart and the joints. There are two types: acute rheumatic fever and rheumatic heart disease.

Acute rheumatic fever: Rheumatic fever caused by beta-hemolytic streptococci and characterized by polyarthritis, erythema, subcutaneous nodules, chorea, and carditis. It is more common in children.

Rheumatic heart disease: A disease that causes stenosis or insufficiency of the mitral valve.

Shock: The collapse of the cardiovascular system—a dangerous reduction of blood flow throughout the body tissues. It is a life-threatening emergency that can be caused by sepsis, hemorrhage, heart failure, respiratory distress, or anaphylaxis. (For more information see chapter 21).

Cardiac tamponade: Accumulation of fluid, such as blood, in the pericardial sac.

Cardiogenic shock: Shock resulting from extensive myocardial infarction.

Aneurysm: A dilation or saclike formation in a weakened blood vessel wall. A common cause is atherosclerotic plaque. Other causative agents include trauma, inflammation or infection, and congenital factors.

Abdominal aortic aneurysm: The most common form of aneurysm.

Thrombophlebitis: Also called phlebitis, the inflammation of a vein, often accompanied by the formation of a clot. It occurs most commonly in the lower legs.

Varicose vein: An enlarged, twisted superficial vein, usually in the lower leg, caused by incompetent valves. It is very common, especially in women.

Buerger's disease (thromboangiitis obliterans): An occlusion and inflammation of the peripheral vascular circulation, usually in the leg or foot. The primary cause is a long history of smoking tobacco.

Raynaud's disease: Episodic vasospasm of the small cutaneous arteries, usually occurring in the fingers. It is often aggravated by cold temperatures.

Anemia: A reduction in the quantity of either RBCs or hemoglobin in a measured volume of blood. There are several forms of anemia, including iron-deficiency anemia, pernicious anemia, and aplastic anemia.

Iron-deficiency anemia: The most common type of anemia. It results from greater demand on stored iron than can be supplied. RBC count may be normal, but there is insufficient hemoglobin.

Pernicious anemia: Chronic anemia caused by decreased hydrochloric acid in the stomach, lack of intrinsic factor, and a vitamin B_{12} deficiency.

Aplastic anemia: A congenital form of anemia, also called Fanconi syndrome. The bone marrow stops producing erythrocytes, leukocytes, and platelets. It is caused by exposure to excessive radiation, certain drugs, and industrial toxins.

Sickle cell anemia: A condition in which abnormal hemoglobin causes RBCs to change to a sickle (crescent) shape. These sickle-shaped red blood cells get stuck in capillaries.

Polycythemia: An increase in the number of circulating erythrocytes and the amount of hemoglobin. There are three types: polycythemia vera, secondary polycythemia, and relative polycythemia. Complications may include thrombosis, cerebrovascular accident, peptic ulcers, leukemia, and hemorrhage.

Agranulocytosis: Also called neutropenia, a condition in which the number of leukocytes is very low.

Lymphedema: An abnormal collection of lymph, commonly in the extremities. Congenital lymphedema is known as Milroy's disease.

Lyme disease: A tickborne disease characterized by skin lesions, malaise, fatigue, arthritis, carditis, encephalitis, meningitis, loss of memory, numbness, and facial palsy. The incubation period is 3 to 33 days after a tick bite.

Plague: A highly fatal disease characterized by high fever, mental confusion, prostration, delirium, shock, and coma. There are three types: bubonic, septicemic, and pneumonic. Caused by *Yersinia pestis*, a gram-negative, nonmotile bacillus. The incubation period is 2 to 6 days.

Pneumonic plague: A disease characterized by extensive involvement of the lungs. It is very contagious and usually fatal.

Bubonic plague: An acute or severe infection characterized by the formation of buboes, which are inflamed and swollen lymph nodes. It is transmitted by infected rats and squirrels. In the Middle Ages, it was also known as the Black Death.

Diseases and Disorders of the Endocrine System

Hypoglycemia: Low blood sugar.

Hyperglycemia: High blood sugar.

Ketosis: The accumulation of ketone bodies in the blood and urine as a result of abnormal utilization of carbohydrates.

Gigantism: Excessive size and stature of the body, usually caused by the hypersecretion of growth hormone. It is usually the result of a tumor (adenoma) of the anterior pituitary and generally occurs before puberty.

Acromegaly: A disease caused by an excess of growth hormone in an adult. The bones of the hands, feet, and face can be enlarged. It is generally due to a tumor.

Dwarfism: A growth hormone deficiency that results in the abnormal underdevelopment of the body, or hypopituitarism, mainly in children. It causes extreme shortness of stature.

Hyperthyroidism: Hypersecretion of the thyroid gland that results in protrusion of the eyeballs, tachycardia, goiter, and tumor.

Hypothyroidism: Hyposecretion of the thyroid gland that results in sluggishness, slow pulse, and obesity.

Goiter: An enlargement of the thyroid gland, possibly due to a lack of iodine in the diet, thyroiditis, inflammation from infection, tumors, or hyperfunction or hypofunction of the thyroid gland.

Graves' disease: A condition of severe hyperthyroidism, possibly with an autoimmune base. A sudden exacerbation of symptoms may signal thyrotoxicosis.

Thyrotoxicosis: A toxic condition caused by hyperactivity of the thyroid gland and characterized by rapid heartbeat, tremors, nervous symptoms, and weight loss.

Hashimoto's disease: An inflammatory autoimmune disease that attacks the thyroid gland. It is more common in women and is the leading cause of non-simple goiter and hypothyroidism.

Myxedema: The acquired form of severe hypothyroidism. It is more common in females and occurs in adulthood.

Cushing's syndrome: Hyperactivity of the adrenal cortical gland that develops from an excess of the glucocorticoid hormone. The individual experiences fatigue, weakness, fat deposits in the scapular area (buffalo humps), protruding abdomen, hypertension, edema, and hyperlipidemia.

Addison's disease: A life-threatening condition resulting from chronic hypoadrenalism. Symptoms include weakness, nausea, abdominal discomfort, anorexia, and weight loss, among many others.

Diabetes insipidus: A metabolic disorder caused by injury to the neurohypophyseal system. The disease results from antidiuretic hormone deficiency.

Diabetes mellitus: A chronic disorder of carbohydrate, fat, and protein metabolism resulting from inadequate production of insulin by the pancreas. This disorder results in hyperglycemia.

Gestational diabetes: A type of diabetes that occurs during pregnancy and often resolves after the birth of the baby.

Hyperinsulinism: A condition resulting from excessive insulin in the blood, causing hypoglycemia, fainting, and convulsions.

Diseases and Disorders of the Sensory System

Diseases and Disorders of the Eye

Myopia: A severe form of nearsightedness that results when light rays entering the eye focus in front of the retina. Myopia occurs when the eyeball is abnormally long.

Hyperopia: A severe form of farsightedness that occurs when light rays entering the eye focus behind the retina. The eyeball is abnormally short.

Presbyopia: The inability to focus with the lens because of loss of its elasticity. It commonly develops with advancing age, usually beginning in the mid 40s.

Nystagmus: Involuntary, rhythmic movement of the eyes. Brain tumors or cerebrovascular lesions may cause nystagmus.

Astigmatism: An irregular focusing of the light rays entering the eye. The cornea is not spherical, and vision is typically blurred.

Strabismus: A disorder in which the visual axes of the eyes are not directed at the same point. Hence, the eyes are crossed. The main symptom is diplopia.

Conjunctivitis: Inflammation of the conjunctiva caused by bacterial or viral infection, allergy, or environmental factors. Red eyes, thick discharge, and sticky eyelids in the morning are the most common signs and symptoms.

Hordeolum: Also called stye, an infection of the hair follicles of the eyelids.

Cataract: A clouding of a normally clear lens of the eye. The most common cause is aging.

Glaucoma: One of the most common and severe ocular diseases, characterized by increased intraocular pressure, which can result in damage to the optic nerve. It is more common in people 60 and older.

Retinal detachment: An elevation of the retina from the choroid. Extremely nearsighted people are more susceptible to retinal detachments.

Uveitis: Inflammation of the uveal tract, including the iris, ciliary body, and choroid. It can be caused by autoimmune disorders or by infections such as tuberculosis, toxoplasmosis, syphilis, or histoplasmosis.

Diseases and Disorders of the Ear

Otalgia: Earache.

External otitis: Also known as swimmer's ear, an infection of the ear canal, commonly caused by *Escherichia coli*, *Pseudomonas aeruginosa*, *Proteus vulgaris*, *Staphylococcus aureus*, or *Aspergillus* (a genus of fungi).

Otitis media: An infection of the middle ear. It is most common in children younger than 8. The bacteria that most often cause otitis media are *Haemophilus influenzae*, *Streptococcus pneumoniae*, *Streptococcus pyogenes*, and *Staphylococcus aureus*.

Tympanitis: Inflammation of the eardrum.

Conductive hearing loss: Loss of hearing caused by an interruption in the transmission of sound waves to the inner ear.

Sensorineural hearing loss: Hearing loss caused by damage to the inner ear, to the nerve from the ear to the brain, or to the brain itself, so that the brain does not perceive sound waves as sound.

Anacusis: Total hearing loss.

Tinnitus: Ringing or buzzing in the ear.

Vertigo: Dizziness.

Diseases and Disorders of the Urinary System

Dysuria: Painful urination.

Enuresis: Involuntary discharge of urine, most often due to a lack of bladder control.

Incontinence: Involuntary discharge of urine, feces, or semen.

Urethritis: Inflammation of the urethra.

Cystitis: Inflammation of the urinary bladder. It is more common in women.

Urinary tract infection (UTI): Bacteria or other organisms in the urethra and bladder, causing dysuria and malaise.

Renal failure: In acute cases a sudden and severe reduction in renal function. Causes include complications from surgery, shock after an incompatible blood transfusion, severe dehydration, and trauma or kidney disease. Renal failure results in uremia.

Uremia: Excess of urea and other waste in the blood as a result of kidney failure.

Glomerulonephritis: Inflammation of the glomerulus in the kidney. There are three types: acute, chronic, and subacute.

Acute glomerulonephritis: A common disease, primarily affecting children and young adults, marked by protein and blood in the urine and edema with no pus formation. It is a type of allergic disease caused by an antigen-antibody reaction.

Chronic glomerulonephritis: A slowly progressive, noninfectious disease that may result in irreversible renal damage and renal failure. Uremia is common with this condition.

Nephrotic syndrome: Referred to as the protein-losing kidney, a condition characterized by protein in the urine, hypoalbuminemia, hypertension, and hyperlipidemia.

Pyelonephritis: A diffuse pyogenic infection of the renal pelvis. It is the most common type of renal disease, and it may be acute or chronic. It is commonly caused by infection, calculi, pregnancy, tumors, or benign prostatic hypertrophy.

Hydronephrosis: Distention of the pelvis and calyces of the kidney by urine that cannot flow past an obstruction in the ureter. The obstruction may be a result of urinary calculi, a tumor, an enlarged prostate gland, or pregnancy.

Polycystic renal disease: A congenital anomaly that affects children and adults and results in kidney failure due to the presence of multiple cysts in the kidney tubules.

Renal calculus: Better known as a kidney stone, a deposit that can block urine flow in the ureter, resulting in renal colic with chills, fever, hematuria, and a frequent need to urinate. Kidney stones can be treated with smooth muscle relaxants that help pass the stones and offer some pain relief. If the stones don't pass and they continue to block urine flow, surgery must be performed, or the stones can be destroyed with ultrasound.

Diseases and Disorders of the Reproductive System

Gonorrhea: A contagious inflammation of the genital mucous membrane of both sexes caused by the gram-negative gonococcus bacterium. It may also affect other parts of the body, including the heart, rectum, and joints, and in women it may cause pelvic inflammatory disease.

Genital warts: An infection caused by any of a group of human papillomaviruses (HPVs). In women, genital warts may be associated with cancer of the cervix.

Chlamydial infection: The most prevalent sexually transmitted disease in the United States. It is a leading cause of pelvic inflammatory disease in women. In men, chlamydia may cause urethritis and penile discharge. Chlamydia is caused by the *Chlamydia trachomatis* bacterium, and it is sometimes called the silent STD because the symptoms may be very mild. Chlamydia left untreated can lead to infertility and sterility.

Syphilis: One of the most serious sexually transmitted diseases. The causative organism is a spirochete, *Treponema pallidum*. Infection in pregnant women can cause congenital defects in the fetus (such as mental retardation, physical deformities, deafness, and blindness), the death of the fetus, and spontaneous abortion.

Genital herpes: A very painful, recurring, incurable viral disease that involves the mucous membranes of the genital tracts. During pregnancy, it can cause spontaneous abortion and premature delivery, and it can be transmitted to the newborn. It can also develop into cervical cancer and spread to the lungs, brain, liver, and spleen.

HIV: The human immunodeficiency virus, which is transferable by direct sexual contact (homosexual or heterosexual), by contaminated intravenous needles and syringes, and by blood transfusion with contaminated blood or other blood products. It is also transplacental and can be transferred from mother to child. The first signs of infection include fever, malaise, rashes, arthralgia, and lymphadenopathy. As the disease progresses, there is a steady drop in the number of T cells in the blood. Diagnosis is determined by the detection of HIV antibodies in the blood.

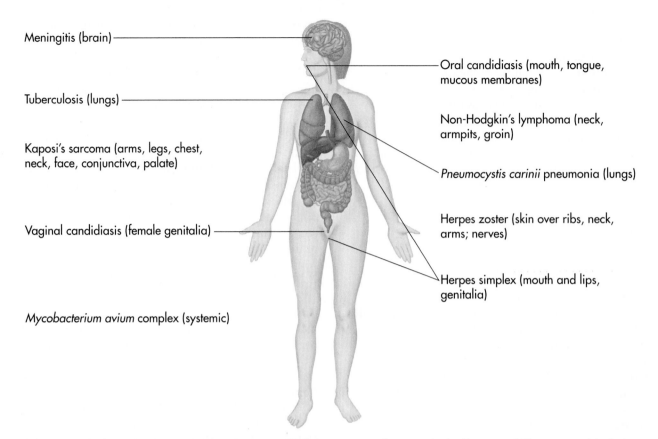

Meningitis (brain)

Tuberculosis (lungs)

Kaposi's sarcoma (arms, legs, chest, neck, face, conjunctiva, palate)

Vaginal candidiasis (female genitalia)

Mycobacterium avium complex (systemic)

Oral candidiasis (mouth, tongue, mucous membranes)

Non-Hodgkin's lymphoma (neck, armpits, groin)

Pneumocystis carinii pneumonia (lungs)

Herpes zoster (skin over ribs, neck, arms; nerves)

Herpes simplex (mouth and lips, genitalia)

Figure 4-2 *An individual with AIDS may contract a variety of opportunistic infections, which affect many different parts of the body.*

AIDS: Acquired immunodeficiency syndrome, the ultimate result of infection with HIV. It is currently a fatal disease of the immune system. AIDS is marked by opportunistic infections that would otherwise be eliminated by a healthy individual's immune responses. These infections include candidiasis, herpes, Kaposi's sarcoma, recurrent pneumonia, and lymphoma. The typical course of HIV is defined by three phases: primary infection phase, usually lasting between a few days and 2 weeks; chronic asymptomatic or latency phase, lasting an average of 10 years; and overt AIDS phase, that can lead to death (without antiretroviral therapy) within 2 to 3 years. See Figure 4-2.

Diseases and Disorders of the Female Reproductive System

Pelvic inflammatory disease: Inflammation and serious infection of organs in the pelvic cavity, including the fallopian tubes, ovaries, and endometrium. The infection can occur after miscarriage, childbirth, or abortion, but it is most common in young nulliparous females and is not necessarily related to a pregnancy. The causative organism is one that is sexually transmitted or a common vaginal bacterium.

Vaginitis: An inflammation and/or infection of the vaginal tissues. It is common in all age groups and is characterized by various discharge, depending on the

causative agent, from clear and odorless to copious, greenish yellow, and foul smelling.

Toxic shock syndrome: An acute, systemic infection with exotoxin-producing strains of *Staphylococcus aureus.* The syndrome has been associated with menstruating females who use tampons.

Menopause: The cessation of menstrual periods. Many women experience the onset of menopause between the ages of 45 and 55. Hot flashes and night sweats often are reported.

Cervical cancer: A malignancy of the uterine cervix. The biggest risk factor for development of invasive cervical carcinoma is lack of regular cervical Pap smear screening. The other major risk factor is exposure to oncogenic types of HPV, such as 16, 18, 31, and 45. Women should be encouraged to have regular cervical Pap smear screening.

Ovarian cancer: A malignancy that accounts for more deaths than any other gynecological malignancy. Most ovarian cancers occur in women between the ages of 40 and 65.

Endometrial cancer: A malignancy of the lining of the uterus, which undergoes cyclic changes as a result of hormonal stimulation. It is the most common gynecological cancer.

Hydatidiform moles: Tumors of the uterine lining, most of which are benign, that develop after pregnancy or in association with an abnormal pregnancy. These tumors consist of multiple cysts that resemble a bunch of grapes.

Fibroadenoma: The most common benign tumor of the breast. It is a single, movable nodule that occurs at any age. It is painful at the time of the menstrual period.

Amenorrhea: The absence of the onset of menstruation at puberty or the cessation or interruption of menstruation in adulthood.

Menorrhagia: Excessive uterine bleeding that occurs between menstrual periods. Its causes include uterine tumors, pelvic inflammatory disease, and abnormal conditions of pregnancy.

Metrorrhagia: Uterine bleeding at any time other than during menstruation.

Endometriosis: Proliferation of endometrial tissue outside of the uterus. Endometriosis may cause dysmenorrhea, sterility, and dyspareunia.

Ectopic pregnancy: Implantation of the fertilized ovum outside of the uterus, most commonly in the fallopian tubes, rather than on the inside wall of the uterus. It is also called extrauterine pregnancy.

Miscarriage: A spontaneous abortion, commonly as a result of a genetic abnormality.

Preeclampsia: A pathological condition of late pregnancy characterized by edema, protein in the urine, and hypertension. It is also known as the first phase of the toxemia of pregnancy.

Eclampsia: Toxemia of pregnancy resulting in convulsions and coma. It is a potentially life-threatening disorder characterized by severe hypertension, edema, and protein in the urine.

Placenta previa: Implantation of the placenta in the lower uterine segment on the internal cervical os, which causes painless bleeding.

Abruptio placentae: Separation of the placenta from the uterine wall too early during pregnancy. This is a life-threatening emergency that must be treated by an emergent cesarean section.

Diseases and Disorders of the Male Reproductive System

Orchitis: Infection of the testis caused by viral or bacterial infection or injury. It may affect one or both testes, causing swelling, tenderness, and acute pain.

Prostatitis: Acute or chronic inflammation of the prostate gland. It is more common in men older than 50 years of age. The cause of inflammation of the prostate is usually infection but is not always known.

Impotence: Failure to initiate or maintain an erection until ejaculation.

Benign prostatic hyperplasia: Enlargement of the prostate gland. It is common in men over the age of 50. This condition usually progresses to the point of causing compression of the urethra with urinary obstruction.

Prostate cancer: A malignancy of the prostate gland, located below the bladder and anterior to the rectum in males. This is the second leading cause of cancer death in men.

Testicular cancer: A malignancy of the testicle that is one of the most curable solid neoplasms. Nearly all testicular tumor are germ cell tumors. These tumors are most common in males between the ages of 20 and 35.

Cryptorchidism: The failure of the testes to descend into the scrotum from the abdominal cavity. Undescended testes atrophy and may become the potential site of cancer.

Diseases and Disorders Specific to Children

Colic: Abdominal distress of unknown cause in newborns or young infants.

Reye's syndrome: A combination of encephalopathy and fatty infiltration of the internal organs that may follow acute viral infections, most commonly in children under 15 years of age. The condition sometimes arises following infection with influenza A or B viruses or chickenpox and has been linked to the use of aspirin during these infections.

Sudden infant death syndrome (SIDS): Also called crib death, a syndrome that occurs in infants younger than 1 year of age. Death occurs within seconds during sleep. The cause is unknown. However, there are several risk factors, such as stomach sleeping, soft mattress, loose bed covers, room temperature too warm, and low birth-weight.

Erythroblastosis fetalis: A type of hemolytic anemia in newborns that results from maternal fetal blood group incompatibility, specifically involving the Rh factor and the ABO blood groups. Common symptoms include anemia, jaundice, kernicterus, splenomegaly, and hepatomegaly. It is sometimes called hydrops fetalis.

Wilms' tumor: Also called nephroblastoma, a highly malignant neoplasm of the kidney that affects children younger than 5 years. It is the most common kidney tumor of childhood.

STRATEGIES TO SUCCESS

▶ Test-Taking Skills

No tricks, just focus!
Always read all the responses to a question before answering. If you choose an answer too hastily, you might miss the best answer. Don't make any assumptions about the questions and how the writer of the question might be trying to trick you. Use only the information provided in the question and choose the best answer based on your knowledge of the subject matter.

Instructions:

Answer the following questions. Check your answers in the *Answer Key* that follows this section.

1. Chronic glomerulonephritis and renal failure may both result in
   A. Dehydration
   B. Cystitis
   C. Uremia
   D. An enlarged prostate
   E. Hirschsprung's disease

2. Which of the following definitions best explains encephalitis?
   A. Inflammation of the brain
   B. Inflammation of the meninges
   C. Inflammation of the spinal cord
   D. Inflammation of the brain and meninges
   E. Inflammation of the brain and spinal cord

3. What is the name of the condition caused by hypersecretion of growth hormone before puberty?
   A. Myxedema
   B. Acromegaly
   C. Dwarfism
   D. Gigantism
   E. Hyperthyroidism

4. Which of following sexually transmitted diseases is sometimes called the silent STD?
   A. Syphilis
   B. AIDS
   C. Genital warts
   D. Moles
   E. Chlamydial infection

5. Cancer in which of the following sites is the leading cause of cancer death in males?
   A. Prostate
   B. Pancreas
   C. Lung
   D. Colon
   E. Kidney

6. Chronic dilation and distention of the bronchial walls is called
   A. Hemoptysis
   B. Pneumoconiosis
   C. Bronchiectasis
   D. Atelectasis
   E. Bronchitis

7. Failure of the testes to descend into the scrotum from the abdominal cavity is called
   A. Orchitis
   B. Epididymitis
   C. Varicocele
   D. Cryptorchidism
   E. Peyronie's disease

8. Which of the following conditions may result in a lack of melanin pigment in the body?
   A. Color blindness
   B. Achondroplasia
   C. Albinism
   D. Galactosemia
   E. Rubella

9. Acute glomerulonephritis is marked by all of the following except
   A. Edema
   B. Hematuria
   C. Pus formation
   D. Protein in the urine
   E. Blood in the urine

10. The most common cyanotic cardiac defect is
    A. Patent ductus arteriosus
    B. Angina pectoris
    C. Ventricular septal defect
    D. Coarctation of the aorta
    E. Tetralogy of Fallot

11. Which of the following is the most common disease or condition of the urinary system?
    A. Hydronephrosis
    B. Renal failure
    C. Pyelonephritis
    D. Renal atrophy
    E. Nephrotic syndrome

12. Diabetes insipidus results from the lack or deficiency of which of the following?
    A. Insulin
    B. Thyroxine
    C. Aldosterone
    D. Antidiuretic hormone
    E. Glucose

13. Diverticulosis occurs particularly in the
    A. Lungs
    B. Cecum
    C. Ileum
    D. Anus
    E. Colon

14. Vitiligo is a condition that affects which of the following body systems?
    A. Respiratory
    B. Reproductive
    C. Endocrine
    D. Integumentary
    E. Digestive

15. All of the following are causative factors for pernicious anemia except
    A. Vitamin B_{12} deficiency
    B. Folic acid deficiency
    C. Lack of intrinsic factor
    D. Decreased hydrochloric acid in the stomach
    E. Regional entertitis (Crohn's disease)

16. The failure of bone marrow to produce erythrocytes, leukocytes, and platelets is called
    A. Leukemia
    B. Leukoplakia
    C. Hemolytic anemia
    D. Aplastic anemia
    E. Sickle cell anemia

17. Tetanus is commonly called
    A. Lockjaw
    B. Sleeping sickness
    C. Hydrophobia
    D. Hydronephrosis
    E. Both A and C

18. Which of the following is not an obvious sign of Parkinson's disease?
    A. Tremor
    B. Rigidity
    C. Seizure
    D. Slowness of movement
    E. They are all signs of the disease

19. Which of the following fractures of the bone is common in children?
    A. Comminuted
    B. Open
    C. Incomplete
    D. Compound
    E. Greenstick fracture

20. All of the following are symptoms of nephrotic syndrome <u>except</u>
    - A. Hyperlipidemia
    - B. Hypoalbuminemia
    - C. Proteinuria
    - D. Hypertension
    - E. Hypotension

21. The absence of the onset of menstruation at puberty is called
    - A. Metrorrhagia
    - B. Amenorrhea
    - C. Dysmenorrhea
    - D. Miscarriage
    - E. Eclampsia

22. Undescended testes may become the potential site of
    - A. Infection
    - B. Lymphedema
    - C. Gangrene
    - D. Polyposis
    - E. Cancer

23. Which of the following terms means "inflammation of the tening membrane of the heart"
    - A. Valnulitis
    - B. Vasculitis
    - C. Pericarditis
    - D. Endocarditis
    - E. Pericarditis

24. A prolapse of one section of the intestine into the lumen of another segment, causing intestinal blockage, is called
    - A. Intussusception
    - B. Diverticulosis
    - C. Volvulus
    - D. Crohn's disease
    - E. Luminescence

25. Episodic vasospasm of the small cutaneous arteries, usually located in the finger, is known as
    - A. Buerger's disease
    - B. Raynaud's disease
    - C. Phlebitis
    - D. Varicose veins
    - E. Thrombosis

26. The most common type of anemia in the U.S. is
    - A. Sickle cell
    - B. Pernicious
    - C. Folic acid deficiency
    - D. Iron-deficiency
    - E. None of the above

27. Which of the following is a fungal infection of the skin that forms a ringlike pattern?
    - A. Sehorrfea
    - B. Psoriasis
    - C. Impetigo
    - D. Tinex
    - E. Impetigo

28. Which of the following cells can release histamine and heparin?
    - A. Lymphocytes
    - B. Kupffer cells
    - C. Erythrocytes
    - D. Neurons
    - E. Mast cells

29. The most common causative organism of meningitis in adults is
    - A. *Herpes zoster*
    - B. *Streptococcus pneumoniae*
    - C. Poliovirus
    - D. *Neisseria meningitidis*
    - E. *Escherichia coli*

Microb

MEDICAL ASS

COMPETENCY

Clinical

Apply principles of a:
hand washing

Practice Standard Pre

General/Legal/Pro

Use appropriate med

30. Trisomy 21 is also called
   A. Galactosemia
   B. Turner's syndrome
   C. Down syndrome
   D. Polydactyly
   E. Klinefelter's syndrome

31. Thrombophlebitis occurs most commonly in the
   A. Lower legs
   B. Lower arms
   C. Lower abdomen
   D. Neck
   E. Lungs

32. The sudden onset of a disease marked by intensity is described as
   A. Critical
   B. Aplastic
   C. Chronic
   D. Morbid
   E. Acute

33. A patient with Addison's disease should be examined by which of the following types of specialist?
   A. Neurologist
   B. Radiologist
   C. Nephrologist
   D. Endocrinologist
   E. Immunologist

34. Serum sickness is what type of hypersensitivity?
   A. I
   B. II
   C. III
   D. IV
   E. V

35. An area of dead cells due to lack of oxygen is called
   A. Ischemia
   B. Infarction
   C. Atresia
   D. Gangrene
   E. Placenta previa

36. The condition in which one of the sex chromosomes is missing is called
   A. Klinefelter's syndrome
   B. Turner's syndrome
   C. Down syndrome
   D. Tetralogy of Fallot
   E. Peyronie's disease

37. A cancer of the epithelial cells is called
   A. Carcinoma
   B. Sarcoma
   C. Carcinogen
   D. Metastasis
   E. Endometriosis

38. Athlete's foot is otherwise known as
   A. Tinea cruris
   B. Tinea capitis
   C. Tinea epidermis
   D. Tinea corporis
   E. Tinea pedis

39. The biggest risk factor for invasive cervical cancer is which of the following?
   A. Cigarette smoking
   B. Absence of menstrual periods
   C. Pain associated with menstruation
   D. Lack of regular sexual intercourse
   E. Lack of regular cervical Pap smears

40. Which of the following organisms commonly causes toxic shock syndrome?
   A. *Myconacterium leprae*
   B. *Staphylococcus aureus*
   C. *Haemophilus ducreyi*
   D. *Neisseria meningitidis*
   E. *Neisseria gonorrhoeae*

ANSWER K

1. C
2. A
3. D
4. E
5. C
6. C
7. D
8. C
9. C
10. E
11. C
12. D
13. E
14. D
15. B
16. D
17. A
18. C
19. E
20. E

STRATEGIES TO SUCCESS

▶ Study Skills

Study everywhere and anywhere!
Although it's important to have a regular study place you feel comfortable with, it's also important that you use idle parts of your day to review material. Write definitions of hard-to-remember terms on flash cards and carry them with you. Review them between classes and while you're waiting for a bus or an appointment.

Microorganisms

Microbiology: The study of very small living organisms, including bacteria, algae, fungi, protozoa, and viruses; often called microbes, germs, or single-celled organisms.

Microscope: An instrument used to obtain an enlarged image of a small object and to reveal details of a structure otherwise not distinguishable. Microscopes are routinely used in a modern medical laboratory and magnify anywhere from $10\times$ up to $1000\times$.

Microorganisms: Tiny microscopic entities that are able to carry on all the processes of life, including metabolism, reproduction, and motility. Some microorganisms are pathogenic, and others are either beneficial or neutral in relationship to human beings. There are two main types of microorganisms: eukaryotes and prokaryotes.

Saprophyte: An organism that obtains its nutrients from dead organic matter. Many bacteria and fungi are saprophytes.

Bacteria

Bacteria: Microorganisms, the majority of which are harmless. They vary widely in size, shape, and cell arrangement and include bacilli, cocci, spirilla, diplobacilli, streptobacilli, coccobacilli, and cells that appear curved and comma-like. See Figure 5-1. There are three basic forms of bacteria: bacilli, cocci, and spirilla.

Bacilli: Rod-shaped bacteria, such as *Bacillus anthracis*, coliform bacilli, tubercle bacilli, and typhoid bacilli.

Cocci: Spherical bacteria. Pathogenic cocci are staphylococci, streptococci, and diplococci. See Table 5-1.

Spirilla: Spiral-shaped bacteria.

Diplococci: Any of the spherical or coffee-bean-shaped bacteria that usually appear in pairs.

Streptobacilli: Bacteria in which the rods or filaments tend to fragment into chains.

Coccobacilli: Short bacilli that are thick and somewhat ovoid.

Characteristics of bacteria: Bacteria are classified according to morphology, motility, growth, staining reactions, metabolic activities, pathogenicity, antigen-antibody reactions, and genetic composition.

Stain: A substance used to impart color to tissue or cells in order to study and identify microscopic organisms.

Gram's stain: A staining procedure in which bacteria are stained with crystal violet, treated with strong iodine solution, and decolorized with ethanol. Microorganisms that retain the stain are said to be gram positive, and those that lose the crystal violet stain by decolorization but stain with a counterstain are said to be gram negative.

Gram-positive bacteria: Bacteria with cell walls that are composed of peptidoglycan and teichoic acid. Some of the most important pathogenic gram-positive bacteria are listed in Table 5-2.

Gram-negative bacteria: Bacteria with cell walls that are composed of a thin layer of peptidoglycan covered by an outer membrane of lipoprotein and lipopolysaccharide. Table 5-3 is a summary of some gram-negative bacteria.

Gram stain limitations: The following organisms do not Gram stain well: rickettsia, mycoplasma, treponema, chlamydia, mycobacteria, and *Legionella pneumophila*.

Streptococci: A genus of gram-positive bacteria that occurs in chains. They are classified in four types: the

AT A GLANCE	Arrangement of Cocci	
Arrangement	**Description**	**Pathogenic Form**
Diplococci	Pairs	*Neisseria gonorrhoeae*
Streptococci	Chains	*Streptococcus pyogenes*
Staphylococci	Clusters	*Staphylococcus aureus*

Table 5-1

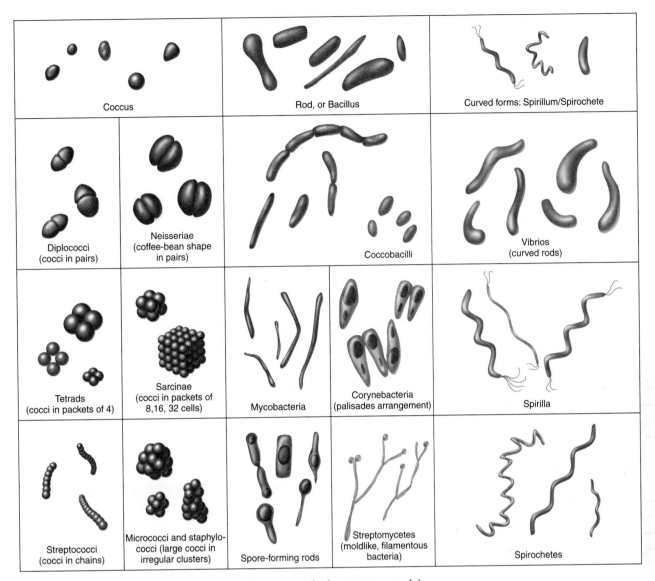

Figure 5-1 *Bacterial shapes and arrangements (not necessarily shown to exact scale).*

pyogenic group, the viridans group, the enterococcus group, and the lactic group.

Staphylococci: A genus of gram-positive bacteria made up of spherical microorganisms and grapelike clusters. See Table 5-4.

Intermediate organisms: Obligate intracellular parasites, which can reproduce only in living cells. There are three groups: rickettsia, chlamydia, and mycoplasma.

Rickettsia: Any of several small intracellular parasites of the genus *Rickettsia* that require a vector (such as fleas, ticks, or lice) to spread disease.

Chlamydia: A gram-negative nonmotile obligate intracellular parasite that is totally dependent on the host cell for energy. The genus *Chlamydia* comprises three species: *C. trachomatis, C. psittaci,* and *C. pneumoniae.* See Table 5-5.

Mycoplasma: A group of bacteria considered to be the smallest free-living organisms. Unlike most other bacteria, they lack a cell wall. Some are saprophytes, some are parasites, and many are pathogens. They cause primary atypical pneumonia and many secondary infections.

Mycobacterium: A genus of bacteria distinguished by a high lipid content that produces resistance to drying, acids, and various germicides. In form, mycobacteria are long, slender, straight or curved rods. Several are highly significant human pathogens that cause tuberculosis, leprosy, granuloma, and skin ulcers.

Legionella pneumophila: The bacterium that causes Legionnaires' disease. Primarily intracellular, it stains by silver stain.

Viruses

Viruses: Infectious agents that are even simpler in nature than bacteria. They are usually not considered cellular. Viruses are composed of a small amount of DNA or RNA wrapped in a protein covering. A virus is visible only with an electron microscope.

Viron: A virus that exists outside a host cell.

Some Important Pathogenic Gram-Positive Bacteria

Bacterium	Type	Diseases Caused
Corynebacterium diphtheriae	Rod, nonmotile	Diphtheria
Staphylococcus aureus	Cocci in clusters	Carbuncles, septicemia, pneumonia, boils
Streptococcus pyogenes	Cocci in chains	Strep throat, rheumatic fever, septicemia, scarlet fever
Streptococcus pneumoniae	Diplococcus	Pneumonia
Mycobacterium tuberculosis	Rod	Tuberculosis
Mycobacterium leprae	Rod	Leprosy
Clostridium tetani	Noncapsulate, sporing, motile	Tetanus
Clostridium botulinum	Spore-forming rod, noncapsulate, motile	Botulism (food poisoning)
Clostridium perfringens	Spore-forming rod, nonmotile, noncapsulate	Gas gangrene, wound infections

Table 5-2

Some Important Pathogenic Gram-Negative Bacteria

Bacterium	Type	Diseases Caused
Escherichia coli	Rod	Urinary infections
Haemophilus influenzae	Rod	Meningitis or pneumonia
Haemophilus ducreyi	Rod	Chancroid
Klebsiella pneumoniae	Rod	Pneumonia
Neisseria gonorrhoeae	Diplococci	Gonorrhea
Neisseria meningitidis	Diplococci	Meningitis
Rickettsia rickettsii	Rod	Rocky mountain spotted fever
Salmonella typhi	Rod	Typhoid fever
Shigella species	Rod	Shigellosis (bacillary dysentery)
Treponema pallidum	Spirochete	Syphilis
Vibrio cholerae	Curved rod	Cholera

Table 5-3

Type	Diseases Caused
S. aureus	Skin infections Osteopyelitis Food poisoning Endocarditis Toxic shock syndrome
S. epidermidis	Infections following instrumentation or implantation
S. saprophyticus	Urinary tract infection

Table 5-4

Type	Diseases Caused	Treatment
C. trachomatis	Urethritis	Tetracycline; ophthalmic antibiotic solution for newborns
C. psittaci (found in bird feces)	Psittacosis	Tetracycline or doxycycline
C. pneumoniae	Pneumonia, bronchitis, sinusitis	Tetracycline or erythromycin

Table 5-5

Bacteriophage or **phage:** A virus that has a bacterial host.

Fungi

Fungi: Eukaryotic organisms with cellulose or chitin cell walls that include mushrooms, molds, and yeasts. Spores, the means of reproduction for fungi, can be carried great distances by the wind and are resistant to heat, cold, acids, bases, and other chemicals.

Mushrooms: A class of true fungi.

Mycelium: A network of filaments or strands in mushrooms.

Molds: Multicellular fungi that are the main source of antibiotics. Some are used to produce large quantities of enzymes (amylases) and citric acid. Molds can also be harmful, and some are toxic.

Aflatoxin: A toxin produced by *Aspergillus* mold on peanuts and cottonseed. Aflatoxin is extremely toxic to humans and farm animals, and it is also carcinogenic.

Yeasts: Single-celled microscopic eukaryotes that produce vitamins and proteins.

Candida albicans: A type of pathogenic yeast that is dimorphous.

Dimorphism: The ability to live in two different forms, such as the few fungi, usually pathogens, that can live either as molds or as yeasts depending on growth conditions.

Protozoa

Protozoa: The lowest forms of animal life. Protozoa have the ability to move, and they are found in water and soil. Most protozoa are saprophytes, living in the soil and feeding off decaying organic material. Some protozoa are pathogenic; these pathogens are summarized in Table 5-6. (The singular form is *protozoon*.)

Microbial Growth

Microbial growth: Growth that is dependent on a source of energy and nutrient chemicals and influenced by temperature, pH (acidity), moisture content, and available nutrients. There are three types of microbial metabolism: fermentation, respiration, and photosynthesis.

Fermentation: The decomposition of complex substances through the action of enzymes produced by microorganisms.

Respiration: The interchange of gases between an organism and the medium in which it lives.

Pathogen	Diseases Caused
Entamoeba histolytica	Amebic dysentery
Dientamoeba fragilis	Diarrhea, fever
Trypanosoma gambiense	Sleeping sickness
Trichomonas vaginalis	Infections of the male and female genital tracts
Giardia lamblia	Gastroenteritis (intestinal infection)
Plasmodium species	Malaria
Pneumocystis carinii	Severe secondary infections in persons with suppressed immune systems (such as those who have AIDS)

Table 5-6

Photosynthesis: A process by which the energy of light is used to produce organic molecules. This process is most often used by plants to manufacture carbohydrates, but some bacteria are also capable of photosynthesis.

Aerobe: A microorganism that lives and grows in the presence of free oxygen. The majority of microbes are aerobes.

Facultative aerobe: An organism that is able to grow under anaerobic conditions but grows most rapidly in an aerobic environment.

Anaerobe: A microbe that grows and lives in the absence of oxygen.

Facultative anaerobe: A microbe that can grow either with or without oxygen but develops most rapidly in an anaerobic environment.

Obligate anaerobe: A microbe that lives only in the absence of oxygen.

Nutritional types: There are two nutritional types of organisms: heterotrophs and autotrophs.

Heterotrophs: Organisms that obtain carbon from organic material.

Autotrophs: Organisms that use inorganic carbon dioxide (CO_2) as their basic carbon source.

Chemotrophs: Organisms that use chemical substances as a source of energy.

Phototrophs: Organisms that use light as a source of energy.

Binary fission: Also called simple fission, the common form of asexual reproduction of bacteria in which each bacterium splits into two similar cells.

Optimum pH: The level of acidity or alkalinity most conducive to functioning. Each microorganism has an optimum pH for growth.

Acidophile: A bacterial organism that grows well in an acid medium.

Exotoxin: A potent toxin that is secreted or excreted by living microorganisms as the result of bacterial metabolism. Exotoxins are the most poisonous substances known to human beings. Bacteria of the genus *Clostridium* are the most frequent producers of exotoxins.

Enterotoxin: An exotoxin that affects cells of the intestinal mucosa, causing vomiting and diarrhea.

Microbes and the Human Body

Medical microbiology: The study of pathogens and the disease process, including epidemiology, diagnosis, treatment, infection control, and immunology. A list of major diseases, including the causative organisms, routes of transmission, and signs and symptoms, is provided in Table 5-7.

Normal flora: Bacteria that are permanent and generally beneficial residents in the human body. The most common normal flora of the body are presented in Table 5-8 on p. 123.

Host: An organism in which another, usually parasitic, organism is nourished and harbored.

Symbiosis: The living together of two organisms of different species. Four major types of symbiotic relationships exist between humans and their flora: mutualism, commensalism, parasitism, and opportunism.

Mutualism: A relationship in which both organisms benefit. For example, certain normal flora living in the human intestine synthesize vitamin K, biotin, riboflavin, pantothenate, and pyridoxine.

Commensalism: A one-sided relationship in which one member benefits and neither is harmed. Yeast, *Candida albicans,* is one of the normal flora that has a commensal relationship with the skin.

System	Disease	Causative Organism	Route of Transmission	Signs and Symptoms
Integumentary System	Anthrax	*Bacillus anthracis*	Inhalation or ingestion of spores; consumption of contaminated food	Fever, chills, night sweats, cough, shortness of breath, fatigue, muscle aches, sore throat
	Skin infections	*Staphylococcus aureus*	Direct contact of individuals colonized or infected with this bacteria; hand hygiene is the single most important step in controlling spread of these bacteria	Minor: pimples, boils Major: septicemia, surgical wound infection, necrotizing fasciitis
	Chickenpox	*Varicella zoster*	Droplets spread through coughing and sneezing	Skin rash of blister-like lesions, usually on the face, scalp, or trunk
Respiratory System	Pneumonia	*Haemophilus influenzae* *Streptococcus pneumoniae* *Mycoplasma pneumoniae*	Direct contact with respiratory droplets	Fever, decreased breath sounds, shortness of breath, increased heart rate (tachycadia), increased respiratory rate (tachypnea)
	Legionellosis • Legionnaire's disease (severe form) • Pontiac fever (mild form)	*Legionella pneumophila*	Breathing water mists contaminated with *Legionella* bacteria (spa, air conditioner, shower)	Fever, chills, and a cough; muscle aches, headache, tiredness, loss of appetite, and occasionally diarrhea
	Tuberculosis	*Mycobacterium tuberculosis*	Respiratory droplet spread	A bad cough that lasts longer than 2 weeks, pain in the chest, coughing up blood or sputum (phlegm from deep inside the lungs), weakness, fatigue, weight loss, lack of appetite, chills, fever and night sweats
	Pertussis	*Bordetella pertussis*	Contact with respiratory droplets	Typically manifested in children with paroxysmal spasms of severe coughing, whooping, and posttussive vomiting
	Diptheria	*Corynebacterium diphtheriae*	Person-to-person spread through respiratory tract secretions	Sore throat; low-grade fever; adherent membrane of the tonsils, pharynx, or nose; neck swelling

Table 5-7

System	Disease	Causative Organism	Route of Transmission	Signs and Symptoms
	Influenza	Influenza A and B virus	Respiratory droplet spread	Fever (usually high), headache, extreme tiredness, dry cough, sore throat, runny nose, and muscle aches; gastrointestinal symptoms include nausea, vomiting, and diarrhea
	Common cold	Rhinoviruses	Respiratory droplet spread	Runny nose; sneezing; sore throat; mild, hacking cough
	Severe acute respiratory syndrome (SARS)	SARS-associated coronavirus (SARS-CoV)	Close person-to-person contact	High fever (temperature greater than 100.4°F [38.0°C]), headache: overall feeling of discomfort: and body aches, dry cough, pneumonia
Gastrointestinal System	Salmonellosis	*Salmonella enteritidis*	Consumption of contaminated food (raw eggs, chicken, or beef)	Fever, abdominal cramps, diarrhea beginning 12–72 hours after consuming a contaminated food or beverage
	Typhoid fever	*Salmonella typhi*	Fecal oral	Sustained high fever (103°F–104°F), weakness, stomach pains, headache, loss of appetite
	E.coli diarrhea	*Escherichia coli* O157:H7	Eating contaminated foods (ground beef, raw milk)	Severe bloody diarrhea, abdominal cramps
	Cholera	*Vibrio cholerae*	Drinking contaminated water or eating contaminated food	Profuse watery diarrhea, vomiting, leg cramps, dehydration, shock
	Botulism	*Clostridium botulinum*	Consuming improperly canned food contaminated with botulinum	Double vision, blurred vision, drooping eyelids, slurred speech, difficulty swallowing, dry mouth, muscle weakness
	Mumps	Mumps virus (paramyxovirus)	Airborne and direct contact with infected respiratory droplets	Fever, headache, muscle ache, swelling of the lymph nodes close to the jaw

Table 5-7, continued

System	Disease	Causative Organism	Route of Transmission	Signs and Symptoms
	Hepatitis A Hepatitis B Hepatitis C	Hepatitis A virus Hepatitis B virus Hepatitis C virus	Hepatitis A: fecal oral Hepatitis B: blood and body fluids Hepatitis C: blood and body fluids	Symptoms are similar for each: jaundice, fatigue, abdominal pain, loss of appetite, nausea, diarrhea fever, joint pain, dark urine
Genitourinary System	Chlamydia	*Chlamydia trachomatis*	Sexual contact	Usually silent; can have mild symptoms of abnormal vaginal discharge or a burning sensation when urinating
	Gonorrhea	*Neisseria gonorrhea*	Sexual contact	Mucopurulent endocervical or urethral exudates
	Syphilis	*Treponema pallidum*	Sexual contact; can be passed to the fetus from an infected woman	Single sore, usually firm, round, small, and painless, that appears at the spot where syphilis entered the body
	Genital herpes	Herpes simplex viruses type 1 (HSV-1) and type 2 (HSV-2)	HSV-1: oral and genital contact HSV-2: sexual contact	Genital sores: flu-like symptoms, including fever swollen glands
Nervous System	Meningitis	*Neisseria meningitidis Streptococcus pneumoniae Haemophilus influenzae*	Direct contact with respiratory secretions from a carrier	High fever, headache, stiff neck, nausea, vomiting, photophobia, confusion, sleepiness
	Toxoplasmosis	*Toxoplasma gondii*	Accidental ingestion of cat feces; ingestion of contaminated raw or undercooked meat, or contaminated water	Swollen lymph glands or muscle aches and pains that last for a month or more
	Poliomyelitis	Polioviruses 1, 2, and 3	Person-to-person, fecal or oral	Ranges from asymptomatic to symptomatic, including acute flaccid paralysis, quadriplegia, respiratory failure, and, rarely, death
	Rabies	Rabies virus	Bite of a rabid animal	Fever, headache, confusion, sleepiness, or agitation

Table 5-7, continued

System	Disease	Causative Organism	Route of Transmission	Signs and Symptoms
Blood and Immune System	Plague	*Yersinia pestis*	Flea-borne from infected rodents to humans; respiratory droplets from cats and humans with pneumonic plague	Bubonic plague: enlarged, tender lymph nodes, fever, chills, prostration Septicemic plague: fever, chills, prostration, abdominal pain, shock, bleeding into skin and other organs Pneumonic plague: fever, chills, cough, and difficulty breathing; rapid shock
	Rocky Mountain spotted fever	*Rickettsia rickettsii*	Tick-borne ixodid ticks infected with *R. rickettsii*	Fever, nausea, vomiting, severe headache, muscle pain, lack of appetite, rash, abdominal pain, joint pain, diarrhea
	Lyme disease	*Borrelia burgdorferi*	Tick-borne deer ticks infected with *Borrelia burgdorferi*	Fever, headache, fatigue, myalgia
	Mononucleosis	Epstein-Barr virus	Contact with saliva of infected person	Fever, sore throat, swollen lymph glands
	HIV/AIDS	Human immuno-deficiency virus	Blood and body fluids	The following *may be* warning signs of infection with HIV: rapid weight loss; dry cough; recurring fever or profuse night sweats, profound and unexplained fatigue, swollen lymph glands in the armpits, groin, or neck; diarrhea that lasts for more than a week, white spots or unusual blemishes on the tongue, in the mouth, or in the throat, pneumonia, red, brown, pink, or purplish blotches on or under the skin or inside the mouth, nose, or eyelids; memory loss, depression, and other neurological disorders
	Malaria	*Plasmodium: P. falciparum, P. vivax, P. ovale,* or *P. malariae*	Mosquito-borne from Anopheles mosquito infected with *P. malariae*	Fever and influenza-like symptoms, including chills, headache, myalgias, and malaise

Table 5-7, concluded

Source: Centers for Disease Control, Health Topics A to Z. Atlanta, Georgia, 2003. www.cdc.gov/health/default.htm

Body Part	Normal Flora
Skin	*Staphylococcus epidermidis*
Nose	*Staphylococcus aureus, S. epidermidis*
Nasopharynx (upper respiratory tract)	*Streptococcus pneumoniae, Neisseria meningitidis, Haemophilus influenzae*
Eye	*Staphylococcus epidermidis*
Stomach	Because of the stomach's acidic pH, it contains very few microorganisms
Intestine	The distal portion of the small intestine and the entire large intestine have the largest microbial population in the body. The most common microbes in the large intestine are *Bacteroides fragilis, Escherichia coli, Proteus mirabilis,* and *Candida albicans.*
Genital tract	*Lactobacillus*

Table 5-8

Parasitism: A one-sided relationship between a host and a parasite.

Parasite: An organism that lives in, on, or at the expense of another organism without contributing to the host's survival.

Obligate intracellular parasite: A parasite that is completely dependent on its host and must be in a living cell in order to reproduce.

Opportunism: A relationship in which a usually harmless organism becomes pathogenic when the host's resistance is impaired.

Opportunistic microbe: A harmless microorganism that causes disease only if it invades the body when the immune system is weakened and unable to defend against it.

Pathogens: Disease-causing microorganisms. Only a small percentage of microbes are pathogenic; the others are considered harmless or beneficial.

Pathogenicity: The ability of a pathogenic agent to cause a disease.

Virulence: The degree of pathogenicity or relative power of an organism to produce a disease.

Infective dose: The number of organisms required to cause a disease in a susceptible host.

Contagious disease: A disease that is transmitted from one person to another. The following factors influence the cycle involved in the spread of infectious disease: means of transmission, means of entrance, susceptible host, reservoir host, and means of exit. To prevent infection any part of this cycle must be broken. See Figure 5-2.

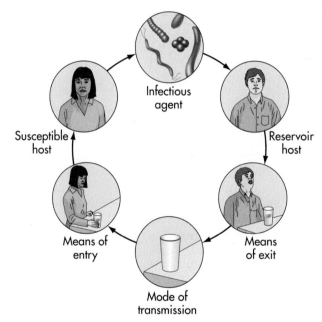

Figure 5-2 *The cycle of infection must be broken at some point to prevent the spread of disease.*

Breaking the cycle of infection: Medical assistants can help break the cycle of infection by proper handwashing, maintaining strict housekeeping standards, adhering to government guidelines to protect against diseases, and educating patients about hygiene, health promotion, and disease prevention.

Vector: A carrier of pathogenic organisms, especially one that can transmit a disease. See Table 5-9.

Carrier	Diseases
Dogs, raccoons	Rabies
Mosquitoes	Malaria, encephalitis
Ticks	Rocky Mountain spotted fever, Lyme disease

Table 5-9

Biological vector: An animal in which the infecting organism multiplies or develops before becoming infectious.

Resistance: The body mechanisms that oppose infection. The host's state of health and other factors, including race, age, sex, and occupation, affect the ability of a pathogen to cause disease. Resistance is also the ability of a microorganism to live in the presence of antibiotics, antimicrobial agents, and phages.

Microbial Control and Asepsis

Microbial control: The prevention of infectious diseases by using heat, steam, fire, and chemicals to control the growth of microbes.

Asepsis: Freedom from infection or infectious material.

Medical asepsis: Destruction of organisms after they leave the body.

Office asepsis procedures: Procedures that can include cleaning the office regularly, enforcing a strict no-eating and no-drinking policy, emptying the trash often, and asking patients to use tissues for coughs and sneezes.

Aseptic hand washing: The most important aseptic procedure for a medical assistant. Wash hands regularly, including at the beginning of the day; before and after lunch; before using gloves, handling specimens or waste, and handling clean and sterile supplies; before and after seeing each patient; after blowing your nose and coughing; after breaks; and before leaving for the day. Remove all jewelry, use warm water and liquid soap, and scrub vigorously for at least 2 minutes. Make sure that you clean all surfaces of your hands, including under the nails and cuticles (use a nailbrush). Rinse well and make sure that your hands don't touch the sink or faucet. Dry with a clean paper towel, and turn off the faucets by using a paper towel, not your hands.

Surgical asepsis: Destruction of organisms before they enter the body.

Sterilization: Complete destruction of all microorganisms and spores. Sterilization will be discussed in chapter 16.

Sterile or **surgical scrub:** A procedure that differs from aseptic hand washing in several important respects: A sterile scrub brush is used instead of a nailbrush, both the hands and the forearms are washed, hands are kept above the elbows to prevent water from running from the arms onto washed areas, sterile towels are used instead of paper towels, and sterile gloves are put on immediately after the hands are dried.

Sanitization: Reduction of the number of microorganisms on an object to a fairly small and safe level.

Disinfection: The process of removing or killing pathogens. Common disinfectants include various chemicals, boiling water, and steam.

Antiseptic: A substance, such as hydrogen peroxide, used externally to prevent or inhibit the growth and reproduction of microorganisms.

Bactericidal or **bacteriocidal:** Destructive to or destroying bacteria.

Bacteriostatic: Inhibiting the growth of bacteria.

Antisepsis: Inhibition, usually through a topical application, of the growth and multiplication of microorganisms.

Biohazardous waste containers: Leakproof, puncture-resistant containers that are color-coded or labeled with special symbols to show that they contain biohazardous materials such as blood and other body fluids, human tissue, or equipment that is no longer sterile. These containers are used to store and dispose of contaminated supplies and equipment.

Instructions:

Answer the following questions. Check your answers in the *Answer Key* that follows this section.

1. An organism that obtains its nutrients from dead organic matter is called
   A. Diplococcus
   B. Chlamydia
   C. Saprophyte
   D. Mycoplasma
   E. Protozoon

2. Which of the following microorganisms is a grape-like cluster?
   A. Streptococci
   B. Spirochete
   C. *Neisseria gonorrhoeae*
   D. *Vibrio cholerae*
   E. Staphylococci

3. Which of the following organisms requires a vector?
   A. Chlamydia
   B. Mycoplasma
   C. Rickettsia
   D. Saprophyte
   E. Diplococcus

4. Bacteria that are permanent and beneficial residents in the human body are called
   A. Pathogens
   B. Hosts
   C. Normal flora
   D. Parasites
   E. Normal fauna

5. The smallest organisms are called
   A. Viruses
   B. Chlamydia
   C. Rickettsia
   D. Acidophiles
   E. Bacteria

6. Aseptic hand washing techniques include all of the following <u>except</u>
   A. Removing all jewelry
   B. Using a nailbrush to scrub under the nails and cuticles
   C. Using liquid soap
   D. Turning off the faucet with the hands
   E. Scrubbing vigorously

7. If a virus has a bacterial host, it is called
   A. A bacteriophage
   B. Bacteriostatic
   C. Bactericidal
   D. Either B or C
   E. None of the above

8. Microbes that can grow either with or without oxygen are called
   A. Anaerobes
   B. Facultative anaerobes
   C. Aerobes
   D. Obligate anaerobes
   E. Aerobic

9. Hydrogen peroxide is an example of a(n)
   A. Sepsis
   B. Aseptic
   C. Antisepsis
   D. Antiseptic
   E. Bacteriostatic agent

10. Any close relationship that exists between two different species is known as
    A. Sebum
    B. Symbionts
    C. Syncope
    D. Synergism
    E. Symbiosis

11. All of the following factors may influence the cycle involved in the spread of infectious disease <u>except</u>
    A. Means of transmission
    B. Susceptible host
    C. Interferons
    D. Means of entrance
    E. Means of exit

12. The degree to which an organism is pathogenic is known as
    A. Infective dose
    B. Pathogen
    C. Tetany
    D. Resistance
    E. Virulence

13. A substance that inhibits the growth of bacteria is said to be
    A. Sterile
    B. Anaerobic
    C. Bactericidal
    D. Bacteriostatic
    E. Symbiotic

14. Which of the following is <u>not</u> true of the Gram staining procedure?
    A. It works for all bacteria
    B. The stain used is crystal violet
    C. It differentiates between gram-positive and gram-negative bacteria
    D. Some bacteria lose the stain by decolorization
    E. They are all true

15. Sterilization is
    A. The process of preventing infectious disease
    B. A substance that destroys or kills bacteria
    C. A technique for destroying microorganisms
    D. A substance for inhibiting the growth of microorganisms
    E. None of the above

16. Biohazardous waste containers
    A. Are color-coded or labeled
    B. Are leakproof
    C. Are puncture-resistant
    D. Can contain blood and other body fluids
    E. Are all of the above

17. Disinfection is
    A. The process of removing or killing pathogens
    B. The process of reducing the number of microorganisms to a safe level
    C. Complete destruction of all microorganisms
    D. Both A and C
    E. All of the above

18. Spiral-shaped bacteria are called
    A. Cocci
    B. Spirilla
    C. Bacilli
    D. Diplococci
    E. Sarcinae

19. Streptococci appear in
    A. Clusters of cocci
    B. Pairs of cocci
    C. Chains of cocci
    D. Spirilla
    E. Capsulate and spore forms

20. The bacterium *Escherichia coli* can cause
    A. Urinary infections
    B. Pneumonia
    C. Gonorrhea
    D. Chancroid
    E. Arthritis

21. A carrier of causative organisms that can transmit diseases to noninfected individuals is called a
    A. Viron
    B. Bacterium
    C. Virus
    D. Vector
    E. Protozoon

22. Viruses are

    A. Simpler than prokaryotes
    B. Visible to the naked eye
    C. Complex disease-causing organisms
    D. The same thing as bacteria
    E. The same thing as fungus

23. Which of the following words is misspelled?

    A. Chlamydia
    B. Myecobacteria
    C. Staphylococci
    D. Eukaryote
    E. Rickettsia

24. A medical assistant needs to wash his or her hands

    A. Before seeing each patient
    B. After handling waste
    C. After using gloves
    D. Before leaving for the day
    E. All of the above

ANSWER KEY

1.	C	13.	D
2.	E	14.	A
3.	C	15.	C
4.	C	16.	E
5.	A	17.	A
6.	D	18.	B
7.	A	19.	C
8.	B	20.	A
9.	D	21.	D
10.	E	22.	A
11.	C	23.	B
12.	E	24.	E

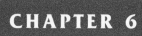

CHAPTER 6

General Psychology

CHAPTER OUTLINE

Basic Principles

Motivation and Emotion

Motivation
Emotions

Personality

Freud
Jung

Humanistic Theory of Personality

Behavioral/Learning Theory of Personality

Psychological Disorders

Aging and Dying

Promoting Health and Wellness

MEDICAL ASSISTING COMPETENCIES

COMPETENCY	CMA	RMA
General/Legal/Professional		
Recognize and respond to verbal and nonverbal communications by being attentive and adapting communication to the recipient's level of understanding.	X	X
Instruct individuals according to their needs.	X	X
Provide patients with methods of health promotion and disease prevention.	X	X
Be impartial and show empathy when dealing with patients.		X

Age	Stage	Characteristics
Birth to 12–18 months	Oral	Interest in oral gratification (sucking, eating, mouthing, biting), in which an infant's center of pleasure is the mouth
12–18 months to 3 years	Anal	Gratification by withholding and expelling feces and getting used to society's controls regarding toilet training, in which a child's pleasure is centered on the anus
3 to 5–6 years	Phallic	Interest in the genitals and coming to terms with the Oedipal conflict (which leads to identification with the same-sex parent); a child's pleasure focuses on the genitals
5–6 Years to Adolescence	Latency	Unimportance of sexual concerns; children's sexual concerns are temporarily put aside
Adolescence to Adulthood	Genital	Reemergence of sexual interests; mature sexual relationships are established or the period from puberty until death, marked by mature sexual behavior (such as sexual intercourse)

Table 6-2

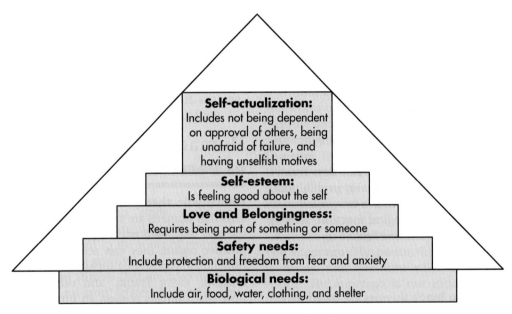

Figure 6-1 *A pyramid illustrates Maslow's hierarchy of human needs.*

Maslow's hierarchy of needs: Abraham Maslow believed that the basic needs of humans must be met before upper level functioning can occur. Maslow's pyramid details how the basics of life are of first concern, and then safety, love, and belonging must be met before humans can begin to become fully actualized. If lower needs in the hierarchy are not met for the most part, then higher motives will not operate. Higher needs lie dormant until the individual has a chance to satisfy immediately pressing lower needs, such as hunger, thirst, and safety. See Figure 6-1.

Personality and culture: Psychologists are accepting the idea that sociocultural factors, such as ethnicity, race, gender, sexual preference, and physical challenges, are important in understanding human personality. One new focus of cross-cultural research has been on the validity of North American concepts of personality in other cultures.

Behavioral/Learning Theory of Personality

Behavioral/learning theory of personality: Learning through operant conditioning (consequences cause a change). Positive reinforcement is achieved when a reward is given. Negative or positive behavior can be reinforced, thereby causing it to be repeated. Other schedules can cause increased learning, such as random intermittent reinforcement schedule, which explains why people gamble. The reward is random and definitely intermittent, which causes the person who has won in the past to try for the reinforcer against all odds. Extinction of the behavior occurs when the reinforcers are no longer given.

Adaptation: The adjustment of a person's sensory capacity after prolonged exposure to a stimulus. For example, viewing excessive violence over a longer period of time does not bring on the same response as during the original sighting.

Behavior modification: A technique used to promote the frequency of a desired behavior while decreasing an undesirable behavior.

Biofeedback: A process whereby the person learns to control internal physiological systems, such as blood pressure, pulse, and respirations, by the use of conscious thought.

Cognitive theory: The theory that a person's emotions are a result of how that person interprets stimuli through his or her belief system. For example, if two people associate the color green with money, the person with the positive belief system about money will be happy when shown the color green. On the contrary, a person who has a negative view of money may react sadly when shown the color green.

Cognitive development: The process through which an infant becomes an intelligent person, acquiring knowledge with growth and improving his or her ability to think, learn, reason, and abstract. Jean Piaget demonstrated the orderly sequence of this process from early infancy through childhood.

Cognition: The intellectual processes through which information is obtained, transformed, stored, retrieved, and otherwise used.

Language: A symbolic code used in communication.

Intelligence: The cognitive abilities of an individual to learn from experience, to reason well, and to cope with the demands of daily living.

Cognitive: Pertaining to the mental processes of comprehension, judgment, memory, and reasoning, as contrasted with emotional and volitional processes.

Cognitive dissonance: The tension that occurs when a person holds two conflicting attitudes about the same event. The anxiety that is generated by the contradictory views causes the person to either change his or her mind about how the event occurred or to deny how he or she really feels about it. One of the typical areas of cognitive dissonance is medical advice. A patient may enjoy smoking but still know that it can cause cancer. With these two contradictory facts, the patient may modify one or both of the cognitions, as follows: modification of one cognition (e.g., "I hardly smoke at all"), addition of cognitions (e.g., "I eat healthily so I am relatively strong"), or outright denial (e.g, "Not all people who smoke get cancer").

Psychological Disorders

Psychological disorders: A mental disorder or disturbance of thought or emotion. It is a disorder of the brain that results in a disruption in a person's thinking, feeling, moods, and ability to relate to others.

Anxiety disorders: Psychological disorders that involve excessive levels of negative emotions, such as nervousness, tension, worry, fright, and anxiety; the occurrence of anxiety without an obvious external cause, affecting daily functioning.

Phobias: Intense, irrational fears of specific objects or situations.

Generalized anxiety disorder: The experience of long-term, persistent anxiety and worry; an uneasy sense of general tension and apprehension that makes the individual highly uncomfortable because of prolonged presence. Sometimes the individual's concerns are about identifiable issues involving family, money, work, or health.

Panic anxiety disorder: A pattern of anxiety in which long periods of calm are broken by an intensely uncomfortable attack of anxiety.

Obsessive-compulsive disorders: Disorders that involve obsessions (anxiety-provoking thoughts that will not go away). Obsessions and compulsions are two separate problems, but they often occur together in the same individuals. Compulsions are irresistible urges to engage in behaviors such as repeatedly touching a spot on one's shoulder or repeatedly washing one's hands.

Dissociative disorders: Disorders that involve the apparent, abrupt, and repeated shifting from one "personality" to another. Formerly, a dissociative disorder was known as *multiple personality.*

Personality disorders: Psychological disorders that are believed to result from personalities that developed improperly during childhood. A number of personality disorders differ widely from one another, but share several characteristics:

- All personality disorders begin early in life
- They are disturbing to the person and to others
- They are very difficult to treat

Somatoform disorders: Disorders in which the individual experiences symptoms of health problems that have psychological rather than physical causes. They are more common in women than in men. They take the form of chronic and recurrent aches, pains, tiredness, and other symptoms of somatic (body) illnesses.

Hypochondriasis: A disorder in which people have a constant fear of illness and a preoccupation with their health.

Conversion disorder: A major somatoform disorder that involves an actual physical disturbance, such as the inability to use a sensory organ or the complete or partial inability to move an arm or leg.

Schizophrenia: A psychological disorder involving cognitive disturbances (delusions and hallucinations), disorganization, and reduced enjoyment and interests. Schizophrenia is an uncommon disorder that affects about 1% of the general population.

Mania: An extended state of intense elation. People experiencing mania feel intense happiness, power, invulnerability, and energy. They may become involved in wild schemes, believing they will succeed at anything they attempt.

Bipolar disorder: A disorder in which a person alternates between periods of euphoric feelings and mania and periods of depression.

Attention deficit disorder: A disorder primarily affecting children and adolescents, characterized by the inability to focus attention, leading to behavior problems and learning disabilities. The condition is more common in boys than in girls and is usually treated with psychotherapy and stimulant drugs.

Autism: A mental disorder characterized by extreme withdrawal and an abnormal absorption in fantasy, accompanied by delusions, hallucinations, and the inability to communicate verbally or otherwise relate to people. Schizophrenic children are often autistic.

Aging and Dying

Erikson's stages of psychosocial development: Erikson believed that as people age, they also go through psychosocial changes. He described a struggle between two forces at each milestone of development,; the resolution of this struggle results in either positive or negative outcomes. Whichever way a person resolves each conflict, his or her identity is formed:

- Birth to $1\frac{1}{2}$ years—the conflict is trust vs. mistrust
  - Positive outcome—ability to trust
  - Negative outcome—fear of others
- $1\frac{1}{2}$ to 3 years—the conflict is autonomy vs. shame and doubt
  - Positive outcome—self sufficiency
  - Negative outcome—lack of independence, self-doubt of one's own abilities

- 3 to 6 years—the conflict is initiative vs. guilt
  - Positive outcome—initiation of actions
  - Negative outcome—guilt from actions and thoughts
- 6 to 12 years—the conflict is industry vs. inferiority
  - Positive outcome—sense of competence
  - Negative outcome—feelings of inferiority
- Adolescence—the conflict is identity vs. role confusion
  - Positive outcome—awareness of one's own uniqueness
  - Negative outcome—inability to identify appropriate roles in life
- Early adulthood—the conflict is intimacy vs. isolation
  - Positive outcome—development of loving sexual relationships and close friends
  - Negative outcome—fear of relationships
- Middle adulthood—the conflict is generativity vs. stagnation
  - Positive outcome—contribution to the continuity of life
  - Negative outcome—feeling that acts are trivial for future generations
- Late adulthood—the conflict is ego-integrity vs. despair
  - Positive outcome—sense of unity with life's accomplishments
  - Negative outcome—regrets over lost opportunities of life

Elizabeth Kübler-Ross' stages of death: Elizabeth Kübler-Ross, a psychiatrist in the late 1960s and early 1970s, gave great insight into the death and dying process. She theorized that people pass through five distinct stages when they learn of their impending deaths and expanded it to include death of a loved one. However, she cautioned that the dying process has very individual reactions and that anyone involved with the dying person should not try to force how he or she experiences the process. The five stages Dr. Kübler-Ross constructed after hundreds of interviews with dying patients are as follows:

1. **Denial:** There are several ways a person may manifest denial of a terminal diagnosis. The person may seek other opinions or say that the doctors and tests are wrong. This is also the stage when a person may seek a "miracle cure" and could fall into a scam or exhaust savings to try to find the "magic pill." Denial is so powerful that the person may simply look as though he or she has ignored the diagnosis and act

as if nothing has changed. Denial is a defense mechanism that patients commonly use to shield themselves from the intense anxiety that can be produced in the medical field.

2. **Anger:** This stage occurs as the denial begins to break down. A common statement that a patient might make is, "Why me?" The patient could also be highly irritable, resentful, and envious of others who are happy. The doctor, nurses, and other staff may be targets of this reaction, but most likely the caregivers will be the ones who experience the most hostility (and will need support from the medical staff to help them through this).

3. **Bargaining:** After the denial and anger have subsided and the person is beginning to deal with the fact that he or she will die, the patient makes a last attempt to change the inevitable. This attempt is to bargain. The bargains are usually religious in nature, and deals are made to extend one's life: "I will faithfully attend church and donate money to the poor if I can live 1 more year."

4. **Depression:** When the bargaining does not come to fruition and the inevitability of the situation sinks in, the patient may lapse into a deep depression. The sense of hope is gone, and the feelings of guilt may overtake the person. The person may regret things he or she has done or said to loved ones and feel guilty over leaving them.

5. **Acceptance:** As the depression lifts, the person gains a sense of peace that death will happen and a quiet state of recognition that all living things die and that this is the person's time. This time is not a happy time, but rather is marked with exhaustion yet free of negative emotions.

Promoting Health and Wellness

Compliance: Strategies to increase compliance are as follows:

- Provide clear instructions to patients regarding medication schedules.
- Maintain good rapport between patients and medical staff.
- Be honest.
- Keep the patient well-informed.
- Frame messages in a positive manner to help the patient with early detection of a disease.
- Frame messages in a negative manner to motivate the patient to prevent disease.

Stress: A person's response to threatening or challenging events. Most people will have a degree of stress when visiting a doctor's office. When a patient is under a high level of stress, he or she may become ill and may be less likely to recover from an illness. It may make the patient less capable of coping with future stressors.

Coping with stress: The ways that a patient attempts to lessen stress through different strategies, such as defense mechanisms. Also, some patients may use alcohol or drugs to cope with stress.

General adaptation syndrome (GAS): Hans Selye's theory that persons under stress experience the same set of physiological reactions regardless of the source of the stress. There are three phases that a person will move through when faced with stress:

- First phase: alarm and mobilization. The patient becomes aware of the stressor, and the nervous system becomes energized.
- Second phase: resistance. If the stress continues, then the patient prepares to fight the stressors. This technique can cause the patient physiological and psychological harm.
- Third phase: exhaustion. If the stressor continues and the patient is unable to adapt or remove the stressor, then the patient will develop negative consequences of physical and psychological symptoms. These symptoms can be manifested in illness, suppressed immune systems, increased irritability, increased substance abuse, and, in some extreme cases, disorientation and loss of touch with reality.
- Aftermath: The patient will be able to lessen the stressor through the exhaustion phase by avoidance. If a person is ill, then he or she can avoid the activity that caused the stress. For example, a person who is overloaded at work cannot go to work if he or she is in the hospital or suffering with a severe condition at home. This serves as a temporary fix to reduce the stressor. If resources are applied during this time, then the patient may be able to handle the stress when he or she re-enters the workplace. If no resources are applied, the patient will return to the stressors and repeat the cycle.

Psychophysiological disorders: Disorders that are real medical conditions influenced by physical, emotional, and psychological difficulties.

Psychophysiological conditions: Common conditions, such as high blood pressure, headaches, backaches, and skin rashes, that may have a link to or are worsened by stress or other psychological difficulties.

Cataclysmic event stressor: Events that happen suddenly and affect many people, simultaneously causing strong stressors for all. For example, the terrorist attacks in New York and the destruction of New Orleans from Hurricane Katrina were cataclysmic events.

Personal stressors: Major events in one's personal life. Life events, whether positive or negative, can cause a great deal of stress, such as death of a spouse, losing one's job, going to war, moving, abuse, having a baby, or getting married. Some victims of high stressors suffer from post-traumatic stress disorder (PTSD), which is the re-experiencing of a traumatic event, and without help can find themselves so overwhelmed that they may harm themselves or others.

Background stressors: Daily annoyances, such as traffic jams, waiting in line, and irritations at work. Alone, these stressors have the least impact on a person but, coupled with other stressors or multiple daily stressors, can result in psychological and physical problems, e.g., colds, flu, backaches, irritability, agitation, and distractibility.

Uplifts: Stress reducers. Minor positive events that can make a person feel good.

Questions 1 to 3 relate to Mr. Martin. He is a 70-year-old male who has been diagnosed with late stage cancer of the stomach. He probably will only live 3 to 6 months. You are the medical assistant at the primary care doctor's office.

1. Mr. Martin has just been told of his diagnosis of cancer and the probability that he will not live too long. According to Kübler-Ross' stages of death, what do you expect to hear from the patient?
   A. A rationalization
   B. A statement of denial
   C. A positive attitude
   D. A sublimation

2. A month later, Mr. Martin returns to the office and snaps back at the receptionist who comments on the nice day. Mr. Martin meets you and is very argumentative and annoyed when you try to help him to get up from the chair. According to Kübler-Ross' stages, what do you think is happening?
   A. Mr. Martin is grumpy because the staff is annoying
   B. Mr. Martin is annoyed because he had to wait
   C. Mr. Martin is realizing that he is dying and is angry
   D. Mr. Martin has reached an acceptance of death and feels an inner peace with his fate

3. Mr. Martin is facing death in his late adulthood and is reviewing his life. According to Erikson's stages of development, what conflict is he trying to resolve?
   A. Identity vs. role confusion
   B. Industry vs. inferiority
   C. Trust vs. mistrust
   D. Ego integrity vs. despair

4. When a person experiences another person's emotional state by viewing it through the other person's eyes, it is known as
   A. Empathy
   B. Sympathy
   C. Denial
   D. Acceptance

5. According to Maslow's hierarchy of needs, which of the following is a physical need?
   A. Approval
   B. Shelter
   C. Love
   D. Award
   E. Self-Esteem

6. Which statement is true about stress?
   A. All stress is from negative sources
   B. Background stressors are events that happen suddenly
   C. Stress can affect the body's ability to fight off illness
   D. All stress causes physiological disorders

7. According to Kübler-Ross, the five stages of grief include denial, bargaining, depression, anger, and which of the following?
   A. Fear
   B. Love
   C. Shock
   D. Acceptance
   E. Repression

8. Your patient was asked to exercise her neck for 3 minutes, six times a day. She told the medical assistant that she could not do the exercises because she had to go to work. Which of the following defense mechanisms is she using?
   A. Regression
   B. Rationalization
   C. Repression
   D. Projection
   E. Displacement

9. A dying patient refuses to eat, refuses visitors, and refuses further medical treatment. According to Elizabeth Kübler-Ross, this stage of dying most likely represents:
   A. Denial
   B. Depression
   C. Anger
   D. Acceptance
   E. Bargaining

10. While recovering from a major surgical pro-
    cedure, a 39-year-old man is laid off from his
    job. He becomes rude and mean-spirited to-
    ward his wife, which is a significant change in
    his behavior. Which of the following defense
    mechanisms is this patient exhibiting?
    A. Displacement
    B. Denial
    C. Sublimation
    D. Rationalization
    E. Regression

11. A 38-year-old woman who has advanced
    breast cancer becomes extremely upset with
    family members when they even talk about
    the disease. The patient refuses to talk about
    the diagnosis and even acts as if she has a
    minor problem. This patient is using which of
    the following defense mechanisms?
    A. Rationalization
    B. Denial
    C. Displacement
    D. Sublimation
    E. Projection

12. A 74-year-old man has severe gangrene of the
    right foot and right lower leg. His physician
    recommends above-the-knee amputation to
    prevent further problems. The patient refuses
    to consider this recommendation and states
    that he will stop smoking to control the condi-
    tion, so that amputation will not be necessary.
    Which of the following defense mechanisms
    is this patient demonstrating?
    A. Denial
    B. Repression
    C. Rationalization
    D. Compensation
    E. Sublimation

13. Major depression and bipolar disorder are
    most characteristic of which of the following
    psychological conditions?
    A. Dissociative disorder
    B. Impulse-control disorder
    C. Mood disorder
    D. Personality disorder
    E. Cognitive disorder

14. An 18-month-old boy temporarily forgets
    potty training when his parents bring his new-
    born sister home from the hospital. This is an
    example of which of the following defense
    mechanisms?
    A. Repression
    B. Regression
    C. Rationalization
    D. Introjection
    E. Suppression

15. A person with a preoccupation toward inner
    thoughts and a lack of responsiveness to oth-
    ers has which of the following conditions?
    A. Paranoia
    B. Mania
    C. Autism
    D. Dysphoria
    E. Dyslexia

16. Which of the following is the most common
    initial reaction to a permanently disabling
    injury?
    A. Guilt
    B. Loss
    C. Denial
    D. Fear
    E. Depression

17. Which of the following is a major life event that commonly causes a high level of stress?
    A. Death of spouse
    B. Getting a raise
    C. Being single
    D. Painting your house
    E. Meeting new friends

18. You observed a patient walking slightly bent over and holding his stomach. What would you chart this as?
    A. A behavior
    B. An emotion
    C. Sympathy
    D. Empathy
    E. None of the above

19. An irritable and complaining patient states to you that everyone around him is negative and irritable. You recognize this defense mechanism as:
    A. Sublimation
    B. Repression
    C. Rationalization
    D. Projection

20. The patient who holds two conflicting attitudes, such as enjoyment of smoking and knowledge that smoking can cause cancer, is suffering from
    A. cognitive dissonance
    B. phobia
    C. obsessive-compulsive disorder
    D. major depression
    E. repression

21. The terms extroversion, introversion, personal unconscious, and collective unconscious are attributed to:
    A. Freud
    B. Skinner
    C. Bantura
    D. Maslow
    E. Jung

22. Mrs. S. shares with you that she is very upset when she has to wait in line or sit in a traffic jam. You recognize this stressor as a:
    A. Posttraumatic syndrome
    B. Cataclysmic stressor
    C. Personal stressor
    D. Background stressor

23. Psychology is the
    A. Scientific study of the mind
    B. Scientific study of behaviors
    C. Scientific study of mental processes
    D. All of the above

24. Biofeedback is a process that can help a person learn to control
    A. Internal physiological systems
    B. External physiological systems
    C. Environmental systems
    D. Other people

ANSWER KEY

1.	B		13.	C
2.	C		14.	B
3.	D		15.	C
4.	A		16.	C
5.	B		17.	A
6.	C		18.	A
7.	D		19.	D
8.	B		20.	A
9.	B		21.	E
10.	A		22.	D
11.	B		23.	D
12.	A		24.	A

CHAPTER 7

Nutrition

CHAPTER OUTLINE

Nutrition

Water

Carbohydrates

Lipids

Protein

Vitamins

    Water-Soluble Vitamins
    Fat-Soluble Vitamins
    Conditions Associated with Vitamins

Minerals

    Major Minerals
    Trace Elements

Nutrition and Diet Needs

Food-Related Diseases

MEDICAL ASSISTING COMPETENCIES

COMPETENCY	CMA	RMA
General/Legal/Professional		
Instruct individual according to their needs	X	X
Provide patients with methods of health promotion and disease prevention	X	X
Use appropriate medical terminology		X

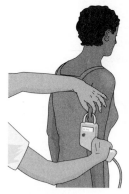
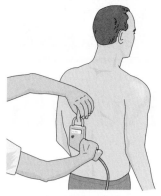

Triceps (back of arm)

Subscapular (below shoulder blade)

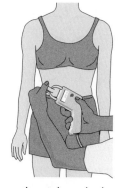
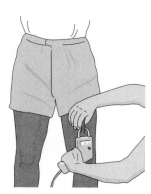

Suprailiac (above hipbone)

Thigh (front)

Figure 7-1 *To estimate an individual's body fat percentage, a professional uses a tool called a caliper to measure the thickness of a fold of skin at one or more points on the body.*

Nutrition

Nutrients: Chemical substances that are necessary for growth, normal functioning, and maintaining life. These substances cannot be synthesized by the body and must be supplied by food. There are six basic groups of nutrients: carbohydrates, fats, proteins, vitamins, minerals, and water. Of these, only carbohydrates, fats, and proteins contain calories that provide the body with energy.

Overweight: Having a body weight that is 10 percent greater than the standard for the person's age, height, and body type.

Obesity: Excessive accumulation of fat in the body. Also, weight 20% higher than that considered desirable for the person's age, height, and bone structure.

Skinfold test: A procedure that determines fat as a percentage of body weight, in which the thickness of a fold of skin measured with a caliper indicates the total percentage of fat. See Figure 7-1.

Malnutrition: Poor nutrition caused by poor diet or by poor utilization of food that may result from an unbalanced, insufficient, or excessive diet.

Metabolism: The use of food as fuel, resulting in the generation of energy and growth and the elimination of waste.

Kilocalorie (Kcal): Commonly known as a calorie and also referred to as a "large calorie," which is equivalent to 1000 "small calories." One kilocalorie is the amount of energy needed to raise the temperature of 1 kg of water by 1°C. Calories measure the amount of energy a food produces in the body.

Energy value: Also called caloric density, the number of calories in food. Energy value is determined by the types and amounts of nutrients each food contains.

Water

Water: Water has no caloric value but contributes about 65% of an individual's body weight, helps maintain fluid balance, dissolves chemicals and nutrients, transports nutrients, lubricates, aids in digestion, flushes out wastes, and regulates body temperature through perspiration.

Amount of water in human cells: Water is the largest single component of the body. Metabolically active cells of the muscle and viscera have the highest concentration, and calcified tissue cells the lowest. Total body water is higher in athletes than in nonathletes and decreases significantly with age because of diminished muscle mass.

Amount of water needed: On average, people should drink 6 to 8 glasses (48 to 64 ounces, or 3 to 4 pints) of water a day to maintain a healthy water balance.

Thirst: Water intake is controlled mainly by thirst. Thirst control centers are located in the hypothalamus.

Absorption of water: Water is ingested as fluid and also as part of ingested food. Water is absorbed rapidly because it moves freely through membranes, mainly by diffusion.

Water loss: Water loss normally occurs through the kidneys in urine, through the gastrointestinal tract in the feces, through the lungs in expired air, and through the skin in sweat that evaporates from the skin. The amount of water taken in daily is approximately equivalent to the amount lost.

Effects of water loss: The loss of 20% of body water may cause death, and the loss of only 10% causes severe disorders. In moderate weather, adults can live up to 10 days without water; children can live up to 5 days. By contrast, it is possible to survive without food for several weeks.

Dehydration: Excessive loss of body water that usually is accompanied by electrolyte balance changes.

Water intoxication: The presence of excess water that causes cells, particularly brain cells, to swell, leading to headache, nausea, vomiting, convulsion, and death. Water intoxication may result from the excessive administration of water when the antidiuretic hormone and the kidney cannot respond, such as after surgery, trauma, or another condition that causes salt and water loss.

Carbohydrates

Carbohydrate: The body's primary source of energy. Carbohydrates provide heat, help metabolize fat, and help reserve protein for uses other than supplying energy. One gram of carbohydrate yields 4 calories. Excess carbohydrates are stored in the liver and muscles as glycogen. According to the current dietary recommendations, carbohydrates should provide 55% to 60% of an individual's total calorie intake. Carbohydrates are classified according to their complexity, from simple sugars to complex saccharides. Fruits, vegetables, pasta, cereal, potatoes, and sugary foods are good sources of carbohydrates.

Starch: A complex carbohydrate that is a major source of energy from plant foods.

Dietary fiber: A nondigestible carbohydrate found in plant cells. It provides bulk and stimulation for the intestines. The main dietary fiber components are cellulose, pectin, lignin, and gums. Some forms are soluble in water; others are not. Dietary fiber is used to treat and prevent constipation, hemorrhoids, diverticular disease, and irritable bowel syndrome. Studies have linked it to reduced levels of blood cholesterol, reduced formation of gallstones, and control of diabetes. Sources of dietary fiber include oats, dry beans, barley, some fruits and vegetables, whole wheat bread, and brown rice.

Lipids

Fats: Also called lipids, fats are not soluble in water but are soluble in some solvents such as alcohol. They provide energy and heat, carry fat-soluble vitamins, protect and support organs and bones, insulate from cold, and supply essential fatty acids. Each gram of fat provides 9 calories. Fats are classified as saturated or unsaturated; unsaturated fats are either monounsaturated or polyunsaturated.

Saturated fats: Fats generally derived from animal sources and usually solid at room temperature. Found in meat, butter, egg yolks, whole milk, and coconut and palm oil, they tend to raise blood cholesterol levels.

Unsaturated fats: Fats that are usually liquid at room temperature and can be monounsaturated or polyunsaturated. They tend to lower blood cholesterol levels.

Monounsaturated fats: Examples include oil from olives, avocados, or cashew nuts.

Polyunsaturated fats: Examples include cooking oils made from sunflower seeds, peanuts, or safflower seeds.

Ketones: Chemical substances that are broken down by fatty acids in the liver.

Ketosis: The abnormal collection of ketones in the blood as a result of excessive breakdown of fats caused by an insufficiency of glucose available for energy.

Cholesterol: A waxy lipid found almost exclusively in foods of animal origin and continuously synthesized in the body. Produced by the liver, cholesterol is essential for the production of vitamin D and bile acid. Because the body produces cholesterol, it is not essential in the diet. Cholesterol is measured by means of a blood test. See Table 7-1.

High-density lipoprotein (HDL): Called "good" cholesterol. It helps transport cholesterol to the liver where it is disposed. It may serve to stabilize very low-density lipoprotein.

Low-density lipoprotein (LDL): Called "bad" cholesterol. A high concentration may result in atherosclerosis and thus puts patients at risk of heart disease.

Cholesterolemia: The presence of an excessive amount of cholesterol in the blood. To reduce cholesterol level, individuals should reduce fat consumption to less than 30% of total caloric intake, with saturated fats providing less than 10% of caloric intake, and should increase consumption of soluble fiber.

AT A GLANCE	Common Nutrition-Related Blood Tests
Test	**Normal Range in Adults**
Cholesterol	Total: 150–200 mg/dl HDL: 25–90 mg/dl LDL: 85–200 mg/dl
Glucose	90–120 mg/dl
Iron	50–175 µg/dl
Triglycerides	200–300 mg/dl

Table 7-1

Triglyceride: One of several combinations of fatty acids and glycerol that circulate in the blood with HDL and LDL. High levels are associated with atherosclerosis.

Protein

Protein: The primary function of protein is to build and repair body tissues. It is the only substance that can make new cells and rebuild tissue. Proteins are also important components of hormones and enzymes. They maintain fluid balance, are essential for the development of antibodies, and can provide energy. Each gram of protein provides 4 calories of energy. Proteins are not as efficient as carbohydrates and fats in providing energy.

Amino acids: Nitrogen-containing compounds that make up proteins, also called the building blocks of protein.

Classification of amino acids: There are about 80 amino acids, of which 20 are necessary for human metabolism and growth. The adult body does not produce nine of them, which must be provided in the diet and are known as essential amino acids. See Table 7-2 for a list of the essential and nonessential amino acids.

AT A GLANCE	Amino Acids
Essential	**Nonessential**
Arginine (in young children)	Alanine
Histidine	Arginine (in adults)
Isoleucine	Asparagine
Leucine	Aspartic acid
Lysine	Cysteine
Methionine	Glutamic acid
Phenylalanine	Glutamine
Threonine	Glycine
Tryptophan	Proline
Valine	Serine
	Tyrosine

Table 7-2

Complete protein: A protein that contains all the essential amino acids and consequently is of high biological value. Casein (milk protein) and egg whites are examples of complete proteins.

Sources of protein: Meat, fish, poultry, eggs, and milk, which are complete proteins, and nuts, dry beans, grains, and vegetables, which are incomplete proteins.

Adequate protein intake: Learning to combine foods containing incomplete proteins in order to obtain all nine essential amino acids is especially important for people who follow vegetarian diets.

Vitamins

Vitamin: An organic compound that does not provide energy but helps in the metabolism of protein, carbohydrates, and fat. Vitamins act as catalysts and body regulators for the bones, skins, glands, nerves, brain, and blood, and they protect against diseases caused by nutritional deficiencies. With a few exceptions, vitamins cannot be produced by the body and must be supplied in the diet. Although they are essential, they should not be overused. There are two types of vitamins: water-soluble and fat-soluble. See Table 7-3.

Water-Soluble Vitamins

Vitamin B_1 (thiamine): Plays a role in carbohydrate metabolism and is essential for normal metabolism of the nervous system, heart, and muscles. Thiamine also promotes good appetite. It is not stored in the body and must be supplied daily. Sources include lean pork, wheat germ, lean meat, egg yolk, and fish. Deficiency causes loss of appetite, irritability, tiredness, sleep disturbance, nervous disorders, beriberi, loss of coordination, paralysis, and Wernicke-Korsakoff syndrome in people severely dependent on alcohol. Deficiency is often associated with alcoholism.

Vitamin B_2 (riboflavin): Is essential for certain enzyme systems in the metabolism of fats and proteins. It can be sensitive to light. Sources include milk, cheddar cheese, cottage cheese, organ meats, and eggs. Deficiency causes impaired growth, weakness, lip sores and cracks at the corners of the mouth, cheilosis, photophobia, cataracts, anemia, and glossitis.

Vitamin B_3 (niacin): Part of two enzymes that regulate energy metabolism. Also called nicotinic acid and nicotinamide, it maintains the health of the skin, tongue, and digestive system. Sources include lean meats, poultry, fish, and peanuts. Deficiency causes pellagra, gastrointestinal disturbance, and mental disturbances.

Vitamin B_6 (pyridoxine): Aids enzymes in the synthesis of amino acids and is essential for proper growth and maintenance of body functions. Sources include yeast, wheat germ, pork, bananas, and oatmeal. Deficiency

Water-Soluble Vitamins	Fat-Soluble Vitamins

Vitamin B complex:
    Thiamine (vitamin B_1)
    Riboflavin (vitamin B_2)
    Niacin (vitamin B_3)
    Pyridoxine (vitamin B_6)
    Folic acid (vitamin B_9)
    Cyanocobalamin (vitamin B_{12})
    Pantothenic acid
    Biotin (formerly vitamin H)
	Vitamin A
	
	Vitamin D
	
	Vitamin E
	
	Vitamin K

Vitamin C	

Table 7-3

causes anemia, neuritis, anorexia, nausea, depressed immunity, and dermatitis.

Vitamin B_9 (folic acid): Is essential for cell growth and the reproduction of RBCs. Also called folacin, it functions in the formation of hemoglobin and aids in metabolism of protein. It is also essential for fetal development, particularly of the neural tube. Sources include liver, kidney beans, lima beans, and fresh dark green leafy vegetables. Deficiency causes anemia and may cause spina bifida in a fetus.

Vitamin B_{12} (cyanocobalamin): Aids in hemoglobin synthesis, is essential for normal functioning of all cells, and is important in energy metabolism. Sources include liver, kidney, milk, eggs, fish, and cheese. Deficiency causes pernicious anemia and neurological disorders.

Pantothenic acid: A part of the vitamin B complex that is essential for fatty acid metabolism, the manufacture of sex hormones, the utilization of other vitamins, the functioning of the nervous system and the adrenal glands, and normal growth and development. Sources include egg yolks, kidney, liver, and yeast. Deficiency causes fatigue, headaches, nausea, abdominal pain, numbness, tingling, muscle cramps, and susceptibility to respiratory infections and peptic ulcers.

Biotin (formerly vitamin H): A water-soluble B-complex vitamin essential for the breakdown of fatty acids and carbohydrates and for the excretion of the waste products of protein breakdown. Good sources include kidney, liver, egg yolks, soybeans, and yeast.

Vitamin C: Also called ascorbic acid, it protects the body against infections and helps heal wounds. Best sources are fruits and vegetables, especially citrus fruits and tomatoes. Deficiency causes scurvy, lowered resistance to infections, joint tenderness, dental caries, bleeding gums, delayed wound healing, bruising, hemorrhage, and anemia. Vitamin C is lost in cooking fresh foods but not in cooking frozen foods.

Fat-Soluble Vitamins

Vitamin A (retinol, carotene): Contributes to the maintenance of epithelial cells and mucous membranes and is important for night vision. Retinol is also necessary for normal growth, development, and reproduction as well as an adequate immune response. Sources include liver, beef, sweet potato, spinach, milk, and egg yolks. Deficiency causes retarded growth, susceptibility to infection, dry skin, night blindness, xeropthalmia, abnormal gastrointestinal function, dry mucous membranes, and degeneration of the spinal cord and peripheral nerves.

Vitamin D: Is essential for the normal formation of bones and teeth. It aids in the reabsorption of calcium and phosphorus and regulates blood levels of calcium. There are two major forms of vitamin D: vitamin D_2, formed in plants, and vitamin D_3, formed in humans from cholesterol in the skin exposed to sunlight or other ultraviolet radiation. Best sources are butter, cream, egg yolks, liver, and fish liver oils. Deficiency causes rickets and osteomalacia.

Vitamin E: An antioxidant, also called tocopherol. It prevents oxidative destruction of vitamin A in the intestine, and it is essential for normal reproduction, muscle development, and resistance of RBCs to hemolysis. Vitamin E also helps maintain normal cell membranes. Sources include seed oil, fruits, vegetables, and animal fats.

Vitamin K: Is essential to blood clotting. There are several fat-soluble compounds of vitamin K. Vitamin K_2 is synthesized in the intestine by bacteria and is also found in animal foods. Vitamin K is found in large amounts in green leafy vegetables (especially broccoli,

Vitamin	Symptoms and Diseases
Vitamin A	Retarded growth, susceptibility to infection, dry skin, night blindness, xeropthalmia, abnormal gastrointestinal function, dry mucous membranes, degeneration of the spinal cord and peripheral nerves
Vitamin B_1	Loss of appetite, irritability, tiredness, nervous disorders, sleep disturbance, beriberi, loss of coordination, paralysis, Wernicke-Korsakoff syndrome
Vitamin B_2	Impaired growth, weakness, lip sores and cracks at the corners of the mouth, cheilosis, photophobia, cataracts, anemia, glossitis (Riboflavin deficiency is believed to be the most common vitamin deficiency in the United States.)
Vitamin B_3	Pellagra, characterized by dermatitis, diarrhea, dementia, and death; gastrointestinal and mental disturbances
Vitamin B_6	Anemia, neuritis, anorexia, nausea, depressed immunity, dermatitis
Viramin B_9 (folic acid)	Anemia, spina bifida in fetal development
Vitamin B_{12}	Pernicious anemia, neurological disorders
Pantothenic acid	Fatigue, headaches, nausea, abdominal pain, numbness, tingling, muscle cramps, susceptibility to respiratory infections and peptic ulcers
Vitamin C	Scurvy, characterized by gingivitis, loose teeth, and slow healing of wounds; lowered resistance to infections; joint tenderness; dental caries; bleeding gums; delayed wound healing; bruising; hemorrhage; anemia
Vitamin D	Rickets and osteomalacia
Vitamin K	Hemorrhage (Extensive oral antibiotic therapy may cause vitamin K_2 deficiency.)

Table 7-4

cabbage, and lettuce) and in fruits. Vitamin K can be used as an antidote for an overdose of an anticoagulant. Deficiency causes hemorrhage.

Conditions Associated with Vitamins

Avitaminosis: Deficiency of vitamins in the diet that causes a disease such as scurvy, rickets, or beriberi. See Table 7-4 for symptoms and diseases caused by vitamin deficiency.

Hypervitaminosis: A condition caused by an overdose of vitamins, especially fat-soluble vitamins. The main symptoms are loss of hair, severe itching, skin lesions, and abnormal tissue growth.

Excessive intake of vitamin A: Can result in a condition called hypervitaminosis A, the symptoms of which include headache, tiredness, nausea, loss of appetite, diarrhea, dry and itchy skin, hair loss, a yellow discoloration, and irregular menstrual periods. Excessive intake during pregnancy may cause birth defects.

Excessive intake of vitamin B_6: May cause neuritis.

Minerals

Minerals: Natural, inorganic substances that the body needs to help build and maintain body tissues and to carry on life functions. There are two separate classes of minerals: major minerals and trace elements. Diseases and symptoms associated with mineral deficiencies are listed in Table 7-5. Deficiencies of calcium, iron, and iodine are the three most common mineral deficiencies.

Mineral	Symptoms and Diseases
Calcium	Rickets, osteomalacia (adult rickets), tetany, osteoporosis
Copper	Anemia, bone disease (Copper deficiency is very rare in adults.)
Fluoride	Tooth decay, possibly osteoporosis
Iodine	Goiter, cretinism (congenital myxedema) (Goiter is more common among women. A thyroid gland dysfunction can cause acquired myxedema, commonly known as hypothyroidism, in adults.)
Iron	Iron-deficiency anemia, nutritional anemia
Phosphorus	Weight loss, anemia, anorexia, fatigue, abnormal growth, bone demineralization (mineral loss)
Potassium	Impaired growth, hypertension, bone fragility, renal hypertrophy, bradycardia, death
Zinc	Dwarfism, delayed growth, hypogonadism, anemia, decreased appetite

Table 7-5

Electrolytes: Compounds, particularly salts, that break up into their separate component particles in water. The particles are called ions, which are electrically charged atoms. Sodium, potassium, and chloride are commonly called electrolytes. Minerals help keep the body's water and electrolytes in balance.

Major Minerals

Calcium (Ca): The body requires calcium for the transmission of nerve impulses, muscle contraction, blood coagulation, and cardiac functions. Calcium also helps build strong bones and teeth and may prevent hypertension. Normal daily requirement: 800–1200 mg. The following factors enhance the absorption of calcium: adequate vitamin D, large quantities of calcium and phosphorus in diet, and the presence of lactose. A lack of physical activity reduces the amount of calcium absorption.

Phosphorus (P): Essential for the metabolism of protein, calcium, and glucose. It helps to build strong bones and teeth and aids in maintaining the body's acid-base balance. Phosphorus is found in dairy foods, animal foods, fish, cereals, nuts, and legumes.

Chloride (Cl): Involved in the maintenance of fluid and the body's acid-base balance. Disturbances in the acid-base balance can result in possible growth retardation and memory loss.

Sodium (Na): Plays a key role in the maintenance of the body's acid-base balance. It transmits nerve impulses and helps control muscle contractions. Toxic levels may cause hypertension and renal disease. The kidney is the chief regulator of sodium levels in body fluids.

Potassium (K): Important in protein synthesis, correction of imbalance in acid-base metabolism, and glycogen formation. It transmits nerve impulses and helps control them. It also promotes regular heartbeat and is needed for enzyme reactions.

Magnesium (Mg): Helps build strong bones and teeth and activates many enzymes. It helps regulate heartbeat and is essential for metabolism and many enzyme activities. It is stored in bone and is excreted mainly by the kidneys.

Trace Elements

Iodine (I): A component of the thyroid hormone thyroxine. Iodine is also used as a contrast medium for blood vessels in CT scans.

Zinc (Zn): Essential for several enzymes, growth, glucose tolerance, wound healing, and taste acuity. Best sources are protein foods.

Iron (Fe): A component of hemoglobin and myoglobin. The major role of iron is to deliver oxygen to the body tissues.

Ferrous sulfate (*Feosol*): The most inexpensive and most commonly used form of iron supplement.

Iron dextran (*Imferon*): An injectable form of iron supplement.

Hemochromatosis: Excessive absorption of iron.

Copper (Cu): An element most concentrated in the liver, heart, brain, and kidneys. It is essential for several important enzymes and for good health. It aids in the formation of hemoglobin. Copper helps in the transportation of iron to bone marrow.

Wilson's disease: A hereditary disease that causes copper accumulation in various organs and can result in degeneration of the brain, cirrhosis of the liver, psychic disturbances, and progressive weakness.

Fluoride: An element that increases resistance to tooth decay. It protects against osteoporosis and periodontal (gum) disease. Excessive amounts of fluoride in drinking water may cause the discoloration of teeth.

Nutrition and Diet Needs

Dietary guidelines: Developed by the U.S. Department of Agriculture and the U.S. Department of Health and Human Services, recommendations to encourage people to eat a balanced diet. Table 7-6 lists the guidelines.

Food pyramid: A diagram introduced by the U.S. Department of Agriculture to show the quantities of food people should consume daily from each of the basic food groups. See Figure 7-2. Also see Table 7-7, which provides information on serving sizes. Some patients may have special dietary preferences or choices. Vegetarians do not eat meat, poultry, and fish. In order to provide vegetarians with guidelines for healthful eating, the American Dietetic Association has developed a Food Guide Pyramid specifically for these individuals. See Figure 7-3.

Therapeutic nutrition: Also referred to as medical nutrition therapy or a therapeutic diet. It may be necessary in order to maintain or improve nutritional status; to correct nutritional deficiencies; to maintain, decrease, or increase body weight; or to eliminate particular foods that may cause allergies.

Nutrition during pregnancy: The protein requirement is increased by 20% for pregnant women. An increase is also recommended in calcium, iron, and folic acid intake. The average energy allowance during the first trimester is 2200 Kcal per day. Lactating women during the first 6 months need 2700 Kcal per day. Doctors recommend that pregnant women gain from 24 to 35 pounds during their pregnancy.

Breastfeeding: The mother's milk provides the infant with temporary immunity to many infectious diseases. It is free from germs and is easy to digest. It usually does not cause allergic reactions. Breastfeeding also stimulates an emotional bond between mother and infant. The American Academy of pediatrics recommends breastfeeding for at least 1 year, and the World Health Organization recommends 2 years. In most cases breastfeeding is the best source of milk for a growing child.

Mechanical soft diet: A diet that consists of soft but otherwise normal foods. It is used by individuals who have difficulty chewing because of a lack of dentures or teeth, inflammation of the oral cavity, or severe dental decay that may cause pain in chewing.

Liquid diet: A diet used by individuals who cannot tolerate solid foods or by patients whose gastrointestinal tract must be free of solid foods. The diet consists of tea, coffee, cream soups, fruit juices, clear broths, and eggnog.

Tube feeding: A diet used for patients with indications such as esophageal obstruction, burns, gastric surgery, or anorexia nervosa.

Bland diet: A diet that is nonirritating to the gastrointestinal tract. It is often prescribed in the treatment of peptic ulcer, ulcerative colitis, gallbladder disease,

AT A GLANCE	**Dietary Guidelines for Americans**
Eat a variety of foods to get the energy, protein, vitamins, minerals, and fiber you need for good health.	
Balance the food you eat with physical activity.	
Choose a diet with plenty of grain products, vegetables, and fruits.	
Choose a diet low in fat, saturated fat, and cholesterol.	
Choose a diet moderate in sugars.	
Choose a diet moderate in salt and sodium.	
If you drink alcoholic beverages, do so in moderation.	

Table 7-6

Anatomy of MyPyramid

One size doesn't fit all

USDA's new MyPyramid symbolizes a personalized approach to healthy eating and physical activity. The symbol has been designed to be simple. It has been developed to remind consumers to make healthy food choices and to be active every day. The different parts of the symbol are described below.

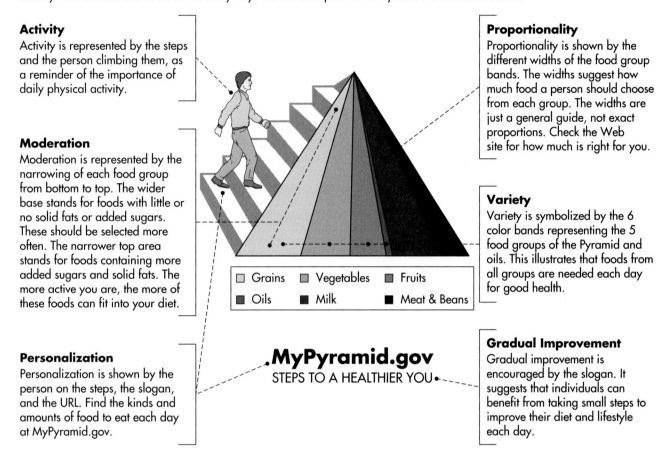

Activity
Activity is represented by the steps and the person climbing them, as a reminder of the importance of daily physical activity.

Moderation
Moderation is represented by the narrowing of each food group from bottom to top. The wider base stands for foods with little or no solid fats or added sugars. These should be selected more often. The narrower top area stands for foods containing more added sugars and solid fats. The more active you are, the more of these foods can fit into your diet.

Personalization
Personalization is shown by the person on the steps, the slogan, and the URL. Find the kinds and amounts of food to eat each day at MyPyramid.gov.

Proportionality
Proportionality is shown by the different widths of the food group bands. The widths suggest how much food a person should choose from each group. The widths are just a general guide, not exact proportions. Check the Web site for how much is right for you.

Variety
Variety is symbolized by the 6 color bands representing the 5 food groups of the Pyramid and oils. This illustrates that foods from all groups are needed each day for good health.

Gradual Improvement
Gradual improvement is encouraged by the slogan. It suggests that individuals can benefit from taking small steps to improve their diet and lifestyle each day.

- Grains
- Oils
- Vegetables
- Milk
- Fruits
- Meat & Beans

.MyPyramid.gov
STEPS TO A HEALTHIER YOU

Figure 7-2 *The U.S. Department of Agriculture's Food Guide MyPyramid can be used to plan a nutritious, well-balanced diet.*

diverticulitis, and gastritis. This diet consists of milk, cream, mashed potatoes, and hot cereal.

High-fiber diet: A diet may be prescribed for atonic constipation, diverticulosis, therapy of gastric ulcers, cancer of the colon, hypercholesterolemia, diabetes, or obesity.

Diabetic diet: A diet prescribed in the treatment of diabetes mellitus. It usually contains limited amounts of simple sugars and increased amounts of proteins, complex carbohydrates, and unsaturated fats. This diet is carefully calculated for each patient to minimize the occurrence of hyperglycemia and hypoglycemia, to maintain body weight, and to promote good health.

Dumping syndrome diet: A diet used for patients who have had a partial gastrectomy or gastric bypass surgery. This diet is low in concentrated sweets and limits fluids at mealtimes to avoid dumping the stomach contents into the small intestine, which results in diarrhea.

Restricted-fat diet: A diet used for patients with diseases of the liver, gallbladder, and pancreas. Generally

40 to 50 grams of fat per day is an adequate and realistic restriction.

Low-cholesterol diet: A diet often recommended for patients with elevated blood cholesterol levels, those with atherosclerosis, and those with elevated triglycerides and low HDL-cholesterol.

High-fat diet: A diet that may be indicated for purposes of weight gain. Ideally, the fat should be monounsaturated. The maximum fat intake is generally 35% to 40% of kilocalories.

Restricted-sodium diet: A diet that is very common for patients with hypertension, renal disease with edema, congestive heart failure, and cirrhosis of the liver with ascites.

Increased-sodium diet: A diet that may be useful in treating Addison's disease.

Restricted-potassium diet: A diet that may be necessary for patients with renal disease.

Increased-potassium diet: A diet used for patients who are on diuretics. Sources of potassium in the diet

MEDICAL ASSISTING COMPETENCIES (concl.)

COMPETENCY	CMA	RMA
General/Legal/Professional		
Be aware of and perform within legal and ethical boundaries	X	X
Determine the needs for documentation and reporting, and document accurately and appropriately	X	X
Demonstrate knowledge of and monitor current federal and state health-care legislation and regulations; maintain licenses and accreditation.	X	X
Follow established policy in initiating or terminating medical treatment		X
Perform risk management procedures		X
Be courtcous and diplomatic		X
Conduct work within scope of education, training, and ability		X
Be impartial and show empathy when dealing with patients		X
Use appropriate medical terminology		X
Receive, organize, prioritize, and transmit information appropriately		X
Unterstand allied health professions and credentialing		X

STRATEGIES TO SUCCESS

▶ Study Skills

Set goals!
   The CMA and RMA exams cover a lot of material, and it's not uncommon to feel stressed in trying to review it all. Try to make your workload easier by prioritizing and setting goals. Create a schedule to review material and set aside time to practice answering exam questions. If there is a certain topic you know you have difficulty with, make sure that you devote more time to review it and less time to something you know you already understand.

Law

Law: A body of regulations that govern society and that people are obligated to observe.

Sources of law: The U.S. Constitution divides the federal government into three equal branches: the Legislative Branch, which passes laws; the Executive Branch, which implements laws; and the Judicial Branch, which interprets laws.

Types of Law

Common law: Law that derives authority from ancient usages and customs affirmed by court judgments and decrees. It is created by the judicial branch through decisions in court cases.

Criminal law: Law dealing with criminal offenses and their punishments.

Private law: The legal rights defining the relationship between private entities.

Public law: The legal rights defining the relationship between the government and the governed.

Case law: Law established by judicial decision in legal cases and used as legal precedent.

The Legal System

Defendant: The person or group accused in a court action.

Plaintiff: A person who files a lawsuit initiating a civil legal action. In criminal actions, the prosecution is the plaintiff, acting on behalf of the people.

Litigant: A party to a lawsuit.

Litigation: A lawsuit or a contest in court.

Jurisdiction: The power, right, and authority given to a court to hear a case and to make a judgment.

Layperson: An individual who does not have training in a specific profession.

Violations of the Law

Crime: An act that violates a criminal law.

Criminal: A person who has committed a crime or who has been proven guilty of a crime.

Accessory: A person who contributes to or aids in the commission of a crime, either by a direct or an indirect act.

Felony: An offense punishable by death or by imprisonment in a state or federal prison. It is a serious crime, such as murder, kidnapping, assault, or rape. Punishment is usually severe: a prison sentence for more than 1 year or, in some cases, death.

Misdemeanor: A crime that is less serious than a felony and consequently carries a lesser penalty. It is punishable by fine or by imprisonment in a facility other than a prison for less than 1 year.

Tort: A civil wrong committed against a person or property, excluding a breach of contract. A tort is the most common civil claim in medical law. When one person intentionally harms another, the law allows the injured party to seek remedy in a civil suit. If the conduct is judged to be malicious, punitive damages may also be awarded.

Intentional torts: Assault, battery, defamation of character, false imprisonment, fraud, invasion of privacy, trespass, and infliction of emotional distress. Intentional torts may also be crimes. Therefore, some civil wrongs may also be prosecuted criminal acts in separate court actions.

Assault: A willful attempt or threat by a person to injure another person with the apparent ability to do so.

Defamation: Spoken or written words about a person that are both false and malicious and that injure that person's reputation or means of livelihood and for which damages can be recovered. Defamation can take the form of libel or slander.

Libel: Defamatory writing, such as published material or pictures.

Slander: Defamatory spoken words.

False imprisonment: The intentional, unlawful restraint or confinement of a person. Refusing to dismiss a patient from a health-care facility upon his or her request or preventing a patient from leaving the facility may be seen as false imprisonment.

Fraud: Dishonest and deceitful practices undertaken in order to induce someone to part with something of value or a legal right.

Invasion of privacy: Intrusion into a person's private affairs and public disclosure of private facts about a person, false publicity about a person, or use of a person's name or likeness without permission. Improper use of or breaching the confidentiality of medical records may be seen as an invasion of privacy.

Infliction of emotional distress: Intentionally or recklessly causing emotional or mental suffering to others.

Battery: The unlawful use of force on a person. Also, nonconsensual or illegal touching of another person.

Trespass: Wrongful injury or interference with the property of another.

Burglary: The act of breaking and entering into a building with intent to commit a felony, especially in order to steal. In a medical building, most burglary attempts are made to steal narcotics.

Misuse of legal procedure: Bringing legal action with malice and without probable cause.

Unintentional torts: The more common torts within the health-care delivery system. Unintentional torts are acts that are not intended to cause harm but are committed unreasonably or with a disregard for the consequences. In legal terms, this constitutes negligence. Negligence is charged when a health care practitioner fails to exercise ordinary care and a patient is injured as a result.

Tortfeasor: A person who commits a tort either intentionally or unintentionally.

The Court System

Court system: There are both federal and state court systems, and each system has two types of court: lower and higher, or inferior and superior. See Figure 8-1.

Supreme court: There are both state and federal supreme courts. A state supreme court is the highest state court. Its decisions are generally final in matters of state law. The federal Supreme Court is the final court of appeal, the highest court in the United States, sometimes also referred to as the court of last resort.

Appeal: A legal proceeding by which a case is transferred from a lower to a higher court for rehearing.

Motion: An application made to a court or judge to obtain an order, ruling, or direction.

Arbitration: The hearing and determination of a case in controversy, without litigation, by a person chosen by the parties involved or appointed under statutory authority.

Summons: An official paper issued by the clerk of the court and delivered with a copy of the complaint to the defendant, directing him or her to respond to the charges.

Subpoena: An official paper ordering a person to appear in court under penalty for failure to do so.

Subpoena *duces tecum*: A legal document requiring the recipient to bring certain records to court to be used as evidence in a lawsuit.

Witness: A person who can testify under oath to events he or she has heard or observed, such as the signing of a will or a consent form.

Testimony: Statements sworn to under oath by witnesses testifying in court and giving depositions.

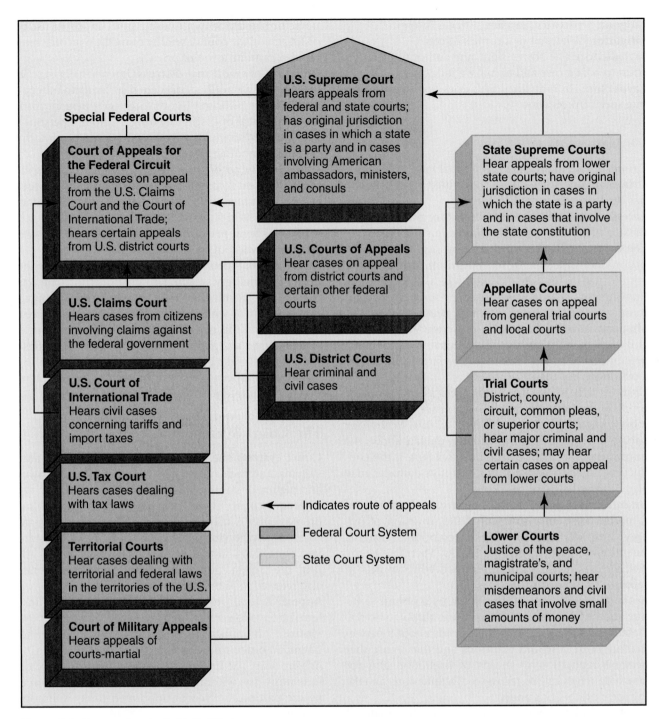

Figure 8-1 *Court systems in the United States.*

Deposition: Sworn pretrial testimony given by a witness in response to written or oral questions and cross-examination. It is made before a public officer for use in a lawsuit, and it may also be presented at the trial if the witness cannot be present.

Perjury: The voluntary violation of an oath to tell the truth; also, a false statement made under oath.

Interrogatory: Formal written questions about a case, addressed to one party by another, that are required to be answered under direction of a court.

Credibility: The quality or power of a witness to inspire belief.

Disposition: The final settlement of a case in criminal law.

Verdict: The finding or decision reached by a jury or judge on the matter submitted to trial.

Bench trial: A trial in which a judge serves without a jury and rules on the law as well as the facts.

Assumption of risk: A legal defense that holds that the defendant is not guilty of a negligent act because the plaintiff knew of and accepted beforehand any risk involved.

Burden of proof: The task of presenting testimony to prove guilt or innocence at a trial.

Plaintiff: The person bringing charges in a lawsuit.

Statute of limitations: The period of time established by state law during which a lawsuit may be filed.

The Law and Medicine

Confidentiality: The principle and practice of treating something as a private matter not intended for public knowledge. Confidentiality protects information so that it is not released to anyone unless such release is required by law. Confidentiality is important because it builds trust and maintains patient dignity. Care should also be taken that any information about a patient cannot be overheard by others. Tables 8-1 and 8-2 present principles for preventing the improper release of information.

Releasing medical records: A release permitted only when authorized in writing by the patient or the patient's legal guardian, when ordered by subpoena, or when dictated by statute to protect public health or welfare. The patient or guardian must sign a legal release form before records can be released to another physician or to an insurance company. The unauthorized disclosure of client information can be considered an invasion of privacy.

Maintaining patients' privacy: Keep these considerations in mind when handling sensitive information about patients:

- Do not leave confidential papers anywhere on the copier.
- Do not discard copies in shared trash containers. Always shred them.
- Always verify the telephone number of the receiving location before faxing confidential material.
- Never fax confidential material to an unauthorized person or in a room where others can observe the material. Use a fax cover sheet with a cautionary statement, "Confidential: To addressee only. Please return by mail if received in error."
- Do not leave a computer monitor unattended if confidential material is displayed on it.
- It is recommended that you not send confidential materials via e-mail.
- Do not print confidential material on a printer shared by other departments or in an area where others can see the printed output.
- Do not leave a printer unattended while printing confidential material.

Privilege: Authority granted to a physician by a hospital governing board to provide patient care in the hospital.

AT A GLANCE	Principles for Preventing Improper Release of Information from a Medical Office

It is the patient's right to keep information confidential. If the patient wants to disclose the information, it is unethical for the physician not to do so.
All patients should be treated with the same degree of confidentiality, whatever the health care professional's personal opinion of the patient might be.
Be aware of all applicable laws, including HIPAA, and of the regulations of agencies such as public health departments.
When it is necessary to break confidentiality, and when there is a conflict between ethics and confidentiality, discuss the matter with the patient. If the law does not dictate what to do in the situation, the attending physician should make the judgment based on the urgency of the situation and any danger that might be posed to the patient or others.
Legally required disclosures include those ordered by subpoena, those dictated by statute to protect public health or welfare, and those considered necessary to protect the welfare of a patient or third party.
Get written approval from the patient before releasing information. For common situations, the patient should sign a standard release of records form.

Table 8-1

of child abuse. In all states, teachers, physicians, and other licensed health-care practitioners are responsible for reporting such cases in person or by telephone and for following up with a written report within a specific time frame, such as 72 hours.

Elder abuse: The physical abuse, neglect, intimidation, or cruel punishment of an elderly individual as defined by the older Americans Act, which created the Administration on Aging and outlined 10 objectives aimed at preserving the rights and dignity of older citizens.

Amendments to the Older Americans Act: A law passed by Congress that defines elder abuse, neglect, and exploitation but that does not deal with enforcement. In 42 states, however, reporting suspected elder abuse is mandatory for physicians; such reporting is voluntary in the other 8 states.

Rape: A sexual assault involving intercourse without consent. Rape is a crime of violence, and the victims are treated for medical and psychological trauma. Rapes are criminal acts that should be reported to local law enforcement officials.

Drug Enforcement Administration (DEA): The agency responsible for enforcing the Comprehensive Drug Abuse Prevention and Control Act of 1970. Requirements for physicians include registration (renewed every 3 years), keeping of records (maintained for 2 years and specifying the patient, the drug, the dosage, the date, and reason for use), inventory (taken on the date of registration and every 2 years following), disposal of drugs (recorded in a log and witnessed), and proper security especially for controlled substances, all of which are major responsibilities of medical assistants.

Business Law

Contracts: Voluntary agreements between two or more parties in which specific promises are made for a consideration. There are three parts to any contract: the offer, the acceptance, and the consideration.

Offer: The beginning of contract process, when one party makes an offer to another. The offer must be communicated effectively and must be made in good faith and not under duress or as a joke. The offer must also be clear enough to be understood by both parties, and it must define what both parties will do if the offer is accepted.

Acceptance: Agreement to the terms of a contract a patient indicates acceptance of the physician's offer of practicing medicine by scheduling appointments, submitting to physical examinations, and allowing the physician to prescribe or perform medical treatment. Acceptance must be absolute and made according to the terms of the offer. If acceptance includes conditions or terms other than the ones made in the original offer, then acceptance actually constitutes a counteroffer for a different contract.

Consideration: Something of value that is bargained for as part of a contract. It is what each party agrees to provide for the other.

Breach of contract: Failure of a party to comply with the terms of a legally valid contract.

Void: Without legal force or effect.

Implied contract: An unwritten and unspoken agreement, the terms of which result from the actions of the parties involved.

Termination of contract: Generally takes place when all treatment has been completed and all bills have been fully paid.

Premature termination of contract: May occur as a result of failure to pay for services, missed appointments, failure to follow the physician's instructions, or obtaining the services of another physician. Figure 8-2 is a sample of a letter sent by a physician who is withdrawing from a case as a result of a patient's failure to follow medical advice.

Liable: Accountable under the law.

Bonding: Insurance against embezzlement for employees who handle financial matters in the medical office.

Licensure: The granting of permission by a competent authority to an individual or organization to engage in a practice or activity that would otherwise be illegal. Licensure is a mandatory credential process established by law. It is the strongest form of regulation. It gives legal permission, granted by state statutes, to perform specific acts.

Registration: The recording of professional qualification information relevant to government licensing regulations.

Certification: A voluntary credential process usually made by a nongovernmental agency. The purpose of certification is to ensure that the standards met are those necessary for safe and ethical practice of the profession.

Reciprocity: The policy under which a professional license obtained in one state may be accepted as valid in other states by prior agreement.

Telemedicine: Remote consultation by patients with physicians or other health professionals via telephone, the Internet, or closed-circuit television. Legal concerns over telemedicine involve matters such as state licenses, reimbursement, confidentiality, and informed consent.

Business structures: Legally, business structures include sole proprietorships, partnerships, and corporations.

Sole proprietorship: A type of medical practice management in which a physician practices alone and is responsible for all profits and liabilities of the business. It is the oldest form of business and is the easiest to start, operate, and dissolve. The advantages are simplicity of organization, being one's own boss, being the sole receiver of all profits, and having fewer government regulations to follow.

Partnership: A type of medical practice management involving the association of two or more individuals

LETTER OF WITHDRAWAL FROM CASE

Dear_____:

I find it necessary to inform you that I am withdrawing from further professional attendance upon you for the reason that you have persisted in refusing to follow my medical advice and treatment. Since your condition requires medical attention, I suggest that you place yourself under the care of another physician without delay. If you so desire, I shall be available to attend you for a reasonable time after you have received this letter, but in no event for more than five days.

This should give you ample time to select a physician of your choice from the many competent practitioners in this city. With your approval, I will make available to this physician your case history and information regarding the diagnosis and treatment which you have received from me.

Very truly yours,

_____ , MD

Figure 8-2 *Physicians are required to inform patients in writing if they wish to withdraw from a case.*
Source: Medicolegal Forms With Legal Analysis, American Medical Association, © 1991.

practicing together under a written agreement specifying the rights, obligations, and responsibilities of each partner. A partnership has more financial strength than a sole proprietorship, but its organization remains relatively simple. There is no limit to the number of partners. The partnership agreement should be written and reviewed by an attorney. A disadvantage of a partnership is that two or more people make the decisions. Each partner is responsible or liable for the business.

Corporation: A body formed by a group of people who are authorized by law to act as a single person. Corporations are governed by state law. There are income and tax advantages to incorporating.

Professional corporation: A corporation designed for professionals such as physicians, dentists, lawyers, and accountants.

Group practice: A medical management system in which a group of three or more licensed physicians share their collective income, expenses, facilities, equipment, records, and personnel. There are single-specialty, multispecialty, and primary care group practices.

Indemnity: A security against loss, hurt, or damage. Indemnity is a traditional form of health insurance that covers the insured against a potential loss of money from medical expenses for an illness or accident.

Managed care: A system in which the financing, administration, and delivery of health care are combined to provide medical services to subscribers for a prepaid fee.

Capitation: A payment method for health-care services in which a fixed amount of money is paid per month or other period to an HMO, medical group, or individual health provider for full medical care of subscribers. The contractual rates are usually adjusted for age, gender, illness, and regional differences.

Liability insurance: Contract coverage for potential damages incurred as a result of a negligent act. Doctors are often required to show proof of coverage up to a predetermined amount before hospitals will grant privileges or before managed care organizations will enter into a contractual agreement.

Workplace Legalities

Employment-at-will: A concept of employment whereby either the employer or the employee can terminate employment at any time and for any reason.

Wrongful discharge: A concept established by precedent whereby an employer risks litigation if he or she does not have just cause for firing an employee.

Legal protections: Laws against wrongful discharge that prevent employers from firing someone for refusing to commit an illegal act, whistleblowing, performing a legal duty, or exercising a private right.

Wagner Act of 1935: A statute that makes it illegal to discriminate in hiring or firing because of union membership or organizing activities.

Fair Labor Standards Act of 1938: A statute that prohibits child labor and the firing of employees for exercising their rights under the act's wage and hour standards. It also provides for overtime pay and a minimum wage.

Equal Pay Act of 1963: A statute that requires equal pay for men and women doing equal work.

Title VII of the Civil Rights Act of 1964: A statute that applies to businesses with 15 or more employees working at least 20 weeks of the year. The act prevents employers from discriminating in hiring or firing on the basis of race, color, religion, sex, or national origin. Some states have laws that also prohibit discrimination based on marital status, parenthood, mental health status, mental retardation, other disabilities, sexual orientation, personal appearance, or political affiliation.

Right-to-know laws: State laws that allow employees access to information about toxic or hazardous substances, employer duties, employee rights, and other workplace health and safety issues.

Documentation and Records Management

SOAP: An approach to documentation that provides an orderly series of steps for dealing with a medical case. SOAP lists (1) the patient's symptoms (*s*ubjective data), (2) the diagnosis (*o*bjective data), (3) an *a*ssessment, and (4) a *p*lan of action.

POMR or POR: A system of *p*roblem-*o*riented *m*edical *r*ecords based on client problems—conditions or behaviors that result in physical or emotional distress or interfere with functioning.

Ownership of medical records: Patients' medical records are considered the property of the owners of the facility where they were created. For example, a physician in private practice owns his or her records; records in a clinic are property of the clinic. These medical records should not be released unless the patient or legal guardian has signed legal release forms, a court has subpoenaed the records, an act or law mandates that the records be released to protect public welfare and safety, or the physician determines that the release is necessary to protect the patient or a third party.

Transferring medical records: Clients who request that their medical records be transferred to another physician should do so in writing. The original record may be retained in the office. No information should be released from the medical record without the approval of the physician and the written permission of the patient. If the client is incompetent, the court-appointed guardian signs the release form.

Children's medical records: The parent or legal guardian may sign the release forms. If the parents are legally separated or divorced, release forms must be signed by the parent who has legal custody.

HIPAA

Health Insurance Portability and Accountability Act (HIPAA): A law passed by the U.S. Congress in August, 1996, to create national guidelines for health privacy protection.

TITLE I, Health-Care Portability: The part of HIPAA that deals with protecting health-care coverage for employees who change jobs. Heath-Care Portability provides the following protection for employees and their families:

- Increases the ability to get health coverage when starting a new job
- Reduces the probability of losing existing health-care coverage
- Helps workers maintain continuous health-care coverage when changing jobs
- Helps workers purchase health insurance on their own if they lose coverage under an employer's group plan and have no other health coverage available

TITLE II, Preventing Health-Care Fraud and Abuse, Administrative Simplification, and Medical Liability Reform: Commonly known as the HIPAA Privacy Rule, the part of HIPAA that provides the first comprehensive federal protection for the privacy of health information. It is designed to provide strong, national privacy protections that do not interfere with patient access to health care or the quality of health-care delivery. The privacy rule is intended to:

- Give patients more control over their health information
- Set boundaries on the use and release of health-care records
- Establish appropriate safeguards that health-care providers and others must achieve to protect the privacy of health information
- Hold violators accountable, with civil and criminal penalties that can be imposed if they violate patients' privacy rights
- Strike a balance when public responsibility supports disclosure of some forms of data (for example, to protect public health)

Individually identifiable health information: An individual's personal information that is gathered in the process of providing health care. Individually identifiable health information includes:

- Name
- Address
- Phone numbers
- Fax number
- Dates (birth, death, admission, discharge, etc.)
- Social Security number
- E-mail address
- Medical record numbers
- Health plan beneficiary numbers

- Account numbers
- Certificate or license numbers
- Vehicle identifiers and serial numbers, including license plate numbers
- Device identifiers and serial numbers
- Web universal resource locators (URLs)
- Internet protocol (IP) address numbers

Protected health information (PHI): Individually identifiable health information that is transmitted or maintained by electronic or other media, such as computer storage devices. This information is protected by the HIPAA Privacy Rule.

Use: As defined by HIPAA, the act of doing any of the following to individually identifiable health information by employees or other members of an organization's workforce:

- Sharing
- Employing
- Applying
- Utilizing
- Examining
- Analyzing

Disclosure: As defined by HIPAA, the act of doing any of the following by the party holding the information so that the information is outside that party:

- Release
- Transfer
- Providing access to
- Divulging in any manner

Treatment, payment, and operations (TPO): The uses that HIPAA authorizes for sharing patient information:

- Treatment—Providers are allowed to share information in order to provide care to patients.
- Payment—Providers are allowed to share information in order to receive payment for the treatment provided.
- Operations—Providers are allowed to share information to conduct normal business activities, such as quality improvement.

Notice of Privacy Practices (NPP): A document given to patients by health-care providers that informs patients of their rights as outlined by HIPAA.

HIPAA Security Rule: The technical safeguards that protect the confidentiality, integrity, and availability of health information covered by HIPAA. The Security Rule specifies how patient information is protected on computer networks, the Internet, disks, and other storage media. See chapter 16.

Ethics

Ethics: The study of values or principles governing personal relationships, including ideals of autonomy, justice, and conduct. The code of ethics for the profession of medical assisting is reproduced in Table 8-4.

Bioethics: A discipline dealing with the ethical and moral implications of biological research and applications, especially as they relate to life and death.

Moral: Conforming to a standard of right behavior or a rule of conduct based on standards of right and wrong. Moral beliefs are usually formed through the influence of family, culture, and society, and they serve as a guide for personal ethical conduct.

Philosophy: A basic viewpoint or system of values, general beliefs, concepts, and attitudes.

Etiquette: Standards of behavior considered appropriate within a profession. Etiquette describes a body of courtesies and manners to be observed in social situations.

Beneficence: Active goodness or kindness.

Nonmaleficence: Abstinence from committing any harm. As human beings, we have an obligation not to harm others.

Duty to improve oneself: As a medical assistant you should always continue your education, learn new competencies and skills, learn from your own mistakes, learn from others you work with, and strive to be a good role model.

Genetics

Genetic: Pertaining to reproduction, birth, or origin or to being produced by genes or attributable to them.

Genetic diseases: Diseases linked to genetic defects. There are as many as 4,000 human genetic diseases. Approximately 500 of them are linked to a defect in a single gene.

Genetic screening: A test for genetic problems that requires a DNA sample from solid tissues, saliva, or blood. Genetic testing is appropriate for prospective parents whose genetic histories indicate an elevated risk for genetic disorders. When a genetic defect is found in the fetus, parents may have to make an ethical decision to request or refuse an abortion. Other ethical concerns include genetic testing by employers and the release of genetic information to insurance companies.

Genetic engineering: Gene splitting, recombinant DNA research, chemical synthesis of DNA, and other technology. It involves numerous ethical issues and requires following stringent ethical guidelines.

Gene therapy: The insertion of a normally functioning gene into cells in which an abnormal or absent element of the gene has caused disease. The goal of gene therapy is to alleviate suffering and disease, not to enhance desirable characteristics or to diminish undesirable characteristics not related to disease.

The Code of Ethics of the AAMA shall set forth principles of ethical and moral conduct as they relate to the medical profession and the particular practice of medical assisting.

Members of the AAMA dedicated to the conscientious pursuit of their profession, and thus desiring to merit the high regard of the entire medical profession and the respect of the general public which they serve, do pledge themselves to strive always to:

A. render service with full respect for the dignity of humanity;

B. respect confidential information obtained through employment unless legally authorized or required by responsible performance of duty to divulge such information;

C. uphold the honor and high principles of the profession and accept its disciplines;

D. seek to continually improve the knowledge and skills of medical assistants for the benefit of patients and professional colleagues;

E. participate in additional service activities aimed toward improving the health and well-being of the community.

Table 8-4
Source: American Association of Medical Assistants.

Cloning: A procedure for producing multiple copies of genetically identical organisms or individual genes.
Eugenics: The study of hereditary improvement achieved by controlling the characteristics of genes.

Pregnancy and Termination of Pregnancy

Artificial insemination: The mechanical injection of viable semen into the vagina. If the donor and the recipient are not married, the recipient will be considered the sole parent of the child except in cases in which both the donor and the recipient agree to recognize a paternity right. Selecting sperm to manipulate the gender of a resulting child is ethical only to avoid a sex-linked inheritable disease.
In vitro fertilization (IVF): Fertilization that takes place outside a woman's body, usually in a test tube. Because of ethical concerns, fertilized human eggs should not be subjected to laboratory research.
Gestation: The length of time after conception during which developing offspring are carried in the uterus. In humans, the duration is approximately 280 days, or 40 weeks. Live birth with a gestation time of less than 37 weeks is considered premature. Beyond 42 weeks, the fetus is considered postmature.
Amniocentesis: An obstetric procedure in which a small amount of amniotic fluid is aspirated for the purpose of analyzing whether a fetus is developing normally.
Amniotomy: The artificial rupture of the fetal membranes. It is performed to stimulate or accelerate the onset of labor. The procedure is painless.

Anencephaly: A congenital deformity in newborns characterized by absence of the brain and spinal cord.
Stillbirth: The death of a fetus before or during delivery. It is known as fetal death if the weight of the fetus is more than 1000g. Stillbirths may require neither birth nor death certificates.
Abortion: The voluntary termination of pregnancy before gestation is complete and, in most cases, before the fetus is viable. Methods include uterine aspiration, dilation and curettage, saline injection, and cesarean section. Its legality as a medical procedure was affirmed by the U.S. Supreme Court in a 1973 case known as *Roe v. Wade* and in several subsequent cases. People's opinions on the controversial subject are based on their own personal ethical and moral values as well as on the law.
Stem cell: Early embryonic cells that have the potential to become any type of body cell. The debate on the therapeutic use of stem cells remains intense because stem cells have shown promise for treating patients with a wide variety of medical problems.

Organ and Tissue Donation and Transplantation

Uniform Anatomical Gift Act: A law adopted by all states. Its provisions are that (1) any person over 18 years may give all or any part of his or her body after death for research, transplantation, or placement in a tissue bank; (2) physicians who accept organs or tissue, relying in good faith on the documents, are protected from lawsuits; and (3) the time of death must be determined by a physician. A uniform donor card is shown in Figure 8-3.

UNIFORM DONOR CARD

Of _____
Print or type name of donor

in the hope that I may help others, I hereby make this anatomical gift, if medically acceptable, to take effect upon my death. The words and marks below indicate my desires.

I give: (a) ☐ any needed organs or parts
        (b) ☐ only the following organs or parts

_____
Specify the organ(s) or part(s)

for the purposes of transplantation, therapy, medical research or education:
        (c) ☐ my body for anatomical study if needed.
Limitations or special wishes, if any: _____

Front of card

Signed by the donor and the following two witnesses in the presence of each other:

Signature of Donor _____
Date of Birth of Donor _____
Date Signed _____
City and State _____
Witness _____
Witness _____

THIS IS A LEGAL DOCUMENT UNDER THE UNIFORM ANATOMICAL GIFT ACT OR SIMILAR LAWS.

Back of card

Figure 8-3 *A sample uniform donor card.*

Transplant: The transfer of an organ or tissue from one person to another or from one part of the body to another. Medical transplants are divided into four categories, depending on the source of the tissue used: autograft, heterograft, homograft, and isograft.

Autograft: Surgical transplantation of a person's own tissue from one part of the body to another location. Autografts are used in several kinds of plastic surgery, most commonly to replace skin lost in severe burns. The term can also be applied to transplants between identical twins.

Heterograft: The transplant of animal tissue into a human. It is also called a xenograft.

Homograft: The nonpermanent transplant of tissue from one body to another (in the same species), such as a tissue transplant between two humans who are not identical twins. It is also called an allograft.

Isograft: Surgical transplantation from genetically identical individuals, such as identical twins.

Death and Dying

Patient Self-Determination Act: A federal law that requires health-care providers to provide written information to patients about their rights under state law to make medical decisions and to execute advance directives. It requires that medical care facilities ask patients whether they have prepared an advance directive for guidance in the event that they are terminally ill.

Advance directives: Documents that make wishes known in the event that individuals are unable to speak for themselves. Examples are living wills, durable powers of attorney, and health-care proxies.

Living will: A document in which an individual expresses his or her wishes regarding medical treatment. It may detail circumstances under which treatment should be discontinued, which treatments to suspend, and which to maintain. A living will is legal only if the person is competent to create such a document and if two witnesses have attested to its accuracy by signing it. Figure 8-4 is a sample living will.

If the time comes when I am incapacitated to the point when I can no longer actively take part in decisions for my own life, and am unable to direct my physician as to my own medical care, I wish this statement to stand as a testament of my wishes. I _____ (name) request that I be allowed to die and not be kept alive through life-support systems if my condition is deemed terminal. I do not intend any direct taking of my life, but only that my dying not be unreasonably prolonged. This request is made, after careful reflection, while I am of sound mind.

_____
(Signature)

_____
(Date)

_____
(Witness)

_____
(Witness)

Figure 8-4 *A sample living will.*

I, _____ , designate and appoint:

Name: _____

Address: _____

Telephone Number: _____

to be my agent for health care decisions and pursuant to the language stated below, on my behalf to:

(1) consent, refuse consent, or withdraw consent to any care, treatment, service or procedure to maintain, diagnose or treat a physical or mental condition, and to make decisions about organ donation, autopsy and disposition of the body;

(2) make all necessary arrangements at any hospital, psychiatric hospital or psychiatric treatment facility, hospice, nursing home or similar institution to employ or discharge health-care personnel to include physicians, psychiatrists, psychologists, dentists, nurses, therapists or any other person who is licensed, certified or otherwise authorized or permitted by the laws of this state to administer health care as the agent shall deem necessary for my physical, mental and emotional well-being; and

(3) request, receive and review any information, verbal or written, regarding my personal affairs or physical or mental health, including medical and hospital records, and to execute any releases of other documents that may be required in order to obtain such information.

In exercising the grant of authority set forth above my agent for health-care decisions shall:

_____

The powers of the agent herein shall be limited to the extent set out in writing in this durable power of attorney for health-care decisions, and shall not include the power to revoke or invalidate any previously existing declaration made in accordance with the natural death act.

The agent shall be prohibited from authorizing consent for the following items:

_____

The durable power of attorney for health-care decisions shall be subject to these additional limitations:

_____

This power of attorney for health-care decisions shall become effective immediately and shall not be affected by my subsequent disability or incapacity or upon the occurrence of my disability or incapacity.

Any durable power of attorney for health-care decisions I have previously made is hereby revoked. This durable power of attorney for health-care decisions shall be revoked in writing, executed, and witnessed or acknowledged in the same manner as required herein.

Executed this _____ , at _____

_____
(Signature of principal)

State _____ County _____ S.S. No. _____

This instrument was acknowledged before me _____ (date) by _____ (name)

_____
(Signature of notary public)

Figure 8-5 *A sample health care proxy.*

be considered inactive, whereas in others the amount of time may be 2 or 3 years.

Closed files: Files of patients who have died or moved away.

Transfer: Removing inactive records from the active files.

Retention period: The amount of time to keep different types of patient records in the office after files have become inactive or closed. Some legal requirements for retaining certain types of information are listed in Table 9-7.

Identical names: When filing identical names, use date of birth, patient identification number, or some other form of identification in order to distinguish between the two patients.

Business and organization records: File business and organization records according to subject and topic.

Filing Equipment

File shelves: An advantage of keeping files on shelves is that it allows several people to retrieve and return files at one time.

File cabinets: Three types of file cabinets are used in the medical office: vertical, lateral, and movable.

Vertical file cabinets: Have from two to five drawers. They are the least efficient type of cabinet because half of the filing time goes into opening and closing drawers. Also, bending, squatting, and stretching to reach files makes these cabinets that much more inefficient.

Open-shelf file cabinets: Take up 50% less space, permit quick access, and have no drawers to open or close. They have the disadvantage of collecting dust.

Movable file units: Allow easy access to large record systems and require less space than vertical or lateral files.

Supplies: Supplies needed for file cabinets are:

File folders designed for the type of cabinet in use.

Identification labels, affixed either along the top of the file folder or along the side of the file folder in open-shelf file cabinets.

Guides and captions: Guides are used to separate the file folders. Captions are used to identify major sections of file folders by more manageable sub-units.

Out guide: A cardboard or plastic sheet kept in place of the patient's chart when the chart is removed from filing storage.

Policies and Procedures

Policy and procedures manual: A written document that covers all office policies and clinical procedures, developed by the physicians and the staff (particularly the medical assistant) for use by permanent and temporary employees.

Policies: Rules or guidelines that dictate the day-to-day workings of an office. Most manuals cover the following policy areas:

- Office purposes, objectives, and goals
- Rules and regulations
- Job descriptions and duties
- Office hours
- Dress code
- Insurance and other benefits
- Vacation, sick leave, and other time away from the office
- Performance evaluations and salary
- Maintenance of equipment and supplies
- Mailings
- Bookkeeping
- Scheduling appointments
- Maintaining patient records
- Health and safety guidelines
- Organizational chart

Procedures: Detailed instructions for maintaining clinical and quality assurance.

Developing a manual: Begins with planning the format and outline, which should be approved by the office manager and physicians. Sources for developing and updating material include journals, product literature, textbooks, and standards publications, among others.

Manual format: Many offices prefer a loose-leaf binder in which pages can be replaced when necessary. Figure 9-13 shows a sample manual page.

STRATEGIES TO SUCCESS

▶ *Test-Taking Skills*

Eliminate wrong answers!
    When answering multiple-choice questions, you can increase your chances of answering correctly by eliminating answers that you know are wrong. As you read the possible answers, put an *X* next to ones you know are incorrect, or cross them out completely. Once you have narrowed down your possible choices, you have a better chance of making an educated guess about the correct answer.

MILLSTONE MEDICAL ASSOCIATES

Policy and Procedures Manual

Procedure for Creating a Medical File for a New Patient

GOAL: To create a complete medical record for each new patient containing all necessary personal and medical information.

PROCEDURE:

1. Establish that the patient is new to the doctor's office.

2. Ask the patient for all necessary insurance information. If the patient has an insurance card, make a photocopy of it for his or her file.

3. Ask the patient to fill out the patient information form. Keyboard the information onto a new patient information form, for legibility.

4. Review all information with the patient, to check for accuracy.

5. Label the new patient's folder according to office procedure. Type either the patient's name (for an alphabetical file) or the correct number (for a numerical file).

6. If filing is done numerically, fill out a cross-reference form on the computer, along with a patient ID card to be stored in a secure location.

7. Add the patient's name to the necessary financial records, including the office ledger, whether on paper or on the computer.

8. After completing the folder label information, place the new patient information form inside the folder, along with any other personal or medical information that pertains to the patient.

9. On the outside of patient's folder, clip a routing slip.

Figure 9-13 *This page from a policy and procedures manual provides the office staff with information about creating a medical file for a new patient.*

Instructions:

Answer the following questions. Check your answers in the *Answer Key* that follows this section.

1. Which of the following is the most widely used filing system for medical practices?
   A. Numeric
   B. Subject
   C. Alphabetical
   D. Chronological
   E. Alphanumeric

2. In appointment scheduling, the matrix indicates
   A. Time available to schedule patients
   B. Time not available to schedule patients
   C. Time open for pharmaceutical representatives
   D. Time open for surgery
   E. Time not available for surgery

3. Financial information
   A. Should always be included in the patient's medical records
   B. Should be included in the patient's medical record if the patient has been delinquent in payments
   C. Should not be included in the patient's medical records
   D. Should be included in the patient's medical record if the patient requests it
   E. Should be included in the patient's medical record if the patient's insurance provider requires it

4. Which of the following terms means the act of articulating and speaking clearly?
   A. Communication
   B. Conversation
   C. Telecommunication
   D. Pronunciation
   E. Enunciation

5. A chronological file used as a reminder is called a(n)
   A. Index file
   B. Tickler file
   C. Active file
   D. Closed file
   E. Timer file

6. The screening and sorting of emergency situations is called
   A. Emergency reception
   B. Documenting emergencies
   C. Telephone emergencies
   D. Incoming emergencies
   E. Emergency triage

7. Scheduling patients so that two come in at the beginning of each hour and the others are scheduled every 10 to 20 minutes is called
   A. Wave scheduling
   B. Appointment time pattern
   C. Modified wave scheduling
   D. Double booking
   E. Advance scheduling

8. Account statements for a medical practice should be sent as
   A. First-Class Mail
   B. Standard Mail (A)
   C. Standard Mail (B)
   D. Special Standard Mail
   E. Express Mail

9. Patients who want to talk about abnormal test results should speak with which of the following medical personnel?
   A. Laboratory technologists
   B. Nurses
   C. Medical assistants
   D. Physicians
   E. Any of the above

10. Which of the following is the most secure service offered by the U.S. Postal Service?
    A. Priority Mail
    B. First-Class Mail
    C. Express Mail
    D. Mail tracing
    E. Registered mail

11. If a patient calls about insurance coverage, the call should be handled by
    A. The physician who performed the test or procedure in question
    B. The medical assistant
    C. The next available physician
    D. The insurance company
    E. An insurance specialist only

12. Which of the following should be included in the patient's medical records?
    A. Physical examination results
    B. Correspondence with and about the patient
    C. Diagnosis and treatment plans
    D. Informed consent forms
    E. All of the above

13. Office policy manuals contain which of the following types of information?
    A. Employee titles
    B. Employee salaries
    C. Employee insurance contributions
    D. Employee health records
    E. Regulations for personal appearance

14. SOAP pertains to
    A. Malpractice
    B. Computer code
    C. Dictation equipment
    D. Asepsis
    E. Patient records

15. According to the Internal Revenue Service, financial records need to be retained for how long?
    A. 2 to 7 years
    B. 10 years
    C. 7 years
    D. 15 years
    E. Permanently

16. According to U.S. Postal Service guidelines, which of the following is the correct state abbreviation for an envelope addressed to Key West?
    A. MS
    B. MA
    C. MT
    D. FL
    E. TX

17. It is important to leave time to complete forms for patients who are
    A. Late for their appointments
    B. New
    C. Poor
    D. Rich
    E. Minors

18. Which one of these is a correct complimentary closing?
    A. Yours Truly,
    B. Very Best,
    C. Best regards,
    D. Yours Sincerely,
    E. Sincerely:

19. Which of the following mail is available 7 days per week?
    A. Priority Mail
    B. First-Class Mail
    C. International mail
    D. Express Mail
    E. Standard Mail (A)

20. When an incoming call is received, the telephone should be answered

    A. Within 1 minute
    B. By the second or third ring
    C. By the third or fourth ring
    D. When there is no patient nearby
    E. After the doctor has been helped

21. If the patient calls in to report that he or she is doing well after surgery, the medical assistant should

    A. Transfer the call to the physician or surgeon
    B. Transfer the call to the attending nurse
    C. Handle the call and make note of the patient's report in his or her medical records
    D. Thank the patient for calling and hang up
    E. Explain to the patient that he or she needs to call only if things are not going well

22. An appointment book is considered

    A. An interpersonal skill
    B. A patient analysis
    C. The doctor's domain
    D. A scheduling system
    E. A legal document

23. The physician should handle calls from patients about which of the following?

    A. Insurance questions
    B. X-ray and laboratory reports
    C. Unsatisfactory progress
    D. Prescription refills previously authorized
    E. Scheduling appointments

24. The words *SPECIAL HANDLING* should appear where on an envelope?

    A. Above the *Attention* line
    B. Above the recipient's address
    C. Below the return address
    D. Below the recipient's address
    E. Below the postage

25. Which of the following is an introductory form that provides demographic data about patients?

    A. Physical examination form
    B. Patient referral form
    C. Patient encounter form
    D. Patient information form
    E. Patient health questionnaire

26. The receptionist who is responsible for opening the medical office must arrive how long before office hours begin?

    A. 45 to 60 minutes
    B. 30 to 45 minutes
    C. 15 to 20 minutes
    D. 5 to 10 minutes
    E. More than 60 minutes

27. What action should a medical assistant take if a caller wants to talk to a physician but refuses to identify himself or herself?

    A. Hang up
    B. Transfer the call to the physician anyway
    C. Advise the person that the physician is not in the office and tell him or her to call back
    D. Ask the person to write a letter to the physician and mark it *Personal*
    E. Transfer the call to another medical assistant

28. Certified mail is used to send

    A. All office mailings
    B. Hazardous materials
    C. Documents, contracts, and bank books
    D. Appointment reminders
    E. Results of medical tests

29. A medical assistant should do all of the following when answering the telephone <u>except</u>
    A. Give the caller the medical assistant's name first and then the name of the office
    B. Identify the caller
    C. Ask "How may I help you?"
    D. Hold the phone's mouthpiece an inch away from the mouth
    E. Use words appropriate to the situation, but avoid using technical terms

30. Which of the following is the most effective way to educate new patients about office policies?
    A. Distribute patient information booklets
    B. Distribute office procedure manuals
    C. Distribute videotapes
    D. Distribute newsletters
    E. Make an appointment for formal patient orientation sessions

31. Through the U.S. Postal Service, a package of books that weighs 90 pounds
    A. Can be sent as Standard Mail (B)
    B. Can be sent as Priority Mail
    C. Cannot be sent because it exceeds weight limits
    D. Can be sent as Express Mail
    E. Can be sent Standard Mail (A)

32. Medical assistants should take all of these actions when opening mail <u>except</u>?
    A. Annotate mail with comments in the margin
    B. Open the physician's personal mail
    C. Date all opened mail
    D. Transmit letters to the physician with the most important ones on the top
    E. Check for enclosures

33. Standard letterhead is
    A. Used in general business correspondence
    B. $5\frac{1}{2}$ inches $\times$ $8\frac{1}{2}$ inches in size
    C. Used for social correspondence
    D. Not used in the medical office
    E. Both B and C

34. The subject line of a letter appears
    A. Two lines below the last line of the body
    B. Two lines below the salutation
    C. One line above the outside address
    D. One line above the inside address
    E. One line below the date

35. In the matrix scheduling system, medical assistants should block off
    A. Physicians' lunch hours
    B. Visits with drug company representatives
    C. Time for performing hospital rounds
    D. Both B and C
    E. All of the above

36. The abbreviation *NP* stands for
    A. Neurological performance
    B. No–show patient
    C. New practice
    D. New physical
    E. New patient

37. Scheduling two or more patients in the same slot is known as
    A. Wave scheduling
    B. Open hours
    C. Modified wave scheduling
    D. Double booking
    E. Either A or C

38. Which of the following is a type of tickler file?

    A. Numerical
    B. Subject
    C. Alphabetical
    D. Geographical
    E. Chronological

39. When dealing with a seriously ill patient, you should

    A. Trivialize the patient's feelings
    B. Judge the patient's statements
    C. Avoid empty promises
    D. Abandon the patient
    E. Isolate the patient

40. Publications and journals are usually sent as

    A. First-Class Mail
    B. Periodicals
    C. Standard Mail (A)
    D. Standard Mail (B)
    E. Priority Mail

41. The proofreaders' mark # represents which of the following?

    A. Delete
    B. Spell out
    C. Transpose
    D. Add a space
    E. Align this line

42. A scheduling method in which patients sign in and are seen on a first-come first-served basis is known as which of the following?

    A. Double booking
    B. Open booking
    C. Stream
    D. Wave
    E. Clustering

ANSWER KEY

1.	B	22.	E
2.	B	23.	C
3.	C	24.	E
4.	E	25.	D
5.	B	26.	C
6.	E	27.	D
7.	C	28.	C
8.	A	29.	A
9.	D	30.	A
10.	E	31.	C
11.	B	32.	B
12.	E	33.	A
13.	E	34.	B
14.	E	35.	E
15.	B	36.	E
16.	D	37.	D
17.	B	38.	B
18.	C	39.	C
19.	D	40.	B
20.	B	41.	D
21.	C	42.	B

CHAPTER 10

Communication in the Medical Office

MEDICAL ASSISTING COMPETENCIES

COMPETENCY	CMA	RMA
General/Legal/Professional		
Respond to and initiate written communications by using correct grammar, spelling, and formatting techniques	X	X
Recognize and respond to verbal and nonverbal communications by being attentive and adapting communication to the recipient's level of understanding	X	X
Demonstrate proper telephone techniques	X	X
Identify and respond to issues of confidentiality by maintaining confidentiality at all times and following appropriate guidelines when releasing records or information	X	X
Explain general office policies and procedures	X	X
Instruct individuals according to their needs	X	X
Project a positive attitude		X
Be a "team player"		X
Adapt to change		X
Evidence a responsible attitude		X
Be courteous and diplomatic		X
Be impartial and show empathy when dealing with patients		X
Serve as a liaison between the physician and others		X
Interview effectively		X
Use appropriate medical terminology		X
Receive, organize, prioritize, and transmit information appropriately		X

STRATEGIES TO SUCCESS

▶ *Study Skills*

Study the things you don't know, not what you do know. As you test yourself, you will find areas that you know very well and those with which you are not as comfortable. Even though it feels good to study those things you know, you should put those subjects aside and spend time with the material you do not know as well. If you study with note cards, make two piles, an "I know that" pile and an "I don't know that" pile. Soon your "I know that" pile will grow larger than your "I don't know that" pile.

Communicating with Patients and Families

Medical assistants play an important role in communicating with patients, their families, and the medical office staff. Your unique communication style is formed by the way in which you attend to individual patient needs, answer questions, explain procedures, and even greet patients. The way that you interact with patients significantly influences how comfortable they feel with being in your medical office, as well as setting the overall tone for their visit.

The 5 Cs of communication:

- Completeness—The message must contain all necessary information.
- Clarity—The message must be free from obscurity and ambiguity.
- Conciseness—The message must not include any unnecessary information.
- Courtesy—The message must be respectful and considerate of others.
- Cohesiveness—The message must be organized and logical.

Developing Good Communication Skills

Attitude: Your confidence and self-esteem can positively affect your success in the medical field. The way you represent yourself is the way others will see you. Communicating a positive attitude begins by doing the following:

- Smiling instead of frowning
- Saying something pleasant instead of complaining
- Using positive statements instead of negative statements

The Communication Cycle

The communication cycle consists of giving and receiving information. As you interact with patients and their families, you will be responsible for giving information and ensuring that the patient understands what you, the physician, and other members of the staff have communicated. You will also be responsible for receiving information from the patient.

Elements of the Communication Cycle

The communication cycle is formed as the sender, or source, sends the message to the receiver and the receiver responds with feedback. The message may be

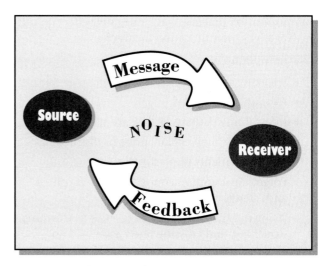

Figure 10-1 *The process of communication involves an exchange of messages through verbal and nonverbal means.*

verbal or nonverbal. This circle of communication may also include noise, which is anything that distorts the message in any way or interferes with the communication process. Noise includes sounds, such as a siren or alarm, and can also include physical discomfort (for example, pain) or personal worries or concerns that may interfere with what is being communicated. Figure 10-1 illustrates the communication cycle.

Types of Communication

Communication can be verbal, nonverbal, or written. It can also be positive or negative.

Positive Communication

Positive communication: Promotes patients' comfort and well-being. Positive communication is essential in the medical office. Some examples of positive communication include:

- Being friendly, warm, and attentive
- Verbalizing your concern for patients
- Encouraging patients to ask questions
- Asking patients to repeat your instructions in order to make sure they understand
- Looking directly at patients when you speak to them
- Smiling naturally
- Speaking slowly and clearly
- Listening carefully

Negative Communication

Negative communication: Most people do not intend to communicate negatively; however, some communication practices have a negative effect on others. Negative communication includes:

- Mumbling
- Speaking sharply or too intensely
- Avoiding eye contact
- Interrupting patients as they are speaking
- Rushing through explanations or instructions
- Treating patients impersonally
- Forgetting common courtesies such as "please" and "thank you"
- Using negative body language, such as frowning, slouching, and crossing one's arms
- Showing boredom

Nonverbal Communication

Body language: Nonverbal communication is also known as body language. In many cases, body language conveys a person's true feelings when words may not. Be aware of your body language, and note the body language of others. Examples of nonverbal communication include the following:

- Facial expressions—These should be nonjudgmental and correspond to your words.
- Hand gestures—This type of body language can emphasize your words.
- Eye contact—Establishing eye contact with others shows interest, attention, and sensitivity.
- Nodding—This gesture acknowledges information and encourages the patient to continue speaking.
- Posture—Turning and leaning your body toward a person helps to communicate your interest in what he or she is saying.
- Attention to personal space—This aspect shows respect for the person's privacy and comfort.
- Touch—This type of body language can communicate sensitivity and empathy. In general, a touch on the shoulder, back, or hand is acceptable. However, not everyone is comfortable being touched. Be aware of cultural and personal differences and adjust your style to the preferences of others.

Improving Your Communication Skills

Listening Skills

Listening is the act of receiving a message. Three different listening patterns are used in a medical office: active, passive, and evaluative.

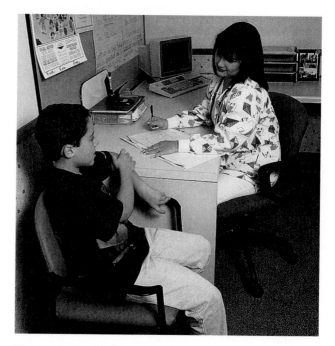

Figure 10-2 *Active listening requires two-way communication and positive body language.*

Active listening: Requires two-way communication, positive body language, asking questions, and offering feedback. See Figure 10-2.
Passive listening: Involves listening without answering and offering feedback.
Evaluative listening: Provides an immediate response and opinion. It is very important to listen to everything a patient says; avoid "selective hearing."

Interpersonal Skills

Interpersonal skills are used when you interact with people. You demonstrate good interpersonal skills when you make a patient feel at ease with your warmth and friendliness. Other valuable interpersonal skills include the following:

- Empathy
- Respect
- Genuineness
- Openness
- Consideration and sensitivity

Therapeutic Communication Skills

Patients in the medical office will come from a variety of backgrounds and will have their own perceptions of the medical office and its staff. It is important to be able to interact with all patients, addressing each of their individual needs and circumstances. Therapeutic communication is the ability to communicate in terms that patients can understand while making them feel at ease and comfortable with what is being said. Therapeutic communication is also the ability to communicate with other health-care professionals by using technical terms appropriate in the health-care setting.

Silence: Periods in which there is no verbal communication. Silence can allow the patient to think without pressure to speak.

Restating: Repeating to a patient what you believe is the main thought or idea expressed. It helps to paraphrase ideas rather than just repeat statements verbatim. In this way you can make sure that you understand what is being communicated.

Reflecting: Encouraging patients to think through and answer their own questions and concerns.

Open-ended questions: General questions that allow patients to elaborate on their answers, providing as much information as they wish to. Open-ended questions lead to better communication.

Focusing: Helping the patient stay on a particular topic with directing questions and statements.

Rapport: Involves a positive and harmonious relationship between a patient and a medical assistant, or between patients and other members of the medical staff. You can build rapport with good communication skills.

Ineffective Therapeutic Communication

Ineffective therapeutic communication includes roadblocks that can interfere with your communication style:

Reassuring: Indicates to the patient that there is no need for anxiety or worry. By doing this, you devalue the patient's feelings and give false hope if the outcome is not positive.

Giving approval: Usually done by overtly approving of a patient's behavior. Giving approval may lead the patient to strive for praise rather than progress.

Disapproving: Done by overtly disapproving of the patient's behavior. This may cause a patient to discontinue communication.

Agreeing/disagreeing: Either one of these is an ineffective way to communicate with patients. When you agree with patients, they will have the perception that they are right because you agree with them. Conversely, when you disagree with patients, you become the opposition to them instead of their caregiver.

Advising: Telling the patient what you think should be done places you outside your scope of practice. You cannot advise patients.

Probing: Discussing a topic that the patient has no desire to discuss.

Defending: Protecting yourself, the medical office, and others from verbal attack. Doing so may make the patient feel the need to discontinue communication.

Requesting an explanation: Involves asking patients to provide reasons for their behavior. "Why" questions may have an intimidating effect on some patients.

Minimizing feelings: Judging or making light of a patient's discomfort or concerns. It is important for you to perceive what is taking place from the patient's point of view, not your own.

Making stereotyped comments: Involves using meaningless clichés when communicating with patients, such as "It's for your own good." Comments of this type are given in an automatic, mechanical way as a substitute for a more reasonable and thoughtful explanation.

Defense Mechanisms

Patients will often develop defense mechanisms, which they are usually not conscious of, to protect themselves from anxiety, guilt, shame, or other uncomfortable situations. It is important for you to observe defense mechanisms when working with patients in order to better understand what they are trying to communicate. The following are some common defense mechanisms that patients may display:

Compensation: Overemphasizing a trait to make up for either a perceived or actual failing.

Denial: An unconscious attempt to reject unacceptable wishes, thoughts, needs, feelings, or external reality factors.

Displacement: The unconscious transfer of unacceptable desires, feelings, or thoughts from the self to a more acceptable external substitute.

Dissociation: Disconnecting emotional significance from specific events or ideas.

Identification: Mimicking the behavior of another person in order to cope with feelings of inadequacy.

Introjection: Adopting the unacceptable feelings or thoughts of others.

Projection: Projecting onto another person one's own feelings, as if they were originally the other person's feelings.

Rationalization: Justifying unacceptable feelings, thoughts, and behaviors into tolerable behaviors.

Regression: Unconsciously returning to more infantile thoughts or behaviors.

Repression: Putting unpleasant events, feelings, or thoughts out of one's mind.

Substitution: Unconsciously replacing an unacceptable or unreachable goal with another more acceptable goal.

Assertiveness Skills

As a professional, you need to be assertive. This means being firm and standing by your principles while still showing respect for others. Being assertive is not the same thing as being aggressive. Aggressive actions make others feel that the aggressive person is trying to impose his position on others or is trying to manipulate others.

Communicating in Special Circumstances

Part of the medical assistant's role includes setting the tone for communications. Medical assistants must therefore be aware of all obstacles that affect communication between human beings. As you interact with patients and their families, you will encounter many different kinds of patients—including those from different cultures, different socioeconomic backgrounds, and different educational levels. In addition, patients' ages will range widely, and some patients may have lifestyles that are very different from your own. Medical assistants must be able to remain professional and diplomatic with all of the patients with whom they communicate.

Communicating with Patients as Individuals

If you make an effort to develop good interpersonal skills, communicating with most patients will be easy. However, some situations can cause difficulties in communication. Sometimes communication problems occur in special circumstances, such as with anxious or angry patients, patients from different cultures, or patients with visual or hearing impairments. Additional problems may be encountered in communicating with patients who are mentally or emotionally disabled, have AIDS or are HIV-positive, are terminally ill, or are elderly or young.

Anxious patients: It is common for patients to become anxious in a health-care setting such as a doctor's office. This reaction is commonly known as the "white-coat syndrome" and can have many different reasons. Some patients, particularly children, may not be able to express in words their feelings of fear or anxiety. You should be alert to signs of anxiety, which include the following:

- Tense appearance
- Increased blood pressure, pulse rate, and rate of breathing
- Sweaty palms
- Reported problems with sleep or appetite
- Irritability
- Agitation

Angry patients: Anger may occur in a medical setting for many different reasons. It may be a way to hide the patient's fear about an illness or a surgical outcome. Anger may come from feelings of being treated unfairly or without compassion. It may be a reaction to an invasion of privacy, feelings of loss of control or self-esteem, disappointment, rejection, or frustration. The medical assistant should help angry patients refocus their emotional energy on solving the problem. The following are some tips for communicating with an angry patient:

1. Learn to recognize anger and its causes.
2. Remain calm and continue to demonstrate respect and genuineness.
3. Focus on the patient's medical and physical needs.
4. Maintain adequate personal space to help the patient feel comfortable.
5. Avoid the feeling of needing to defend yourself or giving reasons that the patient should not be angry.
6. Encourage patients to be specific in describing their feelings, including the cause of their anger and their thoughts about it. Avoid agreeing or disagreeing with the patient. Instead, state what you can and cannot do for the patient.
7. Present your point of view firmly but calmly to help the patient better understand the situation.
8. Avoid a communication breakdown with the patient.
9. If you feel threatened by a patient's anger or if you have concerns about the patient's becoming violent, leave the room and seek assistance from other members of the office staff.

Patients from other cultures: Our cultural background shapes our views of the world, as well as our values, attitudes, beliefs, and use of language. Each culture and ethnic group has its own values, traditions, and behaviors. These differences among cultures should not be viewed as barriers to communication. Remember that these beliefs are neither superior nor inferior to your own beliefs—they are just different.

Patients with visual impairments: Visually impaired patients cannot usually rely on nonverbal clues; therefore, your tone of voice, inflection, and speech volume take on a greater importance when you are communicating with them. Be aware of what you say and how you say it. Use large-print materials whenever possible. Make sure there is adequate lighting in all patient areas. Use a normal speaking voice, talk directly and honestly, and avoid talking down to the patient. The patient's dignity must be preserved in order for effective communication to occur.

Patients with hearing impairments: Communicating effectively with a hearing-impaired patient depends on the degree of impairment and on whether the patient has effective use of a hearing aid. Hearing loss can range from mild to severe. Find a quiet area to talk, and try to minimize background noise. Position yourself close to the patient and face them at all times.

Patients who are mentally or emotionally disturbed: Sometimes you will need to communicate with patients who are mentally or emotionally disturbed. When dealing with these types of patients, you should first determine what level of communication they can understand. The following are some suggestions that can help improve communication with these patients:

- Remain calm if the patient becomes confused or agitated.
- Do not raise your voice or appear to be impatient.
- Ask the patient to repeat what he or she said if you do not understand him or her.

Elderly patients: Medical assistants now spend 50% or more of their time caring for older patients. Elderly patients should not be stereotyped as frail or confused, as most of them are not. Each patient deserves to be treated according to his or her individual abilities. Always treat elderly patients with respect. Use the title "Mr." or "Mrs." to address older patients unless they ask you to call them by their first name.

Terminally ill patients: Because they are often under extreme stress, terminally ill patients can be difficult to treat. Health-care professionals must respect the rights of terminally ill patients and always treat them with dignity. It is also important that medical assistants communicate with the families of terminally ill patients, offering support and empathy as these patients accept their conditions.

Young patients: Children are more receptive to the requests and suggestions made by a medical assistant once they realize that you take their feelings seriously. Explain any procedure in very simple terms, no matter how basic it is. Let the child examine the instruments you will need to use. Use praise for their good behavior, and always be truthful.

Parents: Because parents are naturally concerned about their children, reassuring parents and keeping them calm can also help children relax.

Patients with AIDS and patients who are HIV-positive: Patients with AIDS and patients who have HIV have a very serious illness to deal with. These patients often feel depressed, angry, and guilty about their condition. In communicating effectively with them, you need accurate information about the disease and the risks involved. These patients will have many questions, and part of your role as an effective communicator will be to answer as many questions as you can.

Communicating with Coworkers and Superiors

Communicating with Coworkers

As a medical assistant, you are part of a larger health-care team. The quality of communication that you have with your coworkers is vitally important and influences the development of positive or negative work climates, as well as a team approach to patient care.

Communicating with Superiors

Positive or negative communication affects the quality of your relationship with superiors. Problems arise when communication about your job responsibilities is unclear or when you feel that a superior does not trust or respect you, or vice versa. The following are some suggestions for good communications with superiors:

- Keep superiors informed.
- Ask questions.
- Minimize interruptions.
- Show initiative.

Travel planning: Part of a medical assistant's duties may include helping the physician prepare for a trip. The medical assistant should consult with the person traveling, carefully noting the date and time of departure, destinations, length of stay at each destination, and times of arrival at and departure from each destination. The best resource for travel information is a skilled agent at a reputable travel agency.

Dealing with Conflict

Conflict can arise when the lines of communication break down or when a misunderstanding between staff members or between a medical assistant and a superior occurs. Prejudices and preconceived notions about people, as well as a lack of mutual respect or trust, can also cause conflicts among office staff. The following suggestions can help improve communication among coworkers:

- Do not participate in other people's negative attitudes.
- Try your best at all times to be personable and supportive of coworkers.
- Refrain from passing judgment on others or stereotyping them.
- Do not gossip. Act professionally at all times.
- Do not jump to conclusions. You do not know until you ask.

Managing Stress and Preventing Burnout

Stress can be a communication barrier. Health-care professionals may experience high levels of stress in their daily work environment. Stress can result from feelings of being under pressure, or it can be a reaction to frustration, anger, or a change of routine. You can minimize

- Maintain a healthy balance in your life among work, family, and leisure activities.
- Exercise regularly.
- Eat balanced, nutritious meals and healthful snacks. Avoid foods high in caffeine, salt, sugar, and fat.
- Get enough sleep.
- Allow time for yourself, and plan time to relax.
- Rely on the support that family, friends, and coworkers have to offer. Don't be afraid to share your feelings.
- Try to be realistic about what you can and cannot do. Do not be afraid to admit that you cannot take on another responsibility.
- Try to set realistic goals for yourself.
- Remember that there are always choices, even when there appear to be none.
- Be organized. Good planning can help you manage your workload.
- Redirect excess energy constructively—clean your closet, work in the garden, do volunteer work, have friends over for dinner, exercise.
- Change some of the things you have control over.
- Keep yourself focused. Focus your full energy on one thing at a time, and finish one project before starting another.
- Identify sources of conflict, and try to resolve them.
- Learn and use relaxation techniques, such as deep breathing, meditation, or imagining yourself in a quiet, peaceful place. Choose what works for you.
- Maintain a healthy sense of humor. Laughter can help relieve stress. Joke with friends after work. Go see a funny movie.
- Try not to overreact. Ask yourself if a situation is really worth getting upset or worried about.
- Seek help from social or professional support groups, if necessary.

Table 10-1

stress by maintaining a balance between work, family, and leisure activities, as well as by exercising and eating a healthy diet. It is important to learn how to manage stress in order to prevent burnout. Burnout is an energy-depleting condition that will affect your health and career. Table 10-1 provides tips for reducing stress.

The Policy and Procedures Manual

In the medical office setting, the policy and procedures manual is a key written communication tool. These important documents should be reviewed by all employees for a thorough understanding of their office's rules, standards, and ways of operating.

Policies: Rules or guidelines that determine the daily working of an office. They include:

- Office purposes, objectives, and goals as established by the physician(s)

- Rules and regulations
- Job descriptions and duties of staff personnel
- Office hours
- Dress code
- Insurance and other benefits
- Vacation, sick leave, and other time away from the office
- Salary and performance evaluations
- Maintenance of equipment and supplies
- Mailing
- Bookkeeping
- Scheduling of appointments and maintenance of patient records
- Occupational Safety and Health Administration (OSHA) and HIPAA guidelines

Procedures: Detailed instructions for specific procedures. The instructions include clinical procedures and quality assurance programs.

Administrative Supplies

Appointment books, daybooks
Back-to-school/back-to-work slips
Clipboards
Computer supplies
Copy and facsimile (fax) machine paper
File folders, coding tabs
History and physical examination sheets/cards
Insurance forms: disability, HMO and other third-party payers, life insurance examinations, Veterans Administration, workers' compensation
Insurance manuals

Local welfare department forms
Patient education materials
Pens, pencils, erasers
Rubber bands, paper clips
Social Security forms
Stamps
Stationery: appointment cards, bookkeeping supplies (ledgers, statements, billing forms), letterhead, second sheets, envelopes, business cards, prescription pads, notebooks, notepads, telephone memo pads

Clinical Supplies

Alcohol swabs
Applicators
Bandaging materials: adhesive tape, gauze pads, gauze sponges, elastic bandages, adhesive bandages, roller bandages (gauze and elastic)
Cloth or paper gowns
Cotton, cotton swabs
Culture tubes
50% dextrose solution
Disposable sheaths for thermometers
Disposable tips for otoscopes
Gloves: sterile, examination
Hemoccult test kits
Iodine or Betadine pads
Lancets
Lubricating jelly
Microscopic slides and fixative
Needles, syringes
Nitroglycerin tablets

Safety pins
Silver nitrate sticks
Suture removal kits
Sutures
Thermometer covers
Tongue depressors
Topical skin freeze
Urinalysis test sticks
Urine containers
Injectable medications: diazepam (Valium), diphenhydramine hydrochloride (Benadryl), epinephrine (Adrenalin), furosemide (Lasix), isoproterenol (Isuprel), lidocaine (Xylocaine: 1%, 2%, and plain), meperidine hydrochloride (Demerol), morphine, phenobarbital, sodium bicarbonate, sterile saline, sterile water
Other medicines, chemicals, solutions, ointments, lotions, and disinfectants, as needed

General Supplies

Liquid hypoallergenic soap
Paper cups
Paper towels

Tampons
Tissues: facial, toilet

Table 12-1

the smooth running of the practice. Examples include prescription pads and paper for examinations. To help keep track of supplies, categorize them according to the urgency of need, making sure that vital supplies are readily available.

Incidental supplies: Can be clinical, administrative, or general in nature. The efficiency of the office is not threatened if these supplies run low. Incidental supplies include rubber bands and staples.

Durable items: Pieces of equipment that are used indefinitely, such as telephones or computers, that are not considered supplies.

Expendable items: Items that are used and then must be restocked, also known as consumables. Expendable items are used up within a short period of time, and they are relatively inexpensive.

Capital equipment: Items that are considered major and involve expenditures above a predetermined dollar

Examples of Capital Equipment

General	Administrative	Clinical
Office furnishings	Computers	Examination room furnishings
Carpeting	Copy machines	Examination equipment such as microscopes, autoclaves, and ultrasound machines

Table 12-2

value. Capital equipment includes general, large lab, administrative, and clinical equipment. Table 12-2 lists some examples of capital equipment.

Ordering and Receiving Supplies

Vendors: The medical assistant should obtain recommendations from other medical offices, gather competitive prices, and compare vendors on the basis of price, quality, service, and payment policies. It takes multiple vendors to provide all the supplies for a medical practice.

Local vendors: It is a good idea to establish good credit and business relationships with local vendors, even if they cost a little more. Local vendors may offer special discounts, emergency service, information about sales and specials, and personal assistance.

Catalog services: Can provide ease of availability, competitive pricing, and fast delivery. Many vendors accept telephone, fax, and e-mail orders as well as traditional order forms.

Ordering supplies: Expendable supplies and equipment must be replaced and reordered in time. A copy of the order form should be retained to check against the order when it arrives.

Purchase requisitions: Some practices require approval of a formal request before supplies can be ordered.

Receiving supplies: Orders should be checked for completeness. One person should be responsible for receiving and signing for deliveries. This person must check invoices and/or packing slips against the items delivered, initial and date the invoices as items are received, and distribute goods to the storage room.

Packing slip: A list of supplies packed and shipped, supplied by the vendor in the package with the supplies.

Statement: The monthly bill summarizing invoices. It is a request for payment.

Supply budget: The average medical practice spends from 4% to 6% of its annual gross income on supplies. If costs exceed 6%, you might be required to reevaluate the office's spending practices.

Storage of Supplies

Storage room: Should be arranged with the most commonly used items within easiest reach. Place new stock in the back of the storage area, and move the old

supplies up front so that they will be used first. This practice is referred to as rotating stock. You must know the storage requirements for various kinds of supplies. You must maintain an adequate quantity of supplies in a well-organized storage space to run the office smoothly.

Inventory: A list of articles in stock, with the description and quantity of each. Inventory control requires constant supervision, because a medical office cannot afford to run out of supplies. Most offices maintain an ongoing inventory system, which helps determine when to reorder supplies.

Reminder cards: Many offices develop color-coded re-order reminder cards, which are inserted into the stack of inventory items. When the card comes to the top of the stack, it is time to reorder.

Payment

Invoice: A paper describing a purchase and the amount due. Check the invoice against the original order and the packing slip, mark it to confirm that the order was received, and pay it. The check number, date, and payment amount should then be recorded on the invoice. Invoices should be placed in a special folder until paid.

Payment terms: Many vendors do not charge a handling fee if an order is prepaid. Others offer a discount for enclosing a check with an order. Some delay billing for 30 to 90 days. The vendor's invoice usually describes payment terms.

Records: Copies of all bills and order forms for supplies should be kept on file for 10 years in case the practice is audited by the IRS.

Disbursement: Payment of funds, whether in cash or by check. Usually, you will write a check to the vendor and have the physician sign it. At the time of payment, write the date and check number on the statement, and place it in the paid file. Disbursements can be entered into the accounting records in several ways, depending on the accounting system used.

Purchasing procedure: The purchasing procedure should follow certain standard practices:

- An authorized person should be in charge of purchasing.
- High-quality goods and services should be ordered at the lowest possible prices.

- Receipts of goods should be recorded.
- Shipments received should be checked against packing slips to verify that all goods have been received.
- Invoices should be paid in a timely manner.
- Paid invoices should be kept on file.

Accounting

Accounting: A system of recording, classifying, and summarizing financial transactions.

Account: In bookkeeping terms, a single financial record category or division. It is used to track debit and credit changes, by date, in reference to a specific matter. For example, when a practice accepts a new patient, the patient is assigned an account. As the patient is charged for services and the patient (or third-party payer, such as an insurance company) pays those charges, entries are made in the patient's account.

Account balance: The debit or credit balance remaining in an account.

Accounts payable: Amounts charged with suppliers or creditors that remain unpaid.

Accounts receivable: Amounts owed to a business for services or goods supplied.

Assets: Possessions of value, which in a medical office are inventory, equipment, prepaid rent, and the amounts due from patients.

Liabilities: Amounts owed to creditors, such as a mortgage on the medical building and the accounts payable.

Balance sheet: A financial statement for a specific date or period that indicates the total assets, liabilities, and capital of the business.

Auditing: The review of financial data to verify accuracy and completeness. Medical assistants responsible for bookkeeping must provide required financial records and answer questions about accounting systems used.

Bookkeeping Systems

Bookkeeping: The recording part of the accounting process. Bookkeeping records income, charges, and disbursements. There are three types of manual bookkeeping systems: single-entry, double-entry, and pegboard.

Single-entry system: The oldest bookkeeping system, requiring only one entry for each transaction. This straightforwardness makes it the easiest system to learn and use. Because it is not self-balancing, however, it is the hardest system in which to spot errors. It includes several basic records, such as:

- Daily log to record charges and payments. See Figure 12-1.
- Patient ledger cards
- Payroll records

Dr. _____		Date _____		
Hour	*Patient*	*Service Provided*	*Charge*	*Paid*
	1			
	2			
	3			
	4			
	5			
	6			
	7			
	8			
	9			
	10			
	11			
	12			
	13			
	14			
	15			
	16			
		Totals		

Figure 12-1 *A daily log is used to record charges and payments.*

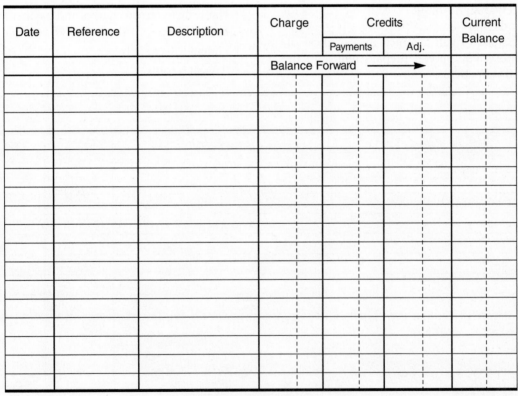

Patient's Name ___Jonathan Jackson_____

Home Phone ___(612) 555-9921____ Work Phone ___(612) 555-1000____

Patient's ID No. ___111-21-4114_____

Employer ___Ashton School District_____

Insurance ___National Insurance Co._____

Policy # ___123-4-56-788_____

Person Responsible for Charges (If Different from Patient) _____

JONATHAN JACKSON
123 Fourth Avenue
Ashton, MN 70809-1222

Date	Reference	Description	Charge	Credits		Current Balance
				Payments	Adj.	
		Balance Forward ⟶				

Please Pay Last Amount in This Column ▲

OV—Office Visit   C—Consultation   EX—Examination
X—X-ray   NC—No Charge   INS—Insurance
ROA—Received on Account   MA—Missed Appointment

Figure 12-2 *Patient ledger cards are used to show how much each patient owes.*

- Cash payment journal
- Petty cash records

Double-entry system: Based on the accounting equation *assets = liabilities + owner equity*. The materials required for a double-entry bookkeeping system are inexpensive, but the system requires more skill and knowledge of accounting procedures than the single-entry system. It is also more time-consuming to use. After each financial transaction, the medical office using a double-entry system must debit one account and credit another account. For example, when the practice charges for a medical service, the patient's account is debited and the appropriate account for the practice is credited.

Pegboard system: A system consisting of daysheets, ledger cards, patient charge slips, and receipt forms or superbills. A pegboard system usually includes a lightweight board with pegs on the left or right edges and is sometimes called a "one-write" system. It is the most commonly used manual medical accounts receivable system and the most expensive to maintain. It used to be the most widely used bookkeeping system in medical practices. This system is now used less commonly in many practices.

A pegboard system has several main advantages:

- The system is efficient and time-saving.
- The daysheet provides complete and up-to-date information about accounts receivable status at a glance.
- The system is easy to learn.

Charge slip: The original record of the doctor's services and the charge for those services.

Posting to Records

General journal: A record of the physician's practice. It includes records of services rendered, charges made, and monies received. The general journal is also known by the names daily log, daybook, daysheet, daily journal, and charge journal. This journal is also called the book of original entry because it is where all transactions are first recorded.

Patient ledger card: A card that contains the patient's name, address, home and work telephone numbers, and the name of the person who is responsible for the charges (if different from the patient). It also contains a record of charges, payment, and adjustments for individual patients or families. See Figure 12-2.

Accounts receivable ledger: Includes all the individual patients' financial accounts on which there are balances.

Posting: The process of copying or recording an amount from one record, such as a journal, onto another record, such as a ledger—or from a daysheet onto a ledger card.

Manual posting: Facilitated by a section at the bottom of each daysheet and a check register page at the end of each month, plus monthly and annual summaries. Accounting records must show every amount paid out, date and check number, and purpose of payment.

Computer posting: Using a computer to keep track of and print accounts receivable and accounts payable. Computers are also used to print checks, as well as payment information.

Accrual basis accounting: Recording income when it is earned and expenses when they are incurred.

Trial balance: A method of checking the accuracy of accounts. It should be done once a month after all posting has been completed and before preparing the monthly statements. The purpose of a trial balance is to disclose any discrepancies between the journal and the ledger.

Account Balances

Equity: The net worth of the medical office. Equity equals the practice's total assets minus the total liabilities.

Balance: The difference between the debit and credit totals.

Adjustment column: An account column, sometimes included to the left of the balance column, used for entering discounts, debits, credits, refunds, and write-offs.

Balance column: The account column on the far right that is used for recording the difference between the debit and credit columns.

Debit: An amount usually representing things acquired for the intended use or benefit of a business. It is recorded in the column to the left of the credit column. In each journal entry, the dollar amount of the debit must be equal to the dollar amount of the credit. A debit is also called a charge. Debits are incurred when the practice pays for something, such as medical supplies.

Credit: An amount constituting an addition to a revenue, net worth, or liability account. It is recorded in the column to the right of the debit column. Credits constitute payments received by the practice, such as from patients or third-party insurance providers.

Credit balance: Money owed to the patient that results when a patient has paid in advance and there has been an overpayment.

Refunds: Debit adjustments. If a patient wishes to have an overpayment refunded, write a check for the amount due and enter the transaction on the daysheet.

Credit bureau: A company that provides information about the creditworthiness of a person seeking credit. If a patient's credit history is in question, you may request a report from a credit bureau. A sample credit bureau report is shown in Figure 12-3.

Equal Credit Opportunity Act: An act that states that credit arrangements may not be denied on the basis of a patient's sex, race, religion, national origin, marital

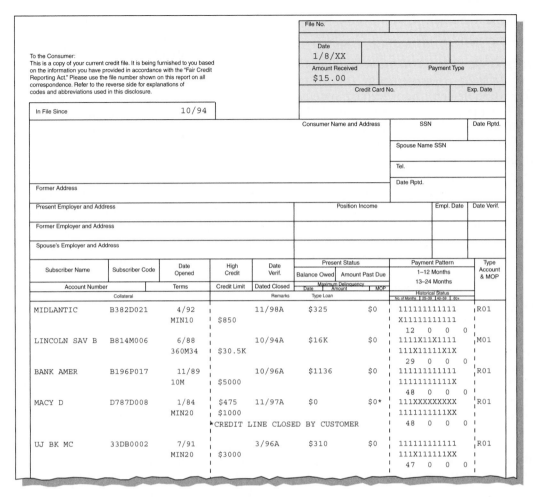

Figure 12-3 *Credit reports are generated by credit bureaus.*

status, or age. Also, credit cannot be denied because the patient receives public assistance or has exercised rights under the Consumer Credit Protection Act, such as disputing a credit card bill or a credit bureau report. Under the Equal Credit Opportunity Act, the patient has a right to know the specific reason that credit was denied.

Payables: Amounts owed to others.

In balance: Accounts are in balance when the total ending balances of patient ledgers equals the total of accounts receivable.

Receipts: Money received.

Petty cash fund: A fund maintained to pay small, unpredictable cash expenses.

Reconciliation of bank statement: The process of verifying that the bank statement and the checkbook balances are in agreement. As you reconcile the bank statement with your accounts, be aware of outstanding checks, outstanding deposits, and any service fees the bank may have charged.

Superbill: A combination charge slip, statement, and insurance reporting form. A superbill includes the charges for services rendered on a day, an invoice for payment or insurance copayment, and all the information for submitting an insurance claim. It is also called an encounter form. See Figure 12-4.

Banking for the Medical Office

Medical business: A medical practice is a business that must produce a profit—that is, its income must exceed its expenses. Bookkeeping and banking are essential and must be 100% accurate.

Absolute accuracy: Necessary when working with bank deposits, reconciliation of statements, and all bookkeeping activities. The medical assistant acts as the agent for the physician.

Banks: Maintain checking and savings accounts for their customers.

Banking functions: Basic bank-related activities carried out by a medical practice include:

- Depositing funds
- Withdrawing funds
- Reconciling statements
- Using auxiliary services

Lakeridge Medical Group
262 East Pine Street, Suite 100
Lakeridge, NJ 07500

☐ PRIVATE   ☐ BLUECROSS   ☐ IND.   ☐ MEDICARE   ☐ MEDI-CAL   ☐ HMO   ☐ PPO

PATIENT'S LAST NAME	FIRST	ACCOUNT #	BIRTHDATE / /	SEX ☐ MALE ☐ FEMALE	TODAY'S DATE / /
INSURANCE COMPANY	SUBSCRIBER		PLAN #	SUB. #	GROUP

ASSIGNMENT: I hereby assign my insurance benefits to be paid directly to the undersigned physician. I am financially responsible for non-covered services. SIGNED: (Patient, or Parent, if Minor) DATE: / /	RELEASE: I hereby authorize the physician to release to my insurance carrers any information required to process this claim. SIGNED: (Patient, or Parent, if Minor) DATE: / /

✔	DESCRIPTION	M/Care CPT/Mod	DxRe	FEE
	OFFICE CARE			
	NEW PATIENT			
	Brief	99201		
	Limited	99202		
	Intermediate	99203		
	Extended	99204		
	Comprehensive	99205		
	ESTABLISHED PATIENT			
	Minimal	99211		
	Brief	99212		
	Limited	99213		
	Intermediate	99214		
	Extended	99215		
	Comprehensive	99215		
	CONSULTATION-OFFICE			
	Focused	99241		
	Expanded	99242		
	Detailed	99243		
	Comprehensive 1	99244		
	Comprehensive 2	99245		
	Dr.			
	Case Management	98900		
	Post-op Exam	99024		

✔	DESCRIPTION	M/Care CPT/Mod	DxRe	FEE
	PROCEDURES			
	Tread Mill (In Office)	93015		
	24 Hour Holter	93224		
	If Medicare (Set up Fee)	93225		
	Physician Interpret	93227		
	EKG w/Interpretation	93000		
	EKG (Medicare)	93005		
	Sigmoidoscopy	45300		
	Sigmoidoscopy, Flexible	45330		
	Sigmoidos. , Flex. w/Bx.	45331		
	Spirometry, FEV/FVC	94010		
	Spirometry, Post-Dilator	94060		
	LABORATORY			
	Blood Draw Fee	36415		
	Urinalysis, Chemical	81005		
	Throat Culture	87081		
	Occult Blood	82270		
	Pap Handling Charge	99000		
	Pap Life Guard	88150-90		
	Gram Stain	87205		
	Hanging Drop	87210		
	Urine Drug Screen	99000		
	SUPPLIES			

✔	DESCRIPTION	M/Care	CPT/Mod	DxRe	FEE
	INJECTIONS/IMMUNIZATIONS				
	Tetanus		90718		
	Hypertet	J1670	90782		
	Pneumococcal		90732		
	Influenza		90724		
	TB Skin Test (PPD)		86585		
	Antigen Injection-Single		95115		
	Multiple		95117		
	B12 Injection	J3420	90782		
	Injection, IM		90782		
	Compazine	J0780	90782		
	Demerol	J2175	90782		
	Vistaril	J3410	90782		
	Susphrine	J0170	90782		
	Decadron	J0890	90782		
	Estradiol	J1000	90782		
	Testosterone	J1080	90782		
	Lidocaine	J2000	90782		
	Solumedrol	J2920	90782		
	Solucortef	J1720	90782		
	Hydeltra	J1690	90782		
	Pen Procaine	J2510	90788		
	INJECTIONS - JOINT/BURSA				
	Small Joints		20600		
	Intermediate		20605		
	Large Joints		20610		
	Trigger Point		20550		
	MISCELLANEOUS				

DIAGNOSIS:

Diagnosis	ICD-9		Diagnosis	ICD-9		Diagnosis	ICD-9		Diagnosis	ICD-9		Diagnosis	ICD-9
Abdominal Pain	789.0		Gout	274.0		C.V.A. - Acute	436.		Electrolyte Dis.	276.9		Herpes Simplex	054.9
Abscess (Site)	682.9		Asthma	493.90		Cere. Vas. Accid. (Old)	438		Fatigue	780.7		Herpes Zoster	053.9
Adverse Drug Rx	995.2		Asthmatic Bronchitis	493.90		Cerumen	380.4		Fibrocys. Br. Dis	610.1		Hydrocele	603.9
Alcohol Detox	291.8		Atrial Fib.	427.31		Chestwall Pain	786.59		Fracture (Site)	829.0		Hyperlipidemia	272.4
Alcoholism	303.90		Atrial Tachi.	427.0		Cholecystitis	575.0		Open/Close			Hypertension	401.9
Allergic Rhinitis	477		Bowel Obstruct.	560.9		Cholelithiasis	574.00		Fungal Infect. (Site)	110.8		Hyperthyroidism	242.9
Allergy	995.3		Breast Mass	611.72		COPD	492.8		Gastric Ulcer	531.90		Hypothyroidism	244.9
Alzheimer's Dis.	290.1		Bronchitis	490		Cirrhosis	571.5		Gastritis	535.0		Labyrinthitis	386.30
Anemia	285.9		Bursitis	727.3		Cong. Heart Fail.	428.9		Gastroenteritis	558.9		Lipoma (Site)	214.9
Anemia - Pernicious	281.0		Cancer, Breast (Site)	174.9		Conjunctivitis	372.30		G.I. Bleeding	578.9		Lymphoma	202.8
Angina	413.9		Metastatic (Site)	199.1		Contusion (Site)	924.9		Glomerulonephritis	583.9		Mit. Valve Prolapse	424.0
Anxiety Synd.	300.00		Colon	153.9		Costochondritis	733.99		Headache	784.0		Myocard. Infarction (Area)	410.9
Appendicitis	541		Cancer, Rectal	154.1		Depression	311.		Headache, Tension	307.81		M.I., Old	412
Arterioscl. H.D.	414.0		Lung (Site)	162.9		Dermatitis	692.9		Migraine (Type)	346.9		Myositis	729.1
Arthritis, Osteo.	715.90		Skin (Site)	173.9		Diabetes Mellitus	250.00		Hemorrhoids	455.6		Nausea/Vomiting	787.0
Rheumatoid	714.0		Card. Arrhythmia (Type)	427.9		Diabetic Ketosis	250.1		Hernia, Hiatal	553.3		Neuralgia	729.2
Lupus	710.0		Cardiomyopathy	425.4		Diverticulitis	562.11		Inguinal	550.9		Nevus (Site)	216.9
			Cellulitis (Site)	682.9		Diverticulosis	562.10		Hepatitis	573.3		Obesity	278.0

DIAGNOSIS: (IF NOT CHECKED ABOVE)

SERVICES PERFORMED AT: ☐ Office ☐ E.R. ☐ ☐	☐ CLAIM CONTAINS NO ORDERED REFERRING SERVICE	REFERRING PHYSICIAN & I.D. NUMBER

RETURN APPOINTMENT INFORMATION: 5 - 10 - 15 - 20 - 30 - 40 - 60 [DAYS] [WKS.] [MOS.] [PRN]	NEXT APPOINTMENT M - T - W - TH - F - S DATE / / TIME:	AM PM	ACCEPT ASSIGNMENT? ☐ YES ☐ NO	DOCTOR'S SIGNATURE

INSTRUCTIONS TO PATIENT FOR FILING INSURANCE CLAIMS:	☐ CASH	TOTAL TODAY'S FEE	
1. Complete upper portion of this form, sign and date. 2. Attach this form to your own insurance company's form for direct reimbursement. **MEDICARE PATIENTS - DO NOT SEND THIS TO MEDICARE. WE WILL SUBMIT THE CLAIM FOR YOU.**	☐ CHECK # _____ ☐ VISA ☐ MC ☐ CO-PAY	OLD BALANCE / TOTAL DUE AMOUNT REC'D. TODAY	

Figure 12-4 *A superbill is a form that can also be used as a charge slip and invoice and can be submitted with insurance claims.*

Types of Bank Accounts

Types of bank accounts: Medical practices typically use three types of bank account:

- Regular checking account
- Interest-earning, or interest-bearing, checking account
- Savings account

Regular checking account: Most medical practices have a regular checking account for office expenses. This account does not pay interest but offers availability and flexibility.

Interest: Money paid to a depositor by a bank or other financial institution for the use of the depositor's money.

Electronic banking: Banking with the use of computers. Electronic banking has several advantages over traditional banking: It can improve productivity, cash flow, and accuracy. The computer screen can display all checks and deposits that were logged into the register in the order they were posted. In electronic banking, someone must still be responsible for recording and physically depositing checks.

Bank statements: All contain certain basic information, including:

- Closing date
- Caption
- List of checks processed
- List of deposits

Caption: A summary of the account activity that has taken place during the month up to the closing date. It includes the beginning balance, total value of checks processed, total amount of deposits made, service charges, and ending balance.

Checks

Check: A written order to a bank to pay or transfer money. It is payable on demand and is considered a negotiable instrument. The person who writes the check is called the payer or drawer.

Types of checks: Cashier's checks, certified checks, money orders, limited checks, traveler's checks, voucher checks, bank drafts, and warrants.

Cashier's check: Written using the bank's own check form and signed by a bank representative. The funds for payment of the check are debited from the payer's account at the time the check is written. A service charge is usually added. Another term for a cashier's check is treasurer's check.

Certified check: Written on the payer's own check form and verified by the bank with an official stamp. The bank withdraws the money from the payer's account when it certifies the check. The stamp indicates that the bank certifies the availability of the funds.

Money order: A certificate of guaranteed payment. It is purchased for the cash value printed on the certificate plus a nominal handling fee. Money orders may be purchased from banks, post offices, and some convenience stores. International money orders can be acquired in U.S. dollars to be cashed in foreign countries.

Limited check: Issued on a special check form that displays a preprinted maximum dollar amount for which the check can be written. This type of check often is used for payroll or insurance payments.

Traveler's check: A check purchased for a small fee for a specified amount of money. It is designed for people who are traveling where personal checks may not be accepted and for people who do not want to carry large amounts of cash. Traveler's checks are also available in foreign currencies. They can be purchased at a bank.

Voucher check: Contains a detachable voucher form. It is frequently used for payroll checks because additional information about the transaction can be supplied to the payee. The voucher portion is used to itemize the purpose of the check, deductions, or other information.

Bank draft: A check written by a bank against its funds in another bank.

Warrant: A nonnegotiable check. It is a statement issued to indicate that a debt should be paid, for example, by an insurance company.

ABA number: Part of a coding system originated by the American Bankers Association (ABA). It is always located in the upper right corner of a printed check to identify the location of the bank at which the check is to be redeemed.

MICR code: Stands for magnetic ink character recognition code, which appears along the bottom of a check and consists of numbers and characters printed in magnetic ink.

Accepting checks: The majority of bills are paid by personal checks drawn on patients' bank accounts. Some checks may be considered risky, such as third-party checks, postdated checks, checks drawn on an out-of-town bank, and checks marked *Paid in full* that do not represent the total due. Accepting such checks should be avoided.

Power of attorney: A directive that grants a person the legal right to handle financial matters for another person who is unable to do so.

Postdated check: A check that bears a date in the future and cannot be cashed until then.

Predated or **backdated check:** A check made out with a date in the past. Predated checks can be accepted as long as the date shown is no more than 6 months before the date on which it is cashed.

Third-party check: A check written by an unknown party to a payee (e.g., your patient) who wishes to release the check to you for payment of an outstanding balance. Government and payroll checks used in this way are also third-party checks.

Canceled check: A check that has been cashed and thus cannot be issued again.

Deposits

Deposits: Cash or checks placed into a bank account. They can be made to either checking or savings accounts. Checks should be deposited promptly for the following reasons:

- They may be lost, misplaced, or stolen.
- There is the possibility of a stop-payment order.
- They may have a restricted time for cashing.

Endorsement: A check must be endorsed to transfer the funds from one person to another. Endorsement is accomplished by signing or rubber-stamping the back of the check, in ink, at the left end. When you accept a check, immediately endorse it and write the words *For deposit only* on the back. See Figure 12-5.

Types of endorsement: There are four principal kinds of endorsement: blank, restrictive, special, and qualified. Blank and restrictive endorsements are the most commonly used.

Blank endorsement: A signature only. Also known as an open endorsement, it is the simplest and most common type of endorsement on personal checks.

Restrictive endorsement: The words *For deposit only* followed by the account number and signature.

Limited endorsement: The words *Pay to the order of* and the name, followed by a signature. A check with a limited endorsement functions as a third-party check. For example, a patient might give you a check that was originally made out to someone else, who used a limited endorsement to sign the check over to the patient. This original payee would become a third-party payer if the practice were to accept the check from the patient.

Qualified endorsement: Used to disclaim future liability of the endorser, generally consisting of the words *Without recourse* above the signature. It is most commonly used by lawyers who accept checks on behalf of clients.

Deposit slip: After endorsing the check, fill out a deposit slip as shown in Figure 12-6.

Methods of deposit: There are three different ways to deposit funds: in person, by mail, or at commercial night depositories. Making deposits in person is the most direct method, and banks immediately provide a receipt to verify transactions. Avoid sending cash through the mail, but if it is absolutely necessary to do so, use registered mail.

Returned checks: Occasionally, the bank returns a deposited check because of problems such as a missing signature or missing endorsement. A check is also returned if the payer has insufficient funds on deposit to cover it.

NSF: Abbreviation for not sufficient funds, meaning that there is not enough money in the account on which a check has been drawn to cover the amount of the check.

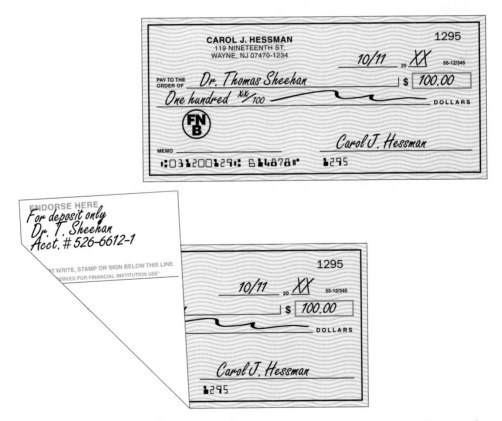

Figure 12-5 *After verifying that a patient's check is correct, immediately endorse it with the words* For deposit only, *the name of the practice, and the bank account number.*

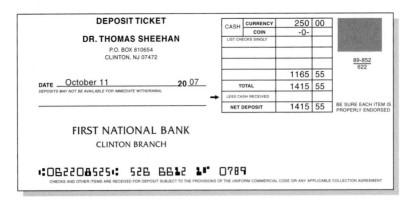

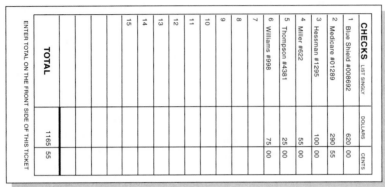

Figure 12-6 *List each check on the deposit slip, including the check number and amount.*

Handling returned checks: If a check is returned, begin by contacting the person who gave you the check. If payment is not made, or if you cannot track down the person, turn the account over to a collection agency.

Bill Payment

Bills: All bills should be paid by check for documentation and control purposes. For small payments, such as public transportation costs, petty cash may be used.

Office banking policy: Should indicate who is responsible for writing and signing all checks. For good control, one person should write the checks, and another person should be authorized to sign them. Sometimes two authorized signatures are required in order to transfer funds from one account to another or to write checks over a certain amount, such as $1,000.

Check writing: Checks are printed on sensitized paper so that erasures are easily noticeable. The bank has the right to refuse payment on any check that has been altered. You must not cross out, erase, or change any part of a check.

Check stub: The part of a check that remains in the checkbook after the check has been written and removed.

Payee: The person to whom the check is payable.

Payer: The person who signs the check to release the funds to the payee.

Lost and stolen checks: Occasionally, an outgoing check may be lost or stolen after it has been issued. You

must report this situation to the bank promptly. The bank will place a warning on the account, and signatures on cashed checks will be carefully inspected to detect possible forgeries. A stop-payment order should be issued, and the stop-payment notice should be attached to the check stub. The amount of the check should be added to the current checkbook balance. A new check can be issued to replace the one lost.

Billing and Collections

Medical Billing

Billing duties of a medical assistant: To be an effective account manager, follow these rules:

- Do not be embarrassed to ask for payment for services. The physician or facility has the right to charge for the care and services provided.

- Practice good judgment.

- Give personal attention and consideration to each patient.

- Show a desire to help patients with financial difficulties.

Payment at the time of service: Every practice should encourage time-of-service collection. There will be no further billing and bookkeeping expenses if patients get into the habit of paying their current charges before they leave the office.

Payment plans and extensions of credit: For procedures and services involving large fees, such as surgery and long-term care, inform patients of:

- What the charges will be
- What services these charges cover
- Credit policies of the facility
  - When payment is due
  - Circumstances in which the practice requires payment at the time of service
  - When or whether assignment of insurance benefits is accepted
  - Whether insurance forms will be completed by the office staff
  - Collection procedures, including circumstances in which accounts will be sent to a collection agency

It is a good idea to have credit policies in writing, for example, included in a new patient brochure.

Balance billing: Billing the patient for the difference between the fee and the amount the insurance company allows. Whether balance billing is acceptable depends on the contract with the insurance company.

Exceptions and rules: Although there will be exceptions, there must be rules, which should be conveyed in writing to the patient at the outset of the relationship. Any patient who needs special consideration can be counseled individually.

Internal billing: In a practice with only a moderate number of accounts, the medical assistant handles the preparation and mailing of statements. A printed statement may be computer-generated, based on a superbill, typewritten, or photocopied from the ledger card.

Statement: Should show the service rendered on each date, the charge for each service, the date on which a claim was submitted to the insurance company, the date of payment, and the balance due from the patient. A regular system of mailing statements should be put into operation. Time limits must also be observed in billing third-party payers. Bills for minors must be addressed to parents or legal guardians.

Cycle billing: A common billing system that bills each patient once a month but spreads the work of billing over the month. In this system, invoices are sent to patients whose names begin with A–D on one day, those whose names begin with E–H on another day, and so on.

Fair Credit Billing Act: A federal law mandating that billing for a balance due or reporting a credit balance of $1 or more must occur every 30 days.

Collection Policies and Procedures

Standard payment period: Normally, people are expected to pay bills within 30 days.

Open-book account: The most typical account for patients of a medical practice, in which the account is open to charges made occasionally. It uses the last date of payment or charge for each illness as the starting date for determining the time limit on that debt.

Written-contract account: An account in which the physician and patient sign an agreement stating that the patient will pay the bill in more than four installments.

Single-entry account: An account with only one charge, as is created, for example, when an out-of-town vacationer consults a local physician for an illness.

Delinquent accounts: Accounts in which payment is overdue. Payment is the most difficult to collect from two groups of patients: those with hardship cases and those who have moved and have not received an invoice.

Hardship cases: Accounts of patients who are poor, uninsured, underinsured, or elderly and on a limited income. Physicians may decide to treat such patients at a deep discount or for free.

Payment collection: Evaluation of the success of collections is based on (1) the collection ratio and (2) the accounts receivable ratio.

Collection ratio: Measures the effectiveness of the billing system. The basic formula for figuring the collection ratio is to divide the total collections by the net charges (gross charges minus any discounts) to reach the percentage figure.

Accounts receivable ratio: Measures how fast outstanding accounts are being paid. The formula for figuring the accounts receivable ratio is to divide the current accounts receivable balance by the average gross monthly charges.

Age analysis: The process of classifying and reviewing delinquent accounts by age from the first date of billing. It should list all patient account balances, when charges were incurred, the most recent payment date, and any notes regarding the account. The age analysis is a tool to show, at a glance, the status of each account. See Figure 12-7.

Reasons for collecting delinquent accounts: The main reasons to try to collect all delinquent accounts are:

- Physicians must be paid for services so that they can pay expenses and continue to treat patients.
- Although a patient cannot be "fired" for nonpayment (in the sense that necessary treatment cannot be withheld because of an inability to pay), failure to collect payment can result in the termination of the established patient-physician relationship.
- Noncollection of medical bills may imply guilt, and a malpractice suit may result.
- Abandoning accounts without collection follow-up encourages nonpayment; as a result, the paying patients indirectly subsidize the cost of medical care for those who can pay but do not.

ACCOUNTS RECEIVABLE–AGE ANALYSIS

Date: October 1, 2007

Patient	Balance	Date of Charges	Most Recent Payment	30 days	60 days	90 days	120 days	Remarks
Black, K.	120.00	5/24	5/24			75.00	45.00	3rd Notice
Brown, R.	65.00	8/30	8/30	65.00				
Green, C.	340.00	8/25						Medicare filed
Jones, T.	500.00	6/1	6/30		125.00	125.00	250.00	3rd Notice
Perry, S.	150.00	7/28	7/28	75.00	75.00			1st Notice
Smith, J.	375.00	6/15	7/1			375.00		2nd Notice
White, L.	200.00	6/24	7/5	20.00	30.00	150.00		2nd Notice

Figure 12-7 *An age analysis organizes delinquent accounts by age.*

Collection techniques: Include telephone collection calls, collection letters or statements, and personal interviews. Send the first letter or statement when the account is 30 days past due, then follow up at 60 days, at 90 days, and again at 120 days. Table 12-3 lists laws governing credit and collections. If you call the patient, make sure that you do so in private and during reasonable hours. Always be respectful and professional, and demonstrate your willingness to help the patient meet his or her financial obligation. Get a definite answer from the patient if you can, and follow up later if the payment has not been received. Do not call the patient's place of work, especially if you do not know whether or not the patient can take personal calls at work. When writing collection letters, make sure that the first few letters simply remind the patient about a possible oversight of debt, and make sure that each letter is specific to the individual situation.

Illegal collection techniques: It is illegal to harass a debtor. Harassment includes making threats or calls late at night (after 9 p.m.). It is also illegal to threaten action that cannot be legally taken or that is not intended to be taken.

Statute of limitations: A statute that limits the time in which rights can be enforced by action. After the statute of limitations expires, no legal collection suit may be brought against a debtor. This time limit depends on the state in which the debt was incurred.

Outside collection assistance: When you have done everything possible internally to follow up on an outstanding account and have not received payment, there are still steps you can take:

- Use a collection agency. If the patient has failed to respond to your final letter or has failed to fulfill a second promise on payment, send the account to the collector without delay. After an account has been released to a collection agency, your office makes no further collection attempts.

- Collect through the court system. Most physicians believe that it is unwise to resort to the courts to collect medical bills unless there are extraordinary circumstances.

Collection agencies: Medical practices should be careful to avoid collection agencies that use harsh collection practices. Once an account has been turned over to an agency, do not send bills or discuss the account with the patient. If the agency is unable to collect the money, the physician should decide whether to write off the debt or to take the matter to court.

Law	Requirements	Penalties for Breaking the Law
Equal Credit Opportunity Act (ECOA)	• Creditors may not discriminate against applicants on the basis of sex, marital status, race, national origin, religion, or age. • Creditors may not discriminate because an applicant receives public assistance income or has exercised rights under the Consumer Credit Protection Act.	• If an applicant sues the practice for violating the ECOA, the practice may have to pay damages, penalties, lawyers' fees, and court costs. • If an applicant joins a class action lawsuit against the practice, the practice may have to pay damages of up to $500,000 or 1% of the practice's net worth, whichever is less. (In a class action lawsuit, one or more people sue a company that wronged all of them in the same way.) • If the Federal Trade Commission (FTC) receives many complaints from applicants stating that the practice violated the ECOA, the FTC may investigate and take action against the practice.
Fair Credit Reporting Act (FCRA)	Credit bureaus are required to supply correct and complete information to businesses to use in evaluating a person's application for credit, insurance, or a job.	• If one applicant sues the practice in federal court for violating the FCRA, the practice may have to pay actual damages, punitive damages (punishment for intentionally breaking the law), court costs, and lawyers' fees. • The FTC may investigate and take action against the practice if it receives too many complaints.
Fair Debt Collection Practices Act (FDCPA)	Debt collectors are required to treat debtors fairly. Certain collection tactics are also prohibited, such as harassment, false statements, threats, and unfair practices.	• If it is sued by a debtor, the practice may have to pay damages, court costs, and lawyers' fees. • In a class action lawsuit, the practice might have to pay damages of up to $500,000 or 1% of the practice's net worth, whichever is less. • The FTC may investigate and take action.
Truth in Lending Act (TLA)	Creditors are required to provide applicants with accurate and complete credit costs and terms, in clear and understandable language.	• If it is sued by a debtor, the practice may have to pay damages, court costs, and lawyers' fees. • The FTC may investigate and take action against the practice if it receives too many complaints.

Table 12-3

Accounts Payable

Accounts payable: Amounts the physician owes to others for equipment and services, including:

- Office supplies
- Medical supplies and equipment
- Equipment repair and maintenance
- Utilities
- Taxes
- Payroll
- Rent

Accounts payable records: Include purchase orders, packing slips, and invoices.

Payroll

Payroll: The total direct and indirect earning of all employees. Federal, state, and local laws require records to be kept of all salaries and wages paid to employees.

Payroll tasks: Include calculating the amount of wages or salaries paid and amounts deducted from employees' earnings. Other payroll tasks involve writing checks, tracking data for payroll taxes, and filling out payroll tax forms.

							Pay Period 6/1–6/14								
Emp. No.	Name	Earnings to?date	Hrly. Rate	Reg. Hrs.	OT? Hrs.	OT Earnings	TOTAL GROSS	Earnings Subject to?Unemp.	Earnings Subject to FICA	Social? Security? (FICA)	Medicare	Federal? W/H	State? W/H	Health Ins.	Net? Pay	Check? No.
0010	Scott, B.	9,823.14	14.00	70.00			980.00	980.00	980.00	60.50	14.10	147.92	15.10	25.00	717.38	11747
0020	Wilson, J.	14,290.38	17.00	70.00	6.50	153.00	1343.00	1343.00	1343.00	83.26	19.47	160.45	15.85	67.50	996.47	11748
0030	Diaz, J.	2,750.26	5.50	46.25			254.37	254.37	254.37	15.77	3.68	38.20	3.75		192.97	11749
0040	Ling, W.	2,240.57	6.80	30.00			204.00	204.00	204.00	12.66	2.96	26.02	3.12		159.54	11750
0050	Harris, E.	2,600.98	10.00	23.50			235.00	235.00	235.00	14.57	3.41	33.52	3.36		180.14	11751

Figure 12-8 *A payroll register is designed to summarize information about all employees and their earnings.*

Retention of payroll records: The physician is required by law to keep payroll data for 4 years. The records should include the following information:

- Employee's Social Security number
- Number of withholding allowances claimed
- Gross salary
- Deductions for Social Security tax; Medicare tax; federal, state, and other tax withholding; state disability insurance; and state unemployment tax

Employer tax identification number (EIN): Every employer, no matter how small, must have an EIN for reporting federal taxes. It is obtained by completing Form SS-4, Application for Employer Identification Number.

Employee identification: Employees are identified for tax purposes by their Social Security numbers.

Payroll register: A list of all employees and their earnings, deductions, and other information. See Figure 12-8.

Employee earnings: Either salaries or wages, plus indirect forms of payment, such as paid time off and employee benefit and service programs.

Salary: A fixed amount paid to an employee on a regular basis regardless of the number of hours worked.

Wages: Pay based on a specific rate per hour, day, or week.

Payroll deductions: Amounts regularly withheld from a paycheck, such as those for federal, state, and local taxes, as well as those for such options as a 401(k) plan, life insurance, or savings bonds.

Methods for calculating payroll checks: Include the manual, the pegboard, and the computer system. Regardless of the accounting system used, attention to accuracy in bookkeeping is necessary. In addition, it is necessary to maintain confidentiality in matters related to employees' wages and salaries.

Net earnings: Gross earnings minus total deductions.

Payroll services: Some offices hire an outside payroll service to process all payroll checks and withholding payments, as well as to keep records.

Tax

Types of tax: The federal government mandates payment of the following taxes through withholding:

- Social Security
- Medicare
- Federal income tax

These taxes are based on a percentage of the employee's total gross income.

Withholding: Amounts of salary held out of payroll checks for the purpose of paying government taxes or for employee benefits.

Form W-4: In order to determine the amount of money to be withheld from each paycheck, each new employee must complete a Form W-4, and each employee should update the W-4 regularly. Figure 12-9 shows a Form W-4, which asks for the (1) employee's name and current address, (2) Social Security number, (3) marital status, and (4) number of allowances the employee claims that should be used in calculating withholding.

Social Security (FICA): The Federal Insurance Contribution Act governs the Social Security system. The employee pays half of the contribution, and the employer pays the other half. IRS *Circular E* lists the FICA tax percentages that should be applied, based on the level of taxable earnings, length of the payroll period, marital status, and number of withholding allowances claimed.

Federal Unemployment Tax Act (FUTA): Requires employers to pay a percentage of each employee's income, up to a specified dollar amount, to fund an account used to pay employees who have been laid off for a specified

Form W-4 (2007)

Purpose. Complete Form W-4 so that your employer can withhold the correct federal income tax from your pay. Because your tax situation may change, you may want to refigure your withholding each year.

Exemption from withholding. If you are exempt, complete **only** lines 1, 2, 3, 4, and 7 and sign the form to validate it. Your exemption for 2007 expires February 16, 2008. See Pub. 505, Tax Withholding and Estimated Tax.

Note. You cannot claim exemption from withholding if (a) your income exceeds $850 and includes more than $300 of unearned income (for example, interest and dividends) and (b) another person can claim you as a dependent on their tax return.

Basic instructions. If you are not exempt, complete the **Personal Allowances Worksheet** below. The worksheets on page 2 adjust your withholding allowances based on itemized deductions, certain credits, adjustments to income, or two-earner/multiple job situations. Complete all worksheets that apply. However, you may claim fewer (or zero) allowances.

Head of household. Generally, you may claim head of household filing status on your tax return only if you are unmarried and pay more than 50% of the costs of keeping up a home for yourself and your dependent(s) or other qualifying individuals.

Tax credits. You can take projected tax credits into account in figuring your allowable number of withholding allowances. Credits for child or dependent care expenses and the child tax credit may be claimed using the **Personal Allowances Worksheet** below. See Pub. 919, How Do I Adjust My Tax Withholding, for information on converting your other credits into withholding allowances.

Nonwage income. If you have a large amount of nonwage income, such as interest or dividends, consider making estimated tax payments using Form 1040-ES, Estimated Tax for Individuals. Otherwise, you may owe additional tax. If you have pension or annuity income, see Pub. 919 to find out if you should adjust your withholding on Form W-4 or W-4P.

Two earners/Multiple jobs. If you have a working spouse or more than one job, figure the total number of allowances you are entitled to claim on all jobs using worksheets from only one Form W-4. Your withholding usually will be most accurate when all allowances are claimed on the Form W-4 for the highest paying job and zero allowances are claimed on the others.

Nonresident alien. If you are a nonresident alien, see the Instructions for Form 8233 before completing this Form W-4.

Check your withholding. After your Form W-4 takes effect, use Pub. 919 to see how the dollar amount you are having withheld compares to your projected total tax for 2007. See Pub. 919, especially if your earnings exceed $130,000 (Single) or $180,000 (Married).

Personal Allowances Worksheet (Keep for your records.)

A Enter "1" for **yourself** if no one else can claim you as a dependent . . . .   **A** _____

B Enter "1" if:
- You are single and have only one job; or
- You are married, have only one job, and your spouse does not work; or
- Your wages from a second job or your spouse's wages (or the total of both) are $1,000 or less.

   B _____

C Enter "1" for your **spouse**. But, you may choose to enter "-0-" if you are married and have either a working spouse or more than one job. (Entering "-0-" may help you avoid having too little tax withheld.) . . . .   **C** _____

D Enter number of **dependents** (other than your spouse or yourself) you will claim on your tax return . . . . .   **D** _____

E Enter "1" if you will file as **head of household** on your tax return (see conditions under **Head of household** above) .   **E** _____

F Enter "1" if you have at least $1,500 of **child or dependent care expenses** for which you plan to claim a credit .   **F** _____
(**Note.** Do **not** include child support payments. See Pub. 503, Child and Dependent Care Expenses, for details.)

G **Child Tax Credit** (including additional child tax credit). See Pub 972, Child Tax Credit, for more information.
- If your total income will be less than $57,000 ($85,000 if married), enter "2" for each eligible child.
- If your total income will be between $57,000 and $84,000 ($85,000 and $119,000 if married), enter "1" for each eligible child plus "1" **additional** if you have 4 or more eligible children.   **G** _____

H Add lines A through G and enter total here. (**Note.** This may be different from the number of exemptions you claim on your tax return.) ▶   **H** _____

For accuracy, complete all worksheets that apply.
- If you plan to **itemize or claim adjustments to income** and want to reduce your withholding, see the **Deductions and Adjustments Worksheet** on page 2.
- If you have **more than one job** or are **married and you and your spouse both work** and the combined earnings from all jobs exceed $40,000 ($25,000 if married) see the **Two-Earners/Multiple Jobs Worksheet** on page 2 to avoid having too little tax withheld.
- If **neither** of the above situations applies, **stop here** and enter the number from line H on line 5 of Form W-4 below.

-    **Cut here and give Form W-4 to your employer. Keep the top part for your records.** -

Form **W-4**

Department of the Treasury
Internal Revenue Service

Employee's Withholding Allowance Certificate

OMB No. 1545-0074

20**07**

▶ Whether you are entitled to claim a certain number of allowances or exemption from withholding is subject to review by the IRS. Your employer may be required to send a copy of this form to the IRS.

1 Type or print your first name and middle initial.   Last name   **2** Your social security number

Home address (number and street or rural route)

3 ☐ Single ☐ Married ☐ Married, but withhold at higher Single rate.
Note. If married, but legally separated, or spouse is a nonresident alien, check the "Single" box.

City or town, state, and ZIP code

4 If your last name differs from that shown on your social security card, check here. You must call 1-800-772-1213 for a replacement card. ▶ ☐

5 Total number of allowances you are claiming (from line **H** above **or** from the applicable worksheet on page 2)   **5** _____

6 Additional amount, if any, you want withheld from each paycheck . . . .   **6** $ _____

7 I claim exemption from withholding for 2007, and I certify that I meet **both** of the following conditions for exemption.
- Last year I had a right to a refund of **all** federal income tax withheld because I had **no** tax liability **and**
- This year I expect a refund of **all** federal income tax withheld because I expect to have **no** tax liability.

If you meet both conditions, write "Exempt" here . . . . ▶   **7** _____

Under penalties of perjury, I declare that I have examined this certificate and to the best of my knowledge and belief, it is true, correct, and complete.

Employee's signature
(Form is not valid unless you sign it.) ▶

Date ▶

8 Employer's name and address (Employer: Complete lines 8 and 10 only if sending to the IRS.)   **9** Office code (optional)   **10** Employer identification number (EIN)

For Privacy Act and Paperwork Reduction Act Notice, see page 2.   Cat. No. 10220Q   Form **W-4** (2007)

Figure 12-9 *Update all Employee's Withholding Allowance Certificates (Forms W-4) at least once a year.*

Service benefit plans: Cover certain medical or surgical services without any additional cost to the insured. There are no scheduled set fees.

Government Plans

Government policies: Government-sponsored insurance coverage for eligible individuals. The federal government provides coverage under Medicare, Medicaid, TRICARE or CHAMPUS, and CHAMPVA.

Medicare Plans

The Original Medicare Plan: Provides health insurance to citizens aged 65 and older and to younger patients who are blind or widowed or who have serious long-term disabilities, such as kidney failure. Medicare Part A covers hospital, nursing facility, home health, hospice, and inpatient care. Those who are eligible for Social Security benefits are automatically enrolled in Medicare Part A. Medicare Part B covers outpatient services, services by physicians, durable medical equipment, and other services and supplies. Medicare Part B coverage is optional. Everyone eligible for Part A can choose to enroll in Part B by paying monthly premiums. Deductibles must be met in Parts A and B before payment benefits begin.

Diagnosis-related groups (DRGs): Groups of procedures or tests related directly to a diagnosis. The fixed fees paid by Medicare Part A are based on DRGs. In other words, Medicare uses DRGs to determine appropriate reimbursement for medical diagnoses and procedures, as do many private insurers. DRGs are assigned in the hospital when a patient is discharged.

Medicare fee schedule (MFS): Providers participating in Medicare must accept the charges listed in this schedule as payment for covered services. The MFS is developed by using the Resource-Based Relative Value Scale. The participating physician may bill the patient for coinsurance and deductibles but may not collect excess charges.

Resource-Based Relative Value Scale (RBRVS): A system used by Medicare since 1992 to determine uniform payments for medical services that take geographic differences into account. A relative value unit is determined for each medical service on the basis of the physician's work, time, and skill and the provider's expenses, such as the costs of running the office and malpractice insurance.

Medicare supplements (Medigap policies): Private insurance contracts that supplement regular Medicare coverage. They are kept uniform in their benefits so as not to be confusing to purchasers. These supplemental plans pay for a beneficiary's deductibles, for coinsurance, and in some cases for services not covered by Medicare. If the subscriber has Medigap insurance, Medicare is still the primary payer, which means that claims must be filed with Medicare first. If a patient has both Medicare and Medicaid, charges must be filed with Medicare first, and Medicaid is the secondary payer.

Medicare + Choice Plans

Medicare also offers a group of plans called the Medicare + Choice Plans. Beneficiaries can choose to enroll in one of three major types of plans instead of the Original Medicare Plan:

1. Medicare Managed Care Plans
2. Medicare Preferred Provider Organization Plans
3. Medicare Private Fee-for-Service Plans

Medicare Managed Care Plans: These plans charge a monthly premium and a small copayment for each office visit, but not a deductible. Like private payer managed care plans, Medicare managed care plans often require patients to use a specific network of physicians, hospitals, and facilities. Some plans offer the option of receiving services from providers outside the network for a higher fee. All plans offer coverage for services not reimbursed in the Original Medicare Plan, such as physical examinations and inoculations. Participants are generally required to select a primary care provider (PCP) from within the network. The PCP provides treatment and manages the patient's medical care through referrals.

Medicare Preferred Provider Organization Plans (PPOs): In these plans, physicians, hospital, and other health-care providers join together and agree to offer services to members of a group (subscribers) at a lower cost or discount. Patients pay less to use doctors within a network, but they may choose to go outside the network for additional costs, such as a higher copayment or higher coinsurance. Patients do not need a PCP, and referrals are not required. This can give the individual more control over his or her health care.

Medicare Private Fee-for-Service Plans: Patients in these plans receive services from the provider they choose, as long as Medicare has approved the provider or facility. The plan is operated by a private insurance company that contracts with Medicare to provide services to beneficiaries. The plan sets its own rates for services, and physicians are allowed to bill patients the amount of the charge not covered by the plan. A copayment may or may not be required.

Medicaid Plans

Medicaid: A health benefit program designed for low-income people (people receiving welfare payments or other forms of public assistance) who cannot pay their medical bills. People covered under Medicaid are categorically needy, medically needy, or medically indigent. Eligibility for coverage might vary from month to month

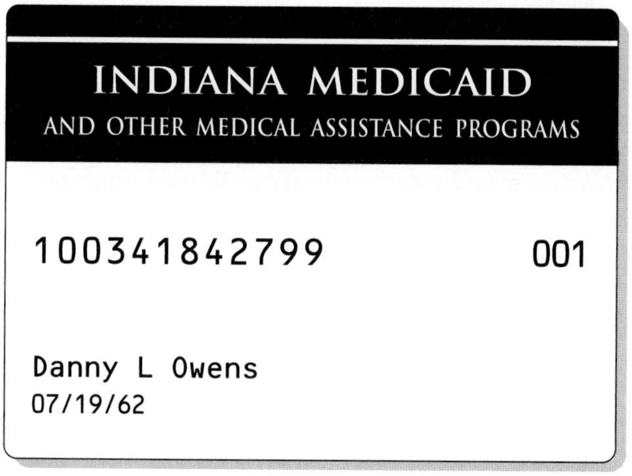

INDIANA MEDICAID
AND OTHER MEDICAL ASSISTANCE PROGRAMS

100341842799   001

Danny L Owens
07/19/62

Figure 13-1 *A Medicaid card gives the patient's name and identification (or Social Security) number.*

based on the recipient's income. Medicaid is a health-cost assistance program, not an insurance program, and physicians may choose to accept or not to accept Medicaid patients. By treating Medicaid patients, physicians accept Medicaid reimbursement for covered services and cannot charge patients for any difference. In some states, Medicaid is known by a different name. For example, in California Medicaid is called MediCal. Always ask for a Medicaid card from patients who state that they are entitled to Medicaid coverage (See Figure 13-1).

Third-party liability: An obligation of a governmental program or insurance plan to pay all or part of a patient's medical costs. Eligibility for Medicaid does not relieve Medicare of its responsibility to cover health-care costs. In other words, Medicaid is always a secondary carrier or a payer of last resort.

Medi/Medi: Older or disabled patients who have Medicare and who cannot pay the difference between the bill and the Medicare payment may qualify for Medicare and Medicaid. This type of coverage is known as Medi/Medi. In such cases, Medicare is the primary payer, and Medicaid is the secondary payer.

State guidelines: Medicaid benefits can vary from state to state. It is important to understand the Medicaid guidelines in your state so that your office's Medicaid reimbursement is prompt and without complications. Here are some suggestions:

- Always ask for a Medicaid card from patients who state that they are entitled to Medicaid.

- Check the patient's Medicaid card, which is issued monthly and shows the patient's eligibility for services or procedures.

- Ensure that the physician signs all claims. Then send them to the state's Medicaid-approved contactor (which pays on behalf of the state) or to the state department that administers Medicaid (for example, the state department of social services or public health).

- Unless the patient has a medical emergency, Medicaid often requires authorization before services are performed.

- Check the time limit on claim submissions. It can be as short as 2 months or as long as 1 year.

- Meet the deadlines. If a Medicaid claim is submitted after the time limit, the claim may be rejected.

- Treat Medicaid patients with the same professionalism and courtesy that you extend to other patients. Simply because a patient qualifies for Medicaid assistance does not mean that the patient is in any way inferior to those with private insurance.

TRICARE and CHAMPVA

TRICARE: TRICARE (formerly CHAMPUS) and CHAMPVA are the most common health-care policies you will encounter when caring for individuals in the military and their families. They are run by the Defense Department. TRICARE is a health-care benefit for families of uniformed personnel and retirees from the uniformed services, including the Army, Navy, Marines, Air Force, Coast Guard, Public Health Service, and National Oceanic and Atmospheric Administration. TRICARE offers families three choices of health-care benefits:

1. TRICARE Prime, a health maintenance organization

2. TRICARE Extra, a managed care network of health-care providers that families can use on a case-by-case basis without a required enrollment

3. TRICARE Standard, a fee-for-service plan

TRICARE for Life: A program aimed at Medicare-eligible military retirees and Medicare-eligible family members. This program offers the opportunity to receive health care at a military treatment facility to individuals aged 65 and older who are eligible for both Medicare and TRICARE.

CHAMPVA: Stands for *Civilian Health and Medical Program of the Veterans Administration.* It covers the expenses of the families of veterans with total, permanent, service-connected disabilities. It also covers surviving spouses and dependent children of veterans who died in the line of duty.

DEERS: Stands for *Defense Enrollment Eligibility Reporting System*, maintained by the Department of Defense. DEERS is a worldwide database of people covered by TRICARE.

Payments under TRICARE and CHAMPVA: Payments on assigned claims are made directly to the physician. As with Medicaid, the physician who does not participate has the option to accept assignment on a case-by-case basis.

Cost-share: The term TRICARE and CHAMPVA use for coinsurance.

Catastrophic cap: The maximum amount a beneficiary might need to pay out as coinsurance within a span of a year. When the cap is reached, TRICARE and CHAMPVA pay all allowed charges for the rest of the year.

Avoiding duplication: TRICARE and CHAMPVA are primary payers when an insured individual also has Medicaid. If the insured is also covered under Medicare, claims must be filed with Medicare first. TRICARE and CHAMPVA also do not pay for illnesses or injuries covered by workers' compensation unless compensation benefits have been exhausted. Claims must be filed within 1 year from date of service.

Private Plans

Coverage with private insurance companies: Physicians and medical societies control neither the premiums paid nor the benefits received from such policies. Insurance payments may be made to the subscriber and not to the physician.

Blue Cross and Blue Shield (BCBS) Association: A nationwide federation of local nonprofit service organizations that offer prepaid health-care services to subscribers. Under a prepaid health coverage plan, the carrier will pay for specified medical expenses if premiums are paid in advance. The Blue Cross part of BCBS covers hospital services, outpatient and home care services, and other institutional care. Blue Shield covers physician services and dental, vision, and other outpatient benefits. Some local BCBS organizations help the government administer Medicare, Medicaid, and TRICARE programs.

Local BCBS organizations: Operate under the laws of the states in which they are located. There are 86 local BCBS plans in the United States, each with its own claim form. Plans make direct payments to member physicians, but payments may be made to the subscriber (patient) if the physician is a nonmember. Many small groups and individuals who may not be able to get coverage elsewhere can join a BCBS Plan. Some plans offer coverage regardless of medical condition during special periods of time. Plans must also get permission from the state to raise their rates.

Blue Card Program: The Blue Card Program is a nationwide program that makes it easy for patients to receive treatment when outside their local service area, and also makes it easy for providers to receive payment when treating patients enrolled in plans outside the provider's services area.

Customary maximum: The term BCBS plans use to describe the fee based on actual fees charged by most physicians in the community.

Fixed fee schedule: A list used by BCBS plans of maximum fees allowed for specific services.

Blue card: An agreement among BCBS plans through which a local plan may provide benefits for any out-of-town BCBS plan subscriber.

Kaiser Foundation Health Plan: A type of prepaid group practice (HMO). The Kaiser Foundation was a pioneer of nonprofit prepaid group practice beginning in California in 1933. The plan owns the medical facilities and directly employs the physicians and other providers.

Workers' compensation: A contract that insures a person against on-the-job injury or illness. The employer is responsible for the premium payment. See Table 13-1 on managing workers' compensation cases. Generally, a workers' compensation plan covers only specific medical bills, such as laboratory bills, physicians' fees, and

AT A GLANCE	Managing Workers' Compensation Cases

If your medical practice accepts workers' compensation cases, you should follow this procedure when contacted by a patient:

- Call the patient's employer to verify that the accident occurred on the employer's premises.

- Obtain the employer's approval to provide treatment.

- Ask the employer for the name of the workers' compensation insurance company.

- Remind the employer to report the accident or injury to the state labor department.

- Contact the insurance company to verify that the employer has a policy in good standing.

- Obtain a claim number from the insurance company.

- Create a patient record.

Table 13-1

other medical services. Lost income is not covered by this policy.

Managed Care

Managed care organizations: Organizations that manage, negotiate, and contract for health care with the goal of keeping costs down. Managed care organizations sign up health-care providers who agree to charge a fixed fee for services. These fixed fees are set by the managed care organization or by the governmental agency responsible for managed care.

Cost-containment practices: Developed by insurance carriers such as managed care organizations to keep premiums as low as possible. Such practices may include, for example, requiring fewer overnight stays after certain surgeries or requiring preauthorization of a service before the procedure is performed.

Health maintenance organization (HMO): A type of managed care program that provides specific services to enrollees. Enrollees are expected to receive treatment only from participating providers, and they may see specialists only when referred by their primary care physicians, who act as gatekeepers.

Group model HMO: Physicians in this type of an arrangement see both members of the HMO and non-member patients, and they remain self-employed. Physicians receive fixed payments from the HMO for each member patient, rather than reimbursement for the services provided. This fixed fee is paid to the physician monthly regardless of the number of times the patient visits the physician. This type of reimbursement is called capitation. Examples of a group model HMO include independent practice associations (IPAs) and network model HMOs.

Staff model HMO: Under this arrangement, the physicians are employees of the HMO and work full time seeing member patients. In this type of HMO, a primary care physician is assigned as the gatekeeper for patients.

Preferred provider organization (PPO): A type of managed care plan in which enrollees receive the highest level of benefits when they obtain services from a physician, hospital, or other health provider designated by their program as a preferred provider. Enrollees receive reduced benefits when they obtain care from a provider who is not designated as a preferred provider by their program. PPO patients may see specialists without prior authorization from their primary care physicians. HMOs offering point-of-service options are more like PPOs.

Point-of-service: An option added to some HMO plans that allows patients to choose a physician outside the HMO network and to pay increased deductibles and coinsurance.

Physician-hospital organization (PHO): An approach to coordinating services for patients, in which physicians join hospitals to create an integrated medical care delivery system. This union then makes arrangements for insurance with a commercial carrier or an HMO.

Fee-for-service: A system of retrospective reimbursement in which the physician or other provider bills for each service that is provided. BCBS is a fee-for-service plan.

Capitation: A system of payment used by managed care plans in which physicians and hospitals are paid a fixed, per capita amount for each patient enrolled over a stated period of time, regardless of the type and number of services provided.

Withhold: A portion of the monthly capitation payment to physicians retained by an HMO until the end of the year to create an incentive for efficient care. If the physician exceeds utilization norms, he or she will not receive this portion.

Relative value scale (RVS): A system of assigning values to medical services on the basis of an analysis of the skill and time required to provide them. Both indemnity plans and many managed care plans are moving to this approach for assigning allowed charges. The RVS assigns numerical values to medical services, which then have to be multiplied by a dollar conversion factor to calculate fees.

Precertification: A call to the patient's insurance carrier to find out whether the treatment, surgery, tests, or hospitalization is covered under the patient's health insurance policy.

Preauthorization: Permission by the insurance carrier that must be obtained before giving a certain treatment to a patient.

Utilization management: A process, based on established criteria, of reviewing and controlling the medical necessity for services and providers' use of medical care resources. In managed care systems such as HMOs, reviews are done to establish medical necessity.

Referrals: In managed care, the primary care physician needs to refer a patient to a specialist before that patient can make an appointment with the specialist. A referral form must be completed, showing the following information:

- Referring physician
- Specialist to whom the patient is being referred
- Diagnosis
- Treatment (past and present, including medications)
- Chart notes
- Minor surgical procedures

Types of referrals: There are three types of referral:

- Regular referral, which usually takes 3 to 10 days.
- Urgent referral, which usually takes 24 hours.
- STAT referral, which can be done on the phone immediately.

Authorization: A referral that is approved.

Insurance claim reimbursement criteria: There are four bases for determining payment:

- UCR charges
- The Medicare RBRVS
- Fee schedules
- DRGs

The most common reason for the return of insurance claim forms is missing or mistyped information. To minimize the chance of errors, it is extremely important always to proofread all claims before submitting them.

Steps in claims processing: Following are the general steps in processing a claim:

1. Gather health insurance information from the patient and verify insurance coverage.
2. Complete the CMS-1500 claim form.
3. Base the claim on the superbill, which lists the name and address of the patient, the name of the insurance carrier, the insurance identification number, a brief description of each service by code number, the fee for the service, the place and date of service, the diagnosis, the physician's name and address, and the physician's signature. You should also have the current editions of the ICD-9-CM and the *Current Procedural Terminology* (CPT), for diagnostic and procedural coding.
4. If possible, use electronic claims submission. Prepare claims on a computer and submit them via modem to the insurance carrier's computer system. Such claims are also called electronic media claims (EMCs).
5. Track insurance claims. Follow up with the insurance company until the claim is paid in a timely manner.
6. Remember that if a claim form is not sufficiently detailed, complete, and accurate, it will be rejected by the insurance company.

Tracing: If after 30 days the insurance company has not paid the claim or responded to a claim, the choices are to bill again or to call the carrier. Because second billings are sometimes rejected as duplicates, the medical office can send a tracer, a letter to the insurance company containing the basic billing information.

Rebilling: Make a copy of the original claim form submitted and write *SECOND BILLING* in red letters at the top. Reasons to rebill include:

- The insurance company is delinquent in responding to a claim.
- A mistake has been made in billing.
- Charges must be detailed to receive maximum reimbursement.

- A claim was overlooked by the physician's office.
- The carrier asked for rebilling because the wrong diagnosis or procedure codes were submitted, some information was incomplete or missing, or the charges did not total properly.

Reasons claims are denied or payments are delayed:

- The claim is not for a covered contract benefit. Bill the patient.
- The patient's preexisting condition is not covered. Bill the patient.
- The patient's coverage has been canceled. Bill the patient.
- Workers' compensation is involved, and the case is under consideration. Check on the claim's progress every 30 days.
- The insurance company considers the physician's procedure to be experimental. Call the carrier to discuss options. Peer review may be requested.
- No preauthorization was obtained. Review the patient's contract and what the sanctions are. Write a letter of appeal if appropriate.
- The physician provided services before the patient's health insurance contract went into effect. Bill the patient.
- The carrier asks for additional information. Send the carrier the requested information and follow up in 30 days.

Claim appeal: A written request to the insurance carrier to review reimbursement. It is usually filed if the preauthorization was not obtained because unusual circumstances exist, the reimbursement was inadequate for a complicated procedure, the physician disagrees that the patient's condition was preexisting, or the patient has unusual circumstances that affect medical treatment.

Medicare claims processing: Guidelines for processing Medicare claims are:

- Providers are required by law to file the CMS-1500 for all eligible patients.
- Providers may be participating or nonparticipating.
- PAR providers accept assignment on Medicare claims and receive the allowed fee.
- NonPAR providers are not required to accept assignment; therefore, the patient is responsible for the balance after Medicare makes its payment. See Table 13-2.
- The allowable payment to nonPAR providers is less than the payment to PAR providers.
- Medicare forms must be signed by both the patient and the physician.

Participating Provider		Nonparticipating Provider	
Physician's standard fee:	$120.00	Physician's standard fee:	$120.00
Medicare PAR fee:	$ 60.00	Medicare nonPAR fee:	$ 57.00
Medicare pays 80% of Medicare fee:	$ 48.00	Medicare pays 80% of nonPAR fee:	$ 45.60
Patient or supplemental plan pays:	$ 12.00	Patient or supplemental plan pays:	$ 11.40
Provider writes off:	$ 60.00	Provider writes off:	$ 63.00

Table 13-2   Note: These charges do not represent realistic or accurate medical service fees. They are used here merely as an example.

- Claims for Medicare must be filed by December 31 of the year following that in which the services were rendered.

Medicaid claims processing: Guidelines for processing Medicaid claims are:

- A physician is free to accept or refuse to treat a patient under Medicaid.
- A patient's eligibility should be verified before the delivery of medical service.
- Preauthorization may be required for the service.
- Claims should be filed on the CMS-1500.
- There is always a time limit for filing claims, according to state regulations.

Medi/Medi claims processing: Guidelines for processing Medi/Medi claims are:

- A physician must always accept assignment.
- A claim form is first processed through Medicare and is then automatically forwarded to Medicaid.
- It is not necessary to prepare two claim forms. The combined claim is sometimes referred to as a crossover claim.

BCBS claims processing: Guidelines for processing Blue card claims are:

- Claims should be submitted as soon as possible after the service is provided.
- Like Medicare, the Blue plans have arrangements with PAR and nonPAR providers. Usually a PAR provider is paid directly for covered services and agrees not to bill the patient for any difference.
- Blue plans have provider manuals that describe coverage and coding features of the plan.

TRICARE claims processing: Guidelines for processing a TRICARE claim are:

- Use the CMS-1500 claim form.
- If the physician accepts assignment (i.e., the physician is a PAR provider), the medical office files the insurance claim and the patient can be billed for the entire deductible and the coinsurance portion of the allowed charge.
- If the physician does not accept assignment, the patient must submit claim forms to the insurance company and is responsible for all charges.
- The claims must be filed no later than December 31 of the year following that in which services were provided.
- PAR providers are paid within 21 days after submitting a claim, and only PAR providers may appeal a claims decision.

CHAMPVA claims processing: CHAMPVA claims follow the same guidelines as TRICARE claims.

Workers' compensation claims processing: Follow these guidelines:

- Records of the workers' compensation case should be kept separate from the patient's regular history.
- The insurance carrier is entitled to receive copies of all records pertaining to the industrial injury.
- The injured person's records must be personally signed by the physician.
- The insurance carrier may supply its own billing forms.
- Payment is usually made on the basis of a fee schedule.

- At the termination of the treatment, a final report and bill are sent to the insurance carrier.
- Do not bill the patient.

Legal Considerations

Legal and ethical issues: There are a variety of legal and ethical issues associated with processing claims:

- Stay current on the laws that affect medicine.
- It is the physician's responsibility to identify the procedures that have been performed. Code only for procedures that appear in the medical records. If you think that a certain procedure has been left out by accident, tell the physician to update the medical records before you file a claim.
- An incorrect code used for billing a service can be considered fraud.
- Obtain patient signatures permitting insurance billing.
- Obtain proper authorization from the insurance carrier whenever required.

Fraud: Occurs when someone intentionally misrepresents facts to receive a benefit illegally. A person who cooperates in a fraudulent situation becomes personally liable, or legally responsible. Some fraudulent actions include:

- Altering a patient's chart to increase the amount reimbursed
- Upgrading or falsifying medical procedures to increase the amount reimbursed
- Billing primary or secondary insurance carriers while at the same time collecting payment from the patient
- Under Medicare law, not attempting to collect a required payment from a Medicare patient

Because an incorrect code can seem like fraud, it is very important to code accurately and keep good records of the coordination of benefits.

STRATEGIES TO SUCCESS

▶ Test-Taking Skills

Circle key words?
Do not get a question wrong just because you misread what it was asking you. Circle key words in the question such as *best, not, except, always, never, all,* and any other words that relate to the main point in the question. Doing so will force you to focus on the central point so that you can untangle even more complicated questions.

Instructions:

Answer the following questions. Check your answers in the *Answer Key* that follows this section.

1. The range of fees charged by most physicians in a community is called the
   - A. Customary fee
   - B. Reasonable fee
   - C. Usual fee
   - D. Premium
   - E. Average fee

2. If a child is covered by both of her parents' insurance and the total medical charges come to $365, $280 of which is covered by the primary insurance, how are the rest of the charges handled?
   - A. The parents are billed for $85
   - B. A claim is submitted to secondary insurance for $85
   - C. A claim is submitted to secondary insurance for $365
   - D. The doctor writes off $85, and no one is charged
   - E. A claim is submitted to secondary insurance for $280

3. Which of the following is an example of fraud?
   - A. Miscoding a diagnosis unintentionally
   - B. Leaving a field blank on the CMS-1500 by mistake
   - C. Altering a patient's chart to increase the amount reimbursed
   - D. Releasing patient's medical records without the patient's consent to the patient's wife because you feel morally obligated to do so
   - E. All of the above

4. A participating provider in a managed healthcare program must write off
   - A. Disallowed charges
   - B. Coinsurance
   - C. Copayments
   - D. Deductibles
   - E. Amounts due from the carrier

5. Which of the following Medicare programs covers hospital charges?
   - A. Part A
   - B. Part B
   - C. Part C
   - D. Both Parts A and B
   - E. None of the above

6. If Medicare sends a check for payment to the medical office, the physician is considered which one of the following parties?
   - A. Participating
   - B. Sponsoring
   - C. Accepting
   - D. Eligible
   - E. Registered

7. Assume that John Smith got an X-ray through Dr. Jones, a participating provider in Mr. Smith's HMO. The allowed charge for such an X-ray is $75, but Dr. Jones's usual fee is $100. John Smith's copayment due for each office visit is $15. How much can Dr. Jones collect from Mr. Smith?
   - A. $25
   - B. $10
   - C. $15
   - D. $0
   - E. $75

8. If a person is covered under both Medicare and Medicaid, to which program should the claim be sent first?
   A. Medicaid
   B. Medicare
   C. Both should get it at the same time
   D. Neither; the patient has to be billed
   E. Neither; claims are sent to an independent government agency to decide

9. The amount due from the patient for covered services from a participating provider is the difference between
   A. The allowed charge and the physician's fee
   B. The allowed charge and the patient's deductible and/or coinsurance
   C. The physician's fee and the coinsurance
   D. The physician's fee and the deductible
   E. The physician's fee and the capitation

10. Which of the following types of medical insurance is designed to offset medical expenses resulting from prolonged injury or illness?
    A. Basic medical
    B. Hospital coverage
    C. Disability protection
    D. Liability insurance
    E. Major medical

11. Which of the following is a third-party health plan that is funded by the federal government?
    A. Blue Cross and Blue Shield
    B. Starmark
    C. Aetna
    D. TRICARE
    E. Physician's Mutual

12. Which of the following is true about Blue Cross and Blue Shield?
    A. It offers prepaid health services
    B. It helps Medicare to determine covered health services
    C. It follows a fee-for-service reimbursement plan
    D. Both A and C
    E. All of the above

13. Capitation is
    A. Payment at the time of service
    B. Fixed prospective payment for services provided
    C. Fixed payment made for each enrolled patient rather than reimbursement based on the type and number of services provided
    D. Various payments for specific services provided during a specified time period
    E. A reduction in payment if services are not provided to a minimum number of enrolled patients

14. Providers are required by law to file which of the following for all eligible Medicare patients?
    A. CMS
    B. HCPCS
    C. ICD-9
    D. RBRVS
    E. CMS-1500

15. If a nonparticipating provider's charge for a service is $65 and the allowed charge is $50, the amount due from the patient is
    A. $10
    B. $65
    C. $50
    D. $15
    E. $115

16. The most common insurance claim form is the
    A. Superbill
    B. Charge sheet
    C. CMS-1500
    D. ICD-9
    E. None of the above

17. If a policy holder of an 80:20 plan had foot surgery that cost $3,600, how much of this bill is the subscriber responsible to pay?
    A. $450
    B. $720
    C. $180
    D. $2,880
    E. $3,600

18. An authorization to the insurance company to make payments directly to the physician is called
    A. HCFA-1500 claim form
    B. Assignment of benefits
    C. Tracker
    D. Coordination of benefits
    E. Service benefit plan

19. The primary difference between an HMO and a PPO is that
    A. An HMO locks patients into receiving services from providers with whom it has contracts whereas a PPO allows patients to choose among providers in return for higher deductibles and copayments
    B. In an HMO patients may select specialists, whereas in a PPO patients must see specialists to whom they were referred
    C. HMOs pay for all services completely except preventive check-ups whereas PPOs do not pay for services completely but do partially cover preventive medicine
    D. An HMO has fee-for-service contracts with providers whereas a PPO has a capitation model for reimbursement
    E. All of the above

20. TRICARE is a health-care benefit program for all of the following except
    A. The Coast Guard
    B. The National Oceanic and Atmospheric Administration
    C. The Navy
    D. Families of uniformed personnel
    E. Families of veterans with service-related disabilities

21. Fee-for-service reimbursement is
    A. Retroactive payment made after services are provided
    B. Fixed prospective payment for services provided during a specified time period
    C. Payment at the time of service
    D. Various payments for specific services provided during a specified time period
    E. Fixed payment made each month for an estimated total of services provided, which is calculated according to the number of member patients

22. A patient's medical fees come to a total of $600 from a participating provider, and the EOB lists the following information:

Charges:	$78
Not Eligible for Payment:	$15
Allowed Charge:	$63
Applied to Deductible:	$ 7
Coinsurance:	$ 5
Amount Due From Carrier:	$51

What amount is the patient required to pay?
    A. $7
    B. $5
    C. $27
    D. $12
    E. Nothing

23. In the point-of-service option,
    A. Plan members can see out-of-network providers for additional fees
    B. Providers are employees of the HMO
    C. The HMO has capitation contracts with provider groups
    D. Contracts exist with an administrative group of physicians that in turn contracts with its provider-members
    E. Physicians receive fixed payments for each nonmember patient rather than reimbursement for the services provided

24. In the group network model,
    A. Providers are employees of the HMO
    B. The HMO has capitation contracts with provider groups
    C. Contracts exist with an administrative group of physicians that in turn contracts with members
    D. Plan members can see out-of-network providers for additional fees
    E. Providers are paid on a fee-for-service basis

ANSWER KEY

1.	A	13.	C
2.	B	14.	E
3.	C	15.	D
4.	A	16.	C
5.	A	17.	B
6.	A	18.	B
7.	C	19.	A
8.	B	20.	E
9.	B	21.	A
10.	E	22.	D
11.	D	23.	A
12.	D	24.	B

Basic Coding

CHAPTER OUTLINE

MEDICAL ASSISTING COMPETENCIES

COMPETENCY	CMA	RMA
Administrative		
Apply managed care policies and procedures	X	X
Analyze and apply third-party guidelines	X	X
Perform procedural and diagnostic coding	X	X
Complete insurance claim forms	X	X
General/Legal/Professional		
Be aware of and perform within legal and ethical boundaries	X	X
Use appropriate medical terminology		X

1. Locate the statement of the diagnosis in the patient's medical record. If needed, decide which is the main term or condition of the diagnosis.

2. Find the diagnosis in the ICD's *Alphabetic Index*. Look for the condition first. Then find descriptive words that make the condition more specific. Read all cross-references to check all the possibilities for a term and its synonyms.

3. Locate the code from the *Alphabetic Index* in the ICD's *Tabular List*. Remember that the number to check is a code number and not a page number. The *Tabular List* gives codes in numerical order. Look for the number in bold-faced type.

4. Read all information to find the code that corresponds to the patient's specific disease or condition. Study the list of codes and descriptions. Be sure to pick the most specific code available. Check for the symbol that shows a five-digit code is required.

5. Record the diagnosis code on the insurance claim and proofread the numbers. Enter the correct diagnosis code on the health-care claim, checking that

   • The numbers are entered correctly.
   • The codes are complete.
   • The highest (most specific) code is used.

Table 14-2

Tabular List—Volume 1

The *Tabular List* has 17 chapters of disease descriptions and codes, with 2 additional types of codes and 5 appendixes. This volume classifies diseases and injuries according to their etiology and organ systems, dividing them into five groups:

1. Anatomical system or type of condition
2. Related groups of codes
3. Third digit (category codes)
4. Fourth digit (subcategory codes)
5. Fifth digit (subclassification codes)

Alphabetic Index—Volume 2

The *Alphabetic Index* of the ICD-9-CM provides the following information:

• An index of the disease descriptions in the *Tabular List*
• An index in table format of drugs and chemicals that cause poisoning
• An index of external causes of injury, such as accidents

Special Codes

In addition to the 17 chapters in Volume 1, 2 supplementary classifications are provided in the ICD-9-CM:

V codes and E codes. When recording a code from these two classifications, always write the alphabetical character first to distinguish the V or E code from a diagnosis code that has the same number of digits but no alphabetical character.

V codes: V codes are used as the primary code to describe an encounter between a provider and an individual without a specific current health-care illness or injury. For example V codes cover screening, such as a mammogram or a colonoscopy; preventive medicines, such as vaccinations; fertility testing and treatments; prenatal checkups; and baby exams. They are used when healthy patients receive services, receive treatment for a current or resolving condition, or are evaluated preoperatively. Some V codes, however, are never primary.

E codes: E codes are used to classify environmental (external) causes of injury, poisoning, or other adverse effects on the body, such as falls, fires, transportation accidents, and accidental poisoning by a drug or other substances. An external cause is not the primary diagnosis of a patient's condition, so E codes are never used alone. These codes are very important, because the event or element that caused the injury may require a different insurance company to pay for these medical expenses.

Symbols: Commonly used ICD-9-CM symbols include the following:

• The square symbol (□) precedes a disease code to indicate that the content of a four-digit category has been moved or modified.

- A bullet point (•) indicates a new entry.
- The triangle symbol (▲) indicates a revision in the *Tabular List* and a code change in the *Alphabetic Index*.
- Facing triangle symbols (▶ ◀) mark both the beginning and the end of new or revised text.

Procedure Codes

After an office visit, each procedure and service performed for a patient is reported on the health-care claim by using a procedure code. The procedure codes (Volume 3 of the ICD) are primarily used in hospitals and other facilities to code the procedures performed in those settings.

Using the CPT

Current Procedural Terminology, commonly known as the CPT, is the most commonly used system of procedure codes. The CPT is published by the American Medical Association (AMA) and is the HIPAA-required code set for physicians' procedures. The CPT is published every year to reflect changes in medical practice. These changes are also available electronically for medical offices that use a computer-based version of the CPT.

Locating Correct Codes

CPT codes are five-digit numbers, organized into six sections (see Table 14-3). Medical offices should have the current year's CPT available for reference. Previous editions of this book should also be kept in case there is a question about already-submitted insurance claims. Figure 14-2 provides examples of CPT codes.

Add-on codes: Used for procedures that are usually carried out in addition to another procedure. A plus sign (+) is used to symbolize these codes. Add-on codes are never reported alone. They are used together with the primary code.

Modifiers: Indicate that a procedure was different from the standard description, but not in a way that changed the definition or required a different code. Modifiers are used primarily in the following instances:

- A service or procedure was performed more than once, or by more than one physician.
- A service or procedure has been increased or reduced.
- Unusual difficulties occurred during the procedure.
- Only part of a procedure was performed.

Symbols: Commonly used CPT symbols include the following:

- A bullet point (•) indicates a new procedure code.
- A triangle (▲) indicates a change in the code's description.
- Facing triangles (▶ ◀) are placed at the beginning and end of new or revised information.
- A plus sign (+) is used for add-on codes, indicating procedures that are usually carried out in addition to another procedure.
- An arrow (→) with a circle around it refers to the CPT Assistant.
- An asterisk (*) indicates a surgical procedure only.

AT A GLANCE	CPT Codes	
Section	**Range of Codes**
Evaluation and Management	99201-99499
Anesthesiology	00100-01999, 99100-99140
Surgery	10040-69990
Radiology	70010-79999
Pathology and Laboratory	80049-89399
Medicine (except Anesthesiology)	90281-99199

Table 14-3

Surgery

General

(10000-10020 have been deleted. To report see 10060, 10061)

10021 Fine needle aspiration; without imaging guidance
➔ *CPT Assistant* Aug 02:10; *CPT Changes: An Insider's View* 2002

10022 with imaging guidance
➔ *CPT Changes: An Insider's View* 2002

(For radiological supervision and interpretation, see 76003, 76360, 76393, 76942)

(For percutaneous needle biopsy other than fine needle aspiration, see 20206 for muscle, 32400 for pleura, 32405 for lung or mediastinum, 42400 for salivary gland, 47000, 47001 for liver, 48102 for pancreas, 49180 for abdominal or retroperitoneal mass, 60100 for thyroid, 62269 for spinal cord)

(For evaluation of fine needle aspirate, see 88172, 88173)

Integumentary System

Skin, Subcutaneous and Accessory Structures

Incision and Drainage

(For excision, see 11400, et seq)

10040 Acne surgery (eg, marsupialization, opening or removal of multiple milia, comedones, cysts, pustules)

10060 Incision and drainage of abscess (eg, carbuncle, suppurative hidradenitis, cutaneous or subcutaneous abscess, cyst, furuncle, or paronychia); simple or single

10061 complicated or multiple

10080 Incision and drainage of pilonidal cyst; simple

10081 complicated

(For excision of pilonidal cyst, see 11770-11772)

10120 Incision and removal of foreign body, subcutaneous tissues; simple

10121 complicated

(To report wound exploration due to penetrating trauma without laparotomy or thoracotomy, see 20100-20103, as appropriate)

(To report debridement associated with open fracture(s) and/or dislocation(s), use 11010-11012, as appropriate)

10140 Incision and drainage of hematoma, seroma or fluid collection
➔ *CPT Changes: An Insider's View* 2002

(If imaging guidance is performed, see 76360, 76393, 76942)

10160 Puncture aspiration of abscess, hematoma, bulla, or cyst
➔ *CPT Changes: An Insider's View* 2002

(If imaging guidance is performed, see 76360, 76393, 76942)

10180 Incision and drainage, complex, postoperative wound infection

(For secondary closure of surgical wound, see 12020, 12021, 13160)

Excision—Debridement

(For dermabrasions, see 15780-15783)

(For nail debridement, see 11720-11721)

(For burn(s), see 16000-16035)

11000 Debridement of extensive eczematous or infected skin; up to 10% of body surface

+ 11001 each additional 10% of the body surface (List separately in addition to code for primary procedure)

(Use 11001 in conjunction with code 11000)

11010 Debridement including removal of foreign material associated with open fracture(s) and/or dislocation(s); skin and subcutaneous tissues
➔ *CPT Assistant* Mar 97:1, Apr 97:10, Aug 97:6

11011 skin, subcutaneous tissue, muscle fascia, and muscle
➔ *CPT Assistant* Mar 97:1, Apr 97:10, Aug 97:6

11012 skin, subcutaneous tissue, muscle fascia, muscle, and bone
➔ *CPT Assistant* Mar 97:1, Apr 97:10, Aug 97:6

11040 Debridement; skin, partial thickness
➔ *CPT Assistant* Fall 93:21, May 96:6, Feb 97:7, Aug 97:6

11041 skin, full thickness
➔ *CPT Assistant* Fall 93:21, May 96:6, Feb 97:7, Aug 97:6

11042 skin, and subcutaneous tissue
➔ *CPT Assistant* Winter 92:10, May 96:6, Feb 97:7, Aug 97:6

11043 skin, subcutaneous tissue, and muscle
➔ *CPT Assistant* May 96:6, Feb 97:7, Apr 97:11, Aug 97:6

11044 skin, subcutaneous tissue, muscle, and bone
➔ *CPT Assistant* Fall 93:21, Mar 96:10, May 96:6, Feb 97:7, Apr 97:11, Aug 97:6

(Do not report 11040-11044 in addition to 97601, 97602)

Figure 14-2 *Examples of CPT codes, surgical section.*
Source: American Medical Association, *Current Procedural Terminology* © 2003.

Sections	Codes
Transportation services	A0000-A0999
Medical and surgical supplies	A4000-A4999
Miscellaneous and experimental	A9000-A9999
Enteral and parenteral therapy	B4000-B9999
Dental procedures	D0000-D9999
Durable medical equipment (DME)	E0000-E9999
Procedures and services, temporary	G0000-G9999
Drugs administered other than by oral method	J0000-J8999
Chemotherapy drugs	J9000-J9999
Temporary codes for durable medical equipment regional carriers	K0000-K9999
Orthotic procedures	L0000-L4999
Prosthetic procedures	L5000-L9999
Medical services	M0000-M9999
Pathology and laboratory	P0000-P9999
Temporary codes	Q0000-Q0099
Diagnostic radiology services	R0000-R5999
Vision services	V0000-V2999
Hearing services	V5000-V5999

Table 14-4

HCPCS

The Health-Care Financing Administration (HCFA) Common Procedure Coding System, commonly referred to as HCPCS, is used to report procedures and services for Medicare patients. This system is also used to report most Medicaid services. HCPCS has three code levels, referred to as Level I, Level II, and Level III.

Level I codes: These codes repeat the CPT's five-number codes for physician procedures and services.

Level II codes: These codes consist of more than 2400 five-digit alphanumerical codes for items that are not listed in CPT-4. Most of these items are supplies, materials, or injections that are covered by Medicare. Level II codes start with a letter followed by four digits, such as J7630. There are 18 sections, each covering a related group of items. See Table 14-4.

Level III codes: Commonly called local carrier codes, these codes are created and used only by the insurance companies that process Medicare for HCFA in the various geographical regions they are assigned.

Avoiding Fraud

Physicians have the ultimate responsibility for proper documentation and correct coding, as well as for compliance with regulations. Medical assistants help ensure maximum appropriate reimbursement for reported services by submitting correct health-care claims. Ensuring that the proper steps are taken to avoid incorrect coding, false claims, and data entry errors helps to ensure that no fraud takes place in the coding and claims submission process.

Fraud: An act of deception used to take advantage of another person or entity. Claims fraud occurs when physicians or others falsely represent services or charges to payers. Examples of fraud include the following:

- A provider who bills for services that were not performed, overcharges for services, or fails to provide complete services under a contract
- A patient who exaggerates an injury to get a settlement from an insurance company, or one who asks a medical assistant to change a date on the patient's chart so that a service is covered by a health plan

Code linkage: The connection between the diagnostic and procedural information on a health-care claim. Insurance company representatives analyze this connection to evaluate the medical necessity of the reported charges.

Coding for coverage: Changing a code to match what the insurance company will pay for, rather than to accurately reflect the procedure that was performed.

Upcoding: Using a code on a claim form that indicates a higher level of service than that which was actually performed.

Double billing: Submitting two claims for one encounter.

Correct Coding Initiative (CCI): A computerized system used by Medicare to prevent overpayment for procedures.

Mutually exclusive codes: Codes that are identified in the coding book as not permitted to be used on the same claim form with other specified codes.

Instructions:
Answer the following questions. Check your answers in the *Answer Key* that follows this section.

1. Which of the following is an example of fraud?
   A. Miscoding a diagnosis unintentionally
   B. Mistakenly leaving a field blank on the CMS-1500 claim form
   C. Altering a patient's chart to increase the amount reimbursed
   D. Releasing a patient's medical records to his wife without the patient's consent because you feel morally obligated to do so
   E. The doctor writes off the amount due as "no charge" to the patient

2. Because coding information is revised annually, medical assistants responsible for coding should
   A. Attend at least one CPT class each year
   B. Attend at least one ICD-9 class every 2 years
   C. Attend at least one ICD-9 and one CPT class every 2 years
   D. Attend at least one CPT and one ICD-9 class each year
   E. Review codes in their spare time; there is no need to attend classes

3. How many digits are assigned to the primary code in the CPT coding system?
   A. 2
   B. 3
   C. 4
   D. 5
   E. 6

4. Which of the following sections of the CPT book refers to Evaluation and Management?
   A. 00100-01999
   B. 70010-79999
   C. 80000-89399
   D. 90701-99199
   E. 99201-99499

5. According to the CPT, when a health-care claim for the removal of a melanoma is coded, the code should be listed under which of the following body systems?
   A. Respiratory
   B. Integumentary
   C. Digestive
   D. Endocrine
   E. Cardiovascular

6. The ICD-9-CM codes for classifying the causes of injuries, poisonings, or adverse drug reactions are
   A. E codes
   B. M codes
   C. G codes
   D. V codes
   E. J codes

7. The Medicare Level II codes are included in which of the following?
   A. Resource-Based Relative Value Scale (RBRVS)
   B. CPT
   C. Diagnosis-related groups (DRGs)
   D. ICD-9-CM
   E. HCPCS

8. Which of the following is a diagnostic coding system that is used to code morbidity?
   A. *Physicians' Desk Reference*
   B. HCPCS
   C. Resource-Based Relative Value Scale (RBRVS)
   D. ICD-9-CM
   E. CPT

9. ICD-9-CM codes are revised, expanded, and refined annually to ensure
   A. Specificity of disease
   B. Speed of claims processing
   C. Bundling of codes
   D. Accuracy of insurance claims
   E. Accuracy of diagnosis

10. Which of the following is indicated by a triangle (▲) placed before a CPT code?

    A. A code has been deleted
    B. A new code has been added
    C. A code description has been changed or modified
    D. A procedure is not subject to the surgical package concept
    E. Multiple procedures have been performed

11. Which of the following is a coding system used by Medicare providers to report supplies and injections?

    A. Relative value scale (RVS)
    B. Resource-based relative value scale (RBRVS)
    C. HCPCS
    D. ICD-9-CM
    E. Diagnosis-related groups (DRGs)

12. When using ICD-9-CM codes, which of the following will occur when the fourth and fifth digits are omitted?

    A. Faster payments
    B. Claim denials
    C. Third-party downcoding
    D. Third-party upcoding
    E. Increased payments

13. Which of the following ICD-9-CM codes indicates the cause of an accident?

    A. V14.6
    B. J1772
    C. E811.0
    D. J49999
    E. V18.8

14. Changing a code to one you know the insurance company will pay for is called

    A. Double billing
    B. Unbundling
    C. Coding for packaging
    D. Coding for coverage
    E. Supporting documentation

15. Which of the following is the most important factor in coding?

    A. Level of codes
    B. Quantity of codes
    C. Accuracy of codes
    D. Speed of coding process
    E. Knowledge and understanding of medical term

16. Which of the following is a coding system used to document the procedure for suturing a laceration?

    A. Relative value studies (RVS)
    B. Resource-based relative value scale (RBRVS)
    C. Diagnostic-related groups (DRGs)
    D. International Classification of Diseases, Clinical Modification (ICD-CM)
    E. Current Procedural Terminology (CPT)

17. A two-digit modifier attached to the five-digit CPT code indicates

    A. The severity of the patient's illness
    B. The time services were performed
    C. A service or procedure has been altered
    D. A surgical procedure was performed
    E. Where services were performed

Contaminated: Exhibiting the presence of blood or other potentially infectious materials.

Biohazard: Anything that poses a risk to the human body or other living organism, such as blood (which can cause the spread of infections), chemical materials, or ionizing radiation.

Biohazard container: A leakproof, puncture-resistant container that is color-coded red or labeled with a biohazard symbol and is used to store and dispose of contaminated supplies and equipment. When a biohazard container is filled to the three-quarter mark, it should be placed in a locked storage area until pickup. All biohazard containers must have a fluorescent orange or orange-red label with the biohazard symbol and the word *BIOHAZARD* in a contrasting color. Every container must have a lid that is replaced after use. These containers are used for disposable gowns, table covers, items contaminated with blood and body fluids, dressings, gloves, needles, and sharp objects.

Sharps: Needles, scalpels, scissors, or other objects that could cause wounds or punctures to individuals handling them.

Needlestick injuries: Accidental skin punctures resulting from contact with hypodermic syringe needles. These injuries can be dangerous, particularly if the needle has been used in a patient with a severe blood-borne infection. Needles should never be recapped or broken. They must be discarded immediately into a biohazard container. If an injury occurs, wash your hands, cover the injury, report and document the injury, and get the injury treated.

Exposure potential: The possibility of bodily contact with a safety hazard, a hazardous chemical, or blood or other potentially infectious material.

Hazardous chemical: A chemical that is explosive, unstable, flammable, carcinogenic, or irritating or that contains toxic agents.

Occupational exposure: Contact with blood or other potentially infected body fluids that occurs as a result of the normal duties of an employee at work.

Disease Profiles

Hepatitis

Hepatitis: Inflammation and infection of the liver that may be caused by several factors, such as drugs, toxins, and microorganisms. The most common cause of hepatitis is a virus. There are six known hepatitis viruses, designated A, B, C, D, E, and G.

Hepatitis A: Inflammation of the liver caused by the hepatitis A virus (HAV), which is transmitted by fecal-oral contamination. Hepatitis A is not generally considered to be an important risk to health-care workers. It is also called acute infective hepatitis.

Hepatitis B: Inflammation of the liver caused by the hepatitis B virus (HBV). It is the main blood-borne hazard for health-care workers. HBV can be transmitted through contaminated serum and plasma; contaminated needles (involved in needlestick injuries or IV drug use); cuts caused by contaminated sharps; sexual contact with an infected person; and splashes of contaminated material onto the eyes, mouth, nose, or broken skin. HBV is also transmitted from infected mothers to newborns. It is a severe infection that may cause a prolonged illness and become a chronic disease resulting in destruction of liver tissues, cirrhosis, or death. It is also known as serum hepatitis. The virus is capable of surviving for at least a week in a dried state on environmental surfaces.

Acute hepatitis B: Approximately one third of all patients are asymptomatic. The initial symptoms, if present, last from 2 to 14 days. No specific treatment or drug kills the hepatitis virus. About 90% of patients recover fully after the acute phase.

Chronic hepatitis B: About 10% of patients who do not recover from the acute phase go on to develop chronic hepatitis. These patients face an increased risk of liver damage, cirrhosis of the liver, liver cancer, or liver failure.

Hepatitis B vaccine: Approximately 90% effective in providing immunity for at least 7 years. The vaccine is recommended as a series of three intramuscular doses in infants, children, adolescents, and adults. Employers must offer this vaccine within 10 days of employment if there is a reasonable expectation of exposure to the virus. At the present time, a routine booster dose is not recommended. The hepatitis B vaccine is recommended for the following individuals:

- Health-care workers in high-risk occupations, such as physicians, dentists, dental hygienists, medical assistants, nurses, and laboratory personnel
- Staff members of residential institutions
- Sexually active homosexual men
- Intravenous drug users
- Persons with hemophilia
- Hemodialysis patients
- Household members or sexual contacts of hepatitis B carriers

Hepatitis C (non-A, non-B hepatitis): A chronic disease transmitted largely by blood transfusion or intravenous drug use (sharing needles). Diagnosis is made by detecting HCV antibodies.

Hepatitis D: Also called delta hepatitis, a form of viral hepatitis that occurs only in patients infected with hepatitis B; consequently, it can be prevented by hepatitis B vaccination. The hepatitis D virus (HDV) is transmitted through needle-sharing and sex. Diagnosis is made by detecting HDV serum antibodies. It is not common in the United States.

Hepatitis E: A common acute infection of the liver, similar to hepatitis A, seen mainly in Southeast Asia,

South America, and Africa. Hepatitis E is frequently seen in the rainy season or after natural disasters because of fecally contaminated water or food. There is no serological test available for the detection of the hepatitis E virus (HEV). The disease is most dangerous in pregnant women and increases the mortality rate among them.

Hepatitis G: Inflammation of the liver caused by the single-stranded RNA flavivirus. Mode of spread is usually blood and possibly semen. Incubation period for hepatitis G may be weeks. There is no vaccine, and the symptoms are usually mild. Viremia may be persistant for months or years.

HIV and AIDS

HIV: The human immunodeficiency virus that causes AIDS. It is passed from one person to another through blood-to-blood and sexual contact. Infected pregnant women can pass the virus to their babies during pregnancy or delivery or by breast-feeding. It is not spread through casual contact. HIV infects and destroys T lymphocytes (T cells) of the immune system.

HIV transmission: HIV has been isolated in blood, semen, saliva, tears, breast milk, cerebrospinal fluid (CSF), amniotic fluid, urine, and vaginal secretions. No cases of AIDS have been reported as a result of exposure to saliva or tears.

AIDS: Acquired immunodeficiency syndrome, caused by HIV. It is a fatal disease that attacks the immune system and is characterized by severe opportunistic infections and rare cancers. Approximately 70% of HIV-infected people develop AIDS within 10 years. An HIV-infected person is diagnosed as having AIDS after development of one of the indicator illnesses or on the basis of certain blood tests.

Risk factors for HIV transmission: The risk factors for HIV transmission are generally the same as the risk factors associated with HBV. People at risk include:

- Those with multiple sexual partners
- Those who have had unprotected anal, vaginal, or oral sex
- Intravenous drug users who share needles
- Sexual partners of an infected person
- Infants born to HIV-positive women

Stages of AIDS: A person who is HIV-positive without any symptoms for months or even years is known as a carrier of HIV. The AIDS virus infection cycle has four stages: acute HIV infection, asymptomatic latency period, AIDS-related complex (ARC), and full-blown AIDS.

Acute HIV infection: An infection that lasts from 3 days to a month. Symptoms are often mistaken for those of other viral infections and include fever, sweats, fatigue, loss of appetite, diarrhea, pharyngitis, myalgia, arthralgia, and adenopathy.

Asymptomatic latency period: A long incubation period, sometimes lasting for years. During this period, the infected individual is asymptomatic. The only evidence of infection during this phase is the body's production of HIV antibodies. These HIV antibodies, however, are unable to destroy the virus. This period is a confounding factor in tests for the presence of HIV infection, because testing may fail to detect HIV for as long as 3 to 6 months after an individual has been infected.

AIDS-related complex (ARC): A syndrome resulting from HIV infection but lacking an opportunistic infection or Kaposi's sarcoma. Patients with ARC often have chronic systemic symptoms, including enlarged lymph nodes, fever, diarrhea, weight loss, fatigue, and dementia. Most people with ARC progress to having full-blown AIDS.

Final stage of AIDS: Full-blown AIDS is characterized by the presence of opportunistic infections and unusual cancers. A severe pneumonia caused by *Pneumocystis carinii* is commonly seen in AIDS patients, and Kaposi's sarcoma, a rare type of cancer, frequently occurs.

Opportunistic infections: Infections that occur when normal immunity is altered. If the immune system cannot respond to a microbe that it would normally eliminate, the infection that results is termed opportunistic. These infections cause most of the morbidity and mortality in AIDS because they attack many different organs of the body. See Figure 15-1. These infections also play a major role in the diagnosis of AIDS. The lungs are the most commonly involved organ system in AIDS and are the principal target for *Pneumocystis carinii* and atypical tuberculous bacteria.

Drug treatments: There is no cure for HIV or AIDS; however, a growing number of drugs are available for the treatment of these diseases. Because more than 20 drugs are available for treatment, an individual with HIV or AIDS who has had no success with one regimen or treatment might find success with another. This is important for increasing life expectancy. Table 15-1 identifies different classifications of drugs currently approved by the FDA for the treatment of diseases associated with HIV infection and AIDS.

Kaposi's sarcoma: A malignancy of the skin and lymph nodes that often occurs in AIDS patients. It is the most common HIV-related cancer and usually appears as painless nodules and reddish purple to dark blue colors on the body.

***Pneumocystis carinii* pneumonia:** A type of pneumonia caused by the parasite *Pneumocystis carinii*, usually seen in patients with HIV infection. Its symptoms include fever, tachypnea, cough, and cyanosis. The diagnosis is not easy to make. The mortality rate in untreated patients is approximately 100%.

Tuberculosis: A disease that is often curable when treatment regimens are followed exactly and completely. However, there has been a rise in the number of cases in recent years as a result of HIV infection and antibiotic resistance. HIV infection is the single largest risk factor for the development of tuberculosis infection into the active form of the disease.

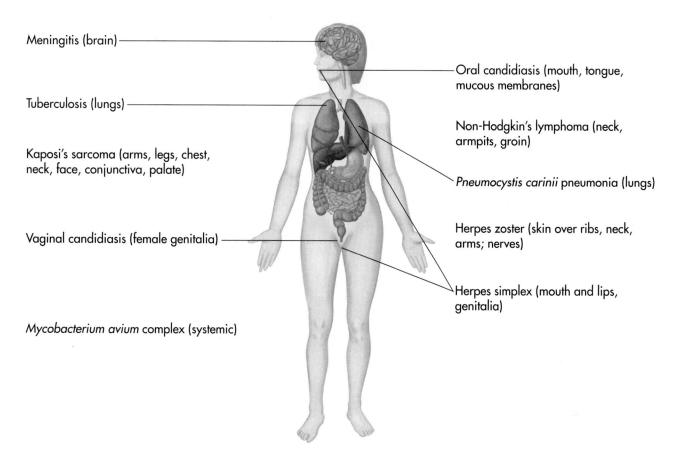

Meningitis (brain)

Tuberculosis (lungs)

Kaposi's sarcoma (arms, legs, chest, neck, face, conjunctiva, palate)

Vaginal candidiasis (female genitalia)

Mycobacterium avium complex (systemic)

Oral candidiasis (mouth, tongue, mucous membranes)

Non-Hodgkin's lymphoma (neck, armpits, groin)

Pneumocystis carinii pneumonia (lungs)

Herpes zoster (skin over ribs, neck, arms; nerves)

Herpes simplex (mouth and lips, genitalia)

Figure 15-1 *The AIDS patient may contract a variety of opportunistic infections, which affect many different parts of the body.*

Serological tests: The only readily available method to detect evidence of HIV infection. There are two serological tests used to detect antibodies to HIV: enzyme-linked immunosorbent assay (ELISA) and western blot technique.

HIV antibody testing: Since 1992, recommendations issued by the Centers for Disease Control and Prevention (CDC) have called for the voluntary testing of people who are at high risk for HIV infection. HIV antibody testing is federally mandated for all military applicants and is also required for those who donate organs, tissue, sperm, or blood.

Inactivation of HIV: HIV is readily destroyed by heat treatment and exposure to disinfectants. The most common disinfectant is 10% NaClO (sodium hypochlorite, the active ingredient in household bleach).

Other Blood-Borne Pathogens

Syphilis: A sexually transmitted disease caused by the spirochete *Treponema pallidum*. The incubation period is 10 to 90 days. There are three stages. The first stage (primary syphilis) is marked by a single lesion, called a chancre. Syphilis can be treated with penicillin.

Malaria: A severe infectious disease caused by one or more of four species of the protozoan genus *Plasmodium*. The disease is transmitted by mosquitoes. It can also be spread by blood transfusion from an infected patient or by the use of an infected hypodermic needle.

Brucellosis: A disease caused by the gram-negative coccobacillus *Brucella*. It is most prevalent in rural areas among farmers, veterinarians, meat packers, and livestock producers. The ingestion of unpasteurized milk from infected stock can also cause brucellosis.

Leptospirosis: An acute infectious disease caused by the spirochete *Leptospira interrogans*, transmitted in the urine of wild or domestic animals, especially dogs and rats. Human infections arise directly from contact with an infected animal's urine or tissue or indirectly from contact with contaminated water or soil.

Toxoplasmosis: An infection caused by *Toxoplasma gondii*, transmitted in cat feces. Pregnant women and AIDS patients should not handle cat litter boxes. During pregnancy, the mother may pass the infection to her fetus through the placenta. Toxoplasmosis can result in spontaneous abortion, retardation, and malformation. It can also cause blindness, deafness, and brain damage.

Cytomegalovirus: One of the most common infections. As many as 80% of adults have been exposed to it. In AIDS patients it may cause severe lung disease. Pregnant women may transmit this infection to the fetus through the placenta, which results in brain damage, mental retardation, blindness, deafness, or death.

Classification & Function	Generic Name (Trade Name)	Major Side Effects
Fusion Inhibitor Blocks viral entrance into the human cell	enfuvirtide; 2003 (Fuzeon®)	Bacterial pneumonia, allergic reaction, injection site infections
Nonnucleoside Reverse Transcriptase Inhibitors (NNRTIs) Block the ability of HIV to make copies of itself	delavirdine; 1997 (Rescriptor®)	Skin rash, eye inflammation, fever, joint or muscle pain, oral lesions, swelling
	efavirenz; 1998 (Sustiva®)	Skin rash, depression
	nevirapine; 1996 (Viramune®)	Skin rash, liver disease, chills and fever, sore throat, oral lesions
Nucleoside Reverse Transcriptase Inhibitors (NRTIs) Block the ability of HIV to make copies of itself	abacavir sulfate; 1998 (Ziagen®)	Fatal hypersensitivity reaction, liver disease
	abacavir + lamivudine + Zidovudine; 2000 (Trizivir®)	Fatal hypersensitivity reaction, liver disease
	didanosine; 1991 (Videx®)	Severe gastralgia, nausea, vomiting; burning, numbness, or tingling of the hands, arms, feet or legs; visual disturbances
	emtricitabine; 2003 (Emtirva®)	Nausea, vomiting, abdominal pain, anorexia, weight loss, dyspnea, fatigue
	lamivudine; 1995 (Epivir®)	Burning, numbness, pain, or tingling in the hands, arms, feet, or legs; fever muscle aches, nausea, vomiting, skin rash
	lamivudine + zidovudine; 1997 (Combivir®)	Burning, numbness, pain, or tingling in the hands, arms, feet, or legs; fever, muscle aches, nausea, vomiting, skin rash, unusual tiredness or weakness
	stavudine; 1994 (Zerit®)	Burning, numbness, pain, or tingling in the hands, arms, feet, or legs; fever, muscle aches, nausea, vomiting, skin rash
	tenofovir disoproxil fumarate; 2001 (Viread®)	Liver or kidney failure, lactic acidosis, pancreatitis

Table 15-1

Classification & Function	Generic Name (Trade Name)	Major Side Effects
	zalcitabine; 1992 (HIVID®)	Gastralgia, nausea, vomiting; burning, numbness, pain, or tingling in the hands, arms, feet, or legs; skin rash, ulcerative stomatitis
	zidovudine; 1987 (Retrovir, AZT, ZDV®)	Fatigue, weakness, fever, chills, sore throat
Protease Inhibitors (PIs) Block the ability of HIV to make copies of itself	amprenavir; 1999 (Agenerase®)	Severe rash, changes in body fat, increased cholesterol, hyperglycemia
	atazanavir; 2003 (Reyataz®)	Jaundice, heart block, hyperglycemia, diarrhea, nausea; infection, hematuria
	fosamprenavir; 2003 (Lexiva®)	Severe rash, changes in body fat, increased cholesterol, hyperglycemia
	indinavir; 1996 (Crixivan®)	Nephrolithiasis, changes in body fat, hyperglycemia
	lopinavir + ritonavir; 2000 (Kaletra®)	Pancreatitis, hyperglycemia, nephrolithiasis
	nelfinavir; 1997 (Viracept®)	Changes in body fat, hypercholesterolemia, hyperglycemia
	ritonavir; 1996 (Norvir®)	Pancreatitis, hyperglycemia, hyperlipidemia
	saquinavir; 1997 (Fortovase®)	Changes in body fat, hyperglycemia

Table 15-1, concluded

Note: The number following the generic drug name represents the date or dates the drugs were approved for the specified purpose.
Source: U.S. Department of Health and Human Services; Food and Drug Administration and AIDSInfo

Medical and Surgical Asepsis

Medical asepsis: Also referred to as the clean technique, used to maintain cleanliness in order to prevent the spread of microorganisms and to ensure that there are as few microorganisms in the medical environment as possible. This technique is usually used for noninvasive procedures.

Surgical asepsis: Also referred to as the sterile technique, used to create a completely sterile environment without the presence of any microorganisms. This procedure is used for invasive or surgical techniques. When you are performing the sterile technique, it is important that nothing interrupts this process and that things are done in the correct order. If there is any question that an area might be contaminated, consider it contaminated and sterilize again.

Aseptic Precautions

Office procedures: The following procedures help promote asepsis:

- Separate areas in the waiting room for well and sick patients

Remove all jewelry, except plain gold wedding bands.
Use a paper towel to turn on faucets, and adjust the temperature to moderately warm.
Wet your hands and apply liquid soap. Liquid soap in a foot pump dispenser is less likely to accumulate dirt.
Work the soap into a lather, and make sure that both of your hands are covered in lather. Rub vigorously in circular motions for at least 2 minutes. Keep your hands lower than your forearms so that the dirty water flows into the sink instead of back onto your arms. Interlace your fingers, and clean the palms and between the fingers.
Use a nailbrush or orange stick to dislodge dirt from the cuticles and nails.
Rinse your hands well, keeping your hands lower than your forearms and not touching the sink or faucets.
With the water still running, dry your hands with clean, dry paper towels, and then use clean, dry paper towel to turn off the faucets. Discard the paper towels.

Table 15-2

- Maintenance of a well-lit, well-ventilated, draft-free office with a room temperature of approximately 72°(F)
- Prohibition of eating and drinking in the office
- Disposal of trash as often as needed
- Elimination of insects from the office
- Signs asking patients to use tissues, put waste in the trash cans, report safety or health hazards, and tell the receptionist if they are nauseated or need to use the restroom

Cross-contamination: Perform procedures in a way that avoids cross-contamination. For example, do not place the lid of a sterile container face down on a surface, and do not pour tablets or capsules into your hand.

Hand washing: One of the most important methods of medical asepsis. Wash your hands:

- At the beginning of the day
- After breaks
- Before and after using the restroom
- Before and after lunch
- Before and after using gloves
- Before and after handling specimens or waste
- Before and after handling clean or sterile supplies
- Before and after performing any procedure
- After blowing your nose or coughing
- Before leaving for the day

Aseptic hand washing: Removes accumulated dirt and microorganisms that could cause infection. Table 15-2 describes how to perform aseptic hand washing, and Figures 15-2 and 15-3 show two important steps in washing your hands.

Hand hygiene: The CDC has released new recommendation for hand hygiene in health-care settings. *Hand hygiene* is a term that applies to either hand washing or

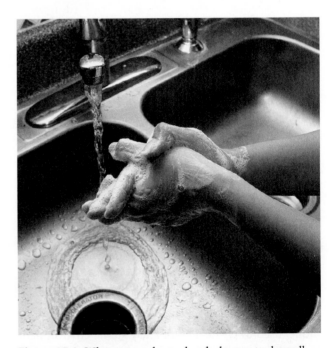

Figure 15-2 *When you wash your hands, be sure to clean all surfaces, including the palms and between the fingers.*

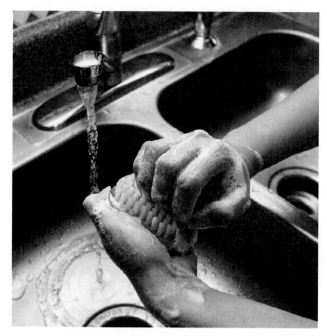

Figure 15-3 *The nails and cuticles require additional attention to ensure that all dirt is removed.*

using an antiseptic hand rub (surgical hand antisepsis. Hand antisepsis with an antiseptic hand rub is more effective in reducing nosocomial infections than plain hand washing.

Surgical scrub: Similar to aseptic hand washing, with the following differences:

- A sterile scrub brush is used instead of a nail brush.
- Hands and forearms are washed.
- Hands are held above the elbows so that water cannot run from the arms onto washed areas.
- Sterile towels are used instead of paper towels.
- Sterile gloves are put on immediately after the hands are dried.

Infection Control

Sanitization: Reducing the number of microorganisms on an object or surface to a fairly safe level by scrubbing it with hot, soapy water. It is used to clean items that touch only healthy, intact skin, such as:

- Blood pressure cuff
- Ophthalmoscope
- Otoscope
- Penlight
- Reflex hammer
- Stethoscope
- Tape measure
- Tuning fork

Ultrasonic cleaning: Used to sanitize delicate instruments and those with moving parts. It involves placing the instruments in a special bath that generates sound waves through a cleaning solution.

Disinfection: The process of destroying infectious agents by chemical or physical means. It is used for instruments that do not penetrate a patient's skin or that come in contact only with a patient's mucous membranes or other surfaces not considered sterile, such as:

- Enamelware
- Endotracheal tubes
- Glassware
- Laryngoscopes
- Nasal specula

Disinfectants: Cleaning products that reduce or eliminate infectious organisms on instruments or equipment. Common disinfectants are chemical germicides, household bleach, boiling water, and steam. Ten percent bleach solution reduces or eliminates infections agents for 24 hours.

Antiseptics: Cleaning products used on human tissues as anti-infection agents.

Germicides: Germ-killing additives. The use of soap in the process of disinfection is less important than the scrubbing and rinsing steps, but germicides may increase the effectiveness of soap.

Sterilization: A destruction of all living microorganisms. It is required for all instruments and supplies that penetrate a patient's skin or come in contact with any normally sterile areas of the body. It is also required for instruments that will be used in a sterile field. Examples of items that need to be sterilized are:

- Curettes
- Needles
- Syringes
- Vaginal specula

Autoclave: A device that forces the temperature of steam above the boiling point of water in order to sterilize instruments and equipment.

Autoclave procedures: Take the following steps when using the autoclave:

1. Wrap sanitized and disinfected instruments and equipment, and label each pack. See Figure 15-4.
2. Clean and preheat the autoclave.
3. Perform quality control procedures.
4. Load the instruments and equipment, allowing adequate space around the items.
5. Set the autoclave for the correct time.
6. Run the autoclave through the cycle, including the drying time.
7. Remove the instruments and equipment.

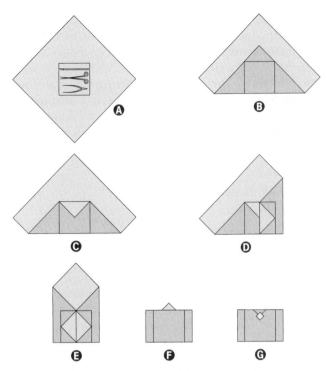

Figure 15-4 *Follow this sequence when you wrap instruments in a paper or fabric pack for sterilization in an autoclave.*

8. Store the instruments and equipment for the next use.
9. Clean the autoclave and the surrounding work area.

Sterilization indicators: Tags, inserts, tapes, tubes, or strips that confirm that the items in the autoclave have been exposed to the correct volume of steam at the correct temperature for the correct length of time.

Chemical sterilization: Used on instruments that would be damaged by prolonged exposure to the high temperatures in a steam autoclave.

Dry heat sterilization: Used on items that would be damaged by immersion in chemical solution or by exposure to steam.

Gas sterilization: Uses ethylene oxide, a hazardous gas. It may be performed only in hospital and manufacturing environments.

Microwave sterilization: The fastest method, using low-pressure steam with radiation.

OSHA Requirements

OSHA: The U.S. Department of Labor's Occupational Safety and Health Administration, which requires basic safety practices, including infection control, and develops federal regulations that aim to protect health-care workers from health hazards on the job, particularly from accidentally acquiring infections.

OSHA Blood-Borne Pathogens Standard of 1991: A set of regulations to protect health-care workers, patients, and other visitors from health hazards. It:

- Requires employers to identify, in writing, tasks, procedures, and job classifications that involve occupational exposure to blood.
- Mandates universal precautions, emphasizing engineering and work practice controls.
- Requires employers to provide and employees to use personal protective equipment.
- Requires a written schedule for cleaning, identifying the method of decontamination to be used, and specifies methods of disposing of regulated waste.
- Specifies procedures to be made available to all employees who have had an exposure incident, including a confidential medical evaluation.
- Requires warning labels, including the biohazard symbol, to be affixed to containers of regulated waste and other containers used to store or transport blood or other potentially infectious materials.
- Mandates training within 90 days of the effective date of assignment and annually thereafter.
- Calls for confidential medical records of employees to be kept for the duration of employment plus 30 years.

Failure to comply with OSHA standards: Could result in a maximum penalty of $7,000 for the first violation, and up to $70,000 for repeated violations. See Table 15-3.

Universal Precautions: An approach to infection control, in which all human blood and certain other human body fluids are treated as if they were known to be infectious for HIV, HBV, and other blood-borne pathogens. Universal Precautions apply to blood and blood products; human tissue; semen and vaginal secretions; saliva from dental procedures; cerebrospinal, synovial, pleural, peritoneal, pericardial, and amniotic fluids; and other body fluids if visibly contaminated with blood or of questionable origin in the body. See Figures 15-5 and 15-6.

Standard Precautions: A combination of Universal Precautions and rules to reduce the risk of disease transmission by means of moist body substances. Standard Precautions apply to blood, other body fluids, secretions, excretions (except sweat), nonintact skin, and mucous membranes. Standard Precautions are used in hospitals for the care of all patients. In medical offices, you use Universal Precautions when dealing with patients.

Work practice controls: Controls that reduce the likelihood of exposure by altering the manner in which a task is performed, such as prohibiting the recapping of needles by using two hands.

Category I tasks: Tasks that expose a worker to blood, body fluids, or tissues, such as assisting with removal of

Infectious Waste Disposal: Penalties for Not Following OSHA Regulations

Type of Violation	Characteristics of Violation	Penalties for Violation
Other than serious violation	Direct relationship to job safety and health but would probably not result in death or serious injury	Fine of up to $7,000 (discretionary)
Serious violation	Substantial probability that death or serious physical harm could result and employer knew or should have known of the hazard	Fine of up to $7,000 (mandatory)
Willful violation	Violation committed intentionally and knowingly	Fine of up to $70,000, with a $5,000 minimum; in the event of the death of an employee, possible additional penalties, including 6 months' imprisonment
Repeated violation	Substantially similar violation found upon reinspection (not applicable if initial citation is under contest)	Fine of up to $70,000
Failure to correct	Initial violation not corrected	Fine of up to $7,000 for each day the violation continues after the date it was supposed to stop

Table 15-3

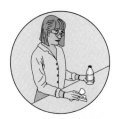 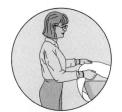 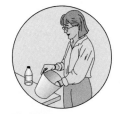 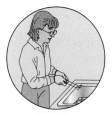 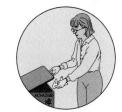

❶ Decontaminate exposed work areas. ❷ Replace exposed protective coverings. ❸ Decontaminate receptacles. ❹ Pick up broken glass. ❺ Discard infectious waste.

Figure 15-5 *Follow these OSHA guidelines to clean and decontaminate the medical environment after each procedure or treatment.*

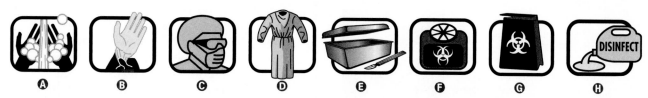

Figure 15-6 *These OSHA guideline icons represent (A) hand washing, (B) gloves, (C) mask and protective eyewear or face shield, (D) laboratory coat or gown, (E) reusable sharps container, (F) sharps disposal, (G) biohazardous waste container, and (H) disinfection.*

a cyst, and tasks that have a chance of spills or splashes. These tasks always require special protective measures.

Category II tasks: Tasks that usually do not involve a risk of exposure but that may involve exposure in certain situations. An example is giving mouth-to-mouth resuscitation. These tasks require precautions to be taken.

Category III tasks: Tasks that involve no exposure to blood, body fluids, or tissues and therefore do not require special protection. An example is giving a patient nose drops.

Postprocedure cleanup: OSHA requires the following steps:

- Decontaminate all exposed work surfaces with bleach or a germ-killing solution.
- Replace protective coverings on surfaces and equipment that have been exposed.
- Decontaminate receptacles.
- Pick up broken glass with tongs.
- Discard all potentially infectious waste materials in appropriate biohazardous waste containers.

Engineering controls: Controls, such as sharps disposal containers and self-sheathing needles, that isolate or remove the hazard of blood-borne pathogens.

Hand-washing facility: A facility providing an adequate supply of running potable water, soap, and single-use towels or hot-air drying machines.

Personal protective equipment: Specialized clothing or equipment worn by an employee for protection against a hazard. It includes gloves, lab coats, protective eyewear, face shields, surgical gowns, and shoe covers. See Figure 15-7.

Hazard warning label: Each hazardous chemical should be identified by a hazard warning label that displays the following information:

- A stated requirement that the chemical be kept in its original container
- A color code (blue for health hazards, red for flammability, yellow for reactivity, and white for specific hazards such as radioactivity)

- A numerical rating superimposed on each colored area of the label indicating a level of hazard from 0 (no hazard) to 4 (extreme hazard)

Decontamination: A term used by OSHA to describe the use of physical or chemical means to remove, inactivate, or destroy blood-borne pathogens on a surface or item to the point at which they are no longer capable of transmitting infection and the surface or item is rendered safe for handling, use, or disposal.

Regulated waste: Liquid or semiliquid blood or other potentially infectious materials contaminated items that would release blood or other potentially infectious materials in a liquid or semiliquid state if compressed items that are caked with blood or other potentially infectious materials and are capable of releasing these materials during handling contaminated sharps and pathological and microbiological wastes containing blood or other potentially infectious materials.

Storing biohazardous materials: OSHA regulations prohibit medical personnel from performing any of the following activities in a room where potentially infectious materials are present:

- Eating
- Drinking
- Smoking
- Chewing gum
- Applying cosmetics
- Handling contact lenses
- Chewing pencils or pens
- Rubbing eyes

You should have separate refrigerators in separate rooms for food and for biohazardous materials.

Refrigerators: To prevent spoilage or deterioration of testing kits and specimens, the temperature of the laboratory refrigerator should be maintained between 36° and 46°F (2° and 8°C).

STRATEGIES TO SUCCESS

▶ Test-Taking Skills

Choose the best answer!
When taking a multiple-choice test such as the CMA or RMA exam, you may find that the choices do not always include the perfect answer or what you think the answer should be. Remember, you must choose the best answer possible. When you return to a difficult question, you should try not to look at any of the given answers. Instead, supply your own answer and then look for the option that is the closest to your response.

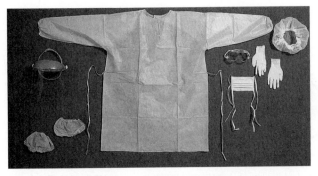

Figure 15-7 *Health-care workers may need to use various types of personal protective equipment, including gloves, masks and protective eyewear or face shields, gowns, and other protective clothing.*

Instructions:

Answer the following questions. Check your answers in the *Answer Key* that follows this section.

1. Potentially infectious body fluids include all of the following <u>except</u>

   A. Blood
   B. Vaginal secretions
   C. Sweat
   D. Cerebrospinal fluid
   E. Semen

2. Which color code for hazard warning labels is <u>not</u> correct?

   A. Blue for health hazards
   B. White for radioactivity hazards
   C. Yellow for radioactivity hazards
   D. Red for flammability
   E. All are correct

3. How long is hepatitis B virus capable of surviving in a dried state on environmental surfaces?

   A. 1 day
   B. 1 week
   C. 2 days
   D. 2 weeks
   E. 1 month

4. Clean technique is another term for

   A. Medical asepsis
   B. Surgical asepsis
   C. Hand washing
   D. Sterilization
   E. Sanitization

5. Instruments that penetrate a patient's skin should be

   A. Sanitized
   B. Disinfected
   C. Sterilized
   D. Treated with antiseptics
   E. Cleaned ultrasonically

6. Instruments that come in contact only with a patient's mucous membranes should be

   A. Sanitized
   B. Disinfected
   C. Sterilized
   D. Treated with antiseptics
   E. None of the above

7. Instruments that touch only healthy, intact skin should be

   A. Sanitized
   B. Disinfected
   C. Sterilized
   D. Treated with antiseptics
   E. Cleaned

8. The vaccine against hepatitis B provides immunity for at least

   A. 3 years
   B. 4 years
   C. 5 years
   D. 6 years
   E. 7 years

9. A syndrome resulting from HIV infection that generally involves chronic systemic symptoms but lacks an opportunistic infection or Kaposi's sarcoma is known as

   A. AIDS-related complex (ARC)
   B. Acute HIV infection
   C. AIDS
   D. Asymptomatic latency period
   E. None of the above

10. Which of the following is the only readily available method to detect evidence of HIV infection?

   A. Patient history
   B. Signs and symptoms
   C. Serological test
   D. Urinalysis
   E. None of the above

11. Which of the following organ systems is the most commonly involved in AIDS?
    A. Kidneys
    B. Ovaries
    C. Lungs
    D. Liver and spleen
    E. Stomach

12. Kaposi's sarcoma is a malignancy of the
    A. Skin and lungs
    B. Skin and brain
    C. Skin and kidneys
    D. Skin and bones
    E. Skin and lymph nodes

13. Anything that poses a risk to the human body or a living organism is called
    A. A pathogen
    B. An occupational exposure
    C. A biohazard
    D. Blood-borne
    E. A virus

14. Which of the following is a possible means of transmission of HIV?
    A. Saliva
    B. Tears
    C. Intact skin
    D. Blood
    E. Hair

15. OSHA standards require which of the following?
    A. A written schedule for cleaning
    B. Cleaning only when needed
    C. Cleaning only after procedures
    D. Cleaning by cleaning staff only
    E. Both A and D

16. Treating all human blood as if it were infectious is known as
    A. Engineering controls
    B. Work practice controls
    C. Asepsis
    D. Universal Precautions
    E. Isolation methods

17. Hand washing is necessary at which of the following times?
    A. Before using gloves
    B. Before leaving for the day
    C. After performing a procedure
    D. After using gloves
    E. All of the above

18. After you have rinsed your hands by using the aseptic hand washing method, what step should you take next?
    A. Using a nailbrush or orange stick, dislodge the dirt from your nails
    B. Turn off the faucets using your hands
    C. Hold your hands above the elbows to prevent water from running onto washed areas
    D. Put on sterile gloves
    E. Dry your hands with clean paper towels and turn off faucets by using a clean paper towel

19. Which of the following is not an example of personal protective equipment?
    A. Gloves
    B. A lab coat
    C. A surgical coat
    D. A uniform
    E. A face shield

20. To dispose of a contaminated needle,

    A. Recap it and drop it into the nearest biohazardous waste container
    B. Drop it into the biohazardous waste container for sharps
    C. Wash it, recap it, and drop it into the biohazardous waste container for sharps
    D. Sterilize it and put it into the biohazardous waste container
    E. Drop it in the nearest trash can

21. Surgical scrub involves washing

    A. Hands and forearms
    B. Hands
    C. Forearms
    D. Hands, forearms, and face
    E. All parts of the body before surgery

22. The autoclave

    A. Is used for instruments that would be damaged by prolonged exposure to high temperatures and steam
    B. Involves the use of soap and scrubbing to disinfect instruments
    C. Forces the temperature of steam above the boiling point of water in order to sterilize equipment
    D. Uses ethylene oxide and may be operated only in the hospital or a manufacturing environment
    E. Is used for items that would be damaged by immersion in a chemical solution or by exposure to steam

23. Standard Precautions are

    A. Used in all medically related fields
    B. Used mainly in hospitals
    C. Used mainly in medical offices
    D. Never used, because they are outdated
    E. The same as Universal Precautions

24. Medical asepsis is defined as which of the following?

    A. Growth of organisms after they leave the body
    B. Growth of organisms before they enter the body
    C. Destruction of organisms after they leave the body
    D. Destruction of organisms before they enter the body

25. Which of the following liquids is used in an autoclave to sterilize instruments and supplies?

    A. Tap water
    B. Distilled water
    C. Sterile water
    D. Alcohol
    E. Bleach

MEDICAL ASSISTING COMPETENCIES

COMPETENCY	CMA	RMA
Clinical		
Apply principles of aseptic techniques and infection control, including hand washing	X	X
Perform sterilization techniques	X	X
Dispose of biohazardous materials	X	X
Practice Standard Precautions	X	X
Obtain specimens for microbiological testing, including throat specimens and wound cultures	X	X
Interview the patient to obtain and record the patient's history	X	X
Prepare and maintain examination and treatment areas	X	X
Prepare the patient for and assist the physician with routine and specialty examinations, treatments, and minor office surgeries	X	X
Screen and follow up on patient test results	X	X
General/Legal/Professional		
Recognize and respond to verbal and nonverbal communications by being attentive and adapting communication to the recipient's level of understanding	X	X
Identify and respond to issues of confidentiality by maintaining confidentiality at all times and following appropriate guidelines when releasing records or information	X	X
Be aware of and perform within legal and ethical boundaries	X	X
Determine the needs for documentation and reporting, and document accurately and appropriately	X	X
Instruct individuals according to their needs	X	X
Provide patients with methods of health promotion and disease prevention	X	X
Perform an inventory of supplies and equipment	X	X
Operate and maintain facilities, and perform routine maintenance of administrative and clinical equipment safely	X	X
Maintain the physical plant		X
Evaluate and recommend equipment and supplies for practice		X
Conduct work within scope of education, training, and ability		X
Be impartial and show empathy when dealing with patients		X
Serve as a liaison between the physician and others		X
Interview effectively		X
Use appropriate medical terminology		X

Review frequently!

   As soon as possible after a lecture, it's important to spend some quiet time organizing and clarifying your notes. Doing so will help you retain and understand material much better than waiting until the night before the exam to take out your notes. Also review by rereading your notes throughout the course of your study. Test yourself on the material you should already know. If your instructor does not give midterm exams, give yourself one to check your progress. As you learn new information, try to link it to things you've already learned. For example, before reading the section on conducting medical interviews, you should go back and review the section on patient communication.

Patient Rights, Responsibilities, and Privacy

It is important to remember that all the data you obtain are subject to legal and ethical considerations. Most states have adopted a version of the American Hospital Association's Patient's Bill of Rights, written in 1973 and revised in 1992. Each state encourages health-care workers to be aware of and follow this document when caring for patients. The statement guarantees the patient's right to:

- Receive considerate and respectful care
- Receive complete and current information concerning his or her diagnosis, treatment, and prognosis
- Know the identity of physicians, nurses, and others involved with his or her care, as well as when those involved are students, residents, or trainees
- Know the immediate and long-term costs of treatment choices
- Receive information necessary to give informed consent before the start of any procedure or treatment
- Have an advance directive concerning treatment or be able to choose a representative to make decisions
- Refuse treatment to the extent permitted by law
- Receive every consideration of his or her privacy
- Be assured of confidentiality
- Obtain reasonable responses to requests for services
- Obtain information about his or her health care, be allowed to review his or her medical record, and have any information explained or interpreted
- Know whether treatment is experimental and be able to consent or decline to participate in proposed research studies or human experimentation

- Expect reasonable continuity of care
- Ask about and be informed of the existence of business relationships between the hospital and others that may influence the patient's treatment and care
- Know which hospital policies and practices relate to patient care, treatment, and responsibilities
- Be informed of available resources for resolving disputes, grievances, and conflicts, such as ethics committees or patient representatives
- Examine his or her bill and have it explained and be informed of available payment methods

Medical assistants should also know that patients have certain responsibilities when they seek medical care. Patients are responsible for:

- Providing information about past illnesses, hospitalizations, medications, and other matters related to their health status. If an incorrect diagnosis is made because a patient fails to give the physician the proper information, the physician is not liable.
- Participating in decision making by asking for additional information about their health status or treatment when they do not fully understand information and instructions.
- Providing health-care agencies with a copy of their written advance directive if they have one.
- Informing physicians and other caregivers if they anticipate problems in following a prescribed treatment.
- Following the physician's orders for treatment. If a patient willfully or negligently fails to follow the physician's instructions, that patient has little legal recourse.
- Providing health-care agencies with necessary information for insurance claims and working with the health-care facility to make arrangements to pay fees when necessary.

Additionally, in April of 2003, the enforcement of the Health Insurance Portability and Accountability Act (HIPAA) began. If this act is not followed, individual health-care workers can be subject to fines up to $250,000 and 10 years in jail. The privacy standards of this act ensure the following:

- Health-care facilities must provide patients with a written notice of their practices regarding the use and disclosure of all individually identifiable health information.
- Health-care facilities may not use or disclose protected health information for any purpose that is not in the privacy notice.
- Patient consent is required when protected information is used or disclosed for purposes of treatment, payment, or health operations.
- Written authorization is required for other types of disclosures.
- Hospitals must make the privacy notice available either before or at the time of the delivery of care
- A privacy notice must be posted in a clear and prominent location within the hospital facility.

Medical Interview

Patient interview: The first step in the examination process. It establishes a relationship between the medical assistant and the patient, and it allows the medical assistant to collect information and data pertinent to the patient's well-being.

The health history form: The medical office usually has a standard medical history form that it uses for all patients. The specific arrangement and wording of items vary from office to office.

Personal data: This information is obtained from the administrative sheet and includes things like the patient's name, Social Security number, birth date, and other basic data.

Chief complaint: Abbreviated as CC, it is the reason the patient came to visit the practitioner. It should be short, specific, and cover subjective and objective data.

History of present illness: This includes detailed information about the chief complaint, including when the problem started and what the patient has done to treat the problem (including any medications taken). For example, a chief complaint might be "sore throat," and the history of the present illness would include when the sore throat started (e.g., 3 days ago), how severe the pain is on a scale of 1 to 10 (e.g., pain scale rating of 6 out of 10), and what treatments have been used (e.g., throat lozenges and 4 to 6 aspirin daily).

Past medical history: The past medical history includes any and all health problems both present and past, including major illnesses and surgery. The past medical history also includes important information about medications and allergies.

Family history: This section includes information about the health of the patient's family members. Many times the family history can help lead a practitioner to the cause of a current medical problem. Obtain specific information about family members' current ages and medical conditions or, if deceased, their age at death and the cause.

Social and occupational history: Information such as marital status, sexual behaviors and orientation, occupations, hobbies, and use of chemical substances help determine a patient's risk for disease. Patients should be asked about their use of alcohol, tobacco, recreational drugs, or other chemical substances.

Six Cs of charting:

- Client's words—The patient's own phrasing must be recorded exactly.
- Clarity—Use precise medical terminology.
- Completeness—The chart must contain all pertinent information.
- Conciseness—Use abbreviations where you can to save time and space.
- Chronological order—Date all entries.
- Confidentiality—Protect the patient's privacy.

Interviewing successfully:

- Do your research before the interview. Review the patient's medical history.
- Plan the interview. Plan what types of questions you want to ask.
- Approach the patient and request an interview. Make the patient feel part of the process.
- Make the patient feel at ease. Use icebreakers and casual conversation.
- Listen to the patient.
- Conduct the interview in private without interruption.
- Deal with sensitive topics with respect.
- Do not diagnose or give a diagnostic opinion. Never go beyond the scope of your knowledge.
- Formulate a general picture. Summarize key points, and let the patient ask questions.

Methods that can further help you collect patient data include asking open-ended and hypothetical questions, mirroring the patient's explicit responses and verbalizing the implied responses, focusing on the patient, encouraging the patient to take the lead, encouraging the patient to provide additional information, and encouraging the patient to evaluate the situation. Make sure that you do not challenge the patient or probe in a manner that invades the patient's privacy.

Detect nonverbal clues: During the preexamination interview, you may note things that patients have not communicated to you verbally, such as anxiety, depression, signs of physical or psychological abuse, and signs of drug or alcohol abuse. If you suspect abuse, bring it to the physician's attention immediately. Provide such patients with support, advice, and the appropriate hotline number for your area if they want to seek help. Please have community resources such as hotline numbers and informative brochures or literature available for such situations.

Physical Examination

Purpose of the physical examination: The determination of the general state of health of the patient and the diagnosis of any medical problems and diseases the patient may have. The physician uses a variety of devices and laboratory tests to complete the physical findings. The majority of physicians usually start at the patient's head and end at the feet. Sometimes the physician may order some additional tests or procedures, such as blood sample testing, the collection of culture specimens, or X-rays.

Complete physical examination: Includes vital signs, examination of the patient's entire body, laboratory tests (complete blood count [CBC] and urinalysis); and diagnostic tests (X-rays).

Duty of a medical assistant: Preparing the room and equipment, getting the patient ready, and assisting the physician.

Emotional preparation: Begin by explaining what will happen during the examination. This step is especially important when dealing with children.

Physical preparation: The medical assistant is responsible for obtaining and recording weight and height, facilitating the examination, asking the patient to empty his or her bladder and bowel, asking the patient to disrobe completely, dressing the patient in a full gown, and providing a drape sheet.

Examination methods: The six methods for examining a patient that are a part of a complete physical examination are inspection, palpation, percussion, auscultation, manipulation, and mensuration.

Inspection: Observing the patient's outer body and certain mental characteristics.

Palpation: Feeling with the fingers or hand to verify data seen during inspection.

Percussion: Tapping with the fingers and listening for sounds, particularly in the abdomen, back, and chest.

Auscultation: Listening to sounds with a stethoscope.

Manipulation: Skillfully using the hands in therapeutic or diagnostic procedures.

Symptoms: Subjective changes in the body felt or observed by the patient, such as headache, blurred vision, or dizziness.

Signs: Objective findings as perceived by another person such as a physician or medical assistant. Examples of signs include fever, blood pressure, and heart murmurs.

Diagnose: To determine the cause and nature of an abnormal condition. It's important to remember that diagnosis is not within the scope or training of a medical assistant. You should never give a diagnosis to a patient. If patients ask you, refer them to the physician.

Clinical diagnosis: Using the signs and symptoms of a disease to determine its cause and nature.

Differential diagnosis: The process of ruling out certain possibilities, used to determine the correct diagnosis when two or more diagnoses are possible.

Prognosis: The outcome of a disorder, or a predication of the probable course of a disease in an individual and the chances of recovery.

Equipment

Examination tables: Usually adjustable to enable the patient to assume various positions. Tables are usually covered with disposable papers that must be changed after each patient.

Surfaces: Must be disinfected with products approved by the Environmental Protection Agency (EPA), such as 10% NaClO (sodium hypochlorite, the active ingredient in household bleach).

Accessibility: The ease with which people can move in and out of a space. The Americans with Disabilities Act of 1990 (ADA) requires:

- A doorway at least 36 inches wide to allow for the use of wheelchairs
- A clear space in rooms and hallways 60 inches in diameter to allow persons using a wheelchair to make a 180-degree turn
- Stable, firm, slip-resistant flooring
- Door-opening hardware that can be grasped with one hand and does not require the twisting of the wrist to use
- Door closers adjusted to allow time for a person in a wheelchair to enter and exit
- Grab bars in the lavatory

Instrument: A surgical device or tool to assist the physician in performing a specific function, such as measuring, examining, grasping, holding, cutting, or suturing. Some commonly used instruments are shown in Figure 16-1.

Gloves: Should always be worn if the hands will come in contact with a patient's nonintact skin, blood, body fluids, or moist surfaces and if the patient is suspected of having an infectious disease.

Tongue depressors: Used in the examination of the mouth and tongue.

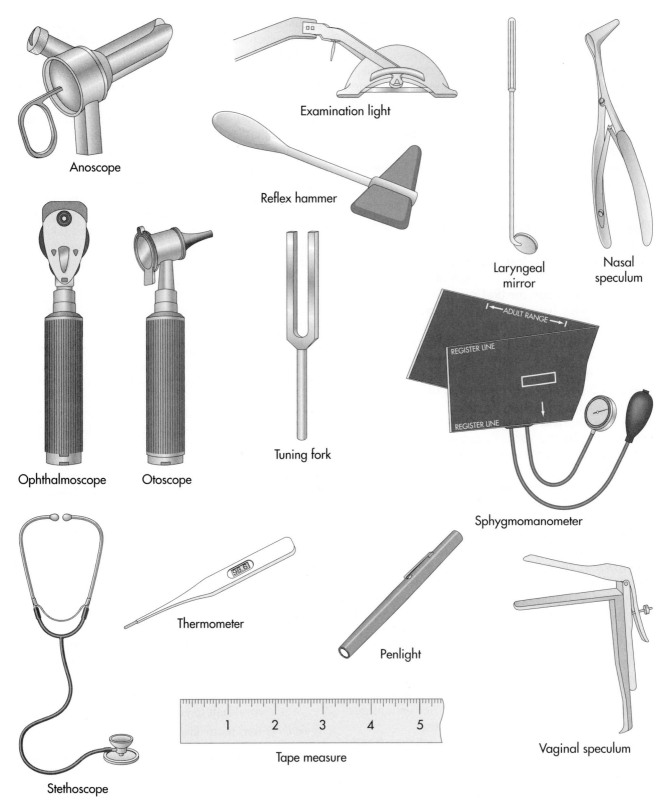

Figure 16-1 *These instruments may be used in a general physical examination.*

Gooseneck lamp: A movable light used to focus on a body area for increased visibility during physical examination.

Penlight: A small flashlight used to provide additional light during an examination, for example, to check pupil response.

Reflex hammer: A percussion mallet with a rubber head, used to tap tendons, nerves, or muscles to elicit reflex reactions.

Lubricants: Used in examination of the rectum and female genitalia.

Anoscope: An instrument used to open the anus for examination.

Speculum: An instrument that expands and separates the walls of a cavity (such as the ear, nose, and vagina) to make examination possible.

Nasal speculum: Used to enlarge the opening of the nose to permit viewing. This type of speculum may consist of a reusable handle with a disposable speculum tip, or it may be a disposable one-piece unit.

Vaginal speculum: Used to enlarge the vagina to make the vagina and the cervix accessible to visual examination and specimen collection.

Thermometer: Used to measure body temperature.

Otoscope: An instrument used to examine the external ear canal and tympanic membrane.

Ophthalmoscope: A handheld instrument, equipped with a light, used to view inner eye structures.

Tuning fork: A small, metal instrument consisting of a stem and two prongs that produces a constant pitch when either prong is struck. It is used by physicians as a screening test of air and bone conduction.

Inspecting and maintaining instruments: Before examination, check all instruments and sanitize, disinfect, and sterilize as appropriate. Also make sure that all of them are in good working order, and replace or repair instruments as necessary.

Arranging instruments: Arrange instruments so the physician may find them easily.

Disposable supplies used in physical examinations: Supplies that are used once and then discarded. They include:

- Cervical scraper
- Cotton balls
- Cotton-tipped applicators
- Curettes
- Disposable needles
- Disposable syringes
- Gauze, dressings, and bandages
- Glass slides
- Gloves, both sterile and nonsterile
- Paper tissues
- Specimen containers
- Tongue depressors

Consumable supplies: Supplies that can be emptied or used up in an examination. They include:

- Sprays (chemical spray used to preserve specimens)
- Isopropyl alcohol (used to cleanse the skin)
- Lubricants

Positioning and Draping

Draping: The placing of a sheet of fabric or paper during an examination to protect and cover all or a part of a patient's body, for the comfort and privacy of the patient.

Positioning: For physical examinations, the patient may need to be placed in a variety of positions to facilitate the examination of various parts of the body. The physician indicates which positions are needed for specific examinations, and the medical assistant helps the patient assume the positions. Cover the patient with a drape that will help keep the patient warm and maintain privacy. The patient can remain draped and gowned until the physician begins the examination, at which time only the part of the body being examined should be uncovered.

Positions: Many positions are used for medical examinations, including sitting, supine, dorsal recumbent, lithotomy, Trendelenburg's, Fowler's, prone, Sims', knee-chest, proctological, jackknife, and standing. See Figure 16-2.

Sitting position: The patient sits at the edge of the examination table without back support. This position is used for examination of the head, neck, chest, heart, back, and arms. In this position, the physician can evaluate the patient's ability to fully expand the lungs and can check the upper body parts for symmetry. The drape is placed across the lap of male patients and the chest and lap of female patients.

Supine position: Also called the recumbent position. The patient lies flat on the back (face up). This position is used for examination of the head, neck, chest, heart, abdomen, and arms and legs. The patient is normally draped from the neck or underarms down to the feet.

Dorsal recumbent: The patient lies face up while flexing the knees, with the soles of the feet flat on the table. This position is the same as the supine position except that the patient's knees are drawn up. It is used for examination of the head, neck, chest, heart, and lower extremities (vaginal, rectal, and perineal areas).

Lithotomy position: The patient lies on the back with the knees sharply flexed and the feet placed in stirrups that are set wide apart and away from the table. This position is used for examination of the vaginal and perineal areas. It is an embarrassing and physically uncomfortable position for most women, so you should not ask the patient to stay in this position any longer than necessary.

Trendelenburg's position: The patient lies flat on the back with the head lower than the legs. This position is used for abdominal surgery and for treatment of patients who are in shock.

Fowler's position: The patient lies face up on the examination table with the head elevated. Although the head of the table can be raised to 90-degrees, the most common position is 45°. This position is used for examination and treatment of the head, neck, and chest. This position is best for people with lower-back injury or for those experiencing shortness of breath.

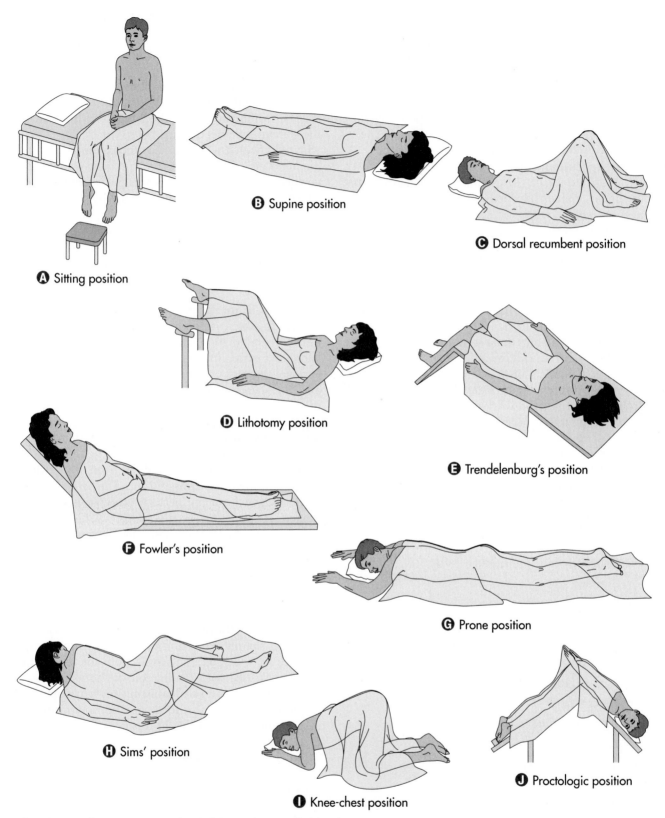

A Sitting position

B Supine position

C Dorsal recumbent position

D Lithotomy position

E Trendelenburg's position

F Fowler's position

G Prone position

H Sims' position

I Knee-chest position

J Proctologic position

Figure 16-2 *These positions may be used during the general physical examination.*

Prone position: The patient lies face down on the table. This position is used for examination of the back and feet. It is not suitable for patients who are obese, pregnant (in the late stage), or elderly or who have difficulties of the respiratory system.

Sims' position: Also called the lateral position. The patient lies on the left side with the left arm placed behind the body and the left leg slightly flexed. The right arm is flexed toward the head, and the right leg is flexed. This position is used for examination of the rectum.

Knee-chest position: The patient rests on the knees and chest with the thighs slightly separated. Patients who have difficulty in maintaining this position can be placed in a knee-elbow position. The knee-chest position is used for examination of rectal, sigmoid, and vaginal areas.

Proctological position: The patient lies face down with both the torso and the legs lowered. The hips of the patient are flexed at a 90-degree angle. Adjustable tables can be raised in the middle with both ends sloping down. This position is used for rectal examination.

Jackknife position: The patient lies face up with both the torso and the legs raised. The hips of the patient are flexed at a 90-degree angle.

Standing position: Used for examination of the musculoskeletal system, the neurological system, hernias, and the peripheral vascular system.

Eye and Ear Examination

Eye

Optometrist: A specialist who measures the eye's refractive power and prescribes correction of visual defects when needed.

Ophthalmologist: A medical doctor who is an eye specialist.

Ophthalmic assistant: Provides administrative and clinical support for an ophthalmologist; works with patients; assists with surgery; keeps instruments and equipment in proper working order; and may conduct distance acuity, near acuity, and color perception tests.

Visual acuity test: Used to measure the degree of clarity or sharpness of vision. There are many types of tests for visual acuity. The test most commonly used in the medical office and performed by the medical assistant is the Snellen eye test.

Snellen letter chart: A chart used to test the distance vision of adults. The distance between the patient and the chart should be 20 feet. Normal vision is recorded as 20/20. Have the patient read the chart, and record the smallest line read. If the patient misses only one or two letters on a line, record the results with a minus sign. For example, if one letter is missed on the 30-foot line from 20 feet away with the right eye, the result would be recorded as O.D. 20/30 –1. See Figure 16-3.

Color blindness: The congenital or acquired inability to distinguish certain colors. Congenital color blindness is more common. This condition is seen in males more frequently than in females.

Color vision acuity test: Measures the patient's ability to determine and differentiate between colors. The medical assistant may be responsible for administering the color vision test. There are two common color tests, Ishihara and Richmond pseudoisochromatic, in which the individual must distinguish a figure made up of colored dots from a background made up of dots of another color. A score of 10 or above indicates

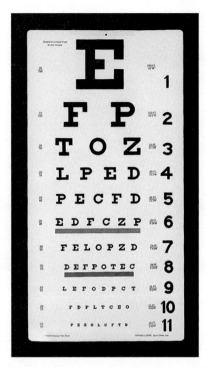

Figure 16-3 *The Snellen letter chart is used to test the ability to see objects that are relatively far away.*

average color vision. A score of less than 7 may represent a color vision deficiency.

Tonometer: An instrument used in measuring tension or pressure of the intraocular region. It is used for the detection of glaucoma.

Eye irrigation: The flushing of foreign materials from the eye with a sterile solution formulated for this purpose.

Ear

Audiologist: A specialist who evaluates and corrects hearing problems.

Hearing loss: An inability to perceive the entire range of sound heard by a person with normal hearing. There are two types: conductive and sensorineural.

Conductive hearing loss: Caused by damage to the middle ear.

Sensorineural hearing loss: Caused by damage to the inner ear (the cochlea or the auditory nerve).

Audiometer: An electronic device that measures hearing acuity by producing sounds in specific frequencies and intensities.

Audiology tests: Tests to determine the presence of conduction defects or nerve impairment. They are used to evaluate hearing loss and disturbances in equilibrium.

Weber's test: A method of evaluating auditory acuity. The test is performed by placing the stem of a vibrating tuning fork against the center of a person's forehead, or the midline vertex. The loudness of the sound is equal in both ears if hearing is normal.

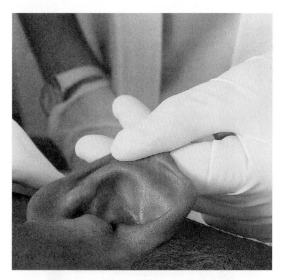

Figure 16-4 *Straighten an adult's ear canal by pulling the auricle upward and outward.*

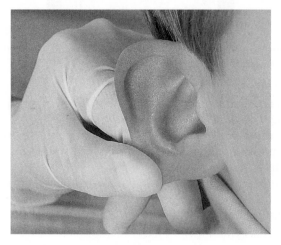

Figure 16-5 *Straighten an infant's or a child's ear canal by pulling the auricle downward and back.*

Rinne test: Compares bone conduction hearing with air conduction hearing. A vibrating tuning fork is held on the mastoid process of the ear until the patient no longer hears it. Then it is held close to the external auditory meatus.

Ear irrigation: Flushing of the ear canal to remove impacted cerumen, to relieve inflammation, or to remove a foreign body. The solution used should be warmed to room temperature before administration. To perform the irrigation for adults, the earlobe should be pulled upward and outward. For infants and children, the earlobe should be pulled down and back. See Figures 16-4 and 16-5.

Ear instillation: Applying eardrops to treat an ear disorder. The medication should be warmed to room temperature before application.

Cardiovascular Examination

Cardiologist: A physician trained in the treatment of heart diseases.

Medical assistant's role: To assist with and perform tests, to keep equipment properly maintained and calibrated, to educate patients about diet and exercise, and to provide emotional support to patients.

General cardiovascular examination: Taking a blood pressure reading, palpating the heart and chest wall and the vessels in the extremities, and recording an electrocardiogram (ECG).

Cardiac stress test: Recording an ECG while a patient is exercising on a treadmill, stationary bicycle, or stair-stepping ergonometer. The test determines the capacity of a patient to respond to an increased demand for energy. Performing this test helps diagnose diseases of the heart.

Echocardiography: The process of obtaining echoes with the use of ultrasound and recording them on paper. It is used to evaluate the inner structures of the heart.

Phonocardiography: A process that graphically records the cardiac cycle sounds as heard through a stethoscope.

Cardiac catheterization: A diagnostic procedure in which a catheter is introduced through an incision into a large vein (in the arm or leg) and sent to the chambers of the heart. The procedure takes about 1 to 3 hours.

Angioplasty: The reconstruction of blood vessels damaged by disease or injury.

Pulse oximeter: A machine that measures the oxygen level of the blood. This device measures the pulse and oxygen saturation of the blood.

Respiratory System Examination

Eupnea: Normal breathing.

Throat culture: A commonly performed diagnostic test for determination of infection.

Sputum culture: Difficult to obtain. The patient must cough deeply and expectorate material from the lungs. Early morning is the best time to collect sputum.

Pulmonary function tests: Tests performed to measure the amount of air a patient can inhale and exhale.

Spirometer: An instrument that measures the air taken into and expelled from the lungs.

Spirometry: The measuring of breathing capacity.

Forced vital capacity (FVC): The greatest volume of air that can be expelled when a person performs rapid, forced expiration.

Total lung capacity (TLC): The total volume when lungs are maximally inflated.

Laryngoscope: An endoscope for examining the larynx.

Bronchoscopy: Visual examination of the tracheobronchial tree by means of the standard rigid, tubular metal bronchoscope. The procedure may also be used for suctioning or biopsy.

Cheyne-Stokes respiration: A breathing pattern marked by a period of apnea lasting 10 to 60 seconds, followed by gradually increasing depth and frequency of respirations.

Gastrointestinal System Examination

Gastroenterologist: A physician who diagnoses and treats disorders of the gastrointestinal tract.

Proctology: The branch of medicine concerned with treating disorders of the colon, rectum, and anus.

Medical assistant's role: To tell patients how to prepare for examinations, to order informational brochures, and to answer patients' questions.

Endoscopy: Visual examination of the interior of cavities and organs of the body with an endoscope. The purpose of this procedure is the diagnosis of disorders. Endoscopy can also be used for biopsy. See Figure 16-6.

Gastroscopy: Examination of the stomach and abdominal cavity with a type of endoscope called a gastroscope.

Sigmoidoscopy: Inspection of the rectum and sigmoid colon with the aid of a sigmoidoscope. The medical assistant should assist the physician with the procedure and clean the equipment.

Colonoscopy: Visual examination of the large intestine by means of a colonoscope inserted through the anus.

Anoscope: A speculum used to examine the anus and lower rectum.

Proctoscopy: Examination of the lower rectum and anal canal by means of a protoscope.

Cholecystogram: An X-ray of the gallbladder, made after injection of a radiopaque substance, usually a contrast medium containing iodine.

Barium swallow: Also called an upper GI series, used to diagnose abnormalities in the esophagus, stomach, and small intestine. The patient swallows a liquid containing barium, and X-rays are taken to record the diagnostic images.

Barium enema: Also called a lower GI series, used to detect abnormalities in the large intestine. Barium is given as an enema.

Gastric lavage: Obtaining a sample of stomach contents with an orogastric tube, which suctions the contents up for analysis.

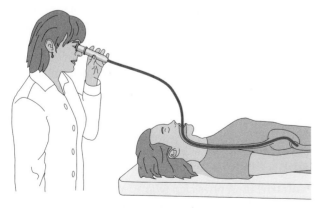

Figure 16-6 *To perform peroral endoscopy, the physician inserts a scope into the patient's mouth.*

Occult blood test: A chemical test or microscopic examination for blood, especially in the feces, that is not apparent on visual inspection.

Laparotomy: Surgical incision into the peritoneal cavity.

Urinary System Examination

Urologist: A physician who specializes in the study of the urinary system.

Medical assistant's role: It is important to be thorough in taking a patient's history in order to obtain information about changes in frequency or urgency of urination, difficulty or pain with urination, and incontinence.

Urinalysis: Physical, chemical, and microscopic examination of urine to find bacteria, blood, or other substances and to monitor for dysfunctions of the prostate gland and for sexually transmitted diseases. The medical assistant collects the urine specimen for chemical or physical analysis.

Urine culture: The placement of urine samples on special media that promote the growth of microorganisms and thus facilitate bacterial analysis. It requires special training and equipment but may be performed in the office.

Cystoscopy: Visual examination of the bladder by means of a special instrument called a cystoscope.

Pyelogram: An X-ray image of the bladder made by using an opaque dye for visualization. The dye may be injected into the patient's vein, or the physician may insert a small catheter into the urethra through a cystoscope and inject the dye through the catheter.

Urinometer: A device for determining the specific gravity of urine. It is also called a urometer.

Vasectomy: A sterilization procedure for men in which a section of each vas deferens is removed.

Gynecology and Obstetrics

Obstetrician/gynecologist (OB/GYN): A physician who specializes in the female reproductive system.

Role of the medical assistant: The medical assistant collects a urine specimen; interviews the patient about her health and any changes in appetite, weight, and emotional status; and asks about the date of the patient's last menstrual period. If the doctor is male, a female medical assistant should be present during the examination not only to assist but also to provide legal protection.

Pelvic examination: The physician checks the external genitalia, cervix, vaginal wall, internal reproductive organs, and rectum via palpation and inspection with a speculum.

Papanicolaou test (Pap test or smear): Used to determine the presence of abnormal or precancerous cells in the cervix and vagina. A Pap test is done during the pelvic examination. The patient is instructed not to douche, use vaginal medications, or have intercourse within 48 hours before the examination. The test should not be done during a patient's menstrual period.

Wet mount: A method of adding liquid, usually saline or formalin, to a specimen on a slide for examination and preservation. The specimen is placed on a slide and one drop of saline (for diagnosis of trichomonas vaginalis) or potassium hydroxide (for diagnosis of vaginal yeast infections) is applied and mixes with the specimen. It is then covered with a coverslip and examined microscopically.

Pregnancy test: A test to determine whether the hormone human chorionic gonadotropin, which is produced during pregnancy, is present in a woman's blood or urine. False negatives and false positives can occur.

Ultrasonography: The process of imaging deep structures of the body by measuring and recording the reflection of pulsed or continuous high-frequency sound waves. It is a valuable tool to diagnose fetal abnormalities, gallstones, heart defects, and tumors. It is also called sonography.

Mammogram: A low-dose X-ray of a woman's breasts to detect early cancer. A mammogram is first taken between the ages of 35 and 40 years.

Colposcopy: The examination of the vagina and cervix with a colposcope.

Schiller's test: Iodine staining of cervical and vaginal areas to diagnose cancer of the cervix or vagina.

Laparoscopy: Examination of the abdominal cavity with a laparoscope through one or more small incisions in the abdominal wall. The incisions are usually at the umbilicus. A general anesthetic is used. This procedure is also called an abdominoscopy.

Skin Examination

Dermatologist: A physician who diagnoses and treats skin diseases and disorders.

Medical assistant's role: To assist with positioning and draping during a skin examination, to take skin scrapings and wound cultures, to administer sunlamp treatments, to apply topical medications, and to instruct patients about caring for a skin condition or wound at home.

Whole-body skin examination: An examination of the entire surface of the skin, including the scalp and the areas between the toes, to look for lesions, especially suspicious moles or precancerous growths.

Wood's light examination: A type of dermatological examination in which a physician inspects the patient's skin under an ultraviolet lamp in a darkened room for certain fungal cultures.

Tuberculin skin test: Administered intradermally, a test performed to detect exposure to tuberculosis. This test is routinely performed on all individuals who have contact with children, on those working in health-care fields, and on patients with a positive X-ray suggestive of infection. The tine test, a common tuberculin skin test, is performed by cleansing the skin on the inside of the forearm and then pressing tuberculin-coated tines

into the skin while pulling the skin taut. The skin is observed for results after 48 to 72 hours.

Scratch test: A test for specific allergies. The skin is scratched with a sterile lancet, and a drop of allergen (antigen) is added to the site. Results are recorded in 30 minutes.

Patch test: A test for hypersensitivity allergy. Antigens are applied to the skin and covered with gauze patches and tape. The site is checked in 48 hours, and results are recorded. This type of test is used to discover the cause of contact dermatitis.

Tissue biopsy: There are three types, or methods: excision biopsy, punch biopsy, and shave biopsy.

Neurology Tests

Neurologist: A physician who diagnoses and treats diseases and disorders of the central nervous system and associated systems.

Medical assistant's role: To ready equipment for use; to position the patient; to hand tools and other items to the physician; to perform visual acuity tests or audiometry; to assist with electroencephalography; and to instruct and educate patients and their families about procedures, disorders, and treatments.

Neurological examination: A complete examination evaluates cognitive function, cranial nerves, the motor system, reflexes, and the sensory system.

Myelogram: An X-ray taken after the injection of a radiopaque medium into the subarachnoid space to demonstrate any distortions of the spinal cord.

Magnetic resonance imaging (MRI): Medical imaging that uses radio-frequency radiation as its source of energy. It has become an important tool in musculoskeletal and pelvic imaging.

Computed tomography (CT): A radiographic technique that produces a film representing a detailed cross section of tissue structure.

Electroencephalogram (EEG): A graphic chart on which is traced the electrical potential produced by the brain, detected by electrodes placed on the scalp. The resulting brain wave patterns are called alpha, beta, delta, and theta rhythms.

Carotid angiogram: A radiographic image of the carotid artery, into which a contrast medium has been injected.

Alpha-fetoprotein (AFP) testing: Measurements of AFP in amniotic fluid are used for early diagnosis of fetal neural tube defects, such as spina bifida and anencephaly.

Lumbar puncture: A diagnostic and therapeutic procedure done by a physician, involving the introduction of a hollow needle and stylet into the subarachnoid space of the lumbar part of the spinal canal.

Infants and Children

Pediatrician: A physician who specializes in the health care of children, monitoring their development and diagnosing and treating their illnesses. Subspecialties include surgery and oncology.

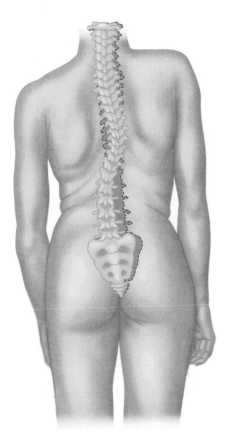

Figure 16-7 *Scoliosis causes the spine to curve into an S shape.*

Medical assistant's role: To prepare the child for examination; to discuss eating habits, sleep patterns, daily activities, immunization schedules, and toilet training with the caregiver or child; to measure the infant's head, length, and weight, and to help relieve the child's fear by calmly explaining procedures.

Well-baby examination: Regular checkups when the infant is 2 weeks, 1 month, 2 months, 4 months, 6 months, 9 months, 1 year, 15 months, and 18 months old. Starting at age 2, children should have checkups every year.

Scoliosis examination: An assessment of a child of 10 years of age or older for abnormal curvature of the spine. See Figure 16-7.

Measurement: Examination and measurement of the circumference of the infant's head to determine normal growth and development. The size of the child's head reflects the growth of the brain. The length and weight measurements in pediatrics are also important. The medical assistant may record and use a physical growth percentile chart to determined the growth value.

Child abuse and neglect: Watch for signs of physical injury, dirty or neglected appearance, hunger, extreme sadness or fear, or inability to communicate. Note suspicions on the chart, and report them to the doctor. Physicians are legally responsible for reporting suspected child abuse or neglect to your community's child protection agency or to the police.

Immunizations: Usually given during routine office visits to protect children against hepatitis B, diphtheria, tetanus, pertussis, poliomyelitis, measles, mumps, rubella, chickenpox, and influenza. The child should not have an illness or fever at the time of immunization.

Minor Surgery

Surgery: The branch of medicine that treats conditions, diseases, deformities, and injury using instruments and operative procedures. Also, the surgical treatment or procedure itself. Generally, the place for major surgery is in a hospital, but minor surgery commonly is performed in a doctor's or dentist's office. Minor surgery may include removal of a sebaceous cyst, wart, or foreign object. Other minor surgeries include circumcision, vasectomy, skin biopsy, dilation and curettage.

Medical assistant's role: To complete forms for insurance; to obtain signed informed consent forms from the patient; to explain the procedure to the patient; to answer questions; to make sure that the doctor is informed about medications the patient is taking; to make sure that the patient knows how to follow presurgical instructions for diet and fluid intake; to make sure that the room is clean; to make sure that all supplies are clean, disinfected, or sterilized, as appropriate, and that all supplies are properly arranged; possibly to assist with the surgery; to help dress the wound and perform other postoperative care; and to clean the room and prepare it for the next patient.

Outpatient surgery: A surgical procedure that requires less than 1 day and for which the patient does not need to stay in the facility overnight.

Ambulatory surgery: A surgical procedure for which the patient is able to walk into and out of the surgical facility on the same day.

Invasive procedure: A diagnostic or therapeutic technique that requires entry into a body cavity or interruption of normal body functions. Examples include the Pap test, sigmoidoscopy, colonoscopy, and intravenous pyelography.

Anesthesia: Partial or complete loss of sensation. It is induced to permit the performance of surgery or other painful procedures. Local anesthesia provides loss of sensation in a particular location without loss of consciousness; it is used for diagnostic procedures or minor surgery. Techniques for administering local anesthetics include topical application, infiltration (injection into tissue), and block (injection into or around a nerve). Types of block anesthesia include regional, spinal, epidural, and saddle, which affect a group of nerves. General anesthesia is used for major surgery.

Anesthetic: A drug or agent used to prevent the sensation of pain and, depending on the situation, to achieve adequate muscle relaxation during surgery, to calm fear and anxiety, and to produce amnesia for the event.

Needle biopsy: The removal of a segment of living tissue for microscopic examination by inserting a hollow needle through the skin or the external surface of an organ or tumor.

Cauterization: The destruction of tissue with a cautery.

Cautery: An agent or device used for scarring, burning, or cutting the skin or other tissues by means of heat, cold, electric current, or caustic chemicals.

Electrocautery: An instrument for directing a high-frequency current through a local area of tissue.

Electrosurgery: The use of electrical current in surgical procedures such as electrocoagulation to cauterize blood vessels and electrocision to excise tissue.

Cryosurgery: The destruction of tissue (e.g., abnormal cells) by the use of freezing temperatures.

Laser: The acronym for *l*ight *a*mplification by *s*timulated *e*mission of *r*adiation. Thermal lasers are used to heat tissue at a microscopic level, causing vaporization and coagulation of the target area.

Surgical Asepsis

Disinfection: The destruction or inhibition of pathogenic organisms by physical means or by chemical germicides. Two common disinfectants are zephrin chloride and chlorophenyl. Contaminated instruments are completely immersed in a germicidal solution for from 1 to 10 hours. The chemical disinfection process is referred to as a "cold" process because no heat is used.

Surgical asepsis: Used when sterility of supplies and the immediate environment is required. This technique is necessary during any invasive procedure. It requires sterile hand washing (surgical scrub), sterile gloves, special handling procedures, and sterilization of materials. Most dangerous bacteria are destroyed at a temperature of 50° to 60°C (122° to 140°F). Pasteurization of a fluid, which is the application of heat at about 60°C, destroys pathogenic bacteria. However, temperatures of 120°C are usually required to destroy spore cells. A sterile object that touches anything nonsterile is automatically considered contaminated and must not be used in surgery.

Surgical scrub: Hand washing to remove all dirt and microorganisms from the surface of the skin and the fingernails. Materials needed include a sterile surgical scrub brush, a dispenser with surgical soap, orange sticks, and sterile towels. The physician or surgical assistant must remove all jewelry, turn on warm water, keep the hands higher than the elbows, use surgical soap, scrub the hands with the scrub brush for 2 minutes, rinse the hands, apply more surgical soap, and again scrub the hands for at least 3 minutes. Total hand-washing time should be approximately 10 minutes.

Sterilization: The process of destroying all microorganisms and their pathogenic products. Methods of sterilization include the application of steam under pressure, dry heat, bactericidal chemical compounds (in liquid or gas form), and radiation.

Moist heat sterilization: A method of sterilization that uses steam under pressure. This method kills all pathogens and spores and is the best and most accepted type of sterilization.

Autoclave: An appliance used to sterilize medical instruments. It allows steam to flow around each article placed in the chamber. The vapor penetrates cloth or paper used to package the articles being sterilized. Autoclaving is one of the most effective methods for destruction of all types of microorganisms. The amount of time and the temperature necessary for sterilization depend on the articles to be sterilized and whether they are wrapped or left directly exposed to the steam under pressure. Wrapped items autoclaved with steam under pressure require 30 pounds of pressure at 132°C (270°F) for 20 minutes. Unwrapped items require only 10 minutes of autoclaving, which is known as flashing. The autoclave chamber must be cleaned after each load.

Dry heat sterilization: A method of sterilization that uses heated dry air at a temperature of 160° to 180°C (320° to 356°F) for 90 minutes to 3 hours.

Sterilization indicator: Any material that undergoes a change in appearance (usually a color shift) when it is exposed to a predetermined combination of temperature, pressure, and time. Indicators are used to confirm that the sterilization process has been completed. The most common forms of indicator include autoclave tape and sterilization indicator strips.

Autoclave indicator: A change of color or the appearance of dots on an indicator strip, tube, tape, or tag shows that steam has entered the chamber, not that the instruments are sterile. Autoclave indicator tape turns black after autoclaving.

Shelf life: The amount of time during which an item may be expected to retain its useful characteristics (such as sterility). Packages that have been autoclaved are stored with the date visible, and the oldest package is placed in front so that it is used first. Sterilized instruments are considered to have a shelf life of approximately 1 month. Autoclaved packages cannot be re-autoclaved without washing, rinsing, drying, and rewrapping the items.

Surgical setup tray: Instruments that may be required for a specific minor surgical procedure should be gathered together into a pack, sterilized, and made ready for use as needed. Specialized trays are used for such procedures as incision, vasectomy, suture removal, and laceration repair. See Figure 16-8.

Clean gloves: Worn to protect health-care personnel from urine, stools, blood, saliva, and drainage from patients' wounds and lesions.

Sterile gloves: Used to prevent contamination of areas that need to be sterile on the patient. See Figures 16-9 to 16-12.

Sterile field: The area immediately around a patient that has been prepared for a surgical procedure. The sterile field includes the scrubbed team members, who are properly attired, and all furniture and fixtures in the area.

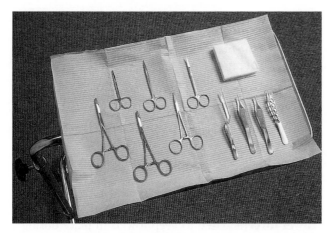

Figure 16-8 *This laceration tray contains scissors, several pairs of forceps, a needle holder, suture material, and sterile gauze.*

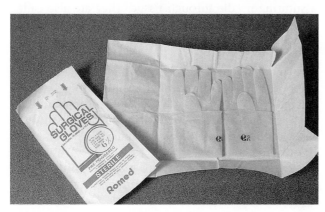

Figure 16-9 *You can put these sterile gloves on without reaching across the sterile surfaces of the gloves or the sterile inner wrap of the pack.*

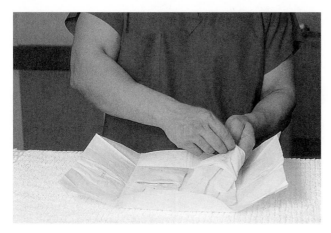

Figure 16-10 *Your palm should face up as you slide your dominant hand into the first glove.*

Formalin: A dilute solution of formaldehyde used to preserve biological specimens.

Instruments

Surgical scissors: A sharp instrument composed of two opposing cutting blades, held together by a central

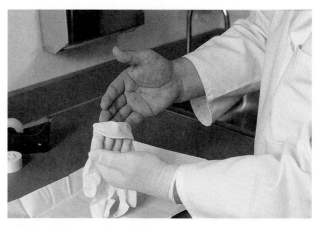

Figure 16-11 *Your gloved fingers secure the remaining glove while you slip it over your nondominant hand.*

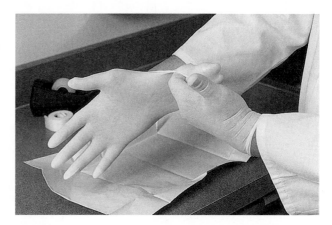

Figure 16-12 *Unfold the cuff over your arm while touching only the sterile surface of the glove.*

pin on which the blades pivot, used to dissect and cut tissues. See Figure 16-13.

Operating scissors: Straight or curved, with a combination of blades such as sharp/sharp (s/s), blunt/blunt (b/b), or sharp/blunt (s/b).

Suture scissors: Used to remove sutures. The hook on the tip aids in getting under a suture, and the blunt end prevents puncturing of the tissues.

Bandage scissors: Inserted beneath a dressing or bandage to cut it for removal.

Scalpel: A small, straight surgical knife consisting of a handle and a sharp blade that has a convex edge used to make surgical incisions. There are both reusable and disposable scalpels. Blades are numbered according to size. A number 15 blade is often used in performing minor surgeries.

Retractors: Used to hold tissue aside to improve the exposure of operative areas. See Figure 16-14.

Probes: Long, slender instruments used to explore wounds or body cavities.

Forceps: A surgical instrument with two handles, each attached to a dull blade, used to grasp, compress, pull, handle, or join tissue, equipment, or supplies. See Figure 16-15. Grasping types include thumb forceps and tissue forceps. (The word *forceps*, like *scissors*, is plural.)

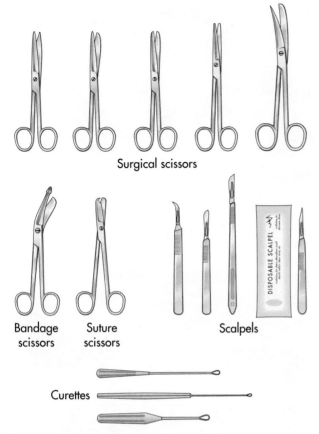

Figure 16-13 *These cutting and dissecting instruments are typically used in minor surgical procedures.*

Thumb forceps: Also called smooth forceps, used to pick up tissue or to grasp tissue between the adjacent surfaces of the blades.

Splinter forceps: Thumb forceps with sharp points that are useful in removing foreign objects.

Tissue forceps: Have teeth to prevent them from slipping. They are used to grasp tissue.

Holding forceps: Have handles that can lock the blades closed.

Dressing forceps: Used in the application and removal of dressings.

Hemostatic forceps or **hemostats:** Used for clamping and grasping blood vessels.

Towel forceps: Used to keep towels in place during a surgical procedure.

Needle holders: Surgical forceps used to hold and pass a suturing needle through tissue. They are also called suture forceps.

Surgical suture needle: A sharp instrument used for puncturing and suturing. The needle carries suture material, also called ligature. Needles vary in their piercing ability (pointed or blunt-tipped), shape (straight or curved), and size, depending on their use. See Figure 16-16. A swaged needle has no eye; instead, the needle and suture material are combined in one length.

Suturing: Using sterile suture material and a needle to close a wound. Ligature (suture material) is of two types: absorbable and nonabsorbable.

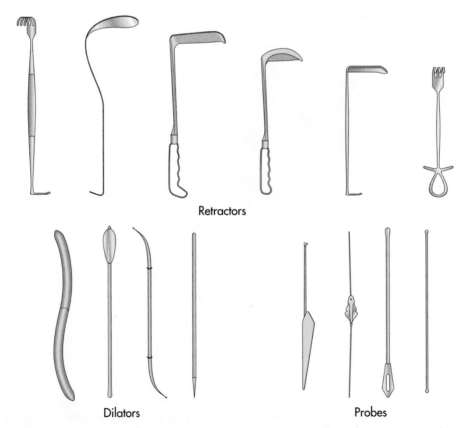

Figure 16-14 *These retracting, dilating, and probing instruments are typically used in minor surgical procedures.*

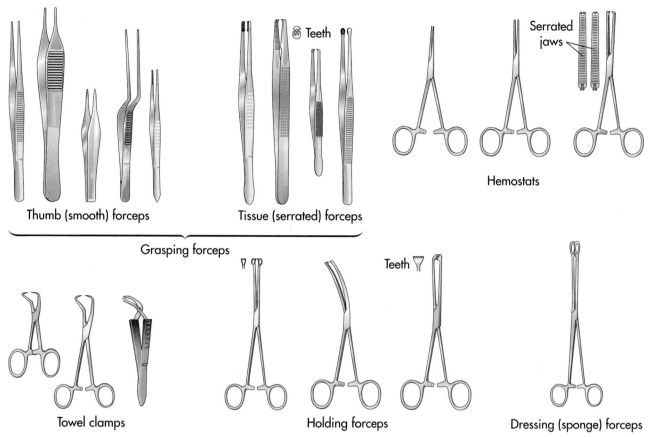

Teeth

Serrated jaws

Hemostats

Thumb (smooth) forceps

Tissue (serrated) forceps

Grasping forceps

Towel clamps

Teeth

Holding forceps

Dressing (sponge) forceps

Figure 16-15 *These grasping and clamping instruments are typically used in minor surgical procedures.*

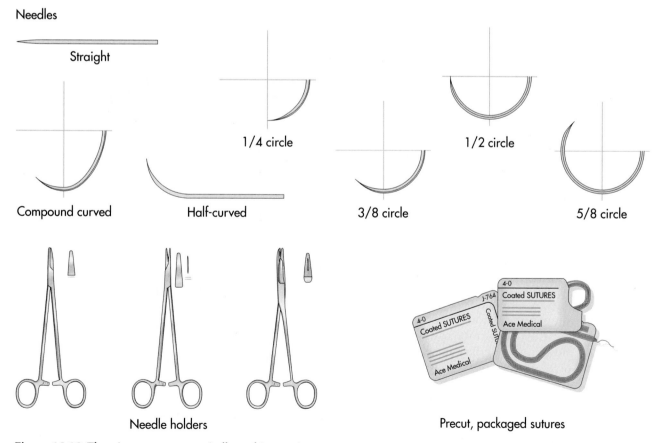

Needles

Straight

1/4 circle

1/2 circle

Compound curved

Half-curved

3/8 circle

5/8 circle

Needle holders

4-0
Coated SUTURES
Ace Medical

4-0   J-764
Coated SUTURES

Coated SUT

Ace Medical

Precut, packaged sutures

Figure 16-16 *These instruments are typically used in suturing.*

Absorbable sutures: Used for internal suturing. They are digested by tissue enzymes and absorbed by the body tissues. Absorption usually occurs 5 to 20 days after insertion. Surgical catgut made from the intestinal lining of sheep is used for the bladder, intestines, and subcutaneous tissue.

Nonabsorbable sutures: Generally used for outer tissues of the body. These types of suture must be removed after the wound begins healing. They may be made of polyester, steel, silk, nylon, and vicryl.

Suture size: In the United States, the size designation of sutures decreases as the thickness (diameter) decreases. Size 7 is the largest generally available. Size 3 is thinner; size 0 is thinner still. Sizes smaller than 0 are indicated by additional 0s: 00 (or 2-0), 000 (or 3-0), and so on. Few sutures are smaller than size 11-0. Sizes 2-0 through 6-0 are the most commonly used.

Staple: A piece of stainless steel wire used to close certain surgical wounds. It is used in major surgery and is the strongest of all suture material.

Suture removal: After surgery, nonabsorbable sutures generally remain in place from 5 to 6 days and then have to be removed. If they are not removed, they can cause infection and skin irritation.

Wounds and Bandaging

Puncture: A wound made by a sharp-pointed object, such as a needle, bullet, carpentry nail, knife, or animal tooth, that pierces the skin layers.

Laceration: A wound in which the tissues are torn apart rather than cut. The edges of the wound are irregular. Dull knife blades and other objects that tear into the skin produce lacerations.

Abrasion: A wound in which the outer layers of the skin are rubbed off, resulting in an oozing of blood from ruptured capillaries. Many falls cause abrasions, such as skinned knees and elbows.

Incision: A clean, smooth cut, as is caused by a sharp knife edge, a razor, or a piece of glass. Also, a cut produced surgically with a sharp instrument that creates an opening into an organ or space in the body. There are two types of incisions: superficial and deep. Generally, a deep incision is accompanied by profuse bleeding with damage to tissues such as muscles, tendons, and nerves.

Contusion: A wound in which the tissues under the skin are injured, as by a blunt object. Blood vessels rupture, allowing blood to seep into the tissue.

Wound healing: The healing process serves to restore the structure and function of the damaged tissue. This process takes place in three phases: lag, proliferation, and maturation.

Lag phase: During the initial phase, bleeding is reduced because of blood vessel constriction.

Proliferation phase: During the second phase, new tissue forms.

Maturation phase: The last phase involves the formation of scar tissue.

Dressing: Sterile material used to cover a surgical or other wound.

Bandage: A strip of woven material used to wrap or cover a part of the body. A bandage causes pressure to control bleeding, protects a wound from contamination, holds a dressing in place, or supports or immobilizes an injured part of the body.

Types of bandage: Three types of bandage are often used in the medical office: roller, elastic, and triangular.

Roller bandages: Long strips of soft material that are coiled to form rolls. They are often used to apply pressure (i.e., as pressure bandages).

Elastic bandages: Made of woven cotton containing elastic fibers. They are typically used on swollen extremities or joints, on the chest to treat empyema, on fractured ribs, and on legs to support varicose veins. They are expensive, but they can be washed and reused.

Triangular bandages: Usually made of muslin and measuring approximately 55 inches across the base and 40 inches along the sides. They are frequently used in first aid.

Tube gauze bandage: Seamless tubular gauze bandage, with or without elastic, is superior material for covering round narrow surfaces such as fingers or toes. It can be used as either a dressing or a bandage. A tubular gauze bandage is applied with a cagelike applicator.

STRATEGIES TO SUCCESS

▶ *Test-Taking Skills*

Answer the easy ones first!

Answering all the questions you know first will give you confidence and momentum to get through the rest of the exam. As you go through the exam, make a mark next to any questions that you want to come back to—questions you are uncertain about or difficult questions you don't want to answer right away. Go back to these questions once you've answered all the questions that you thought were easy. Often you will be surprised how your subconscious mind has continued to work on these questions, or perhaps how something later in the test has jogged your memory, and these hard questions won't seem that difficult any more.

Instructions:

Answer the following questions. Check your answers in the *Answer Key* that follows this section.

1. Which of the following is one of the six Cs of charting?

   A. Clerical
   B. Client's words
   C. Consult
   D. Counsel
   E. Court

2. A small surgical clamp for grasping blood vessels is called

   A. Tissue forceps
   B. Thumb forceps
   C. Smooth forceps
   D. Hemostatic forceps
   E. Dressing forceps

3. Which suture size listed below is the thickest?

   A. 0-0
   B. 5-0
   C. 7-0
   D. 1-0
   E. 15-0

4. The position in which the patient is lying flat on the back is known as

   A. Prone
   B. Sims'
   C. Supine
   D. Fowler's
   E. Lithotomy

5. Needle holders are also called

   A. Staples
   B. Thumb forceps
   C. Suture forceps
   D. Hemostatic forceps
   E. Dressing forceps

6. During the preexamination interview, you notice some cuts on an adult patient's arm that you suspect might be signs of abuse or even of attempted suicide. You try to ask the patient about it, but the patient doesn't want to talk to you. What should you do?

   A. Press the patient and explain how important it is that all your questions be answered
   B. Call the police immediately and report that you have a victim of abuse to whom they need to talk
   C. Tell the examining physician, and prepare a list of community resources that can provide advice and support to the patient even if the patient is not ready to talk to you
   D. Ignore the problem, because the patient obviously does not want to talk about it, and go on with assisting the physician as if you didn't see anything
   E. Transfer the patient to a mental institution and notify immediate family members

7. Which of the following positions is used for vaginal and perineal area examination?

   A. Lithotomy
   B. Fowler's
   C. Supine
   D. Jackknife
   E. Trendelenburg's

8. Which of the following positions requires the examination table to be raised in the middle with both ends pointing down?

   A. Fowler's
   B. Proctological
   C. Knee-chest
   D. Sims'
   E. None of the above

ANSWER KEY

1.	B	14.	B
2.	D	15.	C
3.	A	16.	C
4.	C	17.	E
5.	C	18.	A
6.	C	19.	C
7.	A	20.	B
8.	B	21.	C
9.	A	22.	D
10.	E	23.	A
11.	B	24.	D
12.	D	25.	E
13.	D	26.	B

CHAPTER 17

Vital Signs and Measurement

CHAPTER OUTLINE

Vital Signs

- Temperature
- Pulse Rate
- Respiration Rate
- Blood Pressure

Height and Weight

MEDICAL ASSISTING COMPETENCIES

COMPETENCY	CMA	RMA
Clinical		
Apply principles of aseptic techniques and infection control, including hand washing	X	X
Practice Standard Precautions	X	X
Obtain vital signs	X	X
General/Legal/Professional		
Determine the needs for documentation and reporting, and document accurately and appropriately	X	X
Conduct work within scope of education, training, and ability		X
Use appropriate medical terminology		X

AT A GLANCE	Normal Blood Pressure at Different Ages	
Age	**Average (mm Hg)**	
Newborn	50/25	
6–9 years	95/65	
10–15 years	100/65	
Young adult	118/76	
Adult	$\frac{120 \text{ to } 129}{80 \text{ to } 84}$	

Table 17-5

millimeters (mm) of mercury (Hg). BP readings should routinely be started at the age of 5 years.

Normal BP: Depends on age. The average normal BP in healthy persons of different ages is listed in Table 17-5.

Pulse pressure: The difference between the systolic and the diastolic pressure readings.

Korotkoff's sounds: Heard during the taking of blood pressure by means of a sphygmomanometer and stethoscope. As air is released from the cuff, pressure on the brachial artery is reduced, and the blood is heard pulsing through the artery.

Factors affecting BP: Five physiological factors affect BP: blood volume, peripheral resistance of the vessels, condition of the heart muscle, vessel elasticity, and blood viscosity.

Blood volume and blood viscosity: BP elevates as the blood volume increases. Polycytopenia increases BP. Hemorrhage causes volume and BP to drop.

Peripheral resistance: The relationship of the lumen of the vessel and amount of blood flowing through it. Fatty cholesterol deposits narrow the lumen, resulting in high BP.

Heart muscle condition: The strength of the heart muscle affects the volume of blood flow.

Elasticity of vessels: The ability of blood vessels to expand and contract. It decreases with age.

Hypertension: High BP, defined as systolic pressure consistently above 140 mm Hg and diastolic pressure above 90 mm Hg. According to the American Heart Association, patients with systolic readings from 130 to 139 mm Hg and diastolic readings from 85 to 89 mm Hg are considered prehypertensive. Several factors contribute to hypertension, including hyperthyroidism, heart and liver disease, rigidity of blood vessels, smoking, anxiety, stress, and race. There are two types of hypertension: primary (essential) and secondary (nonessential). Hypertension should be found on

at least two occasions before the patient is placed on medications, unless the diastolic reading is over 120 mm Hg.

Essential hypertension: The vast majority of patients with hypertension (90%) have essential hypertension. The actual cause of essential high BP is not known. It may be genetic.

Nonessential hypertension: Caused by disorders of other organs in the body, such as the kidney, as well as endocrine disorders.

Malignant hypertension: The most fatal form of hypertension. It is characterized by rapidly and severely elevated BP that commonly damages the intima of small vessels, the brain, the retina, the heart, and the kidneys. It is more common among African Americans and may be caused by genetic predisposition, stress, obesity, smoking, the use of contraceptives, and aging.

Hypotension: An abnormal condition in which the BP is not adequate for full oxygenation of the tissues. Several factors may cause hypotension. They include anemia, dehydration, shock, hemorrhage, cancer, starvation, infection, high fever, and certain medications. The common drugs that affect BP and cause hypotension are analgesics, narcotics, antihypertensives, and diuretics. Persistent readings of 90/60 mm Hg or below are usually considered hypotensive.

Orthostatic hypotension: Abnormally and temporarily low BP. It occurs when a patient rapidly moves from a lying to a standing position and is also called postural hypotension. Orthostatic hypotension can cause patients to experience vertigo or syncope. Some medications may cause orthostatic hypotension.

Stethoscope: A diagnostic instrument that amplifies sound, used to detect sounds produced by BP as well as heart sounds. This instrument consists of a chest piece consisting of a diaphragm and/or bell, flexible tubing, binaurals, a spring mechanism, and ear pieces. See Figure 17-4.

Sphygmomanometer: An instrument used to measure BP. The components are the manometer, inflatable rubber bladder, cuff, and bulb. There are three types of sphygmomanometer: mercury, aneroid, and digital (electronic). Mercury sphygmomanometers are being phased out with other mercury-containing medical equipment, such as mercury thermometers. Aneroid and electronic blood pressure measuring devices are more commonly used.

Manometer: A scale that registers the actual BP reading.

BP cuffs: A thigh cuff is available when an adult arm is too large for the large arm cuff. When using a thigh cuff, the popliteal artery is palpated for a pulse.

Measuring BP: Wrap the cuff around the upper arm, just above the pulse point of the brachial artery. Inflate the cuff to the maximum inflation level, then release the air, and listen with the stethoscope as you watch

10. The absence of respiration for
    more than 15 seconds is called

    A. Bradypnea
    B. Hyperpnea
    C. Shock
    D. Cheyne-Stokes
    E. Apnea

11. Blood pressure readings sho
    started at age

    A. 5 years
    B. 10 years
    C. 15 years
    D. 20 years
    E. 25 years

12. Which of the following refers
    determining the circumferer
    head?

    A. Manipulation
    B. Mensuration
    C. Palpation
    D. Inspection
    E. Auscultation

13. Which of the following a
    is the site at which to de
    pulse?

    A. Knee
    B. Ankle
    C. Forearm
    D. Foot
    E. Brachial

14. Which of the following is a
    to amplify sounds?

    A. Tympanoscope
    B. Arthroscope
    C. Stethoscope
    D. Endoscope
    E. Otoscope

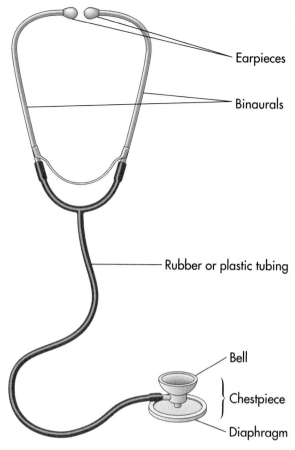

Earpieces

Binaurals

Rubber or plastic tubing

Bell

Chestpiece

Diaphragm

Figure 17-4 *The stethoscope amplifies body sounds.*

the manometer. The point at which the heartbeat is first heard is the systolic pressure; the point at which the sound disappears is the diastolic pressure.

Height and Weight

Mensuration: A general term for the measurement of weight and height. Mensuration for infants also includes measuring the circumference of the head.

First visit: Provides baseline or normal values for the patient's current condition. Weight and height measurements are taken at each office visit. Any sudden changes may be an indication of a medical problem.

Measuring weight (adult): See Figure 17-5.

1. Identify the patient and introduce yourself.
2. Wash your hands and explain the procedure.
3. Check to see whether the scale is in balance by moving all the weights to the left side. The indicator should be level with the middle mark. If you are using a scale equipped to measure both kilograms and pounds, check to see that the scale is set to measure the desired units and that the upper and lower weights show the same units.
4. Place a disposable towel on the scale.

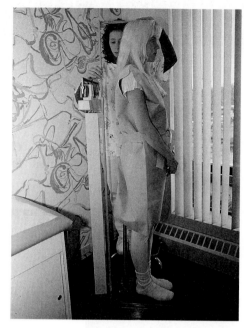

Figure 17-5 *The scale with attached height bar is used for measuring the height and weight of children and adults.*

5. Ask the patient to remove shoes.
6. Ask the patient to step on the center of the scale, facing forward.
7. Place the lower weight at the highest number that does not cause the balance indicator to drop to the bottom.
8. Move the upper weight slowly to the right until the balance bar is centered at the middle mark, adjusting as necessary.
9. Add the two weight measurements together.
10. Record the patient's weight to the nearest quarter of a pound or tenth of a kilogram.

Measuring height (adult):

1. Raise the height bar well above the patient's head and swing out the extension.
2. Ask the patient to step on the center of the scale and stand up straight.
3. Gently lower the height bar until the extension rests on the patient's head.
4. Have the patient step off the scale before you read the measurement.
5. If the patient is fewer than 50 inches tall, read the height on the bottom part of the ruler. If the patient is more than 50 inches tall, read the height on the top, movable part of the ruler. Note that the numbers increase in opposite directions on the top and bottom, so make sure that you read the height in the right direction.
6. Record the patient's height.

Instructions:

Answer the following c
answers in the *Answer*
section.

1. The normal pulse rat
   for adults is
   A. 40–60
   B. 60–100
   C. 80–100
   D. 100–120
   E. 120–140

2. Which of the followii
   sidered the most acc
   temperature?
   A. Oral
   B. Aural or tympani
   C. Axillary
   D. Rectal
   E. Cutaneous

3. The artery most com
   patient's pulse is
   A. Carotid
   B. Apical
   C. Temporal
   D. Celiac
   E. Radial

4. You've taken a patie
   corded it as 96.9° F.
   you to convert this
   What is the patient's
   A. 21.8
   B. 116.8
   C. 36.1
   D. 37.9
   E. 25.8

20. Which of the following arteries is most commonly used to monitor lower limb circulation?
    A. Popliteal
    B. Posterior tibial
    C. Femoral
    D. Common iliace
    E. Dorsalis pedis

21. Which of the following methods of obtaining body temperature is <u>not</u> appropriate for a patient with dyspnea?
    A. Rectal
    B. Aural
    C. Axillary
    D. Oral
    E. Tympanic

22. Which of the following pulses is measured when a medical assistant palpates the fifth intercostal space at the midclavicular line?
    A. Femoral
    B. Apical
    C. Radial
    D. Brachial
    E. Dorsalis pedis

ANSWER KEY

1.	B		12.	B
2.	D		13.	A
3.	E		14.	C
4.	C		15.	E
5.	E		16.	D
6.	C		17.	E
7.	C		18.	D
8.	C		19.	B
9.	B		20.	E
10.	E		21.	D
11.	A		22.	B

CHAPTER 18

Pharmacology

Anticoagulant Drugs
Hypolipidemic Drugs

Pharmacology of the Respiratory System

Antihistamines
Antiallergic Drugs
Asthma Drugs

Pharmacology of the Digestive System

Pharmacology of the Endocrine System

Pharmacology of the Sensory System

Eye Medications
Ear Medications

Pharmacology of the Urinary System

Organic Acid or Loop Diuretics
Thiazide and Thiazide-Like Diuretics
Potassium-Sparing Diuretics

Pharmacology of the Reproductive System

Use of Gonadal Hormones
Impotence

MEDICAL ASSISTING COMPETENCIES

COMPETENCY	CMA	RMA
Clinical		
Apply principles of aseptic techniques and infection control, including hand washing	X	X
Practice Standard Precautions	X	X
Apply pharmacology principles to prepare and administer oral and parenteral (excluding IV) medications as directed by the physician	X	X
Maintain medication and immunization records	X	X
General/Legal/Professional		
Identify and respond to issues of confidentiality by maintaining confidentiality at all times and following appropriate guidelines when releasing records or information	X	X
Be aware of and perform within legal and ethical boundaries	X	X
Determine the needs for documentation and reporting, and document accurately and appropriately	X	X

COMPETENCY	CMA	RMA
General/Legal/Professional		
Demonstrate knowledge of and monitor current federal and state health-care legislation and regulations; maintain licenses and accreditation	X	X
Dispose of controlled substances in compliance with government regulations		X
Perform risk management procedures		X
Instruct individuals according to their needs	X	X
Provide patients with methods of health promotion and disease prevention	X	X
Conduct work within scope of education, training, and ability		X
Use appropriate medical terminology		X

STRATEGIES TO SUCCESS

▶ *Study Skills*

Ask questions!

When you have trouble understanding a concept, don't be afraid to ask your instructor to explain it to you. If you are still unclear about something, go to your local library and try to find the answer in a reference book or check the Internet. The job of a medical assistant is complex, and it's easy to feel overwhelmed. Take control of your own education and success, and seek out the answers you need.

General Pharmacology Terms and Concepts

Pharmacology: The study of the origin, nature, chemistry, effects, and uses of drugs.

Drug: Any substance that may modify one or more of the functions of a living organism. Drugs have several uses, including therapeutic, palliative, preventive, replacement, and diagnostic. Table 18-1 provides information on drug uses. The 50 most commonly dispensed drugs in the United States are listed by category in Table 18-2.

Pharmacy: The art of compounding, preparing, dispensing, and correctly utilizing drugs for medicinal use; also, a drugstore.

Pharmacognosy: The branch of pharmacology dealing with natural drugs or natural products chemistry.

AT A GLANCE | Drugs and Their Uses

Type of Use	Purpose of Use
Therapeutic	To cure disease
Palliative	To relieve symptoms
Preventive	To prevent certain conditions
Replacement	To replace substances that the body is not producing sufficiently
Diagnostic	To diagnose disease

Table 18-1

Category of Pharmacologic Activity	Trade Name	Generic Name
Analgesic	Hydrocodone w/APAP	hydrocodone w/APAP
Analgesic, central acting	Ultram	tramadol
Antianginal, antihypertensive	Norvasc	amlodipine
Antianxiety	Ativan	lorazepam
Antibiotic	Biaxin XL Cipro Levaquin Zithromax	clarithromycin ciprofloxacin levofloxacin azithromycin
Anticoagulant	Coumadin	warfarin
Anticonvulsant	Dilantin Neurontin	phenytoin gabapentin
Anticonvulsant/miscellaneous	Depakote	divalproex
Antidepressant	Lexapro Paxil Wellbutrin SR	escitalopram oxalate paroxetine bupropion HCl
Antidiabetic	Glucophage XR Glucotrol XL	metformin glipizide
Antifungal	Diflucan Nystatin	fluconazole nystatin
Antihistimine	Allegra Zyrtec	fexofenadine cetirizine
Antihyperlipidemic	Lipitor Tricor	atorvastatin fenofibrate
Antihypertensive	Prinivil Toprol-XL	lisinopril metoprolol
Antihypertensive, ace Inhibitor	Accupril Lotensin Monopril	quinapril benazepril hydrochloride fosinopril sodium
Antiplatelet	Plavix	clopidogrel bisulfate
Antiviral	Valtrex	valacyclovir
Beta-adrenergic agonist (Sympathomimetic)	Proventil	albuterol

Table 18-2

Category of Pharmacologic Activity	Trade Name	Generic Name
Calcium channel blocker, antihypertensive	Cartia XT	diltiazem hydrochloride
Cardiac glycoside	Lanoxin	digoxin
Cholinergic blocker	Atrovent	ipratropium/albuterol
Conjugated estrogens	Premarin	conjugated estrogens
Contraceptive	Ortho Tri-Cyclen	norestimate/ethinyl estradiol
Central Nervous System (CNS) stimulant	Concerta	methylphenidate XR
Diuretic	Lasix	furosemide
Erectile dysfunction inhibitor	Viagra	sildenafil citrate
Estrogen receptor modulator	Evista	raloxifene
Gastric acid secretory depressant	Prevacid	lansoprazole
GERD	Nexium	esomeprazole
Glucocorticoid	Flonase Nasonex	fluticasone mometasone
Hypnotic	Ambien	zolpidem
Narcotic analgesic	Oxycontin	oxycodone
NSAID	Celebrex Mobic	celecoxib meloxicam
Osteoclast-mediated inhibitor	Fosamax	alendronate
Sympathomimetic	Serevent	salmeterol/xinafoate
Thyroid hormone	Synthroid	levothyroxine

Table 18-2, concluded

Source: Adapted from "The Top 200 Prescriptions for 2005 by Number of U.S. Prescriptions Dispensed," Rx List: The Internet Drug Index, www.rxlist.com.

Pharmacodynamics: The study of the mechanisms of actions of drugs on living organisms.

Pharmacokinetics: The study of the movement of drugs, metabolism, and action of drugs within the body, especially the processes of absorption, distribution, biotransformation, localization in tissue, and excretion.

Toxicology: The science that deals with poisons.

Prophylactic: An agent used to prevent disease.

Drugs and Their Effects

Drug process: A drug must pass through four basic stages: absorption, distribution, metabolism, and excretion.

Absorption: The process by which a drug is absorbed into circulation.

Distribution: The process by which the circulatory system transports drugs to the affected body parts.

Metabolism: The process by which drugs are broken down into useful by-products by enzymes in the liver. It is also known as biotransformation. The liver is the main body organ involved in the metabolism of drugs.

Excretion: The kidney is responsible for filtering out drugs from the blood. Drugs are also excreted through the lungs, sweat glands, and intestines.

Mechanism of action: The way in which a drug produces its effects.

Drug classification: Drugs are classified according to their effect on the body. See Table 18-3.

Synergism: The joint action of agents in which their combined effect is more intense than the sum of their individual effects.

Cumulation: The compound effect of an agent taken over time in individual small amounts.

Allergic reaction: An acquired, abnormal immune response to a substance that does not normally cause

AT A GLANCE	Common Drug Classifications and Actions
Classification	**Action**
General	
Analgesic	Relieves pain
Antibiotic	Destroys or inhibits bacterial growth
Integumentary System	
Antifungal	Treats fungal infections
Antihidrotic	Prevents or decreases perspiration
Antipruritic	Relieves itches
Musculoskeletal System	
Muscle relaxant	Relaxes muscles on a short-term basis
Nonsteroidal anti-inflammatory drug (NSAID)	Reduces pain, inflammation, and fever
Nervous System	
Antianxiety	Depresses the CNS
Anticonvulsant	Prevents or relieves convulsions
Antidepressant	Prevents or treats mental depression
Antiepileptic	Treats epilepsy
Antihypnotic	Prevents or inhibits sleep
Antiparkinsonian	Treats Parkinson's disease
Antipsychotic	Treats psychosis
Sedative	Creates tranquilizing, soothing effects
Endocrine System	
Antisecretory	Inhibits secretion
Insulin	Treats diabetes
Thyroid agent	Replaces thyroid function
Cardiovascular System	
Antiarrhythmic	Regulates the heartbeat
Anticoagulant	Slows the coagulation process
Antihypercholesterolemic	Prevents or controls high cholesterol
Antihypertensive	Prevents or controls high blood pressure
Vasodilator	Relaxes or dilates blood vessels
Respiratory System	
Antihistamine	Relieves allergies
Antitussive	Relieves or prevents coughs
Decongestant	Reduces mucus production

Table 18-3

Classification	Action
Digestive System	
Antacid	Neutralizes gastric acids
Antiemetic	Controls nausea, vomiting, and motion sickness
Laxative	Promotes evacuation of the intestines
Urinary System	
Diuretic	Increases urine excretion
Reproductive System	
Androgen	Replaces male hormones
Antivenereal	Prevents or controls sexually transmitted (venereal) diseases
Contraceptive	Prevents conception
Estrogen	Replaces female hormones

Table 18-3, concluded

a reaction. It may develop within 30 minutes of administration of therapy. Symptoms of a mild allergic reaction include skin rashes, swelling, itchy eyes and skin, wheezing, and fever. Severe allergic reactions such as anaphylaxis include extreme weakness, nausea, vomiting, cyanosis, dyspnea, hypotension, shock, and cardiac arrest.

Adverse effect: A general term for an undesirable and potentially harmful drug effect.

Anaphylaxis: A severe allergic response to medication, involving respiratory distress.

Side effect: An adverse effect of a drug on another organ system that is not related to the main target of the drug.

Toxic effect: An adverse drug effect that can be harmful or life-threatening.

Antagonism: The combined effect of two drugs that is less than the effect of either drug taken alone.

Tolerance: Increasing resistance to the usual effects of an established dosage of a drug as a result of continued use.

Dependence: A state of reliance on a drug, either psychological or physiological, that may result in withdrawal symptoms if drug use is discontinued.

Idiosyncrasy: An abnormal sensitivity to a drug. It usually refers to an individual patient's unique response to medication.

Factors that affect individual variation in a drug's effect: Age, weight, sex and percentage of body fat, time of day, tolerance, genetic variation, emotional state, placebo effect, presence of a disease, and patient compliance.

Drug indications: Intended uses of any drug.

Contraindications: Situations or conditions under which a certain drug should not be administered.

Drug abuse: The use or overuse of any drug in a manner that deviates from the prescribed pattern.

Prophylaxis: A procedure or medication used to prevent a disease rather than to treat an existing disease.

Half-life: The amount of time required for 50% of the drug to be eliminated from the body.

Teratogen: A drug that causes birth defects. These drugs affect the X chromosome and therefore should not be given to pregnant women.

Placebo: A drug dosage form that has no pharmacological effect because it contains no active ingredients. Placebos are used in controlled clinical trials of new drugs.

Efficacy: A drug's therapeutic value.

Potency: A measure of the strength or concentration of a drug required to produce the desired effect.

Posology: The study of the amount of drug that is required to produce therapeutic effects.

Polypharmacy: Multiple drug prescriptions. This situation is very common for elderly individuals, and it often increases confusion, forgetfulness, and noncompliance. Minimizing polypharmacy should also be an important consideration when trying to avoid harmful drug interactions.

Dosage: The amount of a drug prescribed for a given patient.

Dose: The measured portion of medication to be taken at one time.

Dispense: To distribute a drug in properly labeled containers to a patient.

Administer: To give a drug directly to a patient by injection, by mouth, or by any route that introduces the drug directly into the patient's body.

Lethal dose 50 (LD_{50}): The dose that will kill 50% of the subjects tested.

Effective dose 50 (ED$_{50}$): The dose that will produce an effect in 50% of the subjects tested.

Therapeutic index (TI): The ratio of the LD$_{50}$ to the ED$_{50}$. TI = LD$_{50}$/ED$_{50}$. The ratio gives an estimate of the relative safety of a drug.

Drug names: There are three types of names for any drug: chemical, generic or official, and trade name or brand name.

Chemical name: The chemical structure of a drug that explains the composition of a drug.

Generic name: The official and nonproprietary name of a drug assigned by the U.S. Adopted Names (USAN) council.

Trade name or **brand name:** A word, symbol, or device assigned to a drug (or other product) by its manufacturer, registered by the U.S. Patent Office, and approved by the U.S. FDA.

Prescription: An order written by a physician to be filled by a pharmacist. Physicians must sign their name and title to every prescription. Most prescriptions also contain the DEA number of the item.

Superscription: The part of a prescription that includes the patient's name, address, date, and the symbol *Rx*, which means "take."

Inscription: The part of a prescription containing the names and quantities of the ingredients.

Subscription: The part of a drug prescription that gives directions to the pharmacist about how to prepare the drug.

Signature: The part of a prescription that gives instructions to patients. A signature tells the patient how to take the drug, when to take it, and how much to take.

Over-the-counter (OTC): Available without a prescription.

Drug Forms

Water-Based Solutions

Syrup (syr.): A solution of water and sugar to which a drug is added. Adding flavors can also eliminate the bitter taste of certain drugs. Examples include Robitussin®, a cough syrup.

Emulsion: Liquid medication that contains fats or oils suspended in water. They must be shaken before use. Cod liver oil used as a laxative is an emulsion.

Magma: Heavy particles mixed with water to form a milky liquid. Magmas must be shaken before administration. Examples include milk of magnesia.

Lotion: A suspension of drugs in a water base for external use. Lotions must be patted on the skin for protective, emollient, or antipruritic purposes. Examples include calamine lotion used as an antipruritic for poison ivy.

Liniment: A liquid suspension that is rubbed onto the skin. Liniments relieve pain and swelling. Examples include Ben-Gay®.

Aerosol: A liquid or semiliquid delivered as mist by pressurized gas, as with oral inhalers or nebulizers, which allows rapid absorption into the bloodstream. Examples include Proventil®, a bronchodilator used for asthma.

Alcoholic Solutions

Elixir (elix.): A fluid extract of drugs that are dissolved in various concentrations of alcohol, usually between 10 and 20%. Examples include phenobarbital elixir, an anticonvulsant, and Benadryl® elixir, an antihistamine.

Tincture: A potent solution made with alcohol. Examples include iodine, a strong antiseptic; belladonna tincture, an anticholinergic; and camphorated opium tincture, a laxative.

Injectible Forms

Ampule: A single dose of sterile solution contained in a glass bottle whose seal must be broken to draw up medication.

Vial: A bottle with a rubber stopper or other nonsterile seal. Vials provide multiple doses of medication.

Solids and Semisolids

Ointment: Drugs mixed with lanolin or petrolatum.

Powder: Drugs dried and ground into fine particles. An example is potassium chloride (Kato Powder®).

Tablet (tab.): Drug powders compressed into a convenient form for swallowing.

Troche or **lozenge:** A flattened tablet that is dissolved in the mouth. These medications are often used for colds and sore throats.

Capsule (cap.): A small gelatin enclosure containing powder or liquid drugs. The capsule dissolves in the stomach, releasing the drugs.

Delayed-release: Certain tablets and capsules are treated with special coatings so that various portions of the drug dissolve at different rates. In this way, drug effects can be extended over time.

Enteric-coated: Certain tablets and capsules are coated with an acid-resistant substance so that the drug will be absorbed only in the less acidic portions of the intestine. Enteric-coated products need to be taken on an empty stomach with water, either 1 hour before or 2 hours after a meal.

Spheroidal Oral Drug Absorption System (SODAS): Pellets covered in a gelatin capsule that slowly release the drug, unaffected by food or the acid in the GI tract.

Gastrointestinal Therapeutic System (GITS): A two-compartment tablet. In the GI tract, water is drawn into the tablet forcing the drug out. This system delivers drugs at a constant rate over extended periods of time.

Suppository (supp.): Drugs mixed with a substance (cocoa butter) that will melt at body temperature. Suppositories are inserted into the rectum, urethra, or vagina.

Ointment or **unguent (oint., ung.):** A salve of soft, oily substances to which a drug has been added. It is applied to the skin.

Cream: A thick, smooth, water-based topical medication.

Transdermal: Administered through the skin with a bandage or a patch system. Patches are easy to apply and cause little or no discomfort, and they provide a continuous source of the drug over 24 hours or more.

Sources of Drug Information

Physicians' Desk Reference **(PDR):** The most widely used drug reference publication. It contains an index of manufacturers, a brand name and generic name index, a product category index, and a product identification guide. The brand name and generic name index makes up the pink section, the product classification or category index is the blue section, an alphabetical index by manufacturers is featured in the white section, a generic and chemical name index constitutes the yellow section, and diagnostic product information is found in the green section. The PDR is revised annually.

United States Pharmacopeia Dispensing Information **(USPDI):** Published in three volumes with monthly updates. Volume I provides in-depth information about prescription and OTC medications and nutritional supplements. Volume II contains advice for the patient. Volume III contains state and federal requirements for prescribing and dispensing drugs.

Drug Regulation

Controlled Substance Act of 1970: A law that controls the distribution and use of all drugs of abuse or potential abuse as designated by the DEA. It divides narcotics, stimulants, and some sedatives into five classes, called schedules. See Table 18-4 for examples.

Drug Regulation and Reform Act of 1978: Permits briefer investigation of new drugs, allowing consumers earlier access.

Orphan Drug Act of 1983: Speeds up the availability of drugs for patients with rare diseases.

Record keeping: A doctor's office must maintain two types of records: dispensing and inventory. Dispensing records must indicate to whom, when, and how much

AT A GLANCE   Drug Schedules

Schedule	Abuse Potential	Prescription Requirement	Examples
I	High abuse potential; no accepted medical use	No prescription permitted	Heroin, hallucinogens, marijuana, fenethylline, hashish, lysergic acid diethylamide (LSD), methaqualone (Quaalude®), peyote
II	High abuse potential; an accepted medical use	Prescription required; no refills permitted without a new written prescription	Narcotics, cocaine, morphine, opium, anabolic steroids, hydromorphone hydrochloride (Dilaudid®), amphetamines, short-acting barbiturates
III	Moderate abuse potential; an accepted medical use	Prescription required; 5 refills permitted in 6 months	Moderate-acting barbiturates, butabarbital (Butisol®), secobarbital (Seconal®), glutethimide, most preparations that include codeine combined with something else
IV	Low abuse potential; an accepted medical use	Prescription required; 5 refills permitted in 6 months	Chloral hydrate (Noctec®), diazepam (Valium®), alprazolam (Xanax®), pentazocine HCl (Talwin®)
V	Low abuse potential; an accepted medical use	No prescription required for individuals 18 or older	Cough syrups with codeine (Cheracol® with codeine), guaifenesin (Naldecon Dx®), Lomotil®, Parepectolin®

Table 18-4

of the drug was administered or dispensed. Inventory records involve counting the amount of each drug on hand. The controlled drug inventory must be completed every 2 years, with all the invoice copies from the drug suppliers included.

Registration: Doctor's offices that dispense or administer drugs must register with the DEA with a form called the "Application for Registration Under the Controlled Substances Act of 1970."

Storage: Some medications, such as antibiotics, may need to be refrigerated. All medications should be left in their original containers. Read drug labels and inserts for specific storage directions for each type of drug.

Security: Store controlled substances and prescription pads in a locked area. Be aware of and follow state guidelines and laws about keeping controlled substances secure.

Discarding drugs: Any medication that is out of date or without a label should be discarded. These drugs should be poured down a sink so that no one will be able to take them.

Patient Education

Patient education: Advise patients to provide your medical office with a complete list of drugs they use regularly or periodically—including alcohol and recreational drugs, as well as herbal medicines. Explain to patients how and when to take each drug to ensure safety and effectiveness. Explain how to identify possible adverse effects, and be prepared to answer any questions. Advise patients to report to the physician any adverse reactions or drug interactions.

Poisons

Poisons: All drugs will act as poisons if taken in excess. Only the dose separates the therapeutic effect from a toxic effect.

Antidote: An agent that counteracts a poison. There are four types: chemical, mechanical, physiological, and universal. Antidotes for some of the most common poisons are shown in Table 18-5.

Chemical antidotes: Neutralize the poison by changing its chemical nature.

Physiological antidotes: Counteract the effects of the poison by releasing opposing effects.

Mechanical antidotes: Prevent absorption of the poison.

Universal antidotes: Were supposedly effective against a wide range of toxins. These mixtures were formerly recommended as antidotes when the exact poison was not known. There is, in fact, no known universal antidote.

Drug Administration

Oral route: The drug is swallowed. This is the safest and most convenient route used for most medications. Oral medications may cause nausea and stomach irritation. They also have a slow absorption rate that can be affected by food. Examples include aspirin, sedatives, hypnotics, and antibiotics.

Buccal route (buc): The drug is placed between the gum and cheek and left there until it is dissolved. Examples include Oxytocin®, which induces labor.

Sublingual route (subling, subl, SL): The drug is placed under the tongue and left there until it is dissolved. These drugs are used when rapid effects are needed. Examples include nitroglycerin for angina pectoris and ergotamine tartate (Ergostat®) for migraines.

Topical route (T): The drug is rubbed into, patted on, sprayed on, swabbed on, or rinsed on skin. These drugs are used to soothe irritated areas or to cure local infections. Examples include most creams and ointments.

Transdermal route: A patch is applied to clean, dry, nonhairy skin. This is a convenient form that provides continuous absorption and effects that last over many hours. Estrogen and nitroglycerin can be administered in this way.

Inhalation route, inhalation therapy: The drug is inhaled to achieve local effects within the respiratory tract. Antiasthmatic medications such as epinephrine are administered in this way.

Ophthalmic route: Drops are placed into the eye.

Otic route: Drops are placed into the ear.

Nasal route: Nasal solutions act a locally to treat minor congestion or infection. The medication should be drawn up in the dropper and held just over one nostril,

AT A GLANCE	Poisons and Their Respective Antidotes
Poison	**Antidote**
Acetaminophen	N-acetylcysteine
Benzodiazepines	Flumazenil
Carbon monoxide	Oxygen
Cyanide	Amyl nitrite
Iron	Deferoxamine
Methanol	Ethanol
Opiates	Naloxone
Organophosphates	Atropine or pralidoxime

Table 18-5

and then the required number of nose drops should be administered.

Rectal route (R): A suppository is inserted into the rectum, or a solution is administered as an enema. This method is used when a patient cannot take oral medications or when local effects are desired. Analgesics and laxatives can be administered in this way.

Urethral route: A solution is instilled into the bladder by means of a catheter.

Vaginal route (p.v., vag): A solution is administered as a douche. Other forms are inserted into the vagina with an applicator. Examples include Mycostatin®.

Parenteral route: The drug is injected into the body with a needle and syringe for rapid absorption and controlled dosage. Parenteral administration is divided into four main categories according to the location of the injection: intradermal, subcutaneous, intramuscular, and intravenous.

Intradermal route: The drug is injected into the upper layers of the skin.

Subcutaneous route (SubQ, SC): The drug is injected into the subcutaneous layer of the skin.

Intramuscular route (IM): The drug is injected into a muscle. This method is used when a drug has poor oral absorption, when high blood levels are required, or when rapid effects are desired. Narcotic analgesics and antibiotics are administered in this way.

Intravenous route (IV): The drug is injected or infused into a vein. This method is used when an emergency situation exists, when immediate effects are required, and also when other medications are being administered by infusion. Examples include IV fluids (e.g., dextrose solution), nutrient supplementation, and antibiotics.

Antibiotics

Antibiotic: A chemical substance that destroys or interferes with the development of bacterial microorganisms. Antibiotics are derived from other living microorganisms. These agents are sufficiently nontoxic to the host and are used in the treatment of infectious diseases. They are divided into two groups: bactericidal and bacteriostatic. Some examples of both are shown in Table 18-6.

Bactericidal: Destructive to or killing bacteria.

Bacteriostatic: Inhibiting the growth of bacteria.

Antimicrobial: Killing or inhibiting the growth of microorganisms.

Broad-spectrum: Effective against a wide variety of both gram-positive and gram-negative pathogenic bacteria.

Bacterial resistance: The ability of some bacteria to resist the actions of antibiotics.

Chemotherapy: The use of cytotoxic drugs to kill or to inhibit the growth of infectious organisms or cancerous cells.

AT A GLANCE	Examples of the Two Different Types of Antibiotics
Bactericidal	**Bacteriostatic**
Penicillins	Sulfonamides
Cephalosporins	Tetracyclines
Aminoglycosides	Chloramphenicol
Vancomycin	Clindamycin
Quinolones	Spectinomycin

Table 18-6

Bactericidal Antibiotics

Penicillin: A large group of natural or synthetic antibacterial agents derived from fungi of the genus *Penicillum*. Penicillins were the first true antibiotics, and they are the most widely used class of antibiotics. They interfere with the synthesis of bacterial cell walls. Classifications of penicillin and examples (with generic names and brand names) are seen in Table 18-7. Common uses of penicillin include treatment of otitis media, pneumonia, gonorrhea, syphilis, rheumatic fever, and meningitis. Common side effects of penicillin include diarrhea, nausea, rashes, thrombophlebitis, hyperkalemia, and hypernatremia. When used in high doses, penicillins may cause CNS disturbances, including convulsions. As a drug class, penicillins also cause the highest incidence of drug allergy. Patients must be questioned about the possibility of a penicillin allergy.

Beta-lactamases: Bacterial enzymes that inactivate penicillin and cephalosporin antibiotics.

Penicillinase: An enzyme produced by some bacteria that inactivates penicillin, thus increasing resistance to the antibiotic. It is used in the treatment of reactions to penicillin.

Cephalosporin: One of a large group of broad-spectrum antibiotics from *Cephalosporium*, a genus of soil-inhabiting fungi. Cephalosporins are similar in structure and action to penicillin. Like penicillins, they are classified into four generations. They inhibit cell wall synthesis in bacteria. Common uses of cephalosporins include administration in patients allergic to the penicillins and treatment of certain urinary and respiratory tract infections. Side effects of cephalosporins include oral thrush, diarrhea, rashes, vaginitis, thrombophlebitis, and sometimes electrolyte imbalance. Intramuscular injections of cephalosporins are usually painful and may cause inflammation.

Classification	Example Generic Name (*Brand Name*)	Effectiveness
First Generation Narrow-spectrum	penicillin G (Pentids)	Gram-positive streptococci
Beta-lactamase sensitive	penicillin V (Pen-Vee K®)	Gram-positive streptococci
Beta-lactamase resistant	oxacillin (Prostaphlin®) cloxacillin (Tegopen®) methicillin (Staphcillin®) nafcillin (Unipen®) dicloxacillin (Dynapen®)	Gram-positive streptococci
Second Generation Broad-spectrum	ampicillin (Omnipen®) amoxicillin (Amoxil®)	*Hemophilus* *Escherichia coli* *Neisseria*
Third Generation Extended spectrum	carbenicillin (Geocillin®)	*Pseudomonas*
Fourth Generation Widest spectrum, potent	mezlocillin (Mezlin®) piperacillin (Pipracil®)	Serious infections, *Pseudomonas aeruginosa, Proteus vulgaris, Klebsiella pneumoniae*

Table 18-7

First-generation cephalosporins: Used to treat common gram-positive and gram-negative infections. Examples include cefazolin (Kefzol®), cephalothin (Keflin®), and cephradine (Velosef®).

Second-generation cephalosporins: Used for gram-negative infections. They are more resistant to the actions of penicillinase and cephalosporinase. Examples include cefamamandole (Mandol®), cefotetan (Cefotan®), and cefotixin (Mefoxin®).

Third-generation cephalosporins: Used for serious gram-negative infections. They have longer duration of action and are more potent than the first- or second-generation cephalosporins. Examples include cefotaxime (Claforan®) and ceftriaxone (Rocephin®).

Fourth-generation cephalosporins: Similar in spectrum to third-generation drugs. They have a greater resistance to beta-lactamase-inactivating enzymes. Examples include cefepime (Maxapime®).

Aminoglycoside: One of a group of bacterial antibiotics derived from the genus Streptomyces that irreversibly inhibit protein synthesis. All of the aminoglycosides are highly toxic. Types of aminoglycosides include amikacin (Amikin®), gentamicin (Garamycin®), kanamycin (Kantrex®), neomycin (Neobiotic®), streptomycin, and tobramycin (Nebcin®). Aminoglycosides are used to treat infections caused by gram-negative organisms. They are often given in large doses before abdominal surgery to "sterilize" the bowel. They are also used for the treatment of resistant urinary tract infections. Streptomycin is used to treat tuberculosis, plague, and tularemia. Side effects include nausea, vomiting, diarrhea, ototoxicity (which can result in deafness), and nephrotoxicity. Aminoglycosides may interfere with normal renal function. Aminoglycosides are contraindicated for use during pregnancy.

Quinolone: A general class of broad-spectrum antibiotics that interrupt the replication of DNA molecules in bacteria. They are well absorbed in the GI tract after oral administration. Examples include ciprofloxacin (Cipro®) and nalidixic acid. Common uses include treatment of urinary, GI, respiratory, bone and joint, and soft tissue infections. Common side effects are headache, dizziness, GI disturbances, and rash. Quinolones are contraindicated for pediatric therapy because they cause permanent cartilage damage. Quinolones are also not recommended during pregnancy. Fluoroquinolones are synthetic quinolones.

Vancomycin (Vancocin®): A miscellaneous antibacterial agent that does not fit into any of the preceding categories. Vancomycin interferes with cell wall synthesis and is bactericidal. It is effective only on gram-positive bacteria, particularly staphylococcal infections that are resistant to other antibiotics. It also is prescribed in the treatment of infectious diseases such as pneumonia, meningitis, endocarditis, septicemia, and osteomyelitis. Common side effects include ototoxicity, nephrotoxicity, and a flushing redness of the neck and trunk caused by histamines.

Bacteriostatic Antibiotics

Sulfonamides: Synthetic antibiotics that now have limited uses because of bacterial resistance. They block the synthesis of folic acid, creating a bacteriostatic effect. Examples include mafenide (Sulfamylon®), sulfacetamide (Sulamyd®), and sulfamethizole (Thiosulfil®). Common uses include topical treatment of burns and treatment of urinary and GI tract infections. Common side effects include nausea, vomiting, diarrhea, crystalluria, anemia, leukopenia, and rashes.

Tetracycline: A broad-spectrum antibiotic that is effective against both gram-negative and gram-positive microorganisms. Tetracycline inhibits protein synthesis by bacterial cells. Foods containing calcium, mineral supplements, and antacids interfere with absorption of the tetracyclines. Examples include chlortetracycline (Aureomycin®), doxycycline (Vibramycin®), and tetracycline (Achromycin®). Common uses include treatment of urethritis, cholera, lower respiratory tract infections, meningitis, rickettsiae, and Lyme disease. Common side effects include nausea, vomiting, abdominal cramps, anorexia, and diarrhea. Tetracycline should not be administered in the last half of pregnancy and to children under 8 years of age (because it discolors teeth). It is also secreted in breast milk. The use of outdated tetracycline may cause Fanconi's syndrome.

Chloramphenicol (Chloromycetin®): A broad-spectrum antibiotic with specific therapeutic action against rickettsiae. It is a miscellaneous bacteriostatic antibiotic that does not fit into any of the preceding categories. Chloramphenicol inhibits bacterial protein synthesis, creating a bacteriostatic effect. Common uses include treatment of rickettsial infections, typhoid fever, and meningitis. It is reserved for serious or life-threatening infections. Side effects include aplastic anemia (bone marrow depression), oral thrush, and genital/anal pruritus (itching). Chloramphenicol is potentially a very toxic drug. In most cases, its effects are irreversible. It should not be administered to a newborn less than 2 weeks of age because it can result in a condition known as the gray baby syndrome, involving circulatory collapse, abdominal distention, and respiratory failure.

Clindamycin (Cleocin®): A miscellaneous bacteriostatic antibacterial agent that inhibits protein synthesis. It is used for the treatment of a variety of gram-negative aerobic and gram-positive and gram-negative anaerobic organisms. Common uses include treatment against anaerobic organisms. Side effects include pseudomembranous colitis, severe gastrointestinal disturbances, and hypersensitivity.

Spectinomycin: An antibiotic that is often called by the trademark Trobicin®. It inhibits protein synthesis and is used in the treatment of gonorrhea and certain other infections and in penicillin-allergic patients. Side effects include pain at the injection site and hypersensitivity.

Both Bactericidal and Bacteriostatic Antibiotics

Macrolid: An antibiotic with molecules that have many-membered lacton rings. Macrolids inhibit protein-synthesis in some bacteria. They are bactericidal and bacteriostatic. Examples include erythromycin (E-mycin®), azithromycin (Zithromax®), and clarithromycin (Biaxin®). Common uses include treatment of diseases of the gastrointestinal tract, skin, and respiratory system and of sexually transmitted diseases. Side effects include thrombophlebitis, diarrhea, nausea, vomiting, and abnormal tastes in the mouth.

Antitubercular Agents

Antitubercular agents: A group of drugs used to treat tuberculosis. At least two drugs, and usually three, are required in various combinations in pulmonary tuberculosis therapy. Examples include isoniazid (INH®), rifampin (Rifadin®), ethambutol (Myambutol®), and streptomycin.

Isoniazid (INH®): A synthetic bactericidal drug used to treat tuberculosis. The drug inhibits the production of mycolic acid and thus prevents cell wall synthesis. Common uses include prophylaxis and treatment of tuberculosis. Side effects include peripheral neuritis, hepatitis, numbness, nausea, vomiting, dizziness, ataxia, and hepatotoxicity.

Rifampin (Rifadin®): An antibiotic that prevents RNA synthesis. Common uses include treatment of tuberculosis and prevention of meningococci outbreaks. A common side effect is reddish-orange color in urine, saliva, feces, sputum, sweat, and tears that can permanently discolor soft contact lenses.

Ethambutol (Myambutol®): A bacteriostatic synthetic compound that inhibits the incorporation of mycolic acid into the bacterial cell wall. Side effects include confusion, fever, hallucinations, and blurred vision (red-green color changes).

Antifungal Agents

Antifungal: Destructive to fungi or inhibiting their growth. An antifungal drug is also called antimycotic. See Table 18-8 for a list of antifungal drugs.

Generic Name	Trade Name	Uses
amphoterian B	Fungizone®	Systemic fungal infections, severe progressive fungal infections, cryptococcosis
fluconazole	Diflucan®	Systemic infection, oroesophageal candidiasis
ketoconazole	Nizoral®	Systemic infection
nystatin	Mycostatin®	Candidiasis, skin infections, GI infections
griseofulvin	Grifulvin®	Superficial fungal (dermatophytic) infections
butenafine	Mentax®	Athlete's foot
terconazole	Terazol-3®, Terazol-7®	Vulvovaginal candidiasis

Table 18-8

Antiviral Agents

Amantadine (Symmetrel®): Prevents the virus that causes Asian influenza from penetrating human cells and releasing viral DNA into the cell. When administered after exposure to the flu, it also reduces the severity of the infection. It is recommended for high-risk patients only.

Acyclovir (Zovirax®): Inhibits viral DNA replication. It is used in the treatment of genital herpes and chickenpox. Side effects include kidney damage, headache, confusion, irritability, nausea, and vomiting.

Idoxuridine (Herplex®): Inhibits viral DNA synthesis by blocking incorporation of thymidine. It is used to treat herpes simplex keratitis.

Drugs used against HIV: Didanosine (Videx®), indinavir (Crixivan®), nelfinavir (Viracept®), saquinavir (Invirase®), zalcitabine (Hivid®), and zidovudine (Retrovir®). The frequency of HIV mutation and drug resistance results in poor clinical response.

Pharmacology of the Integumentary System

Anti-inflammatory drugs: Suppress inflammation and relieve itching (pruritus) and swelling (edema). Examples include betamethasone valerate (Valosine®) and hydrocortisone. Anti-inflammatory drugs are classified as steroidal and nonsteroidal.

Astringents: Relieve itching, soothe mild sunburns, and dry the skin. They are used for poison ivy, insect bites, and mild sunburn. Examples include calamine and diphenhydramine (Caladryl®).

Antipruritics: Relieve itching. They also have an antihistamine, sedative, and drying effect. An example is trimeprazine tartrate (Temaril®).

Erythema: Redness caused by an expansion of the capillaries at the skin's surface.

Vasoconstrictors: Reduce swelling and edema (caused by buildup of fluid in the tissues) and increase venous flow. They are used to treat dermal ulcers. Examples include Debrisan® and DuoDERM® hydroactive.

Antiseptics: Kill germs and are used to treat surface infections, burns, minor wounds, and vaginitis. An example is povidone-iodine (Betadine®).

Keratolytics: Swell and soften excess keratin for easy removal and shedding. They are used for warts, corns, calluses, psoriasis, and seborrheic dermatitis. An example is salicylic acid.

Pharmacology of the Musculoskeletal System

Centrally acting skeletal muscle relaxant: Inhibits skeletal muscle contraction by blocking conduction within the spinal cord. Examples include baclofen (Lioresal®), carisoprodol (Rela®, Soma®), and tizandine (Zanaflex®). Common uses include therapy for muscle strain and multiple sclerosis. Side effects include blurred vision, dizziness, lethargy, and decreased mental alertness.

Peripheral skeletal muscle relaxant: Inhibits muscle contraction at the neuromuscular junction or within the contractile process. An example is dantrolene (Dantrium®). It is commonly used during surgical procedures to relax the abdominal muscle, during shock therapy, and during tetanus. Side effects include toxicity-induced paralysis of the respiratory muscles.

Pharmacology of the Nervous System

Central Nervous System

Sedatives and Hypnotic Drugs

Hypnotic: A drug that causes insensitivity to pain by inhibiting the reception of sensory impressions in the brain, causing partial or complete unconsciousness. Sedative and hypnotic drugs produce their effects by increasing the inhibitory activity of gamma-aminobutyric acid (GABA), a neurotransmitter in the CNS.

Sedative: A hypnotic drug that exerts a quieting or tranquilizing effect. The most common sedatives and hypnotics are summarized in Table 18-9.

Barbiturate: A sedative drug that reduces brain activity and promotes sleep. The main sites of action of barbiturates are the reticular formation and the cerebral cortex. Barbiturates are used as sleep aids and as treatment for convulsions or seizures. Common side effects include drowsiness, dry mouth, lethargy, and lack of coordination. An overdose can result in extensive cardiovascular and CNS depression leading to coma, respiratory depression, and death. Prolonged and excessive use of barbiturates can result in tolerance and physical dependence. Patients who have acute intermittent porphyria should not take barbiturates because they may cause nerve damage, pain, and paralysis. Barbiturates should not be taken during pregnancy.

Nonbarbiturate: Any of a diverse group of drugs that produce effects similar to those of barbiturates. Some of these agents were developed with the hope that they would not produce addictions and dependence. Unfortunately, prolonged abuse of these drugs will still result in physical dependence and tolerance. Chloral hydrate is a good example of a nonbarbiturate drug. Its mechanism of action is similar to alcohol, and it is used as a hypnotic, particularly in elderly individuals.

AT A GLANCE	Sedatives and Hypnotic Drugs		
Classification	Uses	Side Effects	Contraindications
• Drug			
Sedative-Hypnotic Barbiturates			
• pentobarbital (Nembutal®, Luminal®) • secobarbital (Seconal®)	Sedation in smaller doses, promotion of sleep in larger doses; treatment of seizure disorders; control of epilepsy	Drowsiness, dry mouth, confusion, incoordination, respiratory depression, coma	Acute intermittent porphyria, pregnancy, suicidal tendencies
Sedative-Hypnotic Nonbarbiturates			
• chloral hydrate (Noctec®, SK-chloral®) • zolpidem (Ambien®)	Treatment of insomnia; sedation in elderly individuals	Nausea, vomiting, diarrhea, gastric irritation, dizziness	
Benzodiazepines			
• flurazepam (Dalmane®) • temazepam (Restoril®) • triazolam (Halcion®)	Treatment of anxiety	Flurazepam: hangover effect after use Triazolam: rebound insomnia and increased daytime anxiety after use	Pregnancy

Table 18-9

Side effects involve excessive CNS depression and gastric irritation.

Benzodiazepines: A class of drugs used in the treatment of anxiety. They are commonly referred to as antianxiety drugs. They depress the reticular activating system to produce sedation and hypnosis. Benzodiazepines are well tolerated and produce few side effects. They do not interfere with REM sleep and produce less tolerance than barbiturates. Flurazepam, a type of benzodiazepine, may cause sedation or a "hangover effect" the following day after use. They are contraindicated during pregnancy.

Antipsychotics

Antipsychotic drugs: Drugs that are used to treat schizophrenia and other psychotic mental disorders characterized by gross impairment in reality testing. Antipsychotic drugs are also referred to as neuroleptics. These drugs are not a cure but a method to control irrational and bizarre behavior and thought associated with psychoses. Most antipsychotics block dopamine D2 receptors. The most important types of antipsychotic drugs are phenothiazines, butyrophenones, and thioxanthenes. See Table 18-10. Common side effects include sedation; dry

AT A GLANCE	Common Antipsychotic Drugs		
Classification	**Uses**	**Side Effects**	**Contraindications**
• Drug			
Phenothiazines			
chlorpromazine (Thorazine®) triflupromazine (Vesprin®)	Antipsychotic; also antihistaminic, anticholinergic, alpha-adrenergic blocking, and antiemetic	Sedation, dry mouth, constipation, visual disturbances, dystonic reactions, akathisia, parkinsonism, tardive dyskinesia, neuroleptic malignant syndrome	Pregnancy
Butyrophenones			
haloperidol (Haldol®)	Treatment of highly agitated and manic patients (more potent than the phenothiazines)	Fewer peripheral (antihistaminic, anticholinergic, etc.) effects but greater movement disturbances	Pregnancy
Thioxanthenes			
thiothixene (Navane®)	Treatment of psychosis; few other pharmacological effects (more selective action than other antipsychotic drugs)	Drowsiness, postural hypotension, disturbances in movement	Pregnancy
Other Antipsychotic Drugs			
clozapine (Clozaril®)	Sedation, hypotension, and anticholinergic effects (atypical in that it blocks serotonin receptors in addition to dopamine receptors)	Reduction in granulocyte count in blood, no extra-pyramidal effects such as parkinsonism or tardive dyskinesia	Pregnancy

Table 18-10

mouth; constipation; visual disturbances; dystonic reactions with muscle spasms; akathisia with continuous body movement and restlessness; parkinsonism with muscular rigidity and tremors; tardive dyskinesia involving involuntary movements of the lips, jaw, tongue, and extremities; and neuroleptic malignant syndrome with hyperthermia, muscular rigidity, catatonia, and autonomic nervous system instability. Antipsychotics are contraindicated during pregnancy.

Clozapine: Atypically blocks both dopamine (D4) and serotonin receptors. It is the second-line drug used for the treatment of schizophrenia and psychosis. Common side effects include a reduction in the number of granulocytes.

Antidepressants, Psychomotor Stimulants, and Lithium

Antidepressant: A drug that prevents or relieves depression. Low levels of norepinephrine and serotonin are associated with mental depression, whereas high levels of norepinephrine and serotonin are involved in mania. Antidepressants increase the level of norepinephrine and serotonin in the brain. There are three major classes of antidepressants: monoamine oxidase (MAO) inhibitors, tricyclic antidepressants (TCAs), and selective serotonin reuptake inhibitors (SSRIs).

Monoamine oxidase (MAO) inhibitors: Increase the concentration of epinephrine, norepinephrine, and serotonin in storage sites in the nervous system. After 2 to 4 weeks of treatment, patients feel an increase in appetite and sleep and an elevation of mood. One of the disadvantages of MAO inhibitors is the dietary restriction of foods containing tyramine (wine, beer, herring, and certain cheeses). A combination of tyramine and MAO inhibitors may cause a hypertensive crisis or cerebral stroke. Other common side effects include postural hypotension, dry mouth, constipation, urinary retention, blurred vision, insomnia, tremors, convulsions, liver damage, and impotence in males. Examples include isocarboxazid (Marplan®), phenylzine (Nardil®), and tranylcypromine (Parnate®).

Tricyclic antidepressant drugs: Block the reuptake of norepinephrine and serotonin into the neuronal nerve endings. These drugs get their name from their characteristic triple-ring structure. In addition to the antidepressant effect, they also produce varying degrees of sedation, anticholinergic effects, and alpha-adrenergic blockade. Common side effects include dry mouth, weight gain, constipation, urinary retention, rapid heartbeat, postural hypotension, blurred vision, drowsiness, restlessness, tremors, convulsion, mania, cardiac arrhythmias, and jaundice. Examples include imipramine (Tofranil®), doxepin (Sinequan®), desipramine (Petrofrane®), and amoxapine (Asendin®).

Selective serotonin reuptake inhibitors: Newer antidepressant drugs that block the reuptake and inactivation of serotonin in the brain. They are the most widely used antidepressants. Fluoxetine (Prozac®) was the first drug of this class to be introduced. Fluoxetine is effective against depression and also obsessive-compulsive disorders. Other examples include fluvoxamine (Luvox®) and sertraline (Zoloft®). Common side effects include headache, nervousness, insomnia, tremors, nausea, diarrhea, dry mouth, weight loss, and anorexia.

Psychomotor stimulants: Include amphetamines and other closely related drugs. They are often used during the first few weeks of depression treatment until other antidepressants, such as the MAO inhibitors or tricyclics, begin their therapeutic effect. They are also used to treat narcolepsy and hyperkinesis. Amphetamines increase the activity of norepinephrine and dopamine in the brain. Common side effects include dry mouth, rapid heartbeat, increased blood pressure, restlessness, and insomnia. Examples include dextroamphetamine (Dexedrine®) and methylphenidate (Ritalin®).

Lithium: An antimanic drug prescribed in the treatment of manic episodes. Lithium decreases the excitability of nerve tissue, increases the reuptake of norepinephrine and dopamine, and decreases the release of neurotransmitters. Clinical use includes the treatment of bipolar affective disorder and acute manic conditions. Lithium also blocks relapse. Common side effects include hypothyroidism, polyuria, polydipsia, tremor, and teratogenesis. Other side effects are nausea, tremors, cardiac arrhythmias, and nephritis. Lithium is contraindicated during pregnancy.

Antiepileptic Drugs

Antiepileptic drugs: Reduce or prevent the severity of epileptic or other convulsive seizures. Antiepileptic drugs decrease the excitability of brain cells. The drug of choice for each type of seizure is shown in Table 18-11. Side effects of antiepileptic drugs are summarized in Table 18-12.

Valproic acid (Depakene®): One of the few drugs that can be used in all types of epilepsy. Its mechanism of action is related to its ability to increase levels of GABA, the inhibitory neurotransmitter in the CNS. Common side effects include nausea, vomiting, diarrhea, tremors, and liver toxicity.

Antiparkinsonian Drugs

Levodopa (Dopar®, Larodopa®): The most effective drug available for Parkinson's disease. In the basal ganglia, levodopa is converted to dopamine, and increased levels of dopamine lessen parkinsonian symptoms. Common side effects include nausea, vomiting, anorexia, orthostatic hypotension or fainting, irregular heartbeat, dystonias, and dyskinesias.

Selegiline (Eldepryl®): Inhibits the metabolism of dopamine in the brain. It slows the progression of Parkinson's disease.

Type of Seizure	Drugs of Choice
Grand mal (tonic-clonic)	phenytoin (Dilantin®), carbamazepine (Tegretol®), phenobarbital (Luminal®)
Status epilepticus	diazepam (Valium®), phenytoin (Dilantin®), phenobarbital (Luminal®)
Complex partial (temporal lobe)	carbamazepine (Tegretol®), phenytoin (Dilantin®), primidone
Petit mal	ethosuximide (Zarontin®), valproic acid (Depakene®), clonazepam (Klonopin®)

Table 18-11

AT A GLANCE | Antiepileptic Drug Toxicities

Drug	Side Effects
Phenobarbital	Sedation, tolerance, dependence
Valproic acid	Nausea, vomiting, diarrhea, tremors, liver toxicity in young patients
Benzodiazepines	Sedation, dependence, tolerance
Phenytoin	Birth defects, gingival hyperplasia, nystagmus, anemias, hirsutism
Carbamazepine	Blood dyscrasias, diplopia, ataxia

Table 18-12

Amantadine (Symmetrel®): An antiviral agent that is often effective in the treatment of Parkinson's disease. Common side effects include dry mouth, GI disturbances, visual disturbances, dizziness, skin discoloration, and confusion.

Atropine and scopolamine: Anticholinergic drugs that relieve some of the symptoms of Parkinson's disease because they decrease the level of cholinergic activity and thus reduce tremors, muscle rigidity, and postural disturbances. Side effects include dry mouth, constipation, urinary retention, rapid heartbeat, and pupillary dilation.

Anesthetics and Analgesics

Anesthetic: A substance that depresses all nervous tissue, inhibits voluntary and involuntary systems, and depresses respiratory function.

General anesthetics: Administered by inhalation or IV injection. Inhalation anesthetics include chloroform, ether, and nitrous oxide. Injectable anesthetics include barbiturates, etomidate, ketamine, midazolam, and propofol; they are usually administered intravenously.

In addition to anesthetic agents, a variety of preanesthetic and postanesthetic medications are used to aid induction of general anesthesia, to counteract side effects, or to make recovery more comfortable. Side effects include dizziness, nausea, mental disorientation, lack of coordination.

Narcotic (opioid) analgesics: Derivatives of opium or synthetic chemicals that relieve severe pain. Certain narcotic analgesics (codeine and dextromethorphan) are also antitussive. All narcotic analgesics produce tolerance and physical dependency with chronic use. Morphine and other narcotic analgesics mimic the effects of endorphins by blocking pain transmission to the brain. For a list of narcotic analgesics, see Table 18-13.

Nonopioid analgesics: The most common drugs used for relieving pain. See Table 18-14.

Autonomic Nervous System

Autonomic nervous system drugs: Drugs that treat the body systems regulated by the autonomic nervous system. They are classified into four groups: adrenergics,

Opioid Analgesics

Drug	Uses	Side Effects	Contraindications
codeine meperidine (Demerol®) morphine pentazocine (Talwin®) propoxyphene (Darvon®, Dolene®)	Relief of severe acute and chronic pain; relief of pain associated with myocardial infarction, posttrauma, cancer, and chronic inflammatory conditions; suppression of coughing (codeine)	Sedation, confusion, euphoria, agitation, headache and dizziness, hypotension, bradycardia, nausea, vomiting, urinary retention, respiratory depression, physical and emotional dependence, convulsions with large doses	Bronchial asthma, heavy pulmonary secretions, convulsive disorders, biliary obstruction, head injuries, pregnancy

Table 18-13

Nonopioid Analgesics

Classification	Uses	Side Effects	Contraindications
Drug			
Salicylates			
aspirin (Bayer®, aspirin, Bufferin®, Anacin®)	Relief of mild to moderate pain and fever; treatment of inflammation; possible reduction in the risk of reinfarction and death following a myocardial infarction	Prolonged bleeding time, bleeding, gastric ulcer and bleeding, tinnitus, renal insufficiency, rash, hepatic dysfunction, stomach irritation, and nausea	GI ulcer and bleeding, asthma, bleeding disorders, influenza-like syndrome in children, pregnancy, vitamin K deficiency
N-Acetyl-P-Aminophenol			
acetaminophen (Tylenol®)	Relief of fever, pain, and discomfort associated with the common cold and flu	Coma, respiratory failure, severe liver toxicity, renal insufficiency, rash	Renal or hepatic disease, anemia, cardiac or pulmonary disease
Synthetic Nonsteroidal Antiinflammatory Drugs (NSAIDs)			
ibuprofen (Advil®, Motrin®, Nuprin®)	Relief of mild to moderate pain (headache, dental extraction, soft tissue injury, sunburn); treatment of chronic osteoarthritis and rheumatoid arthritis	Nausea, GI distress, ulceration, vertigo, confusion	

Table 18-14

AT A GLANCE — Classifications of Autonomic Nervous System Drugs

Adrenergics	Adrenergic Blockers	Cholinergics	Cholinergic Blockers
epinephrine (Adrenalin®) ephedrine	methyldopa (Aldomet®)	neostigmine	atropine
dopamine	guanethidine (Ismelin®)	prostigmim®	scopolamine
norepinephrine	reserpine (Serpasil®)	pilocarpine (Pilomiotin®, Ocusert®) bethanechol (Urecholine®)	homatropine methantheline (Banthine®)
isoproterenol			

Table 18-15

adrenergic blockers, cholinergics, and cholinergic blockers. See Table 18-15.

Sympathetic Nervous System

Adrenergic drugs: Also called sympathomimetic agents, these drugs mimic or stimulate the sympathetic nervous system. They include epinephrine, dopamine, dolutamine, and ephedrine. Adrenergic drugs have two effects: alpha and beta.

Alpha-adrenergic drugs: Cause the contraction of smooth muscle, thereby increasing blood pressure. The prototype alpha-adrenergic drug is norepinephrine. They are commonly used to increase blood pressure in hypotensive states (such as after surgery) and to reduce congestion of nasal and ocular mucosa. Side effects include excessive vasoconstriction of blood vessels, heart palpitations, hypertension, and tissue necrosis. Contraindications include hypertension and cardiac arrhythmias.

Beta-adrenergic drugs: Stimulate the heartbeat and act as bronchodilators. Isoproterenol is the most potent of these drugs; it acts as both a cardiac stimulant and as a bronchodilator. A common use is treatment of acute allergic reactions, such as anaphylaxis. Common side effects include restlessness, tremors, anxiety, overstimulation of the heart, palpitation, and arrhythmias. These drugs should be used with caution in patients with existing heart disease.

Alpha-adrenergic blocking agents: Prevent norepinephrine from producing sympathetic responses resulting in vasodilation and lowered blood pressure. Doxazosin, phentolamine, and prazosin are common alpha-adrenergic blocking drugs. Common uses include treatment of hypertension, treatment of vascular disease, and diagnosis of pheochromocytoma. Common

side effects include nasal congestion, increased GI activity, low blood pressure, and fainting.

Beta-adrenergic blocking agents (beta-blockers): Decrease the activity of the heart. Propranolol is a common beta-adrenergic drug administered for cardiac arrhythmias, angina pectoris, and hypertension. Side effects include nausea, vomiting, diarrhea, bradycardia, and cardiac arrest. Antiadrenergic drugs are contraindicated in patients with asthma or other respiratory conditions.

Parasympathetic Nervous System

Cholinergic: An agent that allows the parasympathetic nerve fibers to liberate acetylcholine. Cholinergics are also called parasympathomimetic drugs. Examples include neostigmine, pilocarpine, and bethanechol. Common uses include treatment of myasthenia gravis (neostigmine), glaucoma (pilocarpine), and nonobstructive urinary retention (bethanechol). Side effects include nausea, vomiting, diarrhea, blurred vision, excessive sweating, weakness, hypotension, bronchospasm, and respiratory depression. Contraindications include asthma, cardiac disorders, peptic ulcer, and benign prostatic hypertrophy.

Cholinergic blocking agents: Drugs that block the action of acetylcholine. These agents, also called anticholinergics or parasympatholytics, may be used by patients who have bradycardia. Examples include atropine, scopolamine, and homatropine. These agents are commonly used as antispasmodics, as preanesthetics, and as antidotes for insecticide poisoning. Common side effects include fever or flushing, blurred vision, dry mouth, urinary retention, and tachycardia. Contraindications include asthma, chronic obstructive pulmonary disease, angle-closure glaucoma, gastrointestinal or genitourinary obstruction, hypertension, hypothyroidism, and hepatic or renal disease.

Pharmacology of the Cardiovascular System

Cardiac Glycosides

Cardiac glycosides: Used in the treatment of congestive heart failure (CHF), atrial fibrillation, and atrial tachycardia to increase the force of myocardial contractions. Glycosides slow and strengthen the heartbeat and increase cardiac output. Major side effects of overdose include arrhythmia, headache, visual disturbances, nausea, vomiting, and diarrhea. Examples include deslanoside (Cedilanid-D®), digitoxin (Puradigin®), and digoxin (Lanoxin®).

Antianginal Drugs

Nitroglycerin: The most common and widely used drug for angina pectoris. Nitroglycerin produces general vasodilation of systemic veins and arteries and decreases the preload and afterload of the heart, thereby reducing cardiac work and oxygen consumption. See Table 18-16.

Antihypertensive Drugs

Antihypertensive agents: Agents that are effective against hypertension. Some antihypertensives, such as calcium antagonists and sympathetic beta-blockers, are also antianginal agents. Some antihypertensive drugs and their side effects are listed in Table 18-17. Other antihypertensive drugs, indications, and contraindications are summarized in Table 18-18.

Antiarrhythmic Drugs

Antiarrhythmic drug: An agent that prevents or alleviates cardiac arrhythmias. Some of these agents are useful in several types of cardiac diseases. There are four classes, which are listed in Table 18-19.

Anticoagulant Drugs

Anticoagulants: The two classes of anticoagulants used most frequently today are coumadin derivatives and heparin. They are employed to prevent venous thrombosis, especially pulmonary embolism. Anticoagulants such as heparin inhibit the function of clotting factors, and anticoagulants such as coumarin derivatives prevent the synthesis of normal clotting factors. They are used in the treatment of myocardial infarction, thrombophlebitis, and stroke. Heparin is the preferred drug to be given to pregnant women because it does not cross the placenta and affect the fetus. Examples include adeparin (Normiflo®), baltepatin (Fragmin®), and heparin.

Hypolipidemic Drugs

Hypolipidemic drug: Used as a dietary control and as a means to reduce cholesterol in the body. There are three main types of hypolipidemic drugs: bile acid sequestrants, HMG-CoA enzyme inhibitors, and drugs that alter lipid and lipoprotein metabolism. Examples include cholestyramine (Questran®), simastatin (Zocor®), and dextrothyroxine (Choloxin®).

Pharmacology of the Respiratory System

Antihistamines

Histamine: A substance that creates a pharmacological reaction when it is released from an injured cell.

Antihistamine: A drug that counteracts the effects of histamine. Antihistamines are used to relieve the symptoms of allergic reactions, such as hay fever and other allergic disorders of the nasal passages. Sometimes antihistamines are also useful in the relief of motion sickness. Others have a sedative and hypnotic action

AT A GLANCE Antianginal Drugs (Vasodilators)	
Drug	**Effects**
nitroglycerin (Nitrol®, Nitrostat®, Nitrong®)	Dilates veins in low doses. In high doses, it also dilates arterioles, so angina may get worse. It increases blood flow in the coronary arteries and thereby decreases angina and hypertension.
isosorbide dinitrate (Isordil®)	Dilates vessels; it is orally active but less potent than nitroglycerin.
nifedipine (Procardia®)	Relaxes arterioles; it is best for coronary artery spasm.
verapamil (Calan®, Isoptin®)	Slows the heart rate; its effect is partially overcome by reflex tachycardia. This drug is also widely used to treat supraventricular arrhythmias.

Table 18-16

AT A GLANCE — Antihypertensive Drugs and Their Side Effects

Drug	Side Effects
Thiazide and Thiazide-like Diuretics	
hydrochlorothiazide (HydroDIURIL®)	Hypokalemia, hyperuricemia, depression, slight hyperlipidemia
Sympathetic Blocking Drugs	
methyldopa (Aldomet®)	Positive Coombs' test, sedation
clonidine (Catapres®)	Dry mouth, sedation
propranolol (Inderal®)	Hypotension, palpitations, bradycardia
Angiotensin-Converting Enzyme (ACE) Inhibitors	
benazepril (Lotensin®)	Headache, dizziness, GI disturbances
captopril (Capoten®)	Leukocytopenia, tachycardia, hypotension
Calcium Antagonists	
diltiazem (Cardizem®)	Lethargy, arrhythmias, bradycardia, hypotension, photosensitivity
verapamil (Calan®)	Dizziness, hypotension, bradycardia
Vasodilator Drugs	
hydralazine (Apresoline®)	Nausea, vomiting, reflex tachycardia, rheumatoid arthritis, systemic lupus erythematosus
minoxidil (Rogaine®)	Myocardial ischemia, pericardial effusion, hirsutism (growth of hair)

Table 18-17

AT A GLANCE — Antihypertensive Drugs and Their Indications and Contraindications

Drug	Indications	Contraindications
Beta-blockers	Angina pectoris, postmyocardial infarction	Diabetes, asthma, peripheral vascular disease
Diuretics	Congestive heart failure, chronic renal failure	Diabetes, hyperlipidemia
Calcium channel blockers	Angina, hypertension, supraventricular tachycardia	Congestive heart failure

Table 18-18

Drug	Mechanism of Action	Uses	Side Effects
Class 1 quinididine (Cardioquin®, Quinidex®)	Depresses the myocardium and the conduction system. Slows the heart rate.	Ventricular arrhythmias, supraventricular tachycardia	Nausea, vomiting, diarrhea, cinchonism due to drug sensitivity or an overdose, hypotension, fatigue
procainamide (Procanbid®)	Depresses the myocardium and the conduction system. Slows the heart rate.	Superventricular arrhythmias, supraventricular tachycardia	Nausea, vomiting, anorexia, skin rashes
lidocaine (Xylocaine®)	Suppresses ectopic foci but does not depress normal impulse conduction. Depresses automaticity.	Ventricular arrhythmias (especially from a myocardial infarction or from surgery); as a local anesthetic	Impaired liver function, convulsions due to stimulation of CNS
phenytoin (Dilantin®)	Appears to increase A-V conduction and may eliminate A-V blockage.	Ventricular arrhythmias induced by digitalis, epileptic seizure	Blurred vision, vertigo, nystagmus, hyperglycemia, gingival hyperplasia
Class 2 propranolol (Inderal®)	Beta-blocker. Depresses cardiac membranes. Slows the heart rate, decreases A-V conduction, and prolongs the refractory period.	Supraventricular and ventricular tachycardia	Hypotension, bradycardia, possible cardiac arrest, skin rashes, mental confusion, visual disturbances
esmolol (Brevibloc®)	Selective beta-blocker.	Supraventricular and ventricular tachycardia	(With overdose): excessive bradycardia, delayed A-V conduction, hypotension
Class 3 amiodarone (Cordarone®)	Very potent local anesthetic. Blocks alpha-adrenergic, beta-adrenergic, and calcium receptors and prolongs the refractory period.	Ventricular tachycardia	Corneal deposits, visual disturbances, dermatitis, skin discoloration, pulmonary fibrosis, liver dysfunction Contraindications: pregnancy, nursing
bretylium (Bretylol®)	Adrenergic neuronal blocker. Prolongs the refractory period of the ventricles	Ventricular tachycardia and ventricular fibrillation	GI disturbances, nausea, diarrhea, hypotension
Class 4 verapamil (Calan®)	Affects pacemaker cells of the heart. Decreases sinoatrial node activity and A-V node conduction.	Supraventricular tachycardia	Headache, dizziness, minor GI disturbances, constipation, hypotension

Table 18-19

MEDICAL ASSISTING COMPETENCIES

COMPETENCY	CMA	RMA
Clinical		
Apply principles of aseptic techniques and infection control, including hand washing	X	X
Dispose of biohazardous materials	X	X
Practice Standard Precautions	X	X
Apply pharmacology principles to prepare and administer oral and parenteral (excluding IV) medications as directed by the physician	X	X
Maintain medication and immunization records	X	X
Screen and follow up on patient test results	X	X
General/Legal/Professional		
Recognize and respond to verbal and nonverbal communications by being attentive and adapting communication to the recipient's level of understanding	X	X
Identify and respond to issues of confidentiality by maintaining confidentiality at all times and following appropriate guidelines when releasing records or information	X	X
Be aware of and perform within legal and ethical boundaries	X	X
Determine the needs for documentation and reporting, and document accurately and appropriately	X	X
Demonstrate knowledge of and monitor current federal and state healthcare legislation and regulations; maintain licenses and accreditation	X	X
Dispose of controlled substances in compliance with government regulations		X
Perform risk management procedures		X
Explain general office policies and procedures	X	X
Instruct individuals according to their needs	X	X
Provide patients with methods of health promotion and disease prevention	X	X
Be a "team player"		X
Evidence a responsible attitude		X
Conduct work within scope of education, training, and ability		X
Be impartial and show empathy when dealing with patients		X

▶ *Test-Taking Skills*

Form study groups!
   Find one or two well-prepared students in your class and arrange to meet for a study or homework session if possible. Working your way through questions and problems with other students will make you feel better about your own difficulties, and it will give you a chance to pose questions to your fellow students and combine your collective knowledge to help you understand material covered in class. You may find that another student can explain something better to you than the instructor could, or you may gain confidence in finding yourself explaining concepts to others that you didn't even realize you knew. During these study sessions, it's important that you know exactly why you are meeting. For example, you may want to work through some difficult practice questions, or you may want to review material covered in a chapter. Don't get bogged down on minor points or stray from the original goal of your meeting.

Drug Classifications

Drug classification: One method of classifying drugs is based on the form in which they are prepared (liquid or solid). See Table 19-1. Please also review this section in Chapter 18, *Pharmacology.*

Measuring Medication and Dosage Calculations

Systems of measurement: Medical assistants must be familiar with the measurement of drug dosage. Three systems of measure are used in the United States for prescribing and administering medication: the metric system, the apothecaries' system, and the household system. They each have units of weight, volume, and length. Several common containers for measuring doses are shown in Figure 19-1.

Metric system: The most commonly used, most accurate, and easiest to use of all the measuring systems. The metric system is used for most scientific and medical measurements, and all pharmaceutical companies now use the metric system for labeling medications. It employs a uniform decimal scale (based on powers of 10). The basic metric units of measurement are the gram, liter, and meter. Prefixes added to the words *gram*, *liter*, and *meter* indicate smaller or larger units in the system. For example, the centimeter is $\frac{1}{100}$ of a meter. For a list of prefixes used in the metric system, see Table 19-2. The unit abbreviations of the metric system are summarized in Table 19-3.

Gram: The basic metric unit of weight (for solids).

Liter: The basic metric unit of volume (for liquids).

Meter: The basic metric unit of length.

Cubic centimeter (cc): The amount of space occupied by 1 milliliter: 1 mL = 1 cc.

Apothecaries' system: An older and less accurate measuring system than the metric system. The basic unit of weight in the apothecaries' system is the grain (gr), derived from the weight of a large grain of wheat. The remaining units of increasing weight are the scruple (scr), dram (dr, ℨ), ounce (oz, ℥), and pound (lb). The pound, which equals 12 apothecaries' ounces, is not generally used in the administration of medication. The smallest unit of measurement of liquid volume is the minim (min), meaning "the least." A minim is approximately equivalent to a volume of water weighing one grain. The remaining units of increasing volume are the fluidram (fl dr), fluid ounce (fl oz), pint (pt), quart (qt), and gallon (gal). Sixty grains equal 1 dram, and 8 drams equal 1 ounce. In the apothecaries' system, dosage quantities are written in lowercase Roman numerals. By convention, the Roman numerals are written with a bar over them after the unit of measurement. For example, gr x̄ means 10 grains.

Household system: More complicated and less accurate for administering liquid medication than the other systems. The only household units of measurement used in the administration of medication are based on volume. The basic unit of liquid volume in the household system is the drop (gt, plural gtt). One drop is approximately equal to 0.6 mL in the metric system and 1 minim in the apothecaries' system. The remaining units, in order of increasing volume, are the teaspoon, tablespoon, ounce, teacup, and glass or cup. See Tables 19-4 and 19-5. (There are also units called the ounce and cup for measuring dry weight; do not confuse them with the units of liquid volume.)

Conversions Between Systems of Measurement

Conversion chart: Lists approximate, not exact, equivalents between systems. Check the chart several times, and place a ruler under the applicable line to be sure that you are reading it correctly. For a list of approximate conversions between the metric and apothecaries' systems, see Table 19-6.

Class	Definition	Example
Liquid		
Aerosol	A pressurized dosage form in which solid or liquid drug particles are suspended in a gas to be dispensed in a cloud or mist	Proventil® inhaler
Elixir	A drug that is dissolved in a solution of alcohol and water	Tylenol® elixir
Emulsion	A mixture of oils in water	Cod liver oil
Liniment	A drug combined with oil, soap, alcohol, or water and applied externally	Camphor liniment
Lotion	An aqueous preparation that contains suspended ingredients	Nutraderm® lotion
Spirit	A drug combined with an alcoholic solution that is volatile	Aromatic spirit of ammonia
Spray	A fine stream of medicated vapor (to treat the nose and throat)	Dristan® nasal spray
Syrup	A drug dissolved in a solution of sugar and water	Robitussin® cough syrup
Tincture	An extract of a therapeutic material in alcohol	Tincture of benzoin
Solid		
Capsule	A drug contained in a gelatin capsule that is water soluble	Benadryl® capsule
Cream	A drug combined in a base that is generally nongreasy, resulting in a semisolid preparation	Aristocort® topical cream
Ointment	A drug combined with an oil base, resulting in a semisolid preparation	Polysporin® ointment
Suppository	A drug mixed with a firm base, such as cocoa butter, that is designed to melt at body temperature	Nupercainal® suppository
Tablet	Powdered drugs that have been pressed into a disc shape	Aspirin tablet

Table 19-1

Ratio method: To convert aspirin gr $\bar{x}$ to metric measurement (e.g., mg), follow these steps:

1. Set up the first ratio:

   unknown quantity : known quantity

   x : 10 gr

2. Set up the second ratio to show the standard equivalence between the desired unit of measurement (mg) and the given unit of measurement (gr). There are 60 mg in 1 grain, so the second ratio is:

   60 mg : 1 gr

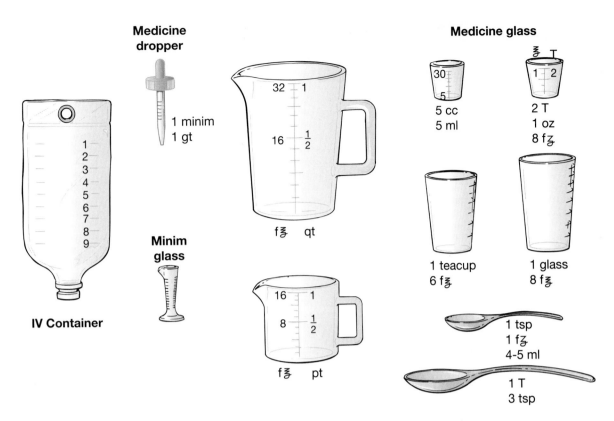

Figure 19-1 *Containers for measuring doses.*

AT A GLANCE		Prefixes in the Metric System	
Prefix	**Meaning**	**Prefix**	**Meaning**
deca-	× 10	kilo-	× 1000
deci-	÷ 10	milli-	÷ 1000
hect- / o	× 100	mega-	× 1,000,000
centi-	÷ 100	micro-	÷ 1,000,000

Table 19-2

3. Create a proportion using the ratios:

   x mg : 10 gr :: 60 mg : 1 gr ("x milligrams are to 10 grains as 60 milligrams are to 1 grain")

   Note that the x, which stands for our unknown measurement in mg, is in the same place in relationship to the 10 gr as the 60 mg is to the 1 gr. Your job now is to solve for x.

4. Multiply the outer and then the inner parts of the proportion and set them equal to each other:

   $x \times 1$ gr $= 10$ gr $\times 60$ mg

5. Divide both sides of the equation by 1 gr, and then do the arithmetic.

   $x = 600$ mg

So 10 grains of aspirin is the same as 600 milligrams of aspirin.

10 gr = 600 mg

Fraction method: To convert 300 mg of aspirin to an apothecaries' measure, follow these steps:

1. Set up a fraction with the known dose as the numerator (on the top) and the unknown amount, representing grains, as the denominator (on the bottom):

   $$\frac{300 \text{ mg}}{x}$$

2. Set up a fraction with the standard equivalent, making sure that the units of measurement are in the same positions as in the first fraction:

   $$\frac{60 \text{ mg}}{1 \text{ gr}}$$

3. Set up a proportion with both fractions; in other words, set the two fractions equal to each other:

   $$\frac{300 \text{ mg}}{x} = \frac{60 \text{ mg}}{1 \text{ gr}}$$

4. Cross multiply:

   $x \times 60$ mg $= 300$ mg $\times 10$ gr

5. Divide both sides of the equation by 60 mg, and then do the arithmetic.

   $x \times 5$ gr

(Notice that the two methods are interchangeable. The ratio method uses : and :: whereas the fraction method uses / and =, and the initial placement of the unknown quantity differs. But the results are the same.)

AT A GLANCE — Metric System Unit Abbreviations

Unit	Abbreviation
Weight	
Microgram	μg
Milligram	mg
Gram	g
Kilogram	kg
Volume	
Milliliter	ml or mL
Cubic centimeter	cc
Liter	l or L
Length	
Millimeter	mm
Centimeter	cm
Meter	m

Table 19-3

AT A GLANCE — Household System Abbreviations

Measurement	Abbreviation
Drop	gt
Teaspoon	tsp, t
Tablespoon	tbs, T
Ounce	oz
Cup	C

Table 19-5

AT A GLANCE — Household System Liquid Equivalents

Measurement	Equivalent
1 teaspoon	60 drops
1 tablespoon	3 teaspoons
1 ounce	6 teaspoons = 2 tablespoons
1 teacup	6 ounces
1 glass or cup	8 ounces

Table 19-4

AT A GLANCE — Approximate Conversions Between the Metric and Apothecaries' Systems

Metric System	Apothecaries' System
2 g (2000 mg)	30 gr
1 g (1000 mg)	15 gr
600 mg (0.6 g)	10 gr
100 mg (0.1 g)	$1\frac{1}{2}$ gr
60 mg (0.06 g)	1 gr
30 mg (0.03 g)	$\frac{1}{2}$ gr
1 mg (0.001 g)	$\frac{1}{60}$ gr
0.1 mg (0.0001 g)	$\frac{1}{600}$ gr

Approximation formulas:

grams × 60 = milligrams

milligrams ÷ 60 = grains

grams × 15 = grains

grains ÷ 15 = grams

Table 19-6

Calculating Drug Doses

Calculating drug doses: On occasion, it is necessary to calculate drug doses when the drug is not available in the exact amount the physician has prescribed. Drug doses can be calculated with either the ratio method or the fraction method.

Ratio method: If a physician orders 500 mg of a drug that comes in tablets of 250 mg, follow these steps to find the number of tablets you will need for the correct dose:

1. Set up a ratio of the unknown quantity (in this case, representing tablets) to the known quantity:

   $x : 500$ mg

2. Set up a ratio of the known conversion equivalence:

   1 tab : 250 mg

3. Put the ratios into a proportion:

   $x : 500$ mg :: 1 tab : 250 mg

4. Multiply the outer and then the inner parts of the proportion:

   $x \times 250$ mg $= 500$ mg $\times 1$ tab

5. To solve for x, divide both sides of the equation by 250 mg, and then do the arithmetic.

   $x = 2$ tabs

Fraction method: If a physician orders 30 mg of a drug that comes in capsules containing only 10 mg, follow these steps:

1. Set up a fraction with the dose ordered and the unknown number of capsules:

   $$\frac{30 \text{ mg}}{x}$$

2. Set up a fraction with the known conversion equivalence. Make sure that the units of measurement are in the same position as in the first fraction:

   $$\frac{10 \text{ mg}}{1 \text{ cap}}$$

3. Set the two fractions equal to each other:

   $$\frac{30 \text{ mg}}{x} = \frac{10 \text{ mg}}{1 \text{ cap}}$$

4. Cross multiply:

   $x \times 10$ mg $= 30$ mg $\times 1$ cap

5. To solve for x, divide both sides of the equation by 10 mg, and then do the arithmetic.

   $x = 3$ caps

Pediatric Dose Calculations

Most pediatric dose calculations are based on the child's age or body weight. The common formulas used for pediatric dose calculations are Clark's rule and Fried's rule.

Clark's Rule

$$\frac{\text{weight of child}}{150 \text{ lbs}} \times \text{adult dose} = \text{child's dose}$$

Fried's Rule

$$\frac{\text{age of child in months}}{150 \text{ lbs}} \times \text{average adult dose}$$
$$= \text{child's dose}$$

Example: Katie has just turned 3 years old and weighs 30 pounds. Her mother wants to know how much cough syrup to give Katie. The directions have worn off the bottle, and she can only make out the dosage for adults: 2 teaspoons every 4 hours. How much cough syrup should Katie receive?

The calculation based on Clark's rule would like this:

$$\frac{30}{150} \times 10 \text{ mL} = \text{Katie's dose}$$

$$\frac{1}{5} \times 10 \text{ mL} = 2 \text{ mL}$$

The calculation based on Fried's rule would look like this:

$$\frac{36}{150} \times 10 \text{ mL} = \text{Katie's dose}$$

$$0.24 \times 10 \text{ mL} = 2.4 \text{ mL}$$

Methods of Administering Medications

"Seven rights" of drug administration: Never deviate from these seven principles: right patient, right drug, right dose, right time, right route, right technique, right documentation.

Right patient: Always check the name on the order, then ask the patient to tell you his or her name.

Right drug: Read the drug label before you take the container off the shelf, before you administer the drug, and before you put the container back on the shelf. Make sure to check the expiration date, and never use a drug that has passed this date.

Right dose: Compare the dose on the order with the dose you prepare.

Right time: If a drug must be taken after a meal, make sure that the patient has eaten recently.

Right route: Make sure that the route you are preparing to use matches the route the doctor ordered.

Right technique: Always use the proper administrative technique.

Right documentation: Document the procedure immediately after administering the drug. Include the date, time, drug name, dose, administration route,

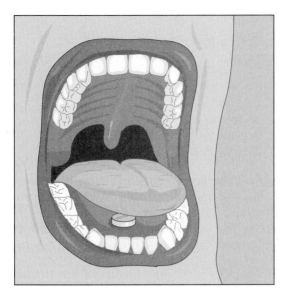

Figure 19-2 *Place a sublingual drug under the tongue.*

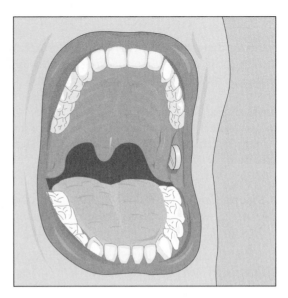

Figure 19-3 *Place a buccal drug between the cheek and gum.*

patient reaction, education of the patient about the drug, and your initials.

Route of administration: Medication may be administered by numerous routes, including oral, sublingual, buccal, inhalation, topical, rectal, urethral, vaginal, parenteral (intramuscular, subcutaneous, intradermal, or intravenous), ophthalmic, and otic.

Oral administration: The drug is given by mouth in either a solid form (tablet, capsule, or powder) or a liquid form (water-based solution, suspension, or alcohol solution). The drug is absorbed into the bloodstream through the lining of the stomach and intestine. This method is easy, safe, and economical, but drug absorption is slow and may be affected by the presence of food. Some medications may also cause nausea or stomach discomfort.

Sublingual administration: The medication must be placed under the tongue until it dissolves. See Figure 19-2. This method is faster than the oral method.

Buccal administration: The medication is placed in the mouth and absorbed in the buccal area. The patient should not chew or swallow the medication. See Figure 19-3.

Inhalation administration: The medication is given in the form of gases, sprays, or aerosol mists (fluid droplets). The respiratory tract absorbs medication more rapidly than any other mucous membrane. One inhalation medication that should be kept in every medical practice is oxygen.

Topical administration: Used in treating skin disorders. The medication is applied directly to affected areas of the skin. Topical medications come in the form of sprays, creams, lotions, ointments, transdermal patches, and compresses.

Transdermal drug delivery (TDD): A method of applying a drug to unbroken skin. The drug is absorbed continuously through the skin and enters the blood-

stream. It is used particularly for the administration of nicotine, nitroglycerin, and scopolamine. To promote adhesion to the skin, the patch should be applied to a clean, dry area without hair.

Rectal administration: Useful if the patient is nauseated, vomiting, or unconscious. The best time to administer a rectal drug is after a bowel movement or the elimination of an enema. A suppository must be inserted about 2 inches above the internal anal sphincter.

Urethral administration: A solution is instilled into the bladder by means of a catheter.

Vaginal administration: A liter or more of a solution of medication in warm water is introduced as a douche into the vagina under low pressure. Other forms of medication are inserted into the vagina with an applicator.

Parenteral administration: A medication is given in the form of an injection. Drugs are absorbed more rapidly and completely than by most other routes. In some cases, injection is the only way a drug can be given (for example, to an unconscious patient). The disadvantages of the parenteral route are that all equipment must be sterile; that the method is often expensive, painful, and awkward for patients to administer themselves; and that there is a danger of injecting a drug incorrectly into a vein, which could cause serious harm or even death.

Intradermal injection: Given into the dermal layer of the skin. A very short needle of small gauge is used. The angle of insertion is 15 degrees, nearly parallel to the skin. Absorption is slow. Only a small amount of medication may be injected (0.01 to 0.2 cc). The anterior forearm is the most common area for injection. See Figure 19-4. The gauge is usually 25 to 27. When an intradermal injection is correctly administered, a small wheal is raised on the skin. See Figure 19-5. The most common uses of intradermal injections are to administer allergy tests and tuberculin skin tests.

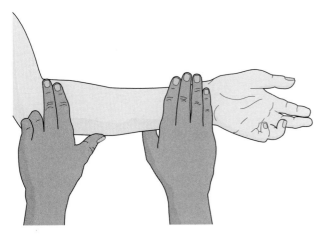

Figure 19-4 *This space is available for intradermal injection sites.*

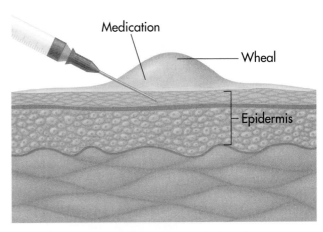

Figure 19-5 *Medication collects under the skin, forming a wheal, during an intradermal injection.*

Subcutaneous (SC) injection: Given into the layer of fatty tissue that lies just below the skin. The most common sites for SC injections are the upper lateral part of the arm, anterior thigh, upper back, and abdomen. See Figure 19-6. The needle length varies from $\frac{1}{2}$ to $\frac{5}{8}$ inch, and the gauge ranges from 23 to 25. The needle should be inserted at a 45-degree angle to the skin. Drugs given subcutaneously must be isotonic, nonviscous, water-soluble, and nonirritating. The amount of drug injected through the SC route should not exceed 2 cc. Medications commonly administered through this route include insulin, local anesthetics, epinephrine, and allergy treatments.

Intramuscular (IM) injection: Given deep into a muscle. Muscles can absorb a greater amount of fluid without discomfort to the patient, and IM injections are preferred for substances that can irritate the skin. The most common muscles used for this method of injection are the deltoid, gluteus medius, and vastus lateralis. See Figure 19-7. For injection of the gluteus muscle site, the patient must be in the prone position. For injection of the vastus lateralis site, the patient may be sitting or in the recumbent position. The needle should be 1 to 3 inches in length or sometimes longer. The gauge of the needle ranges between 18 and 23. The angle of insertion is 90 degrees. Dosage may vary from 0.5 to 5 mL. For medications that are irritating to SC tissue and skin tissue or that may cause discoloration of the skin, the Z-track method should be used. See Figure 19-8. The vastus lateralis muscle in the thigh is the preferred injection site for children under 3 years of age. Penicillin is often injected intramuscularly.

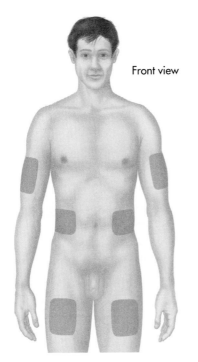

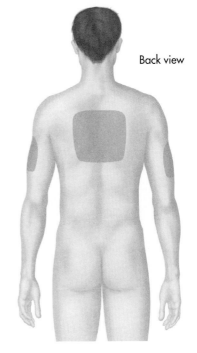

Figure 19-6 *Many sites are available for subcutaneous injections.*

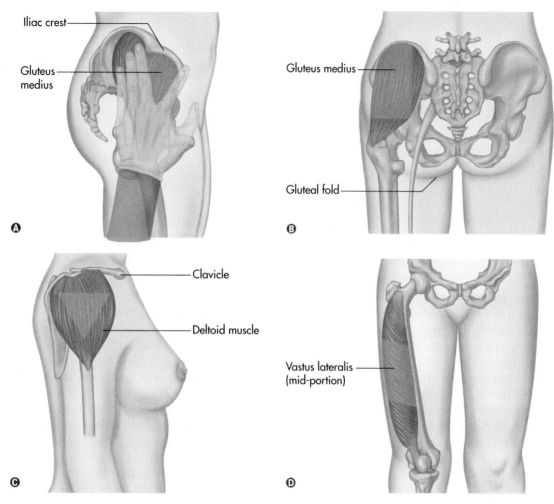

Figure 19-7 *For intramuscular injection in an adult, use (A) the ventrogluteal site, (B) the dorsogluteal site, (C) the deltoid site, or (D) the vastus lateralis site.*

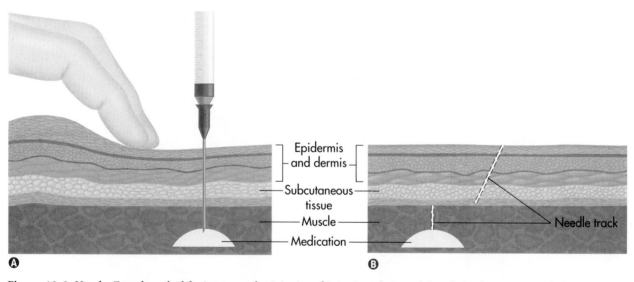

Figure 19-8 *Use the Z-track method for intramuscular injection of irritating solutions. (A) Pull the skin to one side before inserting the needle. (B) After injecting the drug, release the skin to seal off the needle track.*

Intravenous (IV) injection: Given directly into a vein. IV injection is usually used in an emergency situation for an immediate effect. The disadvantage is that painful infection may result. Rotation of the sites is necessary if injections are given repeatedly. Needles are 1 to $1\frac{1}{2}$ inch in length. The gauges are usually between 20 and 21.

IV drip: The insertion into a vein of a tube or a needle through which fluids are slowly added to the bloodstream over a period of time. It is also called infusion. The IV drip should not be confused with IV injection.

Ophthalmic administration: Drugs are placed into the patient's eye.

Otic administration: Drugs are placed into the patient's ear.

Needles and Syringes

Needle: Consists of several parts: hub, shaft, lumen, point, and bevel. See Figure 19-9.

Needle gauge: The inside diameter of the needle. A larger gauge indicates a smaller diameter. The common range for administering medication is between 18 and 27 gauge.

Needle length: Ranges between $\frac{3}{8}$ of an inch and 3 inches. See Table 19-7.

Syringe: Used for inserting fluids into the body. It is usually made of plastic. A syringe consists of three parts: barrel, flange (rim), and plunger. See Figure 19-10.

Hypodermic syringes: Available in 2-, 2.5-, 3-, and 5-cc sizes. They are commonly used to administer IM injections.

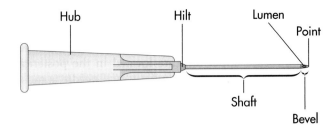

Figure 19-9 *Understanding the parts of a needle will help you use it correctly.*

Insulin syringe: Designed for an insulin injection. It is calibrated in units (U); 100 U = 1 mL. The most commonly used size is the 100 U syringe (with a capacity of 100 units), divided into increments of 2 units. Syringes are also available in 40 U and 80 U sizes.

Tuberculin syringe: Has a capacity of 1 cc. The calibrations are divided into tenths (0.1) and hundredths (0.01) of a cubic centimeter.

Prefilled syringe: Known as a cartridge. It is a sterile, disposable syringe. Needle units are packaged by the manufacturer with a single dose of medication inside, ready to administer.

Ampule: A small, sealed glass container that holds a single dose of medication.

Vial: A closed glass container with a rubber stopper protected by a soft metal cap. There are two types: single- and multiple-dose.

Deltoid muscle: Located at the top of the arm on the upper, outer surface. It is a good site for a small amount

AT A GLANCE	Choosing a Needle	
Type of Injection	**Gauge of Needle**	**Length of Needle**
Intradermal	25–26 gauge	$\frac{1}{6}$–$\frac{1}{2}$ inch
Subcutaneous	23–27 gauge	$\frac{1}{2}$–$\frac{3}{4}$ inch
Intramuscular	18–23 gauge	1–3 inches

Table 19-7

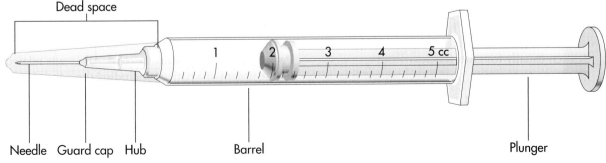

Figure 19-10 *Know the parts of a standard syringe.*

of medicatic
tions of teta
exposure, a
nerves in th
portion of t
frequently u
A 25-gauge,
Gluteus m
deep IM in
tions (antib
This site sh

Medicati

Medication
telling a nur
to adminis
so that ther
situation, w
tions, the o
the physici
the physici
ication sho
Prescriptic
for outpatie
Medication
name, date
the abbrev
time and
which the
refills and
and the ph
for controll

Types of

Routine o
until a disc
fied termin
Standing
the drug is
used in cri
changes ra
PRN orde
the patien
eration or
nata, rough
or "as the
Stat orde
ately, writt

Settin

Diligence
be sure to
tration. G

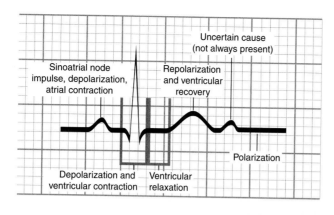

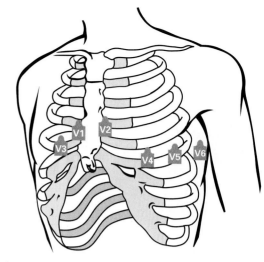

Figure 20-5 *For infants and small children, you may need to place V3 on the right side of the chest to prevent crowding of the chest electrodes. This alternate method of placement is known as V3R and is sometimes used on adults.*

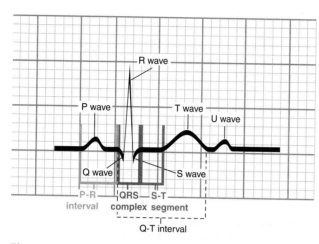

Figure 20-4 *This ECG tracing shows the pattern of one cardiac cycle in a normal heart. These specific electrical impulses (top) represent the cycle of cardiac contraction and relaxation. The waves and lines (bottom) represent specific parts of the pattern.*

repolarization) of Purkinje fibers, as seen in patients who have low potassium levels in their blood. It occurs between the T wave and the following P wave. A U wave taller than 2 mm is considered abnormal and may suggest hypokalemia or the effects of digoxin or quinidine on the conduction system.

P-R interval: Includes the P wave and the straight line connecting it to the QRS complex. It represents the time it takes for the electrical impulse to travel from the sinoatrial (SA) node to the A-V node.

Q-T interval: Includes the QRS complex, S-T segment, and T wave. It represents the time it takes for the ventricles to contract and recover, or repolarize.

S-T segment: Connects the end of the QRS complex with the beginning of the T wave. It represents the time between contraction of the ventricles and recovery.

Asystole: Absence of cardiac electrical activity, represented as a straight (isoelectric) line on the ECG.

Code Blue: The term used for an emergency in a hospital or other health-care facility when a person has a cardiac or respiratory arrest.

Cardiac rate: The pulse rate; the number of beats or contractions per minute.

Deflection: Deviation up or down from zero on the isoelectric line.

Refractory period: The period during repolarization when cells cannot respond normally to a second stimulus.

Cardiac output: The amount of blood ejected by the left ventricle into the aorta in 1 minute.

Amplitude: The height of a waveform on the ECG, showing the degree of voltage variation from zero (the baseline) up or down. It is measured in millimeters and is normally calibrated so that 10 mm represent 1.0 mV.

Pediatric ECG: An ECG for a child is performed with the same lead placement as for an adult. It may be necessary to move the V3 lead to the right side of the chest. This is known as V3 right (V3R). See Figure 20-5.

Troubleshooting

Artifacts: Deflections caused by electrical activity from sources other than the heart. They are irregular and erratic markings caused by poor conduction, outside interference, improper handling of a tracing, a patient's movement (or talking), or dirty sensors. There are several types of artifacts: wandering baseline, flat line, and extraneous marks.

Wandering baseline: A shift in the baseline from the center position for that lead. Its causes include muscle movement and mechanical problems.

Flat line: A flat line on the tracing of one of the leads is typically caused by a loose or disconnected wire. If flat lines occur on more than one lead, two of the wires may have been switched. If flat lines occur on all leads, there are two possible causes: The electrocardiograph unit or the connection to it is faulty, or the patient is in cardiac arrest.

Extraneous marks: Any marks on the paper that are not part of the tracing. The ECG graph paper is sensitive to heat and pressure. It can be easily damaged.

Interpreting the ECG

Heart rate: Can easily be determined by counting the number of QRS complexes in a 6-second strip of the ECG tracing (30 large squares at 25 mm per second) and multiplying by 10.

Heart rhythm: The ECG is the best way to assess heart rhythm and the regularity of the heartbeat. A normal heart rhythm is indicated on the ECG by regularly spaced complexes (repeated intervals, such as between one P wave and the next P wave or between one R wave and the next R wave). The patient's rhythm is usually assessed by viewing the rhythm strip, the ECG tracing from lead II.

Arrhythmia: An irregularity, disturbance, or abnormality in heart rhythm. It is also called a dysrhythmia. Some arrhythmias do not cause problems.

Ectopy: Placement outside the usual location.

Ectopic beat: A beat having an ectopic focus.

Ectopic focus: A site of impulse formation located somewhere other than the SA node.

Bigeminy: A type of arrhythmia in which every other beat is ectopic or premature (or both).

Premature beat or **premature contraction:** A contraction that occurs early. Premature contractions are of three types: premature atrial contractions (PACs), premature junctional contractions (PJCs), and premature ventricular contractions (PVCs).

Premature ventricular contraction (PVC): Can occur normally in healthy persons with apparently normal hearts. Causes of abnormal PVCs include hypoxia; an increase in catecholamines; stimulants such as alcohol, tobacco, and caffeine; acid-base imbalance; electrolyte imbalance; digitalis toxicity; and drugs such as epinephrine, dopamine, phenothiazines, or isoproterenol. PVCs can cause ischemia, myocardial infarction, or congestive heart failure (CHF).

Acardia: The absence of the heart.

Acardiac rhythm: The absence of cardiac rhythm. It is also called asystole.

Bradyarrhythmia: An abnormally slow and irregular cardiac rhythm; irregular bradycardia.

Bradycardia: A heart rate slower than 60 beats per minute.

Tachyarrhythmia: An abnormally fast and irregular cardiac rhythm; irregular tachycardia.

Tachycardia: A heart rate faster than 100 beats per minute.

Atrial fibrillation: Incomplete, irregular, and rapid contraction of the atria between 350 and 500 times per minute. The ventricular rate may also be rapid, or it may be relatively normal.

Atrial flutter: Contraction of the atria between 250 and 350 beats per minute. The ventricular rate varies.

Ventricular fibrillation: Cessation of coordinated ventricular contraction. Untreated ventricular fibrillation leads to cardiac arrest.

Ventricular flutter: Contraction of the ventricles between 150 and 300 times per minute. It is a dangerous rhythm and should be reported immediately.

Sinus rhythm: A heart rhythm established by impulses from the SA node. Irregularities include sinus bradycardia, sinus tachycardia, sinus arrest, and sinus arrhythmia.

Sinus arrest: The failure of the SA node to function. It is also called sinus pause. The complete cardiac complex is absent from the ECG tracing.

Sinus arrhythmia: A usually benign fluctuation of the heart rate occurring within the normal range of 60 to 100 beats per minute, distinguished by a vagally influenced slowing of the cardiac rate during respiratory expiration and an increase in the cardiac rate during inspiration.

Agonal rhythm: The rhythm of a dying heart, usually ventricular, extremely slow and irregular and becoming slower to the point of asystole. A rate of less than 10 beats per minute is common.

Defibrillator: A machine that produces and sends an electrical shock to the heart, intended to correct the electrical pattern of the heart.

Pacemaker (electronic): A device that delivers a small measured amount of electrical energy to cause myocardial depolarization.

Other Tests

Holter monitor: A portable (ambulatory) electrocardiography device that includes a small cassette recorder worn around a patient's waist to record the heart's electrical activity during normal daily activities. This test is given over a 24-hour period. The tape is analyzed by a microcomputer in the physician's office or at a reference laboratory.

Exercise electrocardiography: Assessment of the heart's conduction system during physical exertion such as exercise. It is also known as stress testing. The patient is required to walk on a treadmill, pedal a stationary bicycle, or walk on a stair-stepping ergometer while ECG readings are taken.

Echocardiography: Tests the structure and function of the heart through the use of reflected sound waves, or echoes. The echoes can indicate structural defects and fluid accumulation, among other conditions.

Heart catheterization: A diagnostic method in which a catheter is inserted into a vein or artery in an arm or leg and passed through blood vessels into the heart, so that blood samples may be taken, the pressure in the heart's chambers measured, and/or the heart's motions viewed.

Angiography: The X-ray examination of a blood vessel, after the injection of a contrast medium, to evaluate the function and structure.

Thallium stress test: An invasive type of exercise electrocardiography in which thallium, a radiopapue substance (one that is visible with an X-ray machine), is injected into the body to permit viewing the vessels around the heart.

Cardiac stress test: It is most commonly known as a treadmill stress test because the exercise is usually performed on an exercise treadmill. It is an effective test of diagnosing cardiac disorders. The procedure is performed with a cardiologist or other physician present.

Other Heart Conditions and Procedures

Cardiodynia: Pain in the heart. It is also called cardialgia.

Cardiomegaly: Enlargement of the heart. Cardiomegaly often occur during the course of CHF.

Cardiorrhexis: Rupture of the heart wall.

Dextrocardia: Location of the heart in the right thorax as a result of a congenital defect or displacement by disease.

Cardioptosis: Drooping or falling of the heart at the normal location.

Hypertrophy of the heart: An increase in the size of the heart due to growth of the heart muscle tissue without an increase in the size of the heart chambers.

Heart blocks: Damage to the conduction system of the heart results in abnormal conduction patterns, causing dysrhythmias known as heart blocks. There are four types: first-degree; two variants of second-degree (Wenckebach, or Mobitz I, and Mobitz II); and third-degree, or complete.

Aortic aneurysm: Ballooning of the aorta.

Capture: The successful depolarization of an atrium or ventricle achieved, for example, by an artificial pacemaker.

Cardioversion: The administration of timed electrical shocks for the purpose of correcting certain arrhythmias or restoring normal rhythm, particularly in the ventricular beat.

Cardioplasty: Surgical repair of the heart.

Cardiorrhaphy: The suturing of the heart muscle.

Cardiomyopexy: A surgical procedure in which the blood supply from the nearby pectoral muscles of the chest is diverted directly to the coronary arteries.

STRATEGIES TO SUCCESS

▶ *Test-Taking Skills*

Come prepared!

Always bring all the supplies you need to the exam. Bring a few number 2 pencils with you and a working eraser. Don't depend on someone else to give these supplies to you. Make sure that you have the CMA or RMA admission card you received after registering for the exam. You also need to bring at least two forms of identification, one of which should have a photo.

Instructions:

Answer the following questions. Check your answers in the *Answer Key* that follows this section.

1. The medical term meaning transmission of ECG signals via radio waves is
   A. Telepathy
   B. Telemetry
   C. Telediagnosis
   D. Telocentric
   E. Telecardio

2. On an ECG tracing, an indication of the absence of electrical charge or activity represents
   A. Sinoatrial node
   B. QRS complex
   C. Baseline
   D. Repolarization
   E. None of the above

3. A beat arising from a focus outside the heart is known as
   A. Ectopic beat
   B. Escape beat
   C. Uncontrolled beat
   D. Fusion beat
   E. Bigeminy

4. Which of the following is the epicardium?
   A. Heart muscle
   B. Heart wall
   C. Inner lining of the myocardium
   D. Right atrium
   E. Outermost layer of the heart

5. The sudden rush of blood pushed into the ventricles as a result of atrial contraction is known as
   A. Apex kick
   B. Atrial kick
   C. Acardia
   D. Repolarization
   E. Ventricular contraction

6. The U wave represents
   A. Repolarization
   B. Depolarization
   C. Baseline
   D. Ectopic beat
   E. Contraction

7. Which of the following is not necessary in administering an ECG?
   A. Sterilizing the leads
   B. Activating the standardization control
   C. Washing the patient's skin
   D. Selecting the speed
   E. Both B and D

8. Which type of lead is lead III?
   A. Bipolar limb lead
   B. Unipolar (augmented) limb lead
   C. Precordial lead
   D. Intercostal lead
   E. None of the above

9. Which of the following is represented by the Q-T interval?

  A. Low potassium in the blood
  B. One ventricular contraction and recovery (repolarization)
  C. The depolarization of the atria
  D. The repolarization of the atria
  E. Unusually frequent articular contraction due to high blood sugar

10. Leads aVR, aVL, and aVF are

  A. Standard leads
  B. Limb leads
  C. Intercostal leads
  D. Augmented leads
  E. Both B and D

11. Successful depolarization of the atria or ventricles by an artificial pacemaker is called

  A. Cardioplasty
  B. Capture
  C. Atrial kick
  D. Apex kick
  E. None of the above

12. All of the following are causes of artifacts except

  A. A patient's talking
  B. Clean sensors
  C. Outside interference
  D. Poor conduction
  E. Improper handling of a tracing

13. Augmented leads are also called

  A. Standard leads
  B. Bipolar leads
  C. Unipolar leads
  D. Nonstandard leads
  E. None of the above

14. The QRS complex represents

  A. Contraction of the atria
  B. Recovery of the atria
  C. Contraction of the heart
  D. Recovery of the ventricles
  E. Contraction of the ventricles

15. The coronary sinus empties into the

  A. Left atrium
  B. Right atrium
  C. Left ventricle
  D. Right ventricle
  E. Both B and D

16. The medical term meaning a falling or drooping of the heart is

  A. Cardioplegia
  B. Cardiomyopathy
  C. Cardiomyopexy
  D. Cardioptosis
  E. Cardiolith

17. Which of the following is the measurement of the atrial rate on the ECG tracing?

  A. The PR intervals
  B. The P waves
  C. The R waves
  D. The QRS complexes
  E. None of the above

18. Lead II is a(n)

  A. Chest or precordial lead
  B. Bipolar limb lead
  C. Augmented or unipolar limb lead
  D. Intercostal lead
  E. None of the above

19. The heart's conduction system is measured by which of the following?

    A. Heart catheterization
    B. Angiography
    C. Exercise electrocardiography
    D. Echocardiography
    E. Action potential

20. Which of the patient's limbs serves as an electrical ground?

    A. Right leg
    B. Left leg
    C. Right arm
    D. Left arm
    E. Either arm

21. Depolarization of fast cells is dependent on which of the following electrolytes?

    A. Calcium
    B. Potassium
    C. Magnesium
    D. Chloride
    E. Sodium

22. Which of the following devices may deliver a small amount of electrical energy to cause myocardial depolarization?

    A. Electrocardiography
    B. Electronic pacemaker
    C. Holter monitor
    D. Treadmill
    E. Oscilloscope

ANSWER KEY

1.	B	12.	B
2.	C	13.	C
3.	A	14.	E
4.	E	15.	B
5.	B	16.	D
6.	A	17.	B
7.	A	18.	B
8.	A	19.	C
9.	B	20.	A
10.	E	21.	E
11.	B	22.	B

CHAPTER 21

Radiology

CHAPTER OUTLINE

Terminology

Types of Radiology

Therapeutic Uses of Radiation

Medical Assistant's Role

Safety and Storage

> Safety
> Storage

MEDICAL ASSISTING COMPETENCIES

COMPETENCY	CMA	RMA
Clinical		
Apply principles of aseptic techniques and infection control, including hand washing	X	X
Practice Standard Precautions	X	X
Prepare and maintain examination and treatment areas	X	X
Prepare the patient for and assist the physician with routine and specialty examinations, treatments, and minor office surgeries	X	X
Screen and follow up on patient test results	X	X
General/Legal/Professional		
Be aware of and perform within legal and ethical boundaries	X	X
Instruct individuals according to their needs	X	X
Operate and maintain facilities, and perform routine maintenance of administrative and clinical equipment safely	X	X

Attend every class; read every assignment!

   This tip might seem self-explanatory, but many people don't realize how truly important it is to make sure that you go to every class, read the assigned chapters, and complete any exercises your instructor gives you. In this way you will not fall behind and will have ample time to review for the certification exam. Reading the chapters before you come to class has two advantages: It will enable you to ask more relevant questions in class, and the background information it gives you will make the lecture more comprehensible. In class, try to sit near the front and maintain eye contact with the instructor. Make lists of what your instructor emphasizes in class, and review these lists often. If your instructor points out that certain material is always on the exams, make a point to remember these items. Your instructor and your class time are valuable resources you can use to find answers to questions about topics that seem confusing and to get a feel for what will be covered on the exams.

Terminology

Radiology: The study of the uses of radioactive substances for visualizing the internal structures of the body in order to diagnose and treat disease. It is divided into three specialties: diagnostic radiology, radiation therapy, and nuclear medicine.

X-ray: An electromagnetic wave with a high energy level and short wavelength that can penetrate solid objects. X-rays can be used in diagnosis and therapy.

Magnetism: The ability of certain materials to attract iron and other metals.

Radioactive: Capable of emitting radiant energy; or giving off radiation as the result of the disintegration of the nucleus of an atom.

Nuclear energy: Energy produced by fission of an atomic nucleus.

Radiopaque: Refers to something that does not permit the passage of X-rays. Bones are relatively radiopaque.

Contrast media: Radiopaque substances used in radiography to permit visualization of internal structures. Contrast media include liquids, powders, and gases. They are administered orally, parenterally, and rectally. A positive contrast medium is more dense than the surrounding tissue. A negative contrast medium is less dense than the surrounding area in the body. Barium sulfate and iodine are positive contrast media. Air is a negative contrast medium.

Adverse effects of contrast media: Oral agents may cause skin rash, vomiting, diarrhea, abdominal pain, or constipation. IV agents can cause urticaria, skin reddening, anaphylaxis, or death. Some individuals have allergies to iodine.

X-ray film: A special material with a sensitive emulsion layer that reacts when it is exposed to radiation and thereby produces an image. Single-emulsion film is used to create images of the extremities and the breasts.

Radiograph: An image recorded on film that has been exposed. An older term for radiograph is roentgenogram, named after the discoverer of X-rays.

Film fog: An unwanted increase in the density of the emulsion either before or after exposure to radiation. Heat, light, chemicals, and extraneous radiation can produce fogging, which appears as darkened areas on the finished radiograph.

Artifacts: Extraneous marks and areas of increased or decreased density on film. Artifacts interfere with the diagnostic value of the radiograph.

Cassette: A light-proof container that holds X-ray film and serves to intensify the image.

Contrast: The visible difference between any two areas of radiographic density.

Roentgen: A unit used to measure X-ray dosage in air.

Rem: A unit used to measure X-ray dosage in human beings. It is an abbreviation of *Roentgen equivalent (in) man.*

Rad: A unit used to measure the actual absorbed dose of radiation.

Ionization: The process by which an atom becomes ionized (gains or loses electrons).

Ionizing radiation: Radiation that causes ionization in the tissues that absorb it.

Scan: An image produced on film by a sweeping beam of radiation.

Isotopes: Variants of a single chemical element that have different atomic weights and different charges.

Frequency: The repetition rate of electromagnetic radiation, measured in Hertz.

X-ray machine: Has four basic parts: table, control panel, X-ray tube, and high-voltage generator. The table is usually adjustable. The most important part of the machine is the tube.

Invasive procedure: Some radiological tests are invasive in that they require a radiologist to insert a catheter, wire, or other testing device into a patient's blood vessel or organ through the skin or body orifice. All invasive procedures require surgical aseptic technique.

Types of Radiology

Diagnostic radiology: The use of X-ray technology for diagnostic purposes. It also includes the use of magnetic resonance imaging (MRI), ultrasound, computed tomography (CT), and nuclear medicine technologies, such as positron emission tomography (PET), among others. Table 21-1 provides a list of common radiological tests and the disorders these tests are used to diagnose or treat.

Magnetic resonance imaging (MRI): Uses a combination of nonionizing radiation and a strong magnetic field to produce images of internal structures and soft tissues. It is used for diagnosing cancer and other masses. It is contraindicated in patients with pacemakers or metallic prostheses.

Ultrasound: Directs high-frequency sound waves through the skin and produces an image based on the echoes. Ultrasound has many medical applications, including fetal monitoring, imaging of internal organs, and color imaging of blood vessels.

Tomography: Also called sectional imaging and body-section radiography. It allows the visualization of an organ or the body in cross-section.

Computed tomography (CT) scan: A radiographic technique that shows a detailed, 360-degree cross-section of tissue structure. It is a painless procedure.

Nuclear medicine: A branch of medicine that uses radionuclides in the diagnosis and treatment of disorders.

Positron emission tomography (PET): Involves the injection of isotopes combined with other substances,

AT A GLANCE	Common Radiologic Tests and Disorders Diagnosed
Test	**Disorders Diagnosed/Treated**
Angiography Cardiovascular	Status of blood flow, collateral circulation, malformed vessels, aneurysm, narrowing or blockages of vessels, presence of hemorrhage
Cerebral	Aneurysm, hemorrhage, evidence of cerebrovascular accident, arteriosclerosis
Gastrointestinal (GI)	Upper GI bleeding
Pulmonary	Pulmonary emboli (especially when lung scan is inconclusive), evaluation of pulmonary circulation in some heart conditions before surgery
Renal	Abnormalities of blood vessels in urinary system
Arthrography	Joint conditions
Barium enema (lower GI series)	Obstructions, ulcers, polyps, diverticulosis, tumor, and motility problems of colon or rectum
Barium swallow (upper GI series)	Obstructions, ulcers, polyps, diverticulosis, tumor, and motility problems of esophagus, stomach, duodenum, and small intestine
Cholangiography, cholecystography	Gallstones, gallbladder or common bile duct stones or obstructions, ability of gallbladder to concentrate and store dye
CT	Aortic and heart aneurysms, disorders of liver and biliary systems, renal and pulmonary tumors, brain abnormalities (tumors, blood clots, evidence of cerebrovascular accident, outlines of brain ventricles), GI tract lesions, GI disorders (acute pseudocyst of pancreas, abdominal abscesses, biliary obstruction), breast diseases and disorders, spinal disorders; to guide biopsy procedures

Table 21-1

Test	Disorders Diagnosed/Treated
Fluoroscopy	Structure, process, and function of organs in motion to detect abnormalities
Intravenous pyelography (IVP) (excretory urography)	Urinary system abnormalities, including renal pelvis, ureters, and bladder (for example, kidney stones); abnormal size, shape, or structure of kidneys, ureters, or bladder; space-occupying lesions; pyelonephrosis; hydronephrosis; trauma to the urinary system
KUB (kidneys, ureters, bladder) radiography	Size, shape, and position of urinary organs; urinary system diseases or disorders; kidney stones
MRI	Cancerous tissue, atherosclerotic tissue, blood clots, tumors, and deformities, particularly of the heart valves, brain, spine, and joints
Mammography	Breast tumors and lesions
Myelography	Irregularities or compression of spinal cord
Nuclear medicine (radionuclide imaging)	Abnormal function (defects), lesions, or disorders of bone, brain, lungs, kidneys, liver, pancreas, thyroid, and spleen
Radiation therapy	Treatment of cancer
Retrograde pyelogram	Obstruction of ureters, bladder, or urethra (including tumors, stones, strictures, or blood clots); perinephritic abscess
Stereoscopy	Fractures, dense areas that indicate a tumor or increased pressure within the skull
Thermography	Breast tumors, breast abscesses, fibrocystic breast disease
Ultrasound	Abnormalities of gallbladder, liver, spleen, heart, kidneys, gonads, blood vessels, and lymph system; fetal conditions (including number of fetuses, age and sex of fetus, fetal development, position, and deformities)
Xeroradiography	Breast cancer, abscesses, lesions, calcifications

Table 21-1, concluded

such as glucose. Positrons are emitted and are processed by a computer and displayed on a screen. It is useful for diagnosis of brain-related conditions, such as epilepsy and Parkinson's disease.

Angiography: X-ray visualization of blood vessels after the intravascular introduction of contrast media.

Arthrography: Used for joint conditions. It requires a contrast medium. Arthrography is performed by a radiologist and is usually done for knee, shoulder, or hip injuries. It also requires a local anesthetic.

Barium enema: The rectal infusion of barium sulfate (a radiopaque contrast medium), which is retained in the lower intestinal tract during X-ray studies. It is also called a contrast enema. The digestive tract must be totally empty for this procedure. Patients should thoroughly cleanse their digestive tracts with a series of preparatory steps, including having nothing by mouth for 8 hours before the test except for one cup of clear liquid on the morning of the test.

Barium meal, or **barium swallow:** The ingestion of barium sulfate. It is used for the radiographic examination of the esophagus, stomach, and intestinal tract. Before the test, the patient should have nothing to eat or drink for 12 hours.

Cholecystography: Radiological study of the gallbladder, not as frequently done as in the past. The preceding evening meal must be low fat, and an oral contrast medium is taken 12 to 15 hours before the procedure. The exam takes about 15 minutes.

Cholangiography: Similar to cholecystography and performed by a radiologist. The contrast medium is injected directly into the common bile duct (during gallbladder surgery).

Fluoroscopy: Radiological study, performed by a radiologist, that allows both structural and functional visualization of internal body structures directly on a screen. A contrast medium is needed. It is also called radioscopy.

Intravenous pyelography (IVP): Radiological study of the urinary system in which a series of X-rays is taken after a contrast medium has been injected into a vein. It is also known as excretory urography.

Mammography: Radiological study of the breast. It is used for the early diagnosis of breast cancer.

Myelography: Radiological study of the spinal cord. The radiologist performs a lumbar puncture, removes some cerebrospinal fluid, and injects some radiopaque, water-soluble contrast medium. It is no longer used very often; tomography and MRI have largely replaced it.

Retrograde pyelography: Similar to IVP, except that the radiologist injects the contrast medium through a urethral catheter and takes a series of X-rays.

Sialography: Radiological study of the salivary gland duct. The patient sucks on a lemon wedge to open the duct. A catheter is inserted into the duct, and a contrast medium is introduced. The exam takes about 1 to 2 hours.

Stereoscopy: A rarely used X-ray procedure to study (primarily) the skull.

Thermography: A heat-sensing technique used for the detection of tumors. An infrared camera is used, which records variation in skin temperature. Warm areas appear light, and cool areas appear dark.

Xeroradiography: A diagnostic X-ray technique in which an image is produced electrically rather than chemically. It permits shorter exposure times and lower radiation levels than ordinary X-rays. It is also called xerography. Xeroradiography is used primarily for mammography.

Therapeutic Uses of Radiation

Radiation therapy: The use of radiation to treat diseases such as cancer by preventing cellular reproduction.

Teletherapy: Radiation therapy administered by a machine that is positioned at some distance from the patient. Teletherapy permits deeper penetration and is used primarily for deep tumors. It is done on an outpatient basis.

Brachytherapy: The implanting of radioactive sources into localized tumor tissues that are to be treated for a specific period of time.

Radioiodine: A radioactive isotope of iodine used in nuclear medicine and radiotherapy. It is used especially in the treatment of some thyroid conditions.

Medical Assistant's Role

Extent of participation by the medical assistant: Varies by state. The responsibilities of the medical assistant may involve simply assisting the radiological technologist or radiologist, or they may involve operating certain X-ray equipment.

Timing of procedures: Procedures that require the patient to fast, such as barium enemas, are best scheduled in the morning, so that the patient sleeps through most of the period during which the digestive tract is empty.

Preprocedure care: Involves providing preparation instructions, such as diet restrictions or requirements; explaining the procedure to the patient; obtaining a medication history and other information from the patient; and instructing the patient to remove clothing, jewelry, and any other metals and to put on a gown.

Preparation for arthrography: Ask patients about possible allergies to contrast media, iodine, or shellfish. No other special preprocedure preparations are necessary.

Preparation for barium enema or IVP: Ask the patient about possible allergies to contrast media, iodine, or shellfish. The patient should follow an all-liquid diet starting the morning before the procedure and should take a prescribed amount of electrolyte solution or other laxative on a specified schedule. The patient may have one cup of coffee, tea, or water on the morning of the barium enema but should have no food or liquids after midnight before the IVP.

Preparation for cholecystography: Ask the patient about possible allergies to contrast media, iodine, or shellfish. The patient should eat a fat-free dinner the evening before the examination and should not smoke or have any foods or liquids after midnight. The oral contrast medium should be taken about 2 hours after dinner; tablets should be taken 5 minutes apart.

Preparation for tomography or CT scan: Ask the patient about possible allergies to contrast media, iodine, or shellfish. The patient must lie still while the scans are taken. For a CT scan, the patient may breathe normally, but it is necessary for the patient to hold his or her breath for a tomogram.

Preparation for MRI: If a contrast medium will be used, ask the patient about possible allergies to contrast media, iodine, or shellfish. Ask whether any internal metallic materials are present, such as a pacemaker, clips, shunts, heart valves, or slivers or chips from working with metal. Patients should avoid caffeine for 4 hours before the examination, and they should not wear eye makeup during the procedure.

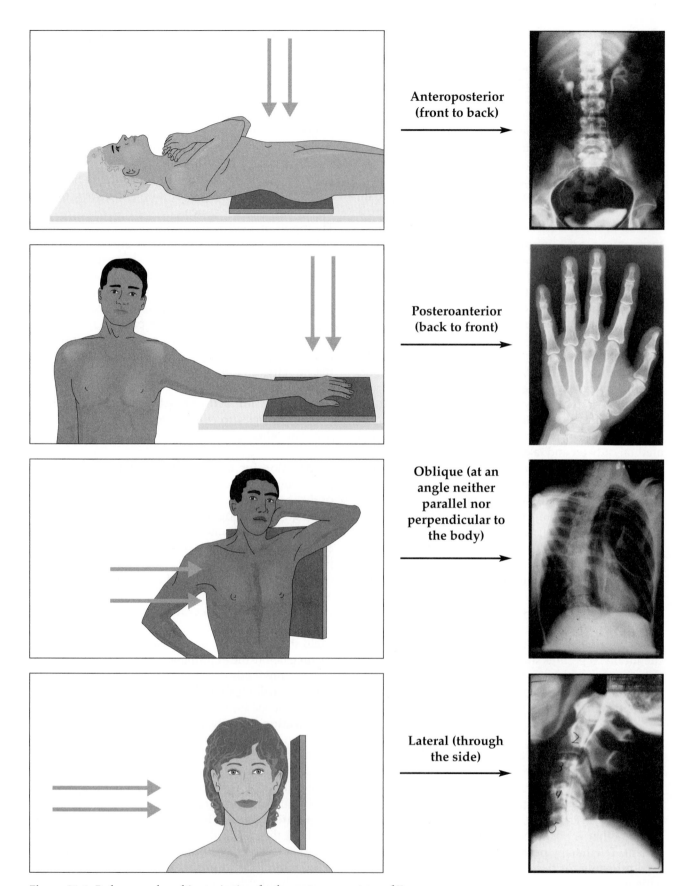

Figure 21-1 *Pathways and resulting projections for the most common types of X-rays.*

Preparation for mammography: Avoiding caffeine for a week or 10 days prior to the procedure will reduce the possibility of swelling and soreness that will heighten discomfort. The patient should not use deodorant, powder, or perfume on the underarm area or breasts before the examination.

Position: Patients need to be positioned in different ways, depending on the specific body part being X-rayed. The most common positions for taking X-rays are anteroposterior, posteroanterior, oblique, and lateral. See Figure 21-1.

Postprocedure care: Have the patient assume a comfortable position while the films are being developed. If the films are satisfactory, have the patient get dressed, and give the patient information on how to find out about the test results.

Safety and Storage

Safety

Radiosensitivity: The susceptibility of cells, tissues, or any living substances to the effects of radiation; also, a biological organism's measure of response to radiation. Immature, nonspecialized cells and cells that are growing rapidly are the most radiosensitive; mature, specialized cells are the most radioresistant.

Exposure: Exposure to radiation is cumulative, meaning that it adds up to a total dosage over the years. The amount of exposure is measured in units called roentgens.

Absorbed dose: The amount of radiation energy absorbed in tissue.

Overexposure: Not likely from routine X-rays, especially if precautions are taken. Overexposure to radiation can produce a variety of symptoms, including nausea, fatigue, and bleeding.

Personnel safety: All medical personnel who work in facilities that perform radiological tests should wear radiation exposure badges, make sure that equipment is in good working order, and wear a lead shield when equipment is operating.

Radiation exposure badge: A sensitized piece of film, in a holder, that indicates the amount of radiation to which the individual has been exposed. The badge should be checked regularly. It is also called a dosimeter.

Patient safety: The medical assistant must follow all rules governing patient safety from radiation exposure, including providing a lead shield. Among the factors to check are how much exposure the patient has received in the past and whether a female patient is pregnant.

Storage

Radiographic film: Sensitive to X-rays, heat, chemical fumes, light, moisture, and pressure. Fresh film must be kept on hand at all times. It must be properly stored and carefully handled.

Sensitometry: The measurement or study of how radiographic film responds chemically to radiation exposure and to processing conditions.

Film storage: Radiographic film should be stored in a cool, dry place. The best temperature for film storage is between 60 and 70°F. The best relative humidity is between 40% and 60%. Store packages on end; do not stack them on top of each other.

Ownership of radiographs: X-ray radiographs are the property of the radiology department where they are taken. They do not belong to the patient.

Documentation: Document the X-ray information on the patient record card or in the record book.

Labeling: Verify that film is labeled with the referring doctor's name, the date, and the patient's name.

Filing: Place the processed film in a film-filing envelope, and file the envelope in the correct place in the filing cabinet.

STRATEGIES TO SUCCESS

▶ Test-Taking Skills

If you must guess, guess!

You should know the material well enough to avoid having to guess on any of the questions. Realistically, however, there will be at least a few questions on the exam that you will be unsure about. When you come across these questions, try to make an educated guess at the correct answer and eliminate any of the answers that you know are wrong. Here are a few tips that will also help you eliminate some answers. However, before you apply them to every question you come across, remember that they are only guidelines, not hard and fast rules, so use them sparingly and only when you have no other option.

- Answers containing absolute terms such as *always, never, none, only, no one,* and *everyone* are often incorrect, because most things cannot be generalized in this way. Conversely, answers that contain relative words such as *generally, most, often, some,* and *usually* are often correct.
- If the answer calls for the completion of a sentence, eliminate the answers that would not form grammatically correct sentences.
- The longest, most complete answer is often correct.
- If two answers are similar except for one or two words, one of these answers is usually the correct one.

Instructions:

Answer the following questions. Check your answers in the *Answer Key* that follows this section.

1. A measurement of the actual absorbed dose of radiation is called
   A. Rem
   B. Rad
   C. Roentgen
   D. Contrast media
   E. Ray

2. An image produced on film by a sweeping beam of radiation is known as
   A. MRI
   B. Cassette
   C. Radioactive
   D. Isotopes
   E. Scan

3. The study of the gallbladder by X-ray with an oral contrast medium is called
   A. Cholecystosonography
   B. Cholecystitis
   C. Cholecystokinin
   D. Cholecystography
   E. Cholangiography

4. Which of the following statements regarding myelography is <u>not</u> correct?
   A. The radiologist performs a lumbar puncture
   B. It is fluoroscopy of the central nervous system
   C. The radiologist removes some cerebrospinal fluid
   D. It is fluoroscopy of the spinal cord
   E. A contrast medium is used

5. Radiation therapy for deeper tumors done on an outpatient basis is known as
   A. Brachytherapy
   B. Cryotherapy
   C. Thermotherapy
   D. Teletherapy
   E. Xeroradiography

6. The best temperature for film storage is between
   A. 40 and 50°F
   B. 50 and 60°F
   C. 60 and 70°F
   D. 70 and 80°F
   E. None of the above

7. Film artifacts are
   A. Areas that interfere with the diagnostic value of the radiograph
   B. Desirable
   C. Films that are beyond their expiration dates
   D. Diagnostic areas of interest
   E. None of the above

8. The frequency of electromagnetic radiation is measured in
   A. Watts
   B. Volts
   C. Rays
   D. Cycles
   E. Hertz

9. Excretory urography is also known as
   A. Sialography
   B. Cystography
   C. Intravenous pyelography
   D. Arthrography
   E. None of the above

10. A type of diagnostic radiology that uses high-frequency sound waves is
    A. Magnetic resonance imaging
    B. X-ray
    C. Tomography
    D. Arthrography
    E. Ultrasound

11. Positions that are neither parallel nor perpendicular to the body are called
    A. Supine
    B. Oblique
    C. Prone
    D. Recumbent
    E. Both A and B

12. The front-to-back position in radiology is known as

    A. Posteroanterior
    B. Lateral
    C. Anteroposterior
    D. Oblique
    E. Supine

13. The process in which an atom may gain or lose electrons is called

    A. Ionization
    B. Radiation
    C. Fractionation
    D. Potential difference
    E. Oxygenation

14. Which of the following statements is <u>not</u> correct in regard to radiosensitivity?

    A. Mature cells are the least radiosensitive
    B. Immature tissues are the most radiosensitive
    C. Cells that are rapidly growing are the most radiosensitive
    D. Nonspecialized cells are the most radiosensitive
    E. Specialized cells are the most radiosensitive

15. Before a mammogram, a woman should

    A. Drink coffee
    B. Use body lotion
    C. Avoid wearing deodorant
    D. Fast after midnight
    E. Avoid exercise

16. In preparing patients for such tests as barium enemas and CT scans, the medical assistant should

    A. Tell them that they will have to hold their breath
    B. Tell them to eat a fat-free dinner the night before
    C. Ask them whether internal metals are present
    D. Ask them whether they are allergic to contrast media, iodine, or shellfish
    E. Ask them whether they are wearing body lotion

17. Safety precautions are necessary because

    A. Radiation exposure is cumulative
    B. Radiation exposure is always fatal
    C. Overexposure is likely from routine X-rays
    D. Both A and C
    E. All of the above

18. Xeroradiography is used primarily for

    A. Cholecystography
    B. Arthrography
    C. Mammography
    D. Intravenous pyelography
    E. Cardiography

ANSWER KEY

1.	B	10.	E
2.	E	11.	B
3.	D	12.	C
4.	B	13.	A
5.	D	14.	E
6.	C	15.	C
7.	A	16.	D
8.	E	17.	A
9.	C	18.	C

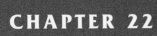

CHAPTER 22

Physical Therapy

CHAPTER OUTLINE

MEDICAL ASSISTING COMPETENCIES

COMPETENCY	CMA	RMA
Clinical		
Apply principles of aseptic techniques and infection control, including hand washing	X	X
Practice Standard Precautions	X	X
Prepare and maintain examination and treatment areas	X	X
Prepare the patient for and assist the physician with routine and specialty examinations, treatments, and minor office surgeries	X	X
Screen and follow up on patient test results	X	X

COMPETENCY	CMA	RMA
General/Legal/Professional		
Recognize and respond to verbal and nonverbal communications by being attentive and adapting communication to the recipient's level of understanding	X	X
Be aware of and perform within legal and ethical boundaries	X	X
Determine the needs for documentation and reporting, and document accurately and appropriately	X	X
Instruct individuals according to their needs	X	X
Provide patients with methods of health promotion and disease prevention	X	X
Be a "team player"		X
Conduct work within scope of education, training, and ability		X

STRATEGIES TO SUCCESS

▶ *Study Skills*

Practice repetition! Practice repetition!
One of the most common ways to remember something is to repeat it often. If you have trouble remembering certain material, use any or all of these strategies: (1) Review your notes on the subject; try reading them aloud to yourself. (2) Create flash cards and test yourself often. (3) Write out summary sheets of the most important terms and concepts you want to remember. The very acts of reading silently, reciting aloud, and writing something over and over again will help you remember it when it's time for the exam.

Terminology

Physical medicine: The branch of medicine that uses physical devices or agents therapeutically for the diagnosis, treatment, management, and prevention of diseases. It is also called physiatry.

Rehabilitation: Restoration of those functions that have been affected by a patient's injuries or disease.

Sports medicine: The branch of medicine that specializes in the prevention and treatment of injuries caused by athletic participation. More than one million people are treated for sports injuries each year in the United States. Most sports injuries involve muscle strains, sprains, and tears. Sports medicine uses a number of different modalities that enable the patient to recover quickly and return to high levels of activity with minimal loss of fitness.

Physiatrist: A physician specializing in physical medicine and rehabilitation.

Fitness: Overall good physical condition, including cardiovascular strength, muscular strength, and flexibility.

Range of motion (ROM): The degree to which a joint is able to move, measured in degrees with a protractor-like device called a goniometer.

Flexion: The bending movement allowed by certain joints of the skeleton, such as the elbow, that decreases the angle between the two adjoining bones.

Extension: The straightening movement allowed by certain joints of the skeleton, such as the knee, that increases the angle between the two adjoining bones.

Hyperextension: The position of maximum extension, or the extension of a body part beyond its normal limits.

Reduction: The correction of a fracture, dislocation, or hernia.

Lordosis: Exaggerated anterior curvature of the lumbar spine.

Kyphosis: Abnormally increased convex curvature of the thoracic spine. It is also colloquially called hunchback or humpback.

Scoliosis: Lateral deviation in the normal vertical curve of the spine.

Osteoporosis: A reduction in the mass of bone per unit of volume that interferes with the mechanical support function of bone, causing bone fractures in situations that would not normally damage the skeleton.

Luxation: Complete dislocation of the bone from the joint.

Subluxation: Incomplete dislocation of the bone from the joint.

Tendonitis: Inflammation of tendons. Tendonitis is one of the most common causes of acute pain in the shoulder.

Quadriplegia: Paralysis of all four extremities of the body and the trunk. This disorder is usually caused by spinal cord injury, especially in the area of the fifth to the seventh cervical vertebrae. Automobile accidents and sporting mishaps are common causes.

Paraplegia: Paralysis of the lower portion of the body, usually caused by spinal cord injury or disease. Paraplegia commonly results from automobile and motorcycle accidents, sporting accidents, falls, and gunshot wounds.

Hemiplegia: Paralysis of one side of the body. The three types of hemiplegia are cerebral, facial, and spastic.

Hemiparesis: Muscular weakness of one half of the body.

Cerebral palsy: Nonprogressive paralysis due to defects in or trauma to the brain, especially at birth. Spastic cerebral palsy is characterized by hyperactive reflexes, rapid muscle contraction, muscle weakness, and underdevelopment of the limbs. Mental retardation, seizure disorders, and impaired speech are also common with this condition. Treatment may include the use of braces, adaptive appliances, and ROM exercises.

Patient Assessment

Gait: A style of walking. A normal gait consists of two phases: stance and swing. See Figure 22-1. Generally, a physician or physical therapist assesses a patient's gait. The patient is asked to walk away, turn around, and walk back. Assessment includes an appraisal of the patient's length of stride, balance, coordination, direction of knees (inward or outward), and direction of feet (inward or outward).

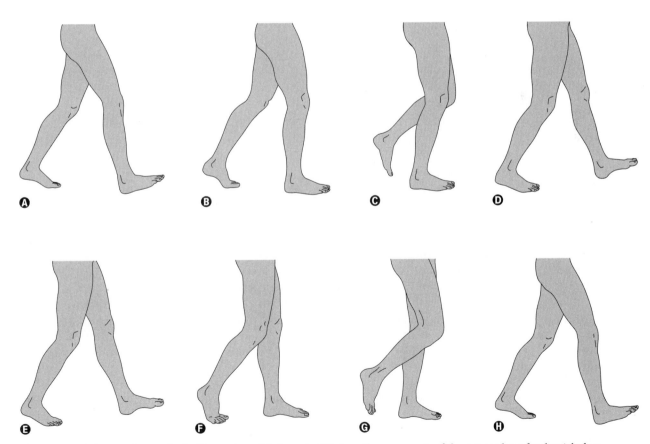

Figure 22-1 *The two phases of gait. Illustrations (A) through (D) show the movements of the stance phase for the right leg; illustrations (E) through (H) show the movements of the swing phase: (A) right heel strike, (B) flat right foot, (C) midstance, (D) push-off with the right foot, (E) right foot poised, (F) left heel strike, (G) midswing, (H) right heel strike.*

Term	Description	Example
Abduction	Movement away from the midline of the body or away from the axis of a limb	Raising an arm straight out to the side
Adduction	Movement toward the midline of the body or toward the axis of a limb	Lowering a raised arm to the side
Circumduction	Circular movement of a body part	Performing arm circles
Dorsiflexion	Upward or backward movement of a body part	Flexing a foot so that the toes point upward
Eversion	Outward movement of a body part	Moving an ankle so that the sole of the foot turns outward
Extension	Movement that spreads two body parts or that opens a joint	Straightening a leg by unbending the knee
Flexion	Movement that brings together two body parts or that closes a joint	Bending a leg at the knee
Inversion	Inward movement of a body part	Moving an ankle so that the sole of the foot turns inward
Plantar flexion	Downward movement of a body part	Flexing a foot so that the toes point downward
Pronation	Twisting movement that brings a palm facing downward	Turning a wrist so that the palm faces downward
Rotation	Movement of a body part around its axis	Turning the head from side to side
Supination	Twisting movement that brings a palm facing upward	Turning a wrist so that the palm faces upward

Table 22-1

Goniometry: The measurement of joint mobility. Goniometric tests are noninvasive. The movements measured by goniometry are explained in Table 22-1.

Goniometer: A device used to measure the degree of joint movement. See Figure 22-2.

Using a goniometer: The medical assistant may be asked to assist with or perform goniometry. Have the patient move each body part in a specified manner, and position the goniometer to measure degrees of movement.

Muscle testing: Consists of ROM tests (with a goniometer), strength tests, and task skill tests.

Muscle strength testing: Determines the amount of muscle force. This test is usually done from head to foot, usually in combination with ROM testing. The patient is asked to resist pressure that the physician

or medical assistant applies to each muscle or group of muscles. Strength is rated according to a five-point scale, as shown in Table 22-2.

Posture testing: The physician looks at the patient's spinal curve from the sides, back, and front; notes the symmetry of alignment of the shoulders, knees, and hips; assesses alignment and degree of straightness as the patient bends at the waist; and assesses knee position by having the patient stand with both feet together.

Electromyography (EMG): A process of electrically recording muscle action potentials. The patient may receive sedation before this test because the electric current can be painful. Abnormal EMG test results can indicate a congenital or an acquired disease condition of the muscles.

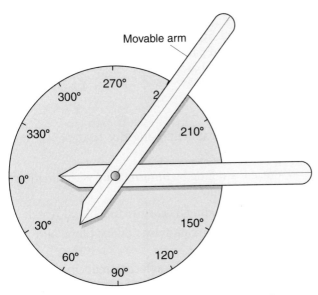

Figure 22-2 *A universal goniometer is a protractor with a movable pointer that measures degrees of joint movement.*

Treatment

Physical therapy: The treatment of disorders with physical agents and methods such as massage, manipulation, therapeutic exercise, cold, heat, hydrotherapy, and electrical stimulation. Physical therapy includes rehabilitative treatment to restore function after an illness or an injury. It is also called physiotherapy.

Physical therapist: An allied health professional who has completed at least a 4-year baccalaureate training program in physical therapy and has received state licensure. He or she deals primarily with movement dysfunction and works with body parts that have been injured by accident, amputation, or disease. As a medical assistant, you may be asked by a physician to assist with some forms of physical therapy, including applying cold and heat; teaching basic exercises; preparing patients; and demonstrating how to use canes, walkers, crutches, and wheelchairs.

Thermotherapy

Thermotherapy: The treatment of disease by the application of heat. Thermotherapy is used to relieve pain, to relax spasms of muscles, to relieve localized swelling, to increase tissue metabolism and repair, and to increase drainage from an infected area. A temperature of 116°F (47°C) or above can cause burning. Heat therapy should not be used on pregnant or menstruating women, and it also should not be used longer than ordered by the physician. Thermotherapy should not be used longer than 30 minutes.

Types of heat therapy: The main types are dry heat, moist heat, and diathermy.

Dry heat therapy: Includes the use of heating pads, hot-water bottles, chemical hot packs, heat lamps, and fluidotherapy.

Heating pad: The physician should specify the heating pad temperature and the length of time the pad should be applied. Cover the pad with a pillowcase or towel, make sure that the cord is not frayed, make sure that the patient's skin is dry, plug the cord into an outlet, and turn on the pad. The patient should not lie on top of a heating pad.

Hot-water bottle: Water temperature should not exceed 125°F for adults and 115°F for children and elderly patients. Fill the bottle halfway, and expel the air. Cover the bottle with a cloth or pillowcase before applying.

Chemical hot pack: A disposable, flexible pack of chemicals that becomes hot when kneaded or slapped. After activating the pack, cover it with a cloth and place it on the patient's skin in the area being treated.

Heat lamp: Uses an infrared or ultraviolet bulb. Place the lamp 2 to 4 feet from the area being treated. Treatment usually lasts 20 to 30 minutes.

Infrared therapy: Treatment by exposure to various wavelengths of infrared radiation. Infrared treatment is performed to relieve pain and to stimulate blood circulation.

AT A GLANCE	Muscle Strength Scale	
Muscle Response	**Rating**	**Meaning**
No response	0	Paralysis
Slight contraction felt	1	Severe weakness
Passive ROM when resistance is removed	2	Moderate weakness
Active ROM against gravity or light resistance	3 or 4	Mild weakness
Active ROM against heavy resistance	5	Normal strength

Table 22-2

Ultraviolet therapy: Used in the treatment of rickets and certain skin conditions such as psoriasis. This therapy is also useful in the control of infectious airborne bacteria and viruses. Ultraviolet ray lamp treatments must be carefully controlled because they can cause severe sunburn and even second- or third-degree burns. The time and the distance of the lamp from the patient must be controlled. Treatment is prescribed by the second, for example, 10 or 20 seconds of exposure. The patient should cover his or her eyes with dark goggles.

Fluidotherapy: A relatively new technique in which the patient places the hand or foot in a container of glass beads that are heated and agitated with hot air.

Moist heat therapy: There are several types of moist heat applications, including hot soaks, hot compresses, hot packs, and paraffin baths.

Hot soak: Usually used on arms or legs. The patient places the body part being treated in a container of plain or medicated water heated to not more than 110°F. A hot soak should last about 15 minutes.

Hot compress: Soak the gauze or cloth in hot water, wring it out, and apply it to the area being treated. Either place a hot-water bottle on top of it or frequently rewarm the compress in hot water.

Paraffin bath: Utilizes a receptacle of heated wax and mineral oil to reduce pain, muscle spasms, and stiffness in patients with arthritis. A thick coat of wax remains on the area for about 30 minutes and then is peeled off.

Diathermy: The production of heat in body tissues for therapeutic purposes by high-frequency currents that are insufficiently intense to destroy tissues. Diathermy is useful in treating muscular disorders, tendonitis, arthritis, and bursitis. Diathermy cannot be used in patients with metal implants, such as hip replacements, because of the electrical field it creates and the consequent danger of burns. Patients must remove all metal jewelry and buckles before treatment, which usually lasts from 15 to 30 minutes. There are three basic methods of diathermy: ultrasound, microwave, and shortwave.

Ultrasound: Projects high-frequency sound waves that are converted to heat in muscle tissue. The most common type of diathermy, it is administered by rubbing a gel-covered transducer over the skin in circular patterns. It is used to treat sprains, strains, and other acute ailments. Ultrasound treatments should not be used in areas where bones are near the skin's surface.

Microwave: Electromagnetic radiation that is converted into heat in tissues. It should not be used on patients with pacemakers, in combination with wet dressings, or near metal implants.

Shortwave: Provides heat deep in the body by means of radio waves that travel between two condenser plates. It is used to treat chronic arthritis, bursitis, sinusitis, and other conditions.

Administering thermotherapy: Place the thermotherapy device on the affected body part. Ask the patient how the device feels. Leave the device in place for as long as ordered by the physician. Check the skin for color, feeling, and pain periodically, and have the physician examine any area that becomes excessively red, blistered, or painful.

Cryotherapy

Cryotherapy: Treatment using dry cold or wet cold applications to

- Prevent swelling by limiting fluid accumulation in body tissue
- Control bleeding by constricting blood vessels
- Reduce inflammation by slowing blood and fluid movement
- Provide an anesthetic effect by reducing inflammation
- Reduce pus formation by inhibiting microorganisms
- Lower body temperature

For best results, cryotherapy should be used frequently, for example, about 20 minutes every hour for acute conditions or injuries (during the first 48 hours).

Dry cold applications: Ice bags (or ice collars) and chemical ice packs.

Ice bag or **ice collar:** Place ice chips or small ice cubes in the device, filling it two-thirds full; compress the container to expel air; dry the container; and cover it with a towel to absorb moisture.

Chemical ice pack: A flat plastic bag containing semifluid chemicals. Most chemical ice packs remain cold for 30 to 60 minutes; some are disposable, and some are reusable. Check the pack for leaks, and shake or squeeze it to activate the chemicals. Cover the pack with a towel.

Wet cold applications: Cold compresses and ice massage.

Cold compress: Place large ice cubes and a small amount of water in a basin. Place a washcloth or gauze square in the basin to moisten it, wring it out, and apply it to the area being treated.

Ice massage: Wrap an ice cube in a plastic bag, or freeze water in a paper cup, then use the device to massage the area.

Administering cryotherapy: Place the cryotherapy device on the affected body part. Ask the patient how the device feels. Leave the device in place for as long as ordered by the physician. Check the skin for color, feeling, and pain periodically, and have the physician examine any area that becomes excessively pale or blue, numb, or painful. After treatment, check for reduced swelling, redness, and pain.

Other Therapy

Hydrotherapy: The use of water in the treatment of various disorders. Hydrotherapy may include continuous tub baths, wet sheet packs, or shower sprays.

Whirlpool: A tank in which water is agitated by jets of air under pressure, used to relax muscles and to increase circulation.

Contrast bath: Two baths, one filled with hot water and the other with cold water. The patient quickly moves the affected body part from one to the other. It is used to induce relaxation, stimulate circulation, and improve mobility.

Underwater exercises: Generally performed in a warm swimming pool by patients with joint injuries, burns, and arthritis.

Exercise therapy: A technique for helping patients prevent deformities, regain body movement, improve muscle strength, stimulate circulation, retain neuromuscular coordination, and resume normal daily activities. Therapeutic exercises are ordered by the physician after complete evaluation of the physical problem.

Medical assistant's role in exercise therapy: To provide information for the patient and family, to provide support and encouragement, to assist with ROM exercises, and to teach the patient how to perform them at home.

Active mobility exercises: Self-directed exercises a patient performs without assistance to increase muscle strength and function. They may require such equipment as a stationary bicycle or treadmill.

Passive mobility exercises: Used for patients with neuromuscular disabilities or weaknesses. The physical therapist or a machine moves the body part.

Aided mobility exercises: Self-directed exercises performed with the help of such devices as exercise machines or therapy pools.

Active resistance exercises: The patient works against resistance, which is provided by a therapist or by an exercise machine, to increase muscle strength.

ROM exercises: Exercises that slowly move each joint through its full range of motion. They may be active (performed by the patient without assistance) or passive (performed with the help of another person or a machine). Typical ROM exercises are shoulder abduction, back rotation, hip flexion, and toe abduction.

Electrical stimulation: The delivery of controlled amounts of low-voltage electric current to motor and sensory nerves to stimulate muscles. It is used to help retrain a patient to use injured muscles.

Massage: The application of pressure with the hands on the soft tissue of the body through stroking, rubbing, kneading, or tapping, in order to increase circulation, improve muscle tone, and relax the patient. It is one of the oldest known methods for promoting healing. The most common sites for massage are the back, knees, elbows, and heels. Stroking is the most common massage modality used in the medical office.

Immobilization: The restriction of movement of a body part in order to promote healing. Devices such as splints and slings are prescribed by the physician and used by the physical therapist to immobilize damaged tissues and bones.

Manipulation: The application of rapid thrusting motions in order to stabilize, stretch, or reposition a joint.

Traction: The process of pulling or stretching a part of the body. It is applied by a physical therapist to create proper bone alignment, reduce joint stiffening and abnormal muscle shortening, correct deformities, relieve compression of vertebral joints, and reduce or relieve muscle spasms.

Mobility-Assisting Devices

Cane: A sturdy wooden or aluminum shaft or walking stick, used to give support and greater mobility to a person who is ambulatory but needs some assistance.

Standard cane: A cane with a single leg, used by someone who needs only a small amount of support in walking.

Tripod and quad-base canes: Canes with bases having three and four legs, respectively, that provide greater support and stability.

Cane height: When the patient is holding the cane and standing up straight, the cane should be level with the top of the patient's femur, and the elbow should be bent at a 30-degree angle.

Teaching a patient to use a cane: The medical assistant may be asked to teach a patient how to use a cane. Table 22-3 explains how to use a cane to stand up, walk, and climb stairs.

Crutch: A metal or wooden staff used to aid a person in walking. It is important that the person be taught how to use the crutch(es) safely and how to achieve a stable and acceptable gait.

Types of crutches: The two basic kinds of crutches are axillary crutches (which reach from the ground almost to the armpit) and forearm crutches (which reach from the ground to the forearm and are also called Lofstrand or Canadian crutches).

Measuring a patient for crutches: Crutches must be measured to fit the patient. Crutches that are too long or too short can cause muscle weakness, back strain, or imbalance. To confirm that the fit is correct, make sure that the patient is wearing the type of shoes that will be worn when walking. When the patient is standing erect, with feet slightly apart, and the crutch tips are positioned 2 inches in front of the feet and 4 to 6 inches to the side of each foot, there should be 2 to 3 fingerwidths between the axillary supports and the armpits (for axillary crutches), and the handgrips should be positioned to create a 30-degree flexion at the elbows.

Using crutches: In teaching patients how to use crutches, emphasize the following points:

- Support body weight with the hands.
- Stand erect.

Standing from a chair

1. Instruct the patient to slide his buttocks to the edge of the chair.
2. Tell the patient to place his right foot against the right front leg of the chair and his left foot against the left front leg of the chair.
3. Instruct the patient to lean forward and use the armrests of the chair to push upward. Caution the patient not to lean on the cane.
4. Have the patient position the cane for support on the strong side of the body.

Walking

1. Teach the patient to hold the cane on the strong side of her body with the tip(s) of the cane 4 to 6 inches from the side of her strong foot. Remind the patient to make sure to keep the tip(s) flat on the ground.
2. Have the patient move the cane forward approximately 12 inches and them move her affected foot forward, parallel to the cane.
3. Next have the patient move her strong leg forward past both the cane and her weak leg.
4. Observe as the patient repeats this process.

Going up stairs

1. Instruct the patient always to start with his strong leg when going up stairs.
2. Advise the patient to keep the cane on the strong side of his body and to use the wall or rail for support on the weak side.
3. After the patient steps on the strong leg, instruct him to bring up his weak leg and then the cane.
4. Remind the patient not to rush.

Going down stairs

1. Instruct the patient always to start with her weak leg when going down stairs.
2. Advise the patient to keep the cane on the strong side of her body and to use the wall or rail for support on the weak side.
3. Have the patient use the strong leg and wall or rail to support her body, bending the strong leg as she lowers her weak leg and cane to the next step. She can move the cane and weak leg simultaneously, or she can move the cane first, followed by the weak leg.
4. Instruct the patient to step down with the strong leg.

Table 22-3

- Look straight ahead.
- Move crutches no more than 6 inches at a time.
- Wear flat, well-fitting, nonskid shoes.
- Remove throw rugs and other unsecured articles from traffic areas.
- Check the tips regularly for wear and wetness.
- Check all wing nuts and bolts for tightness.

Crutch gaits: Begin with the standing or tripod position, in which the patient places the crutch tips 4 to 6 inches in front of the feet and 4 to 6 inches away from the side of each foot. Patients should use a slow gait in crowded areas or when feeling tired.

Four-point gait: A slow gait used by persons who can bear weight on both legs. The patient should begin in the tripod position, then move the right crutch forward, move the left foot forward to the level of the left crutch, move the left crutch forward, and move the right foot forward to the level of the right crutch.

Three-point gait: Used by persons who can bear full weight on one leg and no weight on the other. It requires good muscle coordination and arm strength. The patient begins in the tripod position, moves both crutches and the affected leg forward, then balances weight on both crutches and moves the unaffected leg forward.

Two-point gait: A faster gait used by persons who can bear some weight on both feet and have good muscle coordination and balance. The patient begins in the tripod position, then moves the left crutch and right foot forward at the same time, followed by the right crutch and left foot.

1. Instruct the patient to step into the walker.
2. Tell the patient to place his or her hands on the handgrips on the sides of the walker.
3. Make sure that the patient's feet are far enough apart so that he or she feels balanced.
4. Instruct the patient to pick up the walker and to move it forward about 6 inches.
5. Have the patient move one foot forward and then the other foot.
6. Instruct the patient to pick up the walker again and to move it forward. If the patient is strong enough, explain that he or she may advance the walker after moving each foot rather than waiting until after having move both feet.

Table 22-4

Swing-to gait: A modified three-point gait often used by persons with physical disabilities. The patient begins in the tripod position and then moves both crutches forward at the same time. The patient then lifts the body and swings it to the crutches.

Swing-through gait: Also often used by persons with physical disabilities. It is like the swing-to gait, but the patient swings the body past the crutches.

Walker: An extremely light, movable apparatus, about waist high, made of metal tubing (usually aluminum), used to aid a patient in walking. There are two types: standard (with four widely placed legs ending in rubber tips) and rolling (with wheels).

Walker height: The top of the walker should be just below the patient's waist or at the same height as the top of the hip bone, so that when the patient holds the handgrip, the elbow is bent at a 30-degree angle.

Using a walker: Although a physical therapist usually trains patients in the use of walkers, medical assistants may be asked to do it or to reinforce the information. Table 22-4 provides information on how to teach a patient to use a walker.

Wheelchair: A mobile chair equipped with large wheels and brakes. If long-term use of the chair is expected, a physical therapist may prescribe particular features, such as seat size and height, left- or right-hand propulsion, brake type, armrest height, footrest style (e.g., fixed, swing-away, elevating), and special seat pads.

Using a wheelchair: To get into the wheelchair, the patient should lock the chair and fold back the footplates, then back into the chair, supporting himself or herself on the armrests while lowering the body into the chair.

Transferring a patient from a wheelchair to a table: If the patient is weak, heavy, or unstable, ask for help. Make sure that the wheelchair is in the locked position and that the patient is sitting at the front of the wheelchair seat. Face the patient, spread your feet apart, and bend slightly at the knees. Have the patient hold on to your shoulders, and place your arms around the patient under the arms. At the count of "3," lift and pivot the patient to bring the back of his or her knees against the table. Gently lower the patient into a sitting or supine position on the table.

STRATEGIES TO SUCCESS

▶ *Test-Taking Skills*

Do a mind dump!
    As soon as the exam starts, you may find it helpful to do a mind dump. Briefly look over the questions and quickly write down all the information that is fresh in your head. Write out any lists that you have memorized. All the concepts and formulas that you always had trouble remembering and those that you were still going over and memorizing as the exam began should be written down as soon as possible so that you don't forget them. Then you can focus on the exam with more confidence. A mind dump doesn't work for everyone, and it should not take valuable time away from your exam.

CHAPTER 22 REVIEW

Instructions:

Answer the following questions. Check your answers in the *Answer Key* that follows this section.

1. The branch of medicine that is also a key component of rehabilitation is
   A. Physical therapy
   B. Physiatry
   C. Sports medicine
   D. Manipulation
   E. None of the above

2. The degree to which a joint is able to move is known as
   A. Goniometer
   B. Goniometry
   C. Range of motion
   D. Range of reach
   E. Universal goniometer

3. Lateral deviation in the normal vertical curve of the spine is called
   A. Kyphosis
   B. Lordosis
   C. Scoliosis
   D. Luxation
   E. None of the above

4. Which of the following is paralysis of the lower portion of the body?
   A. Hemiplegia
   B. Paraplegia
   C. Quadriplegia
   D. Hemiparesis
   E. Parapraxia

5. Which of the following is the most appropriate initial treatment of a contusion?
   A. Ultrasonography
   B. Whirlpool therapy
   C. Massage
   D. Application of ice packs
   E. Application of hot soaks therapy

6. In thermotherapy, which of the following temperatures can cause burning?
   A. 105°F
   B. 110°F
   C. 112°F
   D. 114°F
   E. 116°F

7. How long does diathermy usually last?
   A. 5 to 10 minutes
   B. 10 to 15 minutes
   C. 15 to 30 minutes
   D. 60 to 90 minutes
   E. 2 to 3 hours

8. Cryotherapy is used for all of the following purposes <u>except</u>
   A. To lower body temperature
   B. To reduce swelling
   C. To reduce bleeding
   D. To reduce pus formation
   E. To reduce clotting

9. Muscular weakness of one side of the body is called
   A. Hemiparesis
   B. Hemiplegia
   C. Hemimelia
   D. Hemiopia
   E. Hemiphelia

10. Patients instructed on how to use crutches should be told to
    A. Move crutches no more than 6 inches at a time
    B. Look down at the ground to check where they place the crutches
    C. Balance their body weight between their feet and hands
    D. Move crutches approximately a foot at a time
    E. Stand bent over the crutches at a 30-degree angle for increased support

11. Physical therapists are allied health professionals who have completed at least

    A. Medical school
    B. A 4-year baccalaureate training program
    C. A 2-year associate degree program
    D. Postgraduate work
    E. A certificate program

12. Movement allowed by joints to decrease the angle between two adjoining bones is called

    A. Range of motion
    B. Extension
    C. Flexion
    D. Gait
    E. Luxation

13. Correction of a fracture, dislocation, or hernia is called

    A. Reduction
    B. Luxation
    C. Subluxation
    D. Relocation
    E. Casting

14. Electromyography is the process of electrically recording muscle

    A. Contraction
    B. Relaxation
    C. Action potentials
    D. Energy production
    E. Flexion

15. Diathermy is useful in treating all of the following conditions except

    A. Tendonitis
    B. Myocarditis
    C. Muscular disorders
    D. Arthritis
    E. Bursitis

16. How far from the area being treated should a heat lamp be placed?

    A. 6 to 8 feet
    B. 4 to 6 feet
    C. 2 to 4 feet
    D. 1 to 2 feet
    E. Less than 1 foot

17. Which of the following heat therapies uses radio waves to provide heat deep in the body?

    A. Shortwave diathermy
    B. Microwave diathermy
    C. Ultrasound diathermy
    D. Infrared diathermy
    E. Chemical diathermy

18. A way of assessing the patient's walking behavior is called

    A. Muscle strength testing
    B. Walking test
    C. Goniometry
    D. Electromyography
    E. Gait testing

19. When using a chemical hot pack in heat therapy, you should

    A. Place it on the patient's skin on the area being affected
    B. Plug the pack's heating cord into an outlet and turn the pad on
    C. Knead the pad and then cover it with cloth before placing it on the patient
    D. Fill the pack halfway with water, expel the air, and cover it with a pillowcase before applying
    E. Both B and D

20. How high should the top of a cane be?

    A. Axillary height
    B. Waist level
    C. Any height, because patients can use it well regardless of height
    D. 30 inches from the ground
    E. Level with the top of the femur

ANSWER KEY

1.	B		11.	B
2.	C		12.	C
3.	C		13.	A
4.	B		14.	C
5.	D		15.	B
6.	E		16.	C
7.	C		17.	A
8.	E		18.	E
9.	A		19.	C
10.	A		20.	E

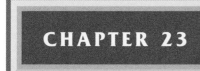

CHAPTER 23

Medical Emergencies and First Aid

CHAPTER OUTLINE

MEDICAL ASSISTING COMPETENCIES

COMPETENCY	CMA	RMA
Clinical		
Apply principles of aseptic techniques and infection control, including hand washing	X	X
Practice Standard Precautions	X	X
Obtain vital signs	X	X
Interview the patient to obtain and record the patient's history	X	X
Recognize emergencies; perform first aid and CPR		X
General/Legal/Professional		
Recognize and respond to verbal and nonverbal communications by being attentive and adapting communication to the recipient's level of understanding	X	X
Be aware of and perform within legal and ethical boundaries	X	X
Determine the needs for documentation and reporting, and document accurately and appropriately	X	X
Instruct individuals according to their needs	X	X
Provide patients with methods of health promotion and disease prevention	X	X
Identify community resources and information for patients and employers	X	X
Project a positive attitude		X
Adapt to change		X
Evidence a responsible attitude		X
Be courteous and diplomatic		X
Conduct work within scope of education, training, and ability		X
Be impartial and show empathy when dealing with patients		X

STRATEGIES TO SUCCESS

▶ *Study Skills*

Rephrase!
   When a concept seems complicated, look up any words you don't understand in a medical dictionary or a reference book, and try rephrasing the definition in your own words. Be sure that you only make the definition clearer and that you are not actually changing what the definition says. Rephrasing will help you understand the subject matter, and the concept will be easier to recall on an exam.

Emergencies

Medical emergency: A situation in which an individual suddenly becomes ill or has an injury that requires immediate attention and help by a health-care professional.

First aid: Immediate care given to a person who has suddenly become injured or ill. First aid can save a life, reduce pain, prevent further injury, reduce the risk of permanent disability, and increase the chance of early recovery.

Emergency Medical Services (EMS): A network of qualified police, fire, and medical personnel who use community resources and equipment to provide emergency care to victims of injury or sudden illness. Post the EMS telephone number, which is 911 in many communities, at every telephone and on the crash cart or first-aid tray.

Involving the EMS: To involve the EMS in an emergency, it is necessary to

1. Recognize that an emergency exists.
2. Decide to act.
3. Call the local emergency telephone number for help.
4. Provide care until help arrives.

Handling Emergencies

Medical assistant's responsibilities: You may be responsible for providing first aid, but you are never responsible for diagnosing or providing other medical care. Note the presence of serious conditions and take the appropriate action. Perform only procedures that you have been trained to perform. See Table 23-1.

Emergency triage: The classification of injuries according to severity, urgency of treatment, and place for treatment. If you receive an emergency call from a patient or patient's family member follow the practice's triage protocols. Stay calm; reassure the patient, and act in a confident, organized manner.

Personal protection: When administering first aid and other emergency treatment, assume that all blood and body fluids are infected with blood-borne pathogens, and follow Universal Precautions, including wearing gloves and other personal protective equipment. Minimize your contact with blood by avoiding touching objects unnecessarily that have been contaminated with blood or other body fluids. Minimize the splattering or spraying of blood. Don't touch your face, eyes, nose, or mouth while providing emergency medical care. If you have been exposed to blood or other body fluids, tell the physician so that you can obtain post-exposure treatment.

Documentation: Document all office emergencies in the patient's chart, including information on assessment, treatment, and response.

Good Samaritan law: Permits emergency care on the condition that it is within the scope of competence of the person administering first aid. It holds individuals giving first aid responsible for any injury they cause as a result of negligence or failure to exercise reasonable care. If the victim is conscious or a family member is present, obtain verbal consent. If the victim is unconscious, consent is implied. State laws also apply.

Crash cart: A rolling cart that contains basic drugs, supplies, and equipment for medical emergencies. Most crash carts also contain a first-aid kit with supplies for managing minor injuries and ailments. See Table 23-2.

AT A GLANCE | **Performing Emergency Assessment**

1. Wash your hands and put on examination gloves if possible.
2. Talk to the patient to determine level of consciousness.
3. If the patient can communicate clearly, ask what happened. If the patient can't talk, ask someone who observed the incident.
4. If you cannot determine the patient's medical history by talking to the patient, check for a medical identification card or a bracelet.
5. Assess the patient's ABCs (airway, breathing, and circulation), and begin rescue breathing or CPR as needed.
6. Assess for injury, observing the body from head to toe. Palpate gently.
7. Observe the skin for pallor (paleness) or cyanosis (a bluish tint). If the patient is dark-skinned, observe for pallor or cyanosis on the inside of the lips and mouth.
8. Check the pulse for regularity and strength.
9. Check the eyes for pupil size. Using a penlight, assess pupil response to light.
10. Document your findings and report them to the doctor or emergency medical technician (EMT).
11. Assist the doctor or EMT as requested.
12. Remove the gloves and wash your hands.

Table 23-1

1. Review the office protocol for a list of items that should be on the crash cart.
2. Check the <u>drugs</u> on the cart against the list. Restock as necessary, and replace any drugs that have passed their expiration date. The following drugs are often included on the cart:
   - Activated charcoal
   - Amobarbital sodium (Amytal Sodium®)
   - Apomorphine hydrochloride
   - Atropine
   - Dextrose 50%
   - Diazepam (Valium®)
   - Digoxin (Lanoxin®)
   - Diphenhydramine hydrochloride (Benadryl®)
   - Epinephrine, injectable
   - Furosemide (Lasix®)
   - Glucagon
   - Glucose paste or tablets
   - Insulin (regular or a variety)
   - Intravenous dextrose in saline and intravenous dextrose in water
   - Isoproterenol hydrochloride (Isuprel®), aerosol inhaler and injectable
   - Lactated Ringer's solution
   - Lidocaine (Xylocaine®), injectable
   - Metaraminol (Aramine®)
   - Methylprednisolone tablets
   - Nitroglycerin tablets
   - Phenobarbital, injectable
   - Phenytoin (Dilantin®)
   - Saline solution, isotonic (0.9%)
   - Sodium bicarbonate, injectable
   - Sterile water for injection
3. Check the <u>supplies</u> on the cart against the list. Restock used items, and make sure that all packaging of supplies on the cart is still intact. Crash cart supplies typically include:
   - Adhesive tape
   - Constricting band or tourniquet
   - Dressing supplies (alcohol wipes, rolls of gauze, bandage strips, bandage scissors)
   - IV tubing, venipuncture devices, and butterfly needles
   - Padded tongue blades
   - Personal protective equipment
   - Syringes and needles in various sizes
4. Check the <u>equipment</u> on the crash cart against the list, and examine everything to make sure that it is in working order. Restock equipment that is missing or broken. The equipment usually consists of:
   - Airways in assorted sizes
   - Ambu-bag™, a trademark for a breathing bag used to assist respiratory ventilation
   - Defibrillator (electrical device that shocks the heart to restore normal breathing)
   - Endotracheal tubes in various sizes
   - Oxygen tank with oxygen mask and cannula
5. Check <u>miscellaneous items</u> on the cart against the list, and restock as needed. These items usually include:
   - Orange juice
   - Sugar packets

Table 23-2

Injuries Caused by Extreme Temperatures

Hypothermia: A medical emergency in which the body temperature is dangerously reduced below the normal range, below 96°F (rectal, child/adult) or 97.5°F (rectal, newborn). Major symptoms include mild shivering, cool skin, and pallor. Minor characteristics include tachycardia, cyanosis, and hypertension. Risk factors include exposure to a cool or cold environment, trauma, malnutrition, consumption of alcohol, specific medications, decreased metabolic rate, aging, and inactivity.

Frostbite: The traumatic effect of extreme cold on skin and subcutaneous tissues, particularly the toes, fingers, ears, and nose. Vasoconstriction of blood vessels causes anoxia, edema, vesiculation, and necrosis. Symptoms include white, waxy, or grayish yellow skin that may feel crusty, with possible softness in the underlying tissue. The body part experiences sensations of cold, tingling, and pain. To treat frostbite, wrap warm clothing or blankets around the affected body part, or place the affected area in warm but not hot water. Do not rub or massage the affected area. Obtain medical assistance.

Hyperthermia: Body temperature elevated above the normal range. Skin is warm to the touch and appears flushed. The patient may experience tachypnea, tachycardia, seizures, or convulsions. Major factors include exposure to a hot environment, vigorous activity, medications or anesthesia, increased metabolic rate, trauma or illness, and dehydration. Individuals who are in poor health, alcoholic, obese, very young, or elderly are less able to tolerate heat waves and constant high temperatures.

Heatstroke: A severe and sometimes fatal condition generally caused by prolonged exposure to high temperatures. Symptoms include hot, dry skin; high body temperature; altered mental state; rapid pulse; rapid breathing; dizziness; and weakness. To treat heatstroke, call the EMS system. Move the patient to a cool place and remove the patient's outer clothing. Cool the patient, using any means available. Keep the patient's head and shoulders slightly elevated.

Heat cramps: Painful spasms of the voluntary muscles in the leg, abdomen, or arm, which may be caused by depletion in the body of both water and salt. It occurs in an extremely hot environment.

Heat exhaustion: Characterized by muscle cramps, weakness, nausea, dizziness, and loss of consciousness, caused by depletion of body fluids and electrolytes. It is the most frequent heat-related injury. Treatment includes moving the patient to a cool place and starting fluid and electrolyte replacement.

Burns

Burn: An injury to the tissues of the body caused by heat, electricity, chemicals, radiation, or gases. The severity of a burn depends on the depth of the burn and the percentage of the body involved. Burns are classified according to the depth of tissue injured. There are three types: first-degree, second-degree, and third-degree. See Figure 23-1.

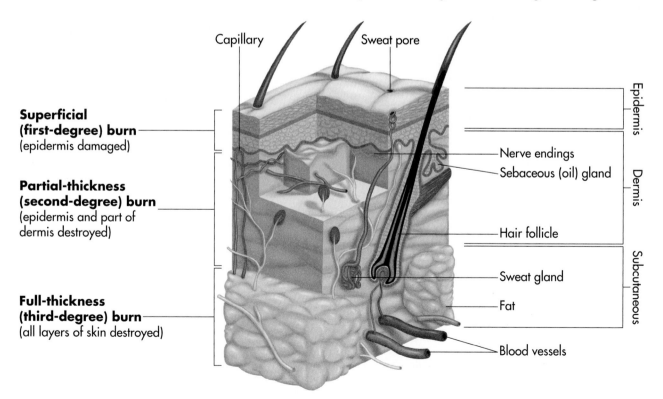

Superficial (first-degree) burn (epidermis damaged)

Partial-thickness (second-degree) burn (epidermis and part of dermis destroyed)

Full-thickness (third-degree) burn (all layers of skin destroyed)

Capillary

Sweat pore

Nerve endings

Sebaceous (oil) gland

Hair follicle

Sweat gland

Fat

Blood vessels

Epidermis

Dermis

Subcutaneous

Figure 23-1 *The depth of skin damage is one factor used to determine the severity of burns.*

Superficial (first-degree) burns: The most common type of burn. They cause pain and make the surrounding skin turn red. A superficial burn damages only the epidermis and causes edema. Sunburn is a common example of a superficial burn. To treat superficial burns, apply cold-water dressings to the burn, or immerse the affected area in cold water. Gently pat the area dry, and apply a dry, sterile dressing. Do not use greasy ointments, butter, or other substances.

Partial-thickness (second-degree) burns: These burns extend deeper into the skin than first-degree burns, damaging the epidermis and dermis. The injured area appears blistered, with redness and pain. The blisters should not be broken. They prevent infection of the burned area. They are usually very painful and heal within 3 to 4 weeks. To treat a partial-thickness burn, immerse the burned area in cold water until the pain subsides, pat the area dry, and apply a dry, sterile dressing. Do not apply antiseptic ointment unless the physician orders it.

Full-thickness (third-degree) burns: These burns involve all layers of skin and completely damage both the epidermis and the dermis, extending into the underlying connective tissues, such as fat, muscle, and even bone. A full-thickness burn is an emergency condition. Spontaneous healing is impossible. These burns require the removal of scars and the application of skin grafts. Victims of full-thickness burns may not feel any pain because of damage to the nerve endings in the skin. The most severe and major complication is infection. To treat a third-degree burn, call the EMS system. While waiting for the EMS team, do not remove charred or adhered clothing. Cover the burns and adhered clothing with thick, sterile dressings; keep the patient warm; and check to see whether the patient is suffering from smoke inhalation. If so, move the patient into a sitting position.

Estimating the extent of the burn: To calculate the amount of skin surface burned on an adult, use the rule of nines. Each of the following parts of the body is considered to be 9% of the body's surface: the head

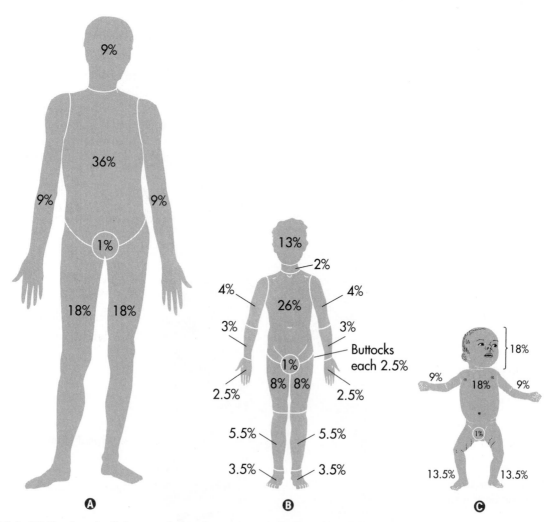

Figure 23-2 *(A) Use the rule of nines to calculate the percentage of body surface affected by burns in adults. Except for the genital region, percentage figures combine front and back surfaces. (B) In children, use the percentages based on the Lund and Browder chart. These numbers take into account that children's body proportions differ from those of adults. (C) In infants, the rule of nines is used. These numbers take into account an infant's properties.*

and neck, each upper limb, the chest, the abdomen, the upper back, the lower back and buttocks, the front of each lower limb, and the back of each lower limb. The remaining 1% is the genital area. See Figure 23-2, which also shows the percentages to use when making calculations in children.

Chemical burns: To treat a chemical burn, flood the area with large amounts of water, and cover it with a dry dressing. Call the EMS system.

Thermal burns: Caused by contact with hot liquids, steam, flames, radiation, excessive heat from fire, or hot objects. Call the EMS system. Use water to cool a burning substance, or use a wet cloth or blanket to put out a flame.

Electrical burns: Injuries from exposure to electrical currents, including lightning. These burns occur at the site where the electricity enters the body and where the current exits the body and enters the ground. Along the current's pathway, extensive tissue damage can occur from heat, followed by chemical changes to nerve, muscle, and heart tissue. Call the EMS team immediately for these types of injuries.

Sunburn: Causes redness, tenderness, pain, swelling, blisters, and peeling skin and can lead to skin damage or cancer. To treat sunburn, soak skin in cool water and apply cold compresses and calamine lotion. Have the patient elevate the legs and arms, drink plenty of water, and take a pain reliever.

Wounds

Wound: A physical injury in which the skin or tissues under the skin are damaged. There are two types of wounds: open and closed.

Open wounds: Include punctures, lacerations, abrasions, and incisions (See Figure 23-3).

Incision: A clean and smooth cut.

Laceration: A cut with jagged edges.

Treating incisions and lacerations: See Table 23-3 for the way to treat minor incisions and lacerations. For deeper wounds that involve muscle, tendons, the face, the genitals, the mouth, or the tongue, control the bleeding with direct pressure to the wound, elevation, and the use of pressure points; contact the physician or EMS system.

Abrasion: A scraping of the skin. Wash with soap and water, making sure to remove all dirt and debris. Use a bandage on a large abrasion. See Figure 23-4.

Puncture: A small hole created by a piercing object. Allow the wound to bleed freely for a few minutes, then clean it with soap and water and apply a dry, sterile dressing. A tetanus immunization may be required.

Closed wound: An injury that occurs inside the body without tearing the skin. Closed wounds are called contusions or bruises. They are caused by a sudden blow or force from a blunt object. Apply cold compresses to reduce swelling.

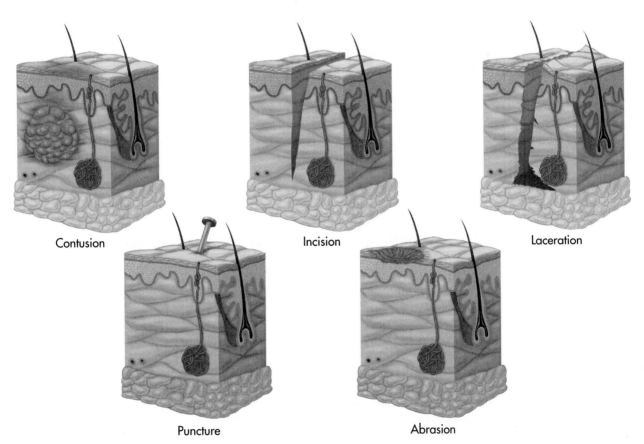

Contusion   Incision   Laceration

Puncture   Abrasion

Figure 23-3 *Different types of wounds produce different degrees of tissue damage.*

1. Wash your hands and put on examination gloves.
2. Dip several gauze squares in a basin of warm, soapy water.
3. Wash the wound from the center outward to avoid bringing contaminants from the surrounding skin into the wound. Use a new gauze square for each cleansing motion.
4. As you wash, remove debris that could cause infection.
5. Rinse the area thoroughly, preferably by placing the wound under warm, running water.
6. Pat the wound dry with sterile gauze squares.
7. Cover the wound with a dry, sterile dressing. Bandage the dressing in place.
8. Properly dispose of contaminated materials.
9. Remove the gloves and wash your hands.
10. Instruct the patient on wound care.
11. Record the procedure in the patient's chart.

Table 23-3

Bites and Stings

Animal bites: May range in severity from minor to serious. A wound that tears the skin should be seen by a physician and may need to be reported to the police, animal control office, and local health department. If the animal can be found, it should be checked for rabies.

Treating animal bites: If the bite is a puncture wound, try to make it bleed to flush out bacteria. Wash the area thoroughly with antiseptic soap and water. Apply an antibiotic ointment and a dry, sterile dressing. The physician will administer a tetanus shot if the patient has not had one for 7 to 10 years.

Rabies: A viral infection normally transmitted through the saliva of rabid animals. Dogs, cats, skunks, squirrels, raccoons, bats, and foxes are more likely to carry rabies than other animals. Prevention involves vaccinating house pets. Immunization of a person who has been exposed to rabies should be started as soon as possible, because treatment is ineffective once clinical symptoms develop. If left untreated, rabies can cause paralysis and death.

Insect sting: An annoyance to most patients, insect stings can be deadly to those who are allergic to the insect venom. The site of an insect sting can become red, swollen, itchy, and painful. To remove the stinger, scrape the skin with a flat, hard, sharp object, being careful not to release more venom. If you cannot remove the stinger, call the physician. Wash the skin with soap and water, apply ice to reduce pain and swelling, and apply a paste of baking soda or a dressing soaked in aloe vera or vinegar to reduce discomfort. Watch for signs of an anaphylactic reaction.

Snakebite: A wound resulting from penetration of the skin by the fangs of a snake. Not all snakebites are poisonous. Symptoms of a poisonous snakebite include puncture marks, pain, swelling, rapid pulse, nausea, vomiting, and possibly unconsciousness and seizures. Bites from snakes known to be nonvenomous are treated as puncture wounds. Bites from poisonous or unidentified snakes require immediate attention. Call a doctor or the EMS system. The bitten area should be immobilized and positioned below heart level, and the patient should not walk. Wash the bite area with soap and water. Do not apply a tourniquet or ice, and do not cut or suction the wound.

Spider bite: A puncture wound produced by the bite of venomous spiders, which in the United States include the black widow and the brown recluse. Symptoms include swelling, pain, nausea, vomiting, rigid abdomen, fever, rash, and difficulty breathing or swallowing. Any patient bitten by a spider should be seen by a doctor. Wash the area thoroughly with soap and water, apply an ice pack, and keep the area below heart level.

Scorpion stings: Of the different scorpion types in the American Southwest, some are more poisonous to young children. Antivenin may be available in some areas. Scorpion stings are treated similarly to spider bites.

Orthopedic Injuries

Strain: Overstretching of muscles or tendons caused by trauma. The neck, back, thigh, and calf are the most common sites for muscle injuries caused by excessive physical force. Strains do not usually cause the intense symptoms associated with fractures, dislocations, and sprains.

Sprain: An acute partial tear of a tendon, muscle, or ligament, characterized by pain and edema. The joints most commonly sprained are ankles, knees, wrists, and fingers. Treatment requires elevation, mild compression, and immediate application of ice. After 24 to 36 hours, application of mild heat is usually indicated. The patient should also rest the affected area.

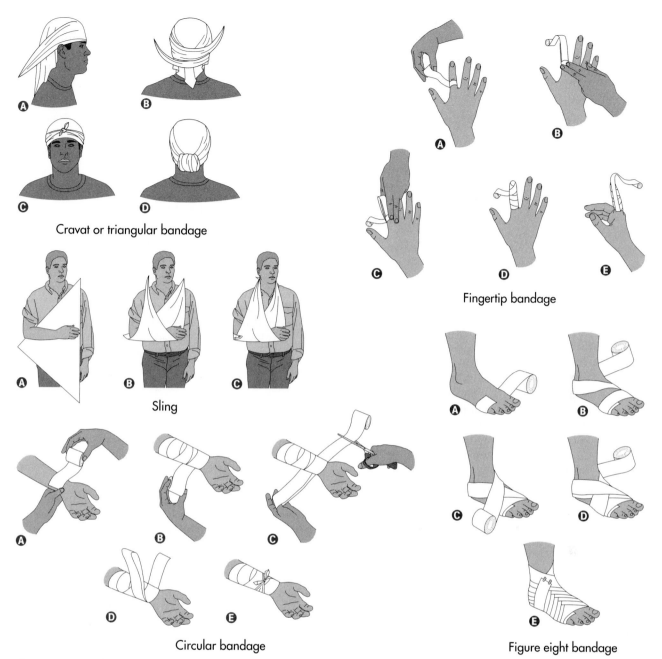

Figure 23-4 *Apply a bandage, as needed, to a wound.*

Dislocation: The displacement of a bone from its normal articulation with a joint. It is caused by a violent pulling or pushing force that tears the ligaments. Symptoms include deformity of the joint, pain, edema, and loss of function.

Fracture: A break in a bone. Review this section in Chapter 4, "Pathophysiology."

Treating fractures and dislocations: To reduce pain and continuing damage to soft tissue, immobilize the body area by the application of a splint or cast. In some cases, it is necessary to move the bone back into the proper position.

Splint: An orthopedic device for immobilization or support of any part of the body. It may be rigid (made

of metal, plaster, or wood) or flexible (made of leather, rolled newspapers, or magazines). The body part should be splinted in the position in which it was found. The splint should immobilize the area above and below the injury.

Cast: A rigid external dressing, usually made of plaster or fiberglass, that is molded to the contours of the body part. The basic elements of cast care, which should be communicated to the patient, are:

- Tell the physician about any pain, swelling, discoloration, lack of pulsation and warmth, or inability to move exposed parts.

- Keep the extremity elevated for the first day.

- Avoid allowing the affected limb to hang down for any length of time.
- Take care to avoid indenting the cast until it is dry.
- Restrict strenuous activity for the first few days.
- Do not put anything inside the cast.
- Keep the cast dry.

Head and Related Injuries

Head injury: Scalp hematoma, scalp laceration, concussion, contusion, fracture, and intracranial bleeding. Some head injuries can be life-threatening.

Scalp hematoma: A bump on the head caused by a buildup of blood under the skin. The swelling can be reduced by applying ice.

Scalp laceration: A wound that usually bleeds profusely. Direct pressure should be applied to stop the bleeding.

Concussion: A jarring injury to the brain, the most common type of head injury. Symptoms include loss of consciousness, temporary loss of vision, pallor, listlessness, memory loss, and vomiting. Symptoms may disappear rapidly or last up to 24 hours. The patient should refrain from strenuous activity and rest, then return to regular activity gradually. Unless the physician approves using other pain medications, only acetaminophen should be used. The patient should eat lightly, and a family member should check on the patient every few hours.

Severe head injuries: Contusions, fractures, and intracranial bleeding. Mortality in severe injury approaches 50% and is only slightly reduced by treatment. Symptoms are more profound than in concussions and also include leakage of clear or bloody fluid from the ears or nose, seizures, and respiratory arrest. The patient requires immediate hospitalization to treat such an injury. Maintain the patient's airway and begin rescue breathing or cardiopulmonary resuscitation (CPR) if needed.

Fainting: A brief loss of consciousness, also called syncope, that can result from a variety of causes. The most common direct cause of syncope is decreased cerebral blood flow. Before fainting, a patient may feel weak, dizzy, cold, or nauseated and may perspire or look pale and anxious. Have the patient lower his or her head between the legs and breathe deeply. Lay a patient who has fainted on his or her back with feet slightly elevated; loosen tight clothing, and apply a cold cloth to the face. Notify the physician.

Convulsions: May be caused by injury, trauma, fever, infection, hypocalcemia, hypoglycemia, or idiopathic factors. Convulsions, also called seizures, usually last only a few minutes. To treat convulsions, remove objects in the environment that may cause injury. Lay the patient on the floor on his or her side. Loosen restrictive clothing. Protect the patient from injury, but do not try to hold the patient still. If necessary, begin rescue breathing.

Cerebrovascular accident (CVA): An abnormal condition of the brain characterized by occlusion by an embolus, thrombus, or cerebrovascular hemorrhage. It is also known as stroke. Possible effects of stroke include paralysis, weakness, speech defects, aphasia, and death. Notify the physician and call the EMS system. Turn the patient's head toward the affected side to maintain the airway. Loosen tight clothing. If directed by the physician, monitor vital signs and administer oxygen.

Diabetic Emergencies

Diabetes: A fairly common disorder of carbohydrate metabolism, diabetes can cause hyperglycemia and hypoglycemia, both of which may become medical emergencies.

Hypoglycemia: A lower-than-normal level of glucose in the blood, usually caused by the administration of too much insulin, excessive secretion of insulin by the pancreas, or dietary deficiency. Symptoms of hypoglycemia include weakness, headache, hunger, ataxia, anxiety, and visual disturbances. Untreated hypoglycemia can result in delirium, coma, and death. The treatment is the administration of glucose in orange juice by mouth; if the patient is unconscious, an IV glucose solution must be started.

Insulin shock: Very severe hypoglycemia. The symptoms include weakness, tachycardia, cold skin, tremors, convulsions, restlessness, confusion, and fainting. The treatment is the administration of some form of sugar.

Hyperglycemia: A higher-than-normal level of blood glucose. Symptoms include dry mouth, intense thirst, muscle weakness, and blurred vision.

Diabetic coma: The end result of severe hyperglycemia. Symptoms are rapid breathing; flushed, warm, dry skin; thirst; acetone breath; and disorientation or confusion. If diabetic coma is suspected, a physician should be notified and the patient transported to a hospital.

Cardiovascular Emergencies

Shock

Shock: A life-threatening state associated with failure of the cardiovascular system. It prevents the vital organs from receiving blood and can bring all normal metabolic functions to a halt. Several types of shock are possible, such as hypovolemic, cardiogenic, neurogenic, septic, and anaphylactic.

Hypovolemic shock: Inadequate intravascular volume producing diminished ventricular filling and reduced stroke volume, which results in decreased cardiac output. It occurs after an injury that causes major fluid loss. Patients should be transported to an emergency facility immediately.

Cardiogenic shock: Results from reduction in cardiac output due to factors other than inadequate intravascular volume (e.g., cardiac tamponade, pulmonary embolism, myocardial infarction, myocarditis, drugs, tachycardia, and bradycardia).

Neurogenic shock: May occur following severe cerebral trauma or hemorrhage.

Septic shock: May be partly due to the effects of endotoxin or other chemical mediators on resistance vessels, resulting in vasodilation and decreased vascular resistance.

Anaphylactic shock: Occurs following allergic reactions. It is also called anaphylaxis.

Symptoms of shock: Restlessness; irritability; fear; rapid pulse; pale, cool skin; and increased respiratory rate.

Treating shock: Elevate the patient's feet 8 to 12 inches, unless there is head injury, in which case, keep the patient flat or elevate the head and shoulders. Monitor airways, breathing, and circulation, and control bleeding if necessary. Wrap the patient in a blanket, and call the EMS system.

Bleeding

Bleeding: The release of blood from the vascular system as a result of damage to a blood vessel. It is also called hemorrhaging and can be minor or very severe. A loss of 25% to 40% of a patient's total blood volume (approximately 2 to 4 pints of blood for the average adult) can be life-threatening and potentially fatal. There are two types of bleeding: external and internal.

Internal bleeding: Hemorrhaging from an internal organ or tissue, such as intraperitoneal bleeding into the peritoneal cavity, or intestinal bleeding into the bowel.

Hematemesis: The vomiting of bright red blood, indicating rapid upper GI bleeding. The most common causes are esophageal varices and peptic ulcer.

Hemoptysis: The coughing up of blood from the respiratory tract.

Controlling internal bleeding: Cover the patient with a blanket, keep the patient quiet and calm, and get medical help immediately.

External bleeding: Bleeding that can be seen outside the body, such as bleeding from wounds, open fractures, and nosebleeds (epistaxis). The type of blood vessel that has been injured determines the classification of external bleeding: arterial, venous, or capillary. The most common type of external bleeding is capillary bleeding. The most serious and least common type of external bleeding is arterial. The correct method of stopping a nosebleed includes: Have the victim sit and tilt head slightly forward with mouth open. Ask the victim to pinch the nostrils together just below the bridge of the nose for 10 minutes. Ask the victim to breathe through the mouth and not speak, swallow, cough, or sniff; then place a cold compress on the bridge of the nose.

Epistaxis (nosebleed): A common type of external bleeding usually caused by trauma, hypertension, exposure to high altitudes, or an upper respiratory infection.

Controlling external bleeding: If time permits, wash your hands and put on personal protective equipment. Apply direct pressure over the wound, using a clean or sterile dressing. Apply an additional dressing on top if blood soaks through. Elevate the body part that is bleeding. If bleeding does not stop, apply pressure over the nearest pressure point between the bleeding and the heart. See Figure 23-5.

Heart Attack

Chest pain: A physical complaint that requires immediate diagnosis and evaluation. Chest pain may be indicative of cardiac disease, such as myocardial infarction, angina pectoris, or pericarditis; of respiratory disorders, such as pleurisy, pneumonia, or pulmonary embolism; or of nonmyocardial infarction. Another source of chest pain can be cocaine use.

Myocardial infarction (MI): Ischemic myocardial necrosis of a portion of the cardiac muscle caused by obstruction in a coronary artery. It is also known as a heart attack. In more than 90% of patients with acute MI, an acute thrombus, often associated with plaque rupture, occludes the coronary artery. Chest pain is the major symptom of a heart attack. The pain may radiate down the left arm or into the jaw, throat, or both shoulders, and it may be accompanied by shortness of breath, sweating, nausea, and vomiting. When symptoms start, notify the physician and EMS system immediately, and do not let the patient walk. Loosen tight clothing, and have the patient sit up. The physician may direct you to administer oxygen. If cardiac arrest occurs, start CPR immediately.

Cardiac arrest: The sudden cessation of cardiac output and effective circulation, usually followed by ventricular fibrillation or ventricular asystole. It is also called cardiac standstill. Immediate initiation of CPR is required to prevent heart, lung, kidney, and brain damage.

Chain of Survival: The term *Chain of Survival* provides useful information for emergency cardiovascular care (ECC). The ECC systems concept summarizes the present understanding of the best approach to the treatment of persons with sudden cardiac arrest. The four links in the adult *Chain of Survival* are:

- Early access
- Early CPR
- Early defibrillation
- Early advanced care

Cardiopulmonary resuscitation (CPR): In collapsed or unconscious persons, the state of ventilation and circulation must be determined immediately. Speed, efficiency, and proper application of CPR directly affect success. Tissue anoxia for more than 4 to 6 minutes

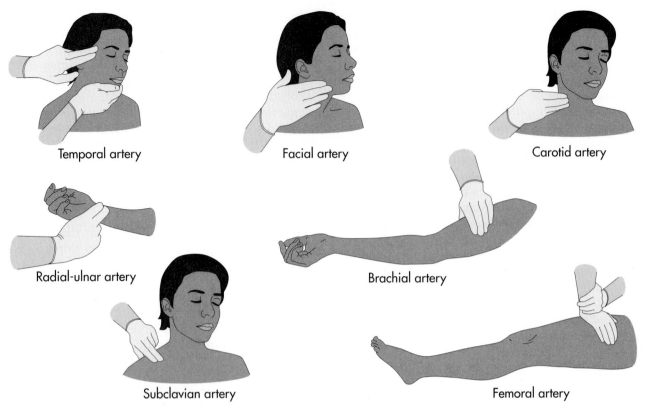

Figure 23-5 *Apply pressure on these pressure points to stop bleeding.*

Temporal artery

Facial artery

Carotid artery

Radial-ulnar artery

Brachial artery

Subclavian artery

Femoral artery

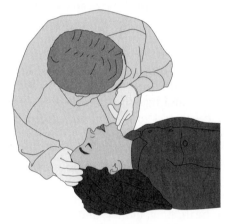

Figure 23-6 *Use the head tilt–chin lift maneuver to open an airway.*

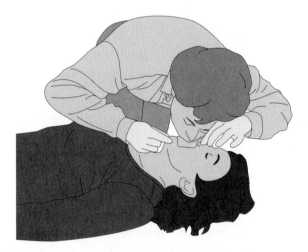

Figure 23-8 *Perform mouth-to-mouth rescue breathing.*

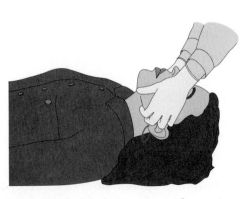

Figure 23-7 *Use the jaw thrust maneuver for a patient with a neck injury.*

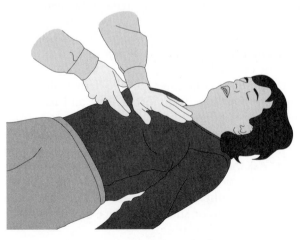

Figure 23-9 *Place your hands at the xiphoid process.*

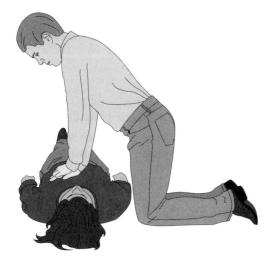

Figure 23-10 *Align your shoulders directly over the victim's sternum, with your elbows locked.*

can result in irreversible brain damage or death. After establishing unresponsiveness of the victim, call for help, note the exact time of arrest, and position the victim horizontally on a hard surface. Do a primary survey by assessing the patient's ABCs: *a*irway, *b*reathing, and *c*irculation. CPR involves three basic components: opening the airway, rescue breathing, and chest compressions. See Figures 23-6 through 23-10. Table 23-4 gives a step-by-step procedure for performing CPR. Table 23-5 gives a summary of steps of CPR for adults, children, and infants. CPR must be continued until the cardiopulmonary system is stabilized, the patient is pronounced dead, or resuscitation cannot be continued (because of rescuer exhaustion). Resuscitation efforts can be divided into basic life support (BLS), which is carried out with techniques and equipment that are immediately available, and advanced cardiac life support (ACLS), which involves drug therapy, cardiac monitoring, and other specialized techniques and equipment.

Defibrillator: A device that delivers an electrical shock at a preset voltage to the myocardium through the chest wall. It is used for restoring the normal cardiac rhythm and rate when the heart has stopped beating or is fibrillating. The office defibrillator is portable and is powered by standard 110V current or batteries.

Modifications to CPR for children: Although the steps for giving CPR to an adult and child are similar, there are a few differences:

- Amount of air for breaths
- Possible need to try more than twice to deliver two breaths that make the chest rise
- Depth of compressions
- Possible use of one-handed chest compressions for very small children
- When to attach an AED
- When to activate the emergency response system.

Note: The American Heart Association (in 2006) has recommended that cycles of compressions and ventilations for adults, children, and infants include the 30:2 ratio.

Respiratory Emergencies

Choking: A condition in which the respiratory passage is blocked by an obstruction, usually food in the trachea. If the victim is coughing forcefully, do nothing but observe. If the victim is conscious but cannot speak, breathe, or cough, use the Heimlich maneuver. Give upward subdiaphragmatic abdominal thrusts until the foreign body is expelled. See Figure 23-11. If the victim loses consciousness, lay the person down slowly on his or her back. Check the mouth for a foreign body, and sweep it out with your fingers if possible. Continue to administer upward abdominal thrusts, with the heel of one hand between the xiphoid process and the navel and the second hand on top of the first, until the foreign body is expelled. If the person is still not breathing independently when the airway is clear, perform CPR. The objectives of emergency treatment are (1) removal of the obstruction and (2) resuscitation if necessary.

Respiratory arrest: Lack of breathing, usually preceded by symptoms of respiratory distress. If a patient shows such symptoms, notify the physician immediately. If the patient develops respiratory arrest, call the physician and the EMS system, and perform CPR.

Asthma: A respiratory disorder characterized by (1) airway constriction that is reversible, either spontaneously or with treatment; (2) airway inflammation; and (3) increased airway sensitivity to a variety of stimuli. If a patient has an asthma attack, notify the physician. If the patient has a respiratory inhaler, help the patient use it.

Hyperventilation: Breathing too rapidly and too deeply, which can cause patients to feel light-headed and as if they cannot get enough air. Move the patient to a quiet area, and have the patient breathe into a paper bag that is held tightly around the nose and mouth. Encourage the patient to take slow, normal breaths.

Poisoning

Poison: A substance that impedes biological functions when taken into the body. The majority of accidental poisonings occur at home in children under the age of 5 years. A poison may enter the body by ingestion, absorption, injection, or inhalation. Clinically, poisons are divided into those that respond to specific antidotes or treatment and those for which there is no specific treatment.

Symptoms of ingested poisons: Abdominal pain; cramping; nausea; vomiting; diarrhea; odor, stains,

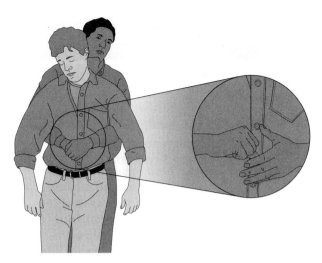

Figure 23-11 *Perform abdominal thrusts on a conscious choking victim.*

Treating absorbed poisons: Call a poison control center. Have the patient remove all contaminated clothing. Wash infected skin thoroughly with soap and water, drench it with alcohol, and rinse well. Apply wet compresses soaked in calamine lotion and suggest a bath in colloidal oatmeal or the application of a paste of baking soda and water to soothe the itching.

Symptoms of inhaled poisons: Headache, tinnitus, angina, shortness of breath, muscle weakness, nausea, vomiting, confusion, dizziness, blurred or double vision, unconsciousness, and cardiac arrest. Carbon monoxide is the most commonly inhaled poison.

Treating inhaled poisons: Get the patient into fresh air. Call the EMS system or a poison control center. Loosen tight-fitting clothing, and wrap the patient in a blanket to prevent shock.

Digestive Emergencies

Abdominal pain: Although many diseases can produce abdominal pain, acute and severe pain nearly always is a symptom of intra-abdominal abnormality (pathology). It may be the most important indication that an emergency operation or treatment is needed, such as for appendicitis, perforated peptic ulcer, intestinal obstruction, general peritonitis, twisted ovarian cyst, or ectopic pregnancy.

Treating abdominal pain: Call for transport, and have the patient lie on the back with the knees flexed. Keep the patient warm and quiet. Do not apply heat. Monitor the patient's pulse and consciousness, and check for signs of shock.

Vomiting: A common symptom of many disorders that can lead to dehydration and electrolyte imbalances. Notify the physician, and use a basin to collect the vomit. Place a cool compress on the patient's forehead, and offer water and a towel to clean the mouth.

Acute diarrhea: Can cause dehydration and electrolyte imbalances and can lead to shock. The patient should lie on his or her back and elevate the legs. The physician may direct you to assist in administering IV fluids.

Melena: Abnormal black, tarry stool that has a distinctive odor and contains digested blood. It usually results from bleeding in the upper GI tract. In adults, it is often a sign of peptic ulcer or small bowel disease.

Reproductive System Emergencies

Vaginal bleeding: If a patient experiences gushing vaginal bleeding, call the EMS system, and have her lie down with her feet elevated.

Emergency childbirth: If a physician is not present, the medical assistant should summon help and begin the procedure. Ask the woman how far apart her contractions are, whether her water has broken, and whether she feels straining or pressure as if the baby is coming. Always explain to the woman what you are doing and reassure her. Do a visual examination of the vagina to see whether there is crowning (a bulging caused by the baby's head). If the head is crowning, childbirth is imminent. Place clean cloths under the woman, and use sterile sheets or towels (if available) to cover her legs and stomach. Wash your hands thoroughly, and put on examination gloves if possible. If a physician is available, position yourself at the woman's head and provide emotional support and help if she vomits. If no physician is available, position yourself at the woman's side so that you can see the vaginal opening. Place one hand below the baby's head as it is delivered. Never pull on the baby. If the umbilical cord is wrapped around the baby's neck, gently loosen it and slide it over the head. If the amniotic sac has not broken, use your finger to puncture the membrane and pull the membranes as well as blood and mucus away from the baby's mouth and nose. After the feet are delivered, lay the baby on his or her side, with the head slightly lower than the body. Keep the baby at the same level as the mother until you cut the umbilical cord. The infant must be breathing independently before you clamp and cut the cord. Wait several minutes until the pulsation of the umbilical cord stops, then use clamps or pieces of string to close off the cord in two places: 6 and 12 inches from the baby. Cut the cord between the two clamps with sterilized scissors. Within 10 minutes of birth, expulsion of the placenta will begin. Keep it in a plastic bag for further examination. Keep the mother and baby warm by wrapping them in towels and blankets. Massage the mother's abdomen just below the navel every few minutes to control internal bleeding.

Bioterrorism

Bioterrorism: The intentional release of a biological agent with the intent to harm individuals. The CDC defines a biological agent as a weapon when it is easy to disseminate, has a high potential for mortality, can cause a public panic or social disruption, and requires public health preparedness. There are numerous biological agents identified as weapons, including anthrax, tularemia, smallpox, plague, and botulism. The CDC maintains an Internet site with current information about identified biological agents at www.bt.cdc.gov.

Physicians' offices will be on the front lines should a biological agent be intentionally released. It will be up to physicians and their staff to sound the alarm to public officials that something may be amiss. Be on the lookout for unusual patterns in affected patients. If you suspect bioterrorism is responsible for an illness, report this to the physician. It is the responsibility of your facility to immediately contact the local public health department. The following is a list of clues of a bioterroristic attack as defined by the American College of Physicians—American Society of Internal Medicine:

- Unusual temporal or geographical clustering of illness
- Unusual age distribution of common disease, such as an illness that appears to be chickenpox in adults but is really smallpox
- A large epidemic, with greater caseloads than expected, especially in a discrete population
- More severe disease than expected
- Unusual route of exposure

- A disease that is outside its normal transmission season or is impossible to transmit naturally in the absence of its normal vector
- Multiple simultaneous epidemics of different diseases
- A disease outbreak with health consequences to humans and animals
- Unusual strains or variants of organisms or antimicrobial resistance patterns

STRATEGIES TO SUCCESS

▶ Test-Taking Skills

Survey the test!

Before you begin answering questions, glance at the exam. Find out how long it is exactly. How many questions are there in each section? Are you missing any pages? Take note of how long you have to complete the exam. Quickly figure out the halfway time and the halfway question number. This information will help you to pace yourself. So on each exam, you actually have less than a minute to answer each question. Make sure that as you are taking the exam, you keep track of your progress. If you fall behind, don't panic. Try to answer questions more quickly, and don't skip questions without answering them. Make educated guesses and move on. Come back to these questions if you finish early.

Instructions:

Answer the following questions. Check your answers in the *Answer Key* that follows this section.

1. What percentage of the body is involved in a burn that covers one arm and the head of an adult?
   A. 1%
   B. 9%
   C. 18%
   D. 36%
   E. 40%

2. The Good Samaritan law explicitly allows medical assistants
   A. To administer first aid within the scope of their competence
   B. To call the EMS system and stay with the victim until EMS personnel arrive
   C. To act freely in an emergency situation to save the victim's life
   D. To diagnose the patient at the scene of an accident or emergency
   E. Only to call the EMS system and wait for authorized personnel but not to touch or communicate with an accident victim

3. In emergency childbirth, at what point should the umbilical cord be tied and cut?
   A. When the infant is fully out
   B. Within 10 minutes of birth
   C. When the infant starts breathing
   D. When the mother and baby get to the hospital
   E. When the baby is ready to nurse

4. To treat frostbite, a medical assistant can
   A. Massage the affected area gently
   B. Rub the affected area with a warmed towel
   C. Keep the patient's head and shoulders slightly elevated
   D. Wash the area with soap and water
   E. Place warm clothing and blankets around the affected area

5. Which of the following are symptoms of heatstroke?
   A. The body tingles, and the patient feels pain
   B. There is a white, waxy, or grayish yellow build-up on the skin, and the patient has a high body temperature
   C. The skin feels moist and hot, and the patient feels dizzy, with a possibly altered mental state
   D. The pulse is rapid, the skin is hot and dry, and the patient feels weak
   E. The patient has a strange metallic taste in his or her mouth and feels hot

6. When treating a second-degree burn, a medical assistant should
   A. Break blisters to relieve the patient's pain
   B. Immerse the burned area in cold water
   C. Remove charred or adhered clothing
   D. Apply medical ointments to the affected area
   E. Apply a wet, sterile dressing

7. When Bill Williams scraped his skin, he most likely got a(n)
   A. Incision
   B. Laceration
   C. Abrasion
   D. Puncture
   E. Bruise

8. Irreversible brain damage can be caused by tissue anoxia lasting
   A. More than 2 minutes
   B. More than 3 minutes
   C. More than 6 minutes
   D. More than 45 minutes
   E. More than 3 hours

9. Which of the following is a correct way to treat a snakebite?
   A. Administer activated charcoal
   B. Walk the patient to a hospital
   C. Suction the wound and apply ice
   D. Immobilize the bitten area and wash it with soap and water
   E. Cut out the affected area

10. If a patient is bleeding from the lower arm and direct pressure and elevation do not stop the bleeding, where should pressure be applied?
    A. Radial-ulnar artery
    B. Brachial artery
    C. Subclavian artery
    D. Carotid artery
    E. Phrenic artery

11. One possible cause of stroke is
    A. Occlusion in the brain by a thrombus
    B. Decreased cerebral blood flow
    C. Ingested poisons
    D. Hypocalcemia
    E. Hyperthermia

12. White, waxy, or grayish yellow skin that also feels crusty and softness in tissue beneath the skin could indicate
    A. Heatstroke
    B. Frostbite
    C. Contusion
    D. Hypothermia
    E. Shock

13. Which of the following is a possible treatment of syncope?
    A. Having the patient lower his or her head between the legs
    B. Laying the patient flat on the patient's back with the feet slightly elevated
    C. Loosening tight clothing and applying a cold cloth to the patient's face
    D. Both B and C
    E. All of the above

14. The Heimlich maneuver is used for which of the following?
    A. Convulsion
    B. Epistaxis
    C. Hematemesis
    D. Shock
    E. Choking

15. Anaphylactic shock occurs following
    A. Hemorrhage
    B. Allergic reaction
    C. Toxemia of pregnancy
    D. Cardiac arrest
    E. None of the above

16. Which of the following should not be done by a patient with a concussion?
    A. Eat
    B. Take aspirin
    C. Take acetaminophen
    D. Rest
    E. Gradually resume normal activities

17. The most severe and major complication for burn victims is
    A. Pain
    B. Anemia
    C. Infection
    D. Malignant fever
    E. Both B and C

18. Which of the following should not be done when a patient complains of abdominal pain?
    A. Have the patient lie on the back
    B. Apply heat to the patient's abdomen
    C. Have the patient flex the knees
    D. Monitor the patient's pulse
    E. Check for signs of shock

19. Closed wounds are called
    A. Bruises or contusions
    B. Lacerations
    C. Abrasions
    D. Scrapes
    E. None of the above

20. When administering CPR, how many compressions should you do?
    A. 15 in 1 minute
    B. 20 in 1 minute
    C. 25 in 2 minutes
    D. 60 in 1 minute
    E. 30 in 2 minutes

21. According to Good Samaritan laws,

    A. Emergency care is required of all medical personnel in all situations
    B. Emergency care is permitted only with the verbal consent of the patient
    C. Emergency care is permitted when it is within the scope of competence of the person
    D. Possible negligence is never a factor in providing emergency care
    E. Both B and D

22. Chest pain might indicate

    A. Cocaine use
    B. Myocardial infarction
    C. Epistaxis
    D. Both B and C
    E. Both A and B

23. When you suspect neck injury, what action should you take to open the patient's airway before administering rescue breathing?

    A. Place your mouth over the patient's nose and blow air into it until the patient's chest rises
    B. Put your fingers behind the jawbone just below the ear and push the jaw forward
    C. Wait for EMS personnel, and do not administer rescue breathing
    D. Hold the patient's neck rigidly while you lift the patient's chin up and push back on the forehead
    E. Open an airway in the patient's neck with a sterile instrument

24. Treat hypoglycemia by

    A. Administering glucose
    B. Giving the patient plain orange juice
    C. Loosening the patient's restrictive clothing and elevating the patient's head
    D. Administering immunization as soon as possible
    E. None of the above

25. What is the best location to check the pulse of a 48-year-old male who is unconscious and not breathing?

    A. At the radial artery of the wrist
    B. At the brachial artery of the arm
    C. At the carotid artery of the neck
    D. On the chest, directly over the heart
    E. At the temples of the head

26. An adult is in sudden cardiac arrest. Which of the following gives the victim the best chance of survival?

    A. CPR performed by EMS personnel immediately upon arrival at the victim's side
    B. Immediate CPR and defibrillation within no more than 3 to 5 minutes
    C. Defibrillation in 10 minutes with or without CPR
    D. Immediate CPR with defibrillation in 10 minutes
    E. Injection of adrenaline followed by CPR

27. Which of the following describes the best way to deliver rescue breaths with a pocket mask, but without additional oxygen?

    A. Reduce the volume and duration of breaths from the volume and duration you would provide with mouth-to-mouth ventilation
    B. Provide approximately the same volume as you would with mouth-to-mouth ventilation (with a volume sufficient to make the chest rise), and deliver the breaths over 2 seconds
    C. Increase your air volume and duration of breaths
    D. Give 3 breaths between series of compressions
    E. Give 10 breaths between series of compressions

28. You are babysitting your infant nephew. You are alone and find the infant unresponsive. Which of the following is the best action?

    A. Check for signs of circulation, and if there are none, phone 911
    B. Phone 911 immediately to ensure that advanced life support is on the way, and then return to the infant to begin the ABCs of CPR
    C. Give 2 rescue breaths; if there is no response to the rescue breaths, then phone 911
    D. Begin the ABCs of CPR and then phone 911 after 1 minute of rescue support
    E. Check for signs of circulation, give 2 rescue breaths, then phone 911

29. A 26-year-old woman has swallowed an overdose of prescribed sleeping pills. She is now unresponsive. When you open her airway, you find that she is gasping for breath and is not breathing normally at all. Using a pocket mask, you provide 2 rescue breaths and check for signs of circulation, including her pulse, which is rapid but weak. What should you do next?

    A. Provide rescue breathing at a rate of one breath every 5 seconds
    B. Begin chest compressions because her pulse is weak
    C. Place the victim in the recovery position
    D. Perform CPR for 1 minute with chest compressions only
    E. Give two more rescue breaths, place the victim in the recovery position, then perform CPR for 2 minutes

30. Which of the following statements best describes the problems that are most commonly present in children or infants whose condition deteriorates to cardiac arrest?

    A. Most cardiac arrests in children are sudden and are caused by an inherited form of heart disease
    B. Most cardiac arrests in children are preceded by severe airway and breathing problems, or shock

    C. Most cardiac arrests in infants and children are caused by electric shock from appliances
    D. Most cardiac arrests in infants and children are caused by severe head injuries
    E. Most cardiac arrests in children develop very slowly over time, usually due to toxins in the environment

31. You are providing rescue breathing to an unresponsive, nonbreathing child who shows signs of circulation. How often should you provide rescue breaths for this child?

    A. Once every 3 seconds (20 breaths per minute)
    B. Once every 4 seconds (15 breaths per minute)
    C. Once every 5 seconds (12 breaths per minute)
    D. Once every 10 seconds (6 breaths per minute)
    E. Once every 12 seconds (5 breaths per minute)

32. You are alone, providing CPR for a 3-year-old child. Which of the following describes the correct technique you should follow in performing chest compressions on this child?

    A. Use both hands, one on top of the other
    B. Use the heel of one hand
    C. Use the tips of two fingers
    D. Use the palm and fingers of one hand
    E. Use the tips of three fingers

33. Which of the following is the correct ratio of compressions to ventilations for child or infant CPR?

    A. 10 to 2
    B. 12 to 2
    C. 5 to 1
    D. 15 to 2
    E. 10 to 1

MEDICAL ASSISTING COMPETENCIES (concl.)

COMPETENCY	CMA	RMA
Clinical		
Obtain specimens for microbiological testing, including throat specimens and wound cultures	X	X
Instruct patients in the collection of a clean-catch midstream urine specimen	X	X
Instruct patients in the collection of fecal specimens	X	X
Perform electrocardiography	X	X
Perform respiratory testing	X	X
Perform selected CLIA-waived tests (i.e., "kit tests")	X	X
Perform urinalysis	X	X
Perform hematological testing	X	X
Perform chemistry testing	X	X
Perform immunology testing	X	X
Perform microbiology testing	X	X
Screen and follow up on patient test results	X	X
General/Legal/Professional		
Identify and respond to issues of confidentiality by maintaining confidentiality at all times and following appropriate guidelines when releasing records or information	X	X
Be aware of and perform within legal and ethical boundaries	X	X
Determine the needs for documentation and reporting, and document accurately and appropriately	X	X
Demonstrate knowledge of and monitor current federal and state health-care legislation and regulations; maintain licenses and accreditation	X	X
Perform risk management procedures		X
Explain general office policies and procedures	X	X
Instruct individuals according to their needs	X	X
Perform quality control procedures	X	X
Conduct work within scope of education, training, and ability		X
Understand allied health professions and credentialing		X

Collecting and Testing Blood

Medical assistant's role: Depending on the laws of the state in which you live, you may collect and process blood specimens, conduct blood tests, and complete necessary paperwork.

Hematology

Hematology: The study of blood and blood-forming tissues.
Functions of blood: To distribute oxygen, nutrients, and hormones to body cells; to eliminate waste products from body cells; to attack infecting organisms or pathogens; to maintain the body's acid-base balance; and to regulate body temperature.
Hematopoiesis: The normal formation and development of blood cells in the bone marrow.
Whole blood: Consists of plasma and the formed elements. In adults, total blood volume normally makes up 7% to 8% of body weight, or 70 mL/kg of body weight in men and about 65 mL/kg in women. Blood is pumped through the body at a speed of about 30 cm per second, with complete circulation in 20 seconds.
Plasma: The liquid in which the other components of blood are suspended. Plasma accounts for 55% of the body's total blood volume. Water makes up about 90% of plasma. About 9% is protein and 1% is other substances, including carbohydrates, fats, gases, mineral salts, protective substances, and waste products. Free of its formed elements and particles, plasma is a clear, yellow fluid. When a tube of blood is centrifuged, the plasma rises to the top.
Formed elements, or **blood cells:** Red cells (erythrocytes), white cells (leukocytes), and platelets (thrombocytes). Blood cells constitute about 45% of the body's total volume of blood. An older term for a formed element is blood corpuscle. See Figure 24-1.
Blood gas: Dissolved gas in the liquid part of the blood. Blood gases include oxygen, carbon dioxide, and nitrogen.
Bone marrow: Found in the cavities of all bones. It may be present in two forms: red and yellow. Yellow marrow is inactive and is composed mostly of fat tissue. Red marrow is active in the production of most types of

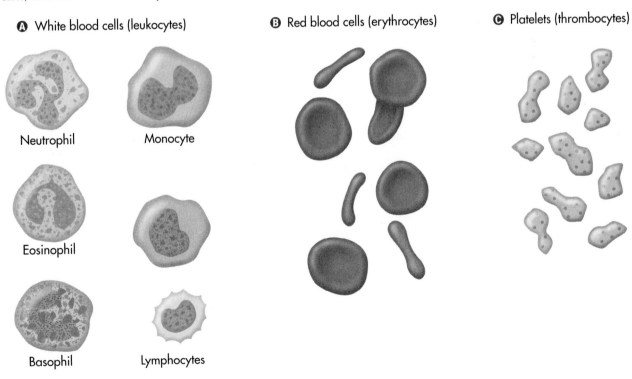

Ⓐ White blood cells (leukocytes)   Ⓑ Red blood cells (erythrocytes)   Ⓒ Platelets (thrombocytes)

Neutrophil   Monocyte

Eosinophil

Basophil   Lymphocytes

Granular   **Nongranular**

Figure 24-1 *The formed elements of the blood are (A) white blood cells, (B) red blood cells, and (C) platelets.*

blood cells. By age 18, red marrow is found only in the vertebrae, ribs, sternum, skull bones, and pelvis.

Erythrocytes

Erythrocyte: Also known as a red blood cell (RBC). A mature RBC is made up of lipids and proteins to which hemoglobin molecules are attached. RBCs play a vital role in internal respiration, the exchange of gases between blood and body cells. They are disk shaped and have concave sides.

Erythropoiesis: The process of erythrocyte production. This process develops in the embryonic yolk sac, liver, and spleen. It is ultimately located in the red bone marrow during late fetal development, childhood, and adult life.

Erythropoietin: A glycoprotein hormone, produced primarily by the kidneys and also secreted by the liver, that stimulates erythropoiesis. It can cross the placental barrier.

Reticulocyte: The last stage of the immature erythrocyte. This cell has a nucleus and is found in both the bone marrow and, often, in peripheral blood.

Transferrin: A specific transport protein in the blood. It binds iron and transports it back to the bone marrow for hemoglobin synthesis.

Hemoglobin: The iron-containing pigment of RBCs that carries oxygen from the lungs to the tissues.

Hemagglutination: The coagulation of erythrocytes.

Hemagglutinin: A type of antibody that agglutinates erythrocytes.

Rouleaux formation: A configuration of RBCs having the appearance of stacked coins.

Leukocytes

Leukocyte: Also known as a white blood cell (WBC). Through phagocytosis, it protects the body against infection. Leukocytes are divided into two groups: granular and nongranular.

Granular leukocytes: Basophils, eosinophils, and neutrophils.

Basophils: Produce histamine, which plays a major role in allergic reactions.

Eosinophils: Capture invading bacteria and antigen-antibody complexes through phagocytosis.

Neutrophils: Attack invaders (specifically target bacteria) and release pyrogens, which cause fever.

Nongranular leukocytes: Lymphocytes and monocytes.

Lymphocytes: The smallest leukocytes, which contain the largest nuclei. They include B cells and T cells. B lymphocytes produce antibodies to combat specific pathogens. T lymphocytes regulate the immune response.

Monocytes: Large leukocytes in the bloodstream with oval or horseshoe-shaped nuclei. Their major functions are phagocytosis and synthesis of various biological compounds, including transferrin, complement, interferon, and certain growth factors.

Macrophages: Monocytes that mature outside the circulatory system, distributed in tissues throughout the body. They have a variety of names (often depending on their location in the body), such as histiocytes, Kupffer cells, osteoclasts, and microglial cells.

Phagocytes: Cells that have the capacity for phagocytosis. Macrophages, as well as most of the leukocytes, are phagocytes. Large phagocytes can destroy worn-out RBCs or bacteria. They are found in the spleen, thymus, and lymphoid tissues.

Phagocytosis: The process by which cells engulf and ingest microorganisms.

Thrombocytes

Platelets: Metabolically active anuclear cell fragments produced in the bone marrow that assist in blood coagulation and clotting. They are also called thrombocytes. Normally, between 130,000 and 400,000 platelets are found in 1 cubic milliliter of blood.

Megakaryocytes: Precursors of platelets. They are the largest cells found in the bone marrow, and they have a nucleus with many lobes. They are normally not present in circulating blood.

Serology and Immunology

Serology: The study of blood serum based on antigen-antibody reactions in vitro.

Serum: The liquid portion of blood that remains after the clotting proteins and cells have been removed. It differs from plasma in that it does not contain fibrinogen, a protein involved in clotting.

Antigen: A substance on cells whose presence in the body stimulates the body's immune response. Antigens produced by the body itself are autoantigens; antigens on other cells are foreign antigens.

Antibody: A protein produced in response to a specific antigen. It defends the body against infection.

Serology abbreviations: Common abbreviations are listed in Table 24-1.

Agglutination: An antigen-antibody reaction in which a solid antigen clumps together with a soluble antibody.

Agglutinin: An antibody that interacts with antigens, resulting in agglutination.

Agglutinogen: Any antigenic substance that causes agglutination.

Opsonization: A process by which antibodies or complements render bacteria more susceptible to phagocytosis by leukocytes. It is also called opsonification.

Immunology: The study of the reaction of immune system tissues to antigenic stimulation.

Immune: Protected by antibodies against infective or allergic disease.

Immune response: A defense function of the body that produces antibodies to destroy invading antigens and cancer cells.

Ab	antibody	Baso	basophil
ABO	classification system for four blood groups	BCA	breast cancer antigen
AcAc	acetoacetate	BJP	Bence Jones protein
ACE	angiotensin-converting enzyme	BT	bleeding time
ACT	activated coagulation time	BUN	blood urea nitrogen
ACTH	adrenocorticotropic hormone	Ca; Ca^{++}	calcium
ADH	antidiuretic hormone	CA	cancer antigen
AFB	acid-fast bacillus	CBC	complete blood (cell) count
AFP	alpha-fetoprotein	CEA	carcinoembryonic antigen
Ag	antigen	CHE	cholinesterase
AG	anion gap	CK	creatine kinase
A/G R	albumin-globulin ratio	CMV	cytomegalovirus
AHF	antihemolytic factor	$CN-$	cyanide anion
Alb	albumin	CO	carbon monoxide
Alc	alcohol	CO_2	carbon dioxide
ALG	antilymphocyte globulin	COHb	carboxyhemoglobin
ALP; alk phos	alkaline phosphatase	Cr	creatinine
ALT	alanine aminotransferase	CrCl	creatinine clearance
ANA	antinuclear antibody	CT	calcitonin
APAP	acetaminophen	DAF	decay accelerating factor
APTT	activated partial thromboplastin time	DHEA	dehydroepiandrosterone, unconjugated
ASA	acetylsalicylic acid (aspirin)	Diff	differential (blood cell count)
AST	aspartate aminotransferase	EBNA	Epstein-Barr virus nuclear antigen
AT-III	antithrombin III	EBV	Epstein-Barr virus
B	blood (whole blood)	EDTA	ethylenediaminetetraacetic acid

Table 24-1

Eos	eosinophil	HDL	high-density lipoprotein
EP	electrophoresis	HDV	hepatitis delta virus
Eq	equivalent	HGH; hGH	human growth hormone
ERP	estrogen receptor protein	HIV	human immunodeficiency virus
ESR	erythrocyte sedimentation rate	HLA	human leukocyte antigen
FBS	fasting blood sugar	HPV	human papilloma virus
FFA	free fatty acids	HSV	herpes simplex virus
FSH	follicle-stimulating hormone (follitropin)	HTLV	human T-cell lymphotrophic virus
FT_4	free thyroxine	Ig	immunoglobulin
FT_4I	free thyroxine index	IgE	immunoglobulin E
GFR	glomerular filtration rate	INH	inhibitor
GH	growth hormone	IV	intravenous
GHRH	growth hormone–releasing hormone	L	liver
GnRH	gonadotropin-releasing hormone	LD; LDH	lactate dehydrogenase
GTT	glucose tolerance test	LDL	low-density lipoprotein
HA	hemagglutination	LH	luteinizing hormone
HAI	hemagglutination inhibition test	LMWH	low-molecular-weight heparin
HAV	hepatitis A virus	Lytes	electrolytes
Hb; Hgb	hemoglobin	MCV	mean cell volume
HbCO	carboxyhemoglobin	MetHb	methemoglobin
HBV	hepatitis B virus	MLC	mixed lymphocyte culture
HCG; hCG	human chorionic gonadotropin	MONO	monocyte
Hct	hematocrit	MPV	mean platelet volume
HCV	hepatitis C virus	MSAFP	maternal serum alpha-fetoprotein

Table 24-1, continued

NE	norepinephrine	RCM	red cell mass
NPN	nonprotein nitrogen	RCV	red cell volume
OGTT	oral glucose tolerance test	RDW	red cell distribution of width
P	plasma	Retic	reticulocyte
PAP	prostatic acid phosphatase	RF	rheumatoid factor; relative fluorescence unit
PB	protein binding	Rh	rhesus factor
PBG	porphobilinogen	RIA	radioimmunoassay
PCT	prothrombin consumption time	rT_3	reverse triiodothyronine
PCV	packed cell volume (hematocrit)	S	serum
P_i	inorganic phosphate	Segs	segmented polymorphonuclear leukocyte
PKU	phenylketonuria	SPE	serum protein electrophoresis
PLT	platelet	T_3	triiodothyronine
PMN	polymorphonuclear (leukocyte; neutrophil)	T_4	thyroxine
PRL	prolactin	TBG	thyroxine-binding globulin
PSA	prostate-specific antigen	TBV	total blood volume
PT	prothrombin time	TG	triglyceride
PTH	parathyroid hormone	TRH	thyrotropin-releasing hormone
PTT	partial thromboplastin time	TSH	thyroid-stimulating hormone
PV	plasma volume	VDRL	Venereal Disease Research Laboratory (test for syphilis)
PZP	pregnancy zone protein	VLDL	very-low-density lipoprotein
RAIU	thyroid uptake of radioactive iodine	WB	Western blot
RBC	red blood cell; red blood (cell) count	WBC	white blood cell; white blood (cell) count
RBP	retinol-binding protein		

Table 24-1, concluded

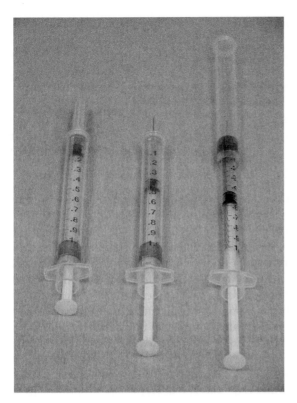

Figure 24-4 *Devices such as the Saf-T Clik needle shield help prevent needle injuries.*

engineered safety devices have been developed. These devices are intended to reduce the possibility of needle-stick injuries (Figure 24-4). According to the National Institute for Occupational Safety and Health (NIOSH), the desired characteristics of engineered safety devices include the following:

- The performance of the device is reliable.
- The device is easy to use, safe, and effective.
- The device should be needleless when possible.
- The device should either not have to be activated by the user or may be activated with only one hand.
- Once the safety feature is activated, it cannot be deactivated.

In certain circumstances, some of these characteristics are not feasible. Drawing blood from an artery or a vein is not possible without the use of a needle. Several types of safety devices for collecting blood specimens have been developed. These include:

- Retracting needles
- Shields that are hinged or sliding that cover phlebotomy needles and winged-steel (butterfly) needles
- Self-blunting phlebotomy and winged-steel needles
- Retractable lancets

In addition to the use of appropriate safety-engineered devices, NIOSH also recommends that health-care workers follow these precautions:

- Recap needles only when absolutely necessary.
- Ensure the safe handling and disposal of sharps before beginning a procedure.
- Dispose of used sharps promptly, using approved sharps containers.
- Report all needlestick injuries.
- Inform their employer of workplace hazards.
- Attend yearly blood-borne pathogen training.
- Follow recommended infection control practices.

Evacuation tube: The most common evacuation system is the Vacutainer® system (manufactured by Becton Dickinson Vacutainer® Systems). It uses a special needle, a needle holder/adapter, and collection tubes that have been sealed to maintain a slight vacuum. See Figure 24-5. Some tubes are prepared with additives needed to process the blood sample for testing, such as anticoagulants. The tube stoppers are color-coded according to the type of additive used. See Table 24-2. Expired tubes may no longer have a vacuum.

Collection tubes: No matter which method is used to collect blood, the samples must immediately be mixed

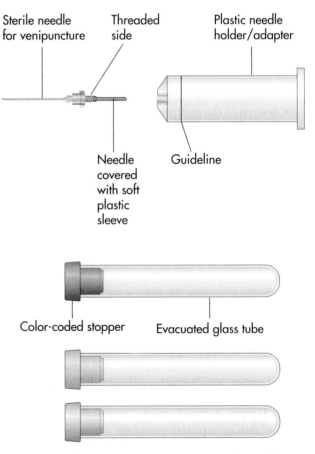

Figure 24-5 *The Vacutainer® system uses interchangeable collection tubes that allow you to draw several blood specimens from the same venipuncture site.*

Color	Additive	Test Types
Yellow	Sodium polyanetholesulfonate	Plasma cultures
Light blue	Sodium citrate (anticoagulant)	Coagulation studies
Red	None	Blood chemistries, AIDS, antibody tests, viral studies, serological tests, blood grouping and typing
Red/black (tiger stripes or marbled)	Silicone serum separator	Tests requiring blood serum
Green	Sodium heparin (anticoagulant)	Electrolyte studies, arterial blood gas tests
Lavender	EDTA (anticoagulant)	Hematology studies, such as complete blood count, WBC differential, and platelet count
Gray	Potassium oxalate or sodium fluoride (anticoagulant)	Blood glucose tests

Table 24-2

with the appropriate additives in the correct collection tubes before they are transported to the laboratory for testing. Each laboratory may choose which tubes to use for a particular test.

Anticoagulants: Substances that prevent blood clotting. Three anticoagulants commonly used in the hematology laboratory are heparin, sodium citrate, and ethylenediaminetetraacetic acid (EDTA).

Heparin: A substance produced naturally by basophils and mast cells. Heparin acts in the body as an antithrombin factor to prevent intravascular clotting. As an additive in blood collection, heparin is used in electrolyte studies and tests for arterial blood gasses. Heparin is also used as an anticoagulant in the prevention and treatment of thrombosis and embolism.

Sodium citrate: A white granular powder, used as an anticoagulant in transfusions and coagulation studies.

EDTA: Used as an anticoagulant additive in hematology studies. It is also used to treat exposure to toxic chemicals; it chemically "grasps" toxic substances, thereby making them nonactive. Excessive EDTA produces a shrinkage of the erythrocytes.

Antiseptic: A substance that inhibits the growth and reproduction of microorganisms. Some examples of antiseptics are 70% isopropyl alcohol, povidone-iodine (Betadine®), and benzalkonium chloride (Zephiran®).

Betadine®: An antiseptic recommended for use in arterial blood gas studies and blood culture draws.

Zephiran®: A trade name for benzalkonium chloride, used in blood collection to detect alcohol levels.

Labeling containers: After blood is drawn, all tubes, slides, and other containers should be labeled with the patient's name, the date and time of collection, the initials of the person who collected the specimen, and any other required information, such as the patient's identification code.

Tube size: Tubes range in size from 15 mL down. Most tubes used for adults range from 3 to 10 mL, and those for children range from 2 to 4 mL. Microcapillary collection tubes hold less than 1 mL.

Order of draw tubes: The National Committee for Clinical Laboratory Standards publishes the recommended order of draw as follow: yellow, light blue, red, red/black (tiger stripes), green, lavender, and gray.

Tourniquet: A device used to control hemorrhage or to distend veins for the withdrawal of blood. A tourniquet increases resistance in the venous blood flow. It should not remain on the patient's arm longer than 1 minute. Tourniquets are available in many materials. They are placed on the upper arm of the patient, 3 to 4 inches above the elbow.

Gloves: Made from a variety of materials, such as vinyl, latex, and nitrile. Latex gloves are the most commonly used, but some individuals are highly allergic to latex. Nitrile gloves are more tear-resistant and feel more comfortable on the hand.

Needle disposal: Needles must be properly disposed of in appropriate biohazard containers. They should not be laid down or placed on any surface and should not be recapped.

Procedures

Assembling equipment and supplies: After reviewing the test order, make sure that you have the appropriate equipment to collect the required samples.

Preparing patients: After greeting the patient, ask for the patient's full name to verify that the patient is the one listed on the order. Confirm that the patient has followed any pretest restrictions, such as fasting before the appointment.

Universal Precautions: It is important to follow Universal Precautions during all phlebotomy procedures. Before collecting blood, make sure to wash your hands and put on examination gloves. When you have finished drawing blood, properly dispose of used supplies and disposable instruments, disinfect the area, remove the gloves, and wash your hands.

Steps in venipuncture or phlebotomy: The following steps describe how to perform venipuncture using the evacuation method:

1. Prepare the needle holder/adapter assembly, and push the collection tube into the open end of the needle holder/adapter. Do not puncture the stopper yet. You usually use a 19–23 gauge needle for venipuncture.

2. Ask the patient which arm he or she prefers you to use, and make sure that the arm is positioned slightly downward.

3. Apply tourniquet to the patient's upper arm.

4. Palpate the site, using your index finger to locate the vein.

5. Clean area with a cotton ball moistened with antiseptic or an antiseptic wipe. Use a circular motion to clean the area, starting at the center and working outward. Let site dry.

6. Remove cap from outer point of the needle.

7. Ask the patient to make a fist.

8. Hold the patient's skin taut above and below the insertion site. Holding the needle at approximately a 15-degree angle, use a steady and quick motion to insert the needle into the vein to a depth of $\frac{1}{4}$ to $\frac{1}{2}$ inch.

9. Seat the collection tube firmly into place over the needle, puncturing the stopper.

10. Once blood is flowing steadily, ask the patient to release the fist, and untie the tourniquet. Switch tubes as needed, using a smooth and steady motion. Fill each tube until the blood stops running. An evacuation tube containing an additive must be filled completely. The last tube must be removed before removing the needle, or bruising will occur.

11. As you withdraw the needle in a smooth and steady motion, place a sterile gauze square over the insertion site. Have the patient hold the gauze in place and keep the arm straight and slightly elevated.

12. If the collection tubes contain additives, invert them slowly several times to mix the chemical with the blood.

13. Check the patient's condition and the puncture site for bleeding, and replace the gauze square with a sterile adhesive bandage.

Steps in capillary puncture: The following steps are taken in capillary puncture using the finger stick method:

1. Examine the patient's hand to determine which finger to use for the procedure. If necessary, warm the hands to improve circulation. Keep the hand below heart level.

2. Prepare the finger by gently rubbing it, and clean the area with a cotton ball and antiseptic or an antiseptic wipe.

3. Hold the patient's finger between the thumb and forefinger of one hand.

4. Hold the lancet at a right angle to the pad of the patient's finger (the part that leaves a fingerprint).

5. Puncture the skin with a quick, sharp motion.

6. Allow a drop of blood to form. If it is slow in forming, apply steady pressure, but do not milk the finger.

7. Wipe away the first droplet of blood.

8. Fill the collection devices.

9. When the samples have been collected, wipe the patient's finger with a sterile gauze square.

10. Check the site for bleeding. If necessary, apply a sterile adhesive bandage.

Chain of custody: A means of ensuring that a specimen obtained from a patient is correctly identified, is under the uninterrupted control of authorized personnel, and has not been altered or replaced. It is established for blood samples drawn for drug and alcohol analysis as well as for specimens taken in cases of medicolegal importance such as rape. Because donating a specimen for drug and alcohol testing is potentially self-incriminating, the patient must sign a consent form for the testing.

Handling an exposure incident: Following Universal Precautions should reduce your risk of exposure, but accidents sometimes still happen. If you suffer a needle stick or other injury that results in exposure to blood or blood products from another person, report the incident to the appropriate staff members immediately. Wash the injured area carefully, and apply a sterile bandage. Record the time, date, and nature of the incident and the names of the people involved. You may have to undergo further blood testing and to receive medications depending on the type of incident. OSHA requires every employer to have an established procedure for handling exposure incidents.

Complications of Blood Collection

Syncope: Fainting, usually caused by pain, fright, and the sight of blood. Syncope lasts only 1 to 2 minutes. If fainting occurs, the procedure must be terminated immediately. The patient should be placed lying down, with legs elevated. The event should be completely documented on the laboratory log. Assistance should be called for, and the patient should never be left alone.

Failure to obtain blood: There are several factors that may make blood collection impossible. It is important to remain calm and to determine the cause of the problem. If you cannot collect a good sample on the second try, do not make a third attempt. Ask for assistance.

Scarred and sclerosed veins: Do not draw blood from injured or diseased areas.

Hematoma: A pooling of blood just under the skin. It is caused by blood leaking into the tissues. When

it happens, pressure should be applied to the area for 3 minutes, and then ice should be applied.

Hemorrhage: Excessive bleeding.

Petechiae: Tiny red spots appearing on the skin as a result of small hemorrhages within the dermal layer. They may be a complication of keeping a tourniquet in place for longer than 2 minutes.

Testing Blood

Hematology

Hematological tests: May be performed on venous or capillary whole blood specimens. These tests include blood cell count, morphological studies, coagulation tests, and the erythrocyte sedimentation rate test. See Table 24-3 for normal ranges of selected blood tests.

Erythrocyte sedimentation rate (ESR, or sed rate) test: Measures the rate at which RBCs settle out in a tube of unclotted blood, expressed in millimeters per hour. The test determines the degree of inflammation

AT A GLANCE	Normal Ranges for Selected Blood Tests	
Test	**Blood Component**	**Normal Range**
Red blood cells	Whole blood	Men: $4.3–5.7 \times 10^6$ cells/μL Women: $3.8–5.1 \times 10^6$ cells/μL
White blood cells	Whole blood	$4.5–11.0 \times 10^3$ cells/μL
Platelets	Whole blood	$150–400 \times 10^3$ cells/μL
Hematocrit (Hct)	Whole blood	Men: 39%–49% Women: 35%–45%
Hemoglobin (Hb, Hgb)	Whole blood	Men: 13.2–17.3g/dL Women: 11.7–16.0 g/dL
Bleeding time	Whole blood	2–7 minutes
Cholesterol, total	Serum, plasma	Men: 158–277 mg/dL Women: 162–285 mg/dL
Glucose (fasting blood sugar [FBS])	Serum	74–120 mg/dL
Insulin	Serum	<17 μU/mL
Iron, total	Serum	Men: 65–175 μg/dL Women: 50–170 μg/dL
Uric acid	Serum	Men: 4.4–7.6 mg/dL Women: 2.3–6.6 mg/dL

Table 24-3

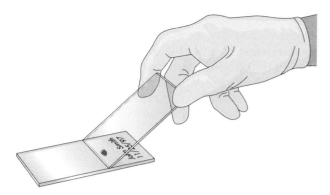

Figure 24-6 *Hold the spreader slide at a 30- to 35-degree angle. Pull the spreader slide toward the frosted end until it touches the drop of blood.*

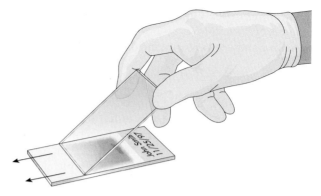

Figure 24-7 *When the drop covers most of the spreader slide edge, push the spreader slide back toward the unfrosted end of the smear slide.*

in the body. There are several testing systems available, and it is important to adhere to the manufacturer's instructions in using each test. Results are sensitive to temperature and freshness of the samples, precise position of the sample tube, and vibrations. The normal rate at which RBCs fall is 1 mm every five minutes. Elevated sedimentation rates are not specific for any disorder but indicate the presence of inflammation. Certain noninflammatory conditions, such as pregnancy, are also characterized by high sedimentation rates.

Bleeding time test: Gives information about the integrity of the patient's platelet function. A prolonged bleeding time indicates such conditions as low platelet count and dysfunction of the platelets. Aspirin impairs the platelets' ability to form aggregates. Antihistamines also interfere with bleeding time.

Blood smears: Used to obtain a differential cell count and to reveal abnormal RBC morphology for anemia. To prepare a blood smear slide, apply a drop of blood to the slide, $\frac{1}{4}$ inch from the frosted end, and use a

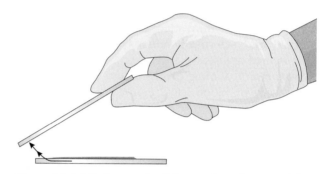

Figure 24-8 *Lift the spreader slide away from the smear slide, maintaining a 30- to 35-degree angle. The smear should be thicker on the frosted end of the slide.*

spreader slide at a 30- to 35-degree angle to spread the blood droplet. See Figures 24-6, 24-7, and 24-8.

Stains: Used to selectively color microscopic objects and tissues for study. Some common stains are listed in Table 24-4.

AT A GLANCE	Common Stains
Stain	**Use**
Acidic	To stain basic elements of cells
Basic	To stain the nucleic or acidic elements of cells
Contrast	To color one part of a tissue or cell
Differential (e.g., Gram's stain)	To differentiate among various types of bacteria
Giemsa's	To stain tissues that include blood cells, Negri bodies, and chromosomes
Wright's	To stain blood smears

Table 24-4

Morphological studies: Used in the examination of a blood smear for the purpose of recording the appearance and shape of cells, with special note made of abnormal cell size, shape, or content and abnormal organization of cells.

Coagulation tests: Used to identify bleeding problems, generally scheduled before surgery or to monitor therapeutic drug levels.

Hemoglobin (Hgb or Hb) tests: Used to measure the concentration of hemoglobin in the blood. Hb testing can be performed on either venous or capillary whole blood specimens. Among the types of hemoglobin are hemoglobin A, hemoglobin F, and hemoglobin S. Hemoglobin level is high at birth but declines during childhood. It then increases at different ages.

Hemoglobin A: Normal adult hemoglobin.

Hemoglobin F (HbF): Fetal hemoglobin, the normal hemoglobin of the fetus and the predominant hemoglobin variety in the fetus and neonate. Most HbF is replaced by hemoglobin A in the first days after birth.

Hemoglobin S: Sickle-shaped hemoglobin, found in sickle cell anemia and also in sickle cell trait. It is found exclusively in persons of African descent. About 8% of African Americans in the United States are affected.

Blood count: The complete blood count (CBC) is the most common laboratory procedure ordered on blood. It includes the red blood count (RBC), white blood count (WBC), differential WBC, and platelet count, as well as a hematocrit determination and a hemoglobin determination.

Hematocrit (Hct): The relative volume of RBCs in a blood sample after the sample has been spun in a centrifuge (packed cell volume), expressed as a percentage. The erythrocytes collect at the bottom of the tube. Above the packed erythrocytes is a layer of leukocytes and thrombocytes. This layer is called the buffy coat. Above the buffy coat is the plasma, which is free of cell elements.

Serology

Serological tests: Used to detect the presence of specific substances in blood serum (e.g., disease antibodies, drugs, hormones, and vitamins) and to determine blood types. See Table 24-5.

AT A GLANCE	**Common Laboratory Blood Tests**	
Substance Identified or Quantified	**Blood Component Tested**	**Indication, Disease, or Disorder**
ABO antigens and Rh factor (indicated by clumping reactions that occur when the blood specimen is mixed with serum containing different antibodies)	Whole blood	Possible transfusion or transplant reaction; hemolytic disease of the newborn
Acetone	Serum, plasma	Diabetic conditions or fasting metabolic ketoacidosis
Antistreptolysin O (ASO) antibodies	Serum	Streptococcal infection (which may indicate rheumatic fever, glomerulonephritis, bacterial endocarditis, or scarlet fever)
Bilirubin	Serum	Liver disease, fructose intolerance, or hypothyroidism
Blood urea nitrogen (BUN)	Serum, plasma	Indicates kidney disorders
Cancer antigens and tumor-associated glycoprotein	Serum	Cancer of a specific type depending on the antigen found
Cholesterol	Serum, plasma	Hyperlipoproteinemia, coronary artery disease, or atherosclerosis

Table 24-5

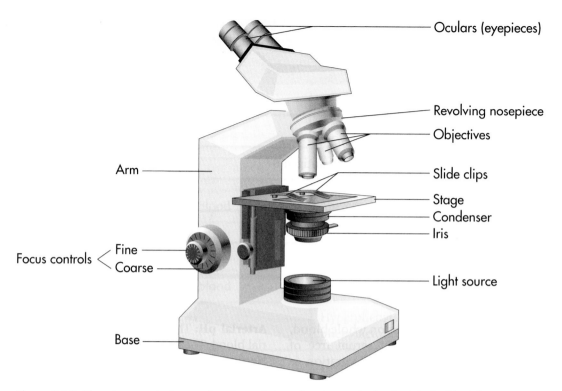

Figure 24-9 *The microscope is the most heavily used piece of equipment in the physician's office laboratory.*

11. Switch to the oil-immersion objective, and examine the specimen. Figure 24-10 shows the pattern to follow for counting leukocytes under the oil-immersion objective.

Oil-immersion objective: The objectives of a microscope contain magnifying lenses that increase the magnification of the oculars by another 10× to 40×. The oil immersion objective is designed to be lowered into a drop of immersion oil placed directly over the prepared specimen under examination. This design eliminates the air space between the microscope slide and the objective, thereby reducing the loss of light and creating images that are sharper and brighter.

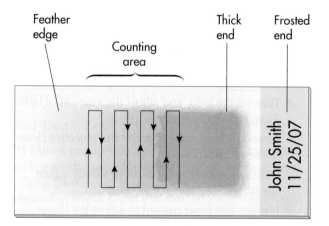

Figure 24-10 *Follow this pattern when counting leukocytes visible in the field under the oil-immersion objective of the microscope.*

Centrifuge: A laboratory machine used to separate particles of different densities within a liquid by spinning them at very high speeds.

Hemocytometer: A special microscope slide used primarily for counting blood cells that can also be used for counting platelets, sperm, and other cells. The most commonly used hemocytometer is the Neubauer type.

Conditions Identified by Blood Testing

Hyperglycemia: A higher-than-normal blood glucose level. The most common cause of hyperglycemia is diabetes mellitus. Other conditions that can cause hyperglycemia are hyperthyroidism, Cushing's syndrome, acromegaly, obesity, severe liver or kidney damage, alcoholism, and elevated levels of the hormones estrogen, epinephrine, or norepinephrine.

Hypoglycemia: Abnormally low levels of glucose in the blood, below 50 mg/dL. The most common cause of hypoglycemia is insulin overdose in patients with unstable insulin-dependent diabetes mellitus.

Hemophilia: A hereditary disorder of clotting factors, in which blood fails to coagulate at a wound site.

Hyperlipidemia: A higher-than-normal level of lipids, especially cholesterol, in the blood.

Visual indications: Hyperlipidemia gives plasma or serum a milky, or turbid, appearance. Sometimes the plasma or serum will have a pale, watery appearance as a result of protein disorders or kidney disease. In certain types of cancers, the color of the serum may be green, attributable to heme (part of hemoglobin).

Extramedullary hematopoiesis: In abnormal circumstances, the spleen, liver, and lymph nodes revert back to producing immature blood cells. This reversion can be the result of aplastic anemia, infiltration by malignant cells, leukemia, or hemolytic anemias.

Anemia: A reduction in the number of circulating RBCs per cubic millimeter. Hemoglobin content is less than that required to provide the oxygen needed by the body.

Abnormal erythrocytes: Vary from the norm in terms of size, shape, and color. Normal mature erythrocytes are biconcave and disc-shaped and lack a nucleus.

Anisocytosis: An abnormal condition characterized by excessive inequality in the size of erythrocytes.

Macrocyte: An abnormally large erythrocyte.

Megalocyte: An erythrocyte that is larger than average.

Microcyte: An abnormally small erythrocyte.

Poikilocytosis: Variation in the shapes of erythrocytes.

Schistocyte or **schizocyte:** An erythrocyte that has been fragmented during circulation.

Ovalocyte: An erythrocyte that is oval in shape. It is also called an elliptocyte.

Spherocyte: An erythrocyte that is spheroid in shape, having a decreased ratio of surface area to volume.

Target cell: An abnormally thin RBC with a dark center and a surrounding ring of hemoglobin. Also called leptocytes, target cells occur in anemia and jaundice.

Sickle cell: An erythrocyte that is sickle- or crescent-shaped. Such cells are produced by the polymerization of hemoglobin and occur in hereditary anemias.

Hypochromia: A condition in which cells have decreased hemoglobin.

Polycythemia: An above-normal concentration of erythrocytes in the circulating blood. It is also called erythrocytosis.

Polycythemia vera: A blood dyscrasia (disease) characterized by abnormally increased levels of erythrocytes, leukocytes, and thrombocytes. It is also called erythremia.

Neutropenia: A severe decrease in the number of neutrophilic granulocytes in the peripheral blood.

Neutrophilia: A significant increase in the number of neutrophilic granulocytes in the peripheral blood.

Leukocytosis: An increase in the number of leukocytes in the blood, generally caused by infection and usually transient.

Leukemia: A neoplastic, proliferative disease characterized by an overproduction of immature or mature cells of various leukocyte types in the bone marrow or peripheral blood.

Lymphoma: A solid, malignant tumor of the lymph nodes and associated tissue or bone marrow.

Infectious mononucleosis (IM): An acute, infectious disease commonly called mono or the kissing disease, in which there is an abnormally high number of mononuclear leukocytes in the blood. Most cases are caused by the Epstein-Barr virus. The most common serological test is the rapid slide test.

Hemolytic disease of the newborn: A neonatal disease generally caused by Rh incompatibility between mother and child, occurring when an Rh− woman carries an Rh+ fetus. Symptoms are anemia, jaundice, liver and spleen enlargement, and generalized edema. It can be controlled during pregnancy but may require intrauterine transfusion or early induced labor.

Bloodletting: The therapeutic opening of an artery or vein to withdraw blood from a particular area. Also called therapeutic phlebotomy, it is sometimes performed to treat polycythemia or congestive heart failure. One pint is collected and discarded.

Blood lavage: The removal of toxic elements from the blood by the injection of serum into the veins.

Collecting and Testing Urine

Role of the medical assistant: To help collect, process, and test urine specimens. These activities involve dealing with potentially infectious body waste, so following Universal Precautions is generally required.

Physical and Chemical Composition and Function

Urinary system or tract: Consists of two kidneys, two ureters, a bladder, and a urethra. The kidneys remove excess water from the body and waste products from the blood in the form of urine, which then drains through the ureters into the urinary bladder. The bladder stores urine until it leaves the body through the urethra.

Nephron: The basic unit of the kidney. See Figure 24-11. Each kidney contains approximately one million nephrons. Nephrons filter blood to produce urine. One of the main functions of the nephron is to remove waste material from the body. It also allows reabsorption of water and some electrolytes back into the blood.

Urinary meatus: The external opening of the urethra.

Chemical composition of urine: Approximately 95% water and 5% waste materials and other components, which include urea, ammonia, uric acid, creatinine, urobilinogen, and a few WBCs & RBCs. The presence of a few sperm cells in the urine of males is normal.

Urea: The end product of protein metabolism after ammonia is broken down by the liver.

Urochrome: The yellow pigment that gives urine its color. It is produced by the breakdown of hemoglobin.

Urination: The act of passing urine. It is also called micturition.

Urgency: An immediate need to urinate.

Urinary retention: The inability to empty the bladder.

Urinary frequency: Increased frequency can often be a symptom of a urinary tract infection, but there may also be other causes.

Incontinence: The inability to prevent release of urine. Some causes include an overfilling of the

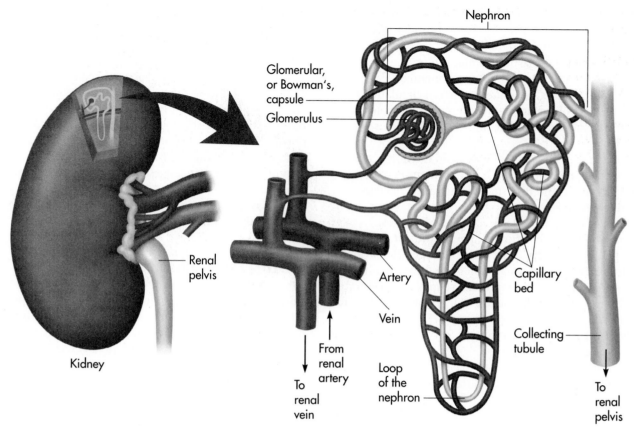

Figure 24-11 *Urine is formed in the nephron, a long tubular structure, during a complex filtering process.*

bladder and stress caused by laughing, sneezing, coughing, or lifting.

Enuresis: The involuntary discharge of urine after the age at which bladder control is normally established.

Nocturnal enuresis: Urinary incontinence during the night, also called bedwetting, which can be a symptom of a neurological disorder.

Dysuria: Painful or difficult urination, symptomatic of cystitis, infection, and many other conditions.

Polyuria: Increased output of urine.

Uropathy: Any disease or abnormal condition of any structure of the urinary tract.

Obtaining Specimens

Urine collection: Urine tests require between 30 and 50 mL of the specimen. When it is collected, it must be properly labeled with the patient's name, the date, and the time. Urine tests for females should be avoided during menstruation. Any medication taken by the patient must be recorded on the laboratory requisition and the patient's chart.

Home collection: Instruct patients on how to obtain the specimen. Tell them to urinate into an appropriate container, one that has a wide opening, and not to add anything else to the container. However, if you provide a container that contains preservative, caution them not to throw out the preservative. Instruct

them to refrigerate the container and to keep the lid on it.

Random specimen: A single urine specimen taken at any time. A random specimen is the most common type of sample. If collection is done in a doctor's office, provide a urine specimen container, show the patient to the restroom, and ask the patient to void a few ounces of urine into the specimen container and leave it on the sink. Transport the specimen to the laboratory immediately, or refrigerate the specimen.

Clean-catch midstream specimen: A method of urine collection that may be ordered to diagnose urinary tract infections or to evaluate the effectiveness of drug therapy. The purpose of this type of collection is to obtain a urine specimen that is free from contamination. Patients completing this procedure independently need written instructions on how to make sure that the container and the urine specimen remain uncontaminated. When assisting patients, use antiseptic towelettes to clean the perineal area or the penis. Make sure that you rinse away any soap residue that might affect the pH of the specimen.

Timed specimen: Collected over a predetermined time period to obtain more specific information. Such specimens are sometimes collected 2 hours after a meal to test for diabetes. The patient should discard the first specimen and then collect all urine for the specified time, making sure that the urine does not mix with stool or toilet paper. The sample should be kept refrigerated until it is brought to the doctor's office or laboratory.

24-hour specimen: Collected to measure the amount of urine output in a 24-hour period. The urine will be tested for substances that are released sporadically into the urine. It is extremely important to avoid using a bedpan, urinal, or toilet tissue, which could retain the substances for which the test is being done. The first specimen should be discarded. Over the next 24 hours, the patient should urinate directly into the small collection container and then pour the urine into the large container. Between two collections, the small container must be sanitized with soap and warm water. This type of collection is helpful in diagnosing renal disease, dehydration, urinary tract obstructions, and pheochromocytoma.

First-voided morning specimen: Collected after a night's sleep. It contains greater concentrations of substances that collect over time than do specimens taken during the day. A urine specimen container or clean, dry jar is used. It is best for pregnancy testing, microscopic examination, and culturing.

Catheterization: Insertion of a sterile plastic tube into the bladder, ureter, or kidney to withdraw urine. It is used to obtain a sterile urine specimen from a patient, to obtain a specimen from a patient who cannot void naturally, or to measure the amount of residual urine in the bladder after normal voiding, among other reasons. Catheterization is not routinely used because it can introduce infection. In some states, the medical assistant may not perform catheterization.

Drainage catheter: Used to withdraw fluids.

Splinting catheter: Used after plastic repair of a ureter.

Urinalysis

Urinalysis: The examination of urine to obtain information about body health and disease, done as part of a general physical examination or for a specific reason. The testing may be physical, chemical, or microscopic. Table 24-7 lists abbreviations common to urine analysis and testing, and Table 24-8 lists normal values for tests done on urine.

Physical testing of urine: Provides information about color, volume, odor, and specific gravity.

Color: Normal urine ranges from pale yellow to dark amber, depending on food and fluid intake, medications and vitamin supplements, and waste products present in the urine.

Clarity: Urine can be clear, or it can range from slightly cloudy to very cloudy. Cloudiness is also known as turbidity and sometimes indicates an abnormal condition. Causes of urine color and cloudiness are listed in Table 24-9.

Urine volume: Normal adult urine output is 600–1800 mL per 24-hour period, with an average of 1250 mL per 24 hours.

Oliguria: Decreased output of urine, often resulting from dehydration, decreased fluid intake, shock, or renal disease.

Anuria: The complete suppression of urine formation by the kidney. It may be a result of renal or urethral obstruction or renal failure.

Urine odor: Can provide clues about the body's condition. Diseases, the presence of bacteria, and certain foods can change the odor.

Urine specific gravity: A measure of the amount or concentration of a substance dissolved in urine. It is calculated by dividing the weight of the sample by the weight of an equal amount of distilled water. The specific gravity of normal urine ranges from 1.005 to 1.030. The specific gravity of urine is lower in cases of chronic kidney disease, diabetes insipidus, overhydration, and systemic lupus.

Measuring specific gravity: Three methods are used to measure specific gravity: urinometer, refractometer, and reagent strip (dipstick).

Urinometer: A sealed glass float with a calibrated scale on the stem that measures specific gravity. At least 15 mL of urine is required. See Figure 24-12.

Refractometer: An optical device that measures the refraction of light as it passes through a liquid. The degree of refraction is proportional to the amount of dissolved material in the liquid. It is faster and easier to use than the urinometer and requires only a drop of urine. It must be calibrated daily. See Figure 24-13.

Reagent strips, or **dipsticks:** Plastic strips to which one or more pads containing chemicals are attached. The pads react to substances in the urine and change color; a chart enables you to interpret the color changes. They are available for many tests: specific gravity, pH, protein, glucose, ketones, leukocytes, erythrocytes, nitrite, bilirubin, urobilinogen, and phenylketones.

Chemical testing of urine specimens: Usually performed with reagent strips. These tests can measure liver or kidney function, metabolism of carbohydrates, acid-base balance, and urinary pH. They also show the presence of drugs or infections, ketone bodies, blood, hemoglobin, myoglobin, bilirubin, urobilinogen, glucose, protein, nitrite, phenylketones, and leukocytes.

Using reagent strips: It is important to follow the directions of the manufacturer. Keep strips in tightly closed containers in a cool, dry area, and do not remove them until immediately before testing. Never use expired strips. A dipstick may be used only once.

Urinary pH: A measure of the acidity or alkalinity (hydrogen ion concentration) of urine. The normal pH of urine is 4.5 to 8.0.

Proteinuria: The presence of protein, such as albumin, in the urine. Protein is not normally found in the urine. Its presence may signal renal disease, heart failure, hypertension, or fever, or it may be the result of heavy exercise.

ADH	antidiuretic hormone	pH	hydrogen ion concentration
BIL; bili; BR	bilirubin	PKD	polycystic kidney disease
BJP	Bence Jones proteins	PKU	phenylketonuria
Ca	calcium	RBCs	red blood cells
CC	clean catch (urine)	SPG; sp gr; sp.gr.	specific gravity
CCMS	clean catch, midstream (urine)	U/A	urinalysis
CL VOID	clean voided specimen (urine)	UBG	urobilinogen
CrCl	creatinine clearance	U/C	urine culture
CSU	catheter specimen (urine)	UC	urinary catheter
Cys	cysteine	UC&S	urine culture and sensitivity
CYS	cystoscopy	UcaV	urinary calcium volume
EMU	early morning urine(s)	UCRE	urine creatinine
HCG; hcg; hCG	human chorionic gonadotropin	UFC	urinary free cortisol
IVP	intravenous pyelogram	UK	urine potassium
K	potassium	Una	urinary sodium
Uosm	urine osmolarity	UV	urinary volume
UTI	urinary tract infection	Vol	volume
UUN	urinary urea nitrogen	WBCs	white blood cells

Table 24-7

Uremia: A high level of urea in the blood. Excessive amounts of urea and other nitrogenous waste products in the blood are seen in renal failure.

Uremic: Pertaining to a toxic level of urea in the blood.

Uric acid: The end product of the metabolism of purine, an important constituent of nucleic acids. A high level of uric acid in the urine may be associated with urinary calculi or gout.

Urobilinogen: A colorless compound formed in the intestines after the breakdown of bilirubin by bacteria. Some of this substance is excreted in feces, and some is reabsorbed and excreted again in bile or urine.

Urobilin: A brown pigment formed by the oxidation of urobilinogen. It is normally found in feces and in small amounts in urine.

Bilirubin: An orange-colored pigment in bile. Jaundice is a result of the accumulation in tissues of excess bilirubin in the blood.

Pyuria: The presence of pus in the urine, which may be evidence of renal disease.

Hematuria: The presence of blood in the urine, which may be a result of menstruation, urinary tract infection, or trauma or bleeding in the kidneys.

Hemoglobinuria: The presence of free hemoglobin in the urine, caused by a transfusion or drug reaction, malaria, snakebite, or severe burn.

Myoglobinuria: The presence of myoglobin in the urine, caused by injured or damaged muscle tissue.

Glycosuria: The presence of sugar (glucose) in the urine.

Nitrite: Occurs in urine when bacteria break down nitrate. It indicates a urinary tract infection.

AT A GLANCE Standard Urine Values

Test	Value
Acetone	None
Albumin, qualitative	Negative
Albumin, quantitative	10–140 mg/L (24 hours)
Bacteria (culture)	< 10,000 colonies/mL
Blood, occult	Negative
Calcium, quantitative	100–300 mg/24 hours
Color	Pale yellow to dark amber
Creatine, nonpregnant women/men	< 6% of creatinine
Creatine, pregnant women	≤ 12% of creatinine
Creatinine, men	1.0–1.9 g/24 hours
Creatinine, women	0.8–1.7 g/24 hours
Crystals	Negative
Ketones	Negative
Lead	0.021–0.038 mg/L
Odor	Distinctly aromatic
pH	4.5–8.0
Phenylpyruvic acid	Negative
Protein	Negative
Specific gravity, single specimen	1.005–1.030
Specific gravity, 24-hour specimen	1.015–1.025
Turbidity	Clear
Volume, adult females	600–1600 mL/24 hours
Volume, adult males	800–1800 mL/24 hours
White blood cells	0–8/high-power field

Table 24-8

Color and Turbidity	Pathological Causes	Other Causes
Colorless or pale straw color (dilute)	Diabetes, anxiety, chronic renal disease	Diuretic therapy, excessive fluid intake (water, beer, coffee)
Cloudy	Infection, inflammation, glomerular nephritis	Vegetarian diet
Milky white	Fats, pus	Amorphous phosphates, spermatozoa
Dark yellow, dark amber (concentrated)	Acute febrile disease, vomiting or diarrhea (fluid loss or dehydration)	Low fluid intake, excessive sweating
Orange-yellow, orange-red, orange-brown	Excessive RBC destruction, bile duct obstruction, diminished liver-cell function, bilirubin	Drugs (such as pyridium and rifampin), dyes

Table 24-9

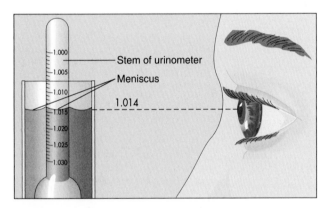

Figure 24-12 *Read the value on the scale where the bottom of the meniscus touches the stem.*

Ketosis: An accumulation of large amounts of ketone bodies in the tissues and body fluids as a result of dehydration, starvation, uncontrolled diabetes, or taking too much aspirin. Ketones are sometimes present after general anesthesia has been administered.

Creatinine: A waste product of the metabolism of creatine. Increased quantities are found in the urine in advanced stages of renal disease.

Pregnancy test: Detects an increase in the concentration of human chorionic gonadotropin (HCG) in the plasma or urine. The presence of increased HCG can also indicate ectopic pregnancy; a hydatidiform mole of the uterus; choriocarcinoma; or cancer of the lung, breast, pancreas, stomach, or colon. The first-voided morning urine has the highest concentration of HCG.

Enzyme immunoassay (EIA) test: A more advanced type of pregnancy testing that uses either urine or serum. In this test, a sample is added through a

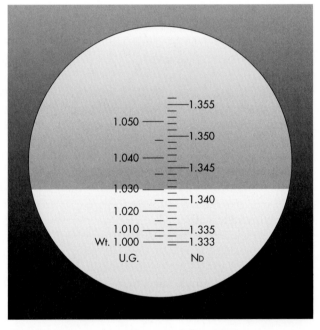

Figure 24-13 *A refractometer uses light refraction to measure specific gravity.*

chamber window where it migrates through the membrane and reacts with the reagents to produce a reaction. The test is easy to set up and interpret, and is designed with a control feature incorporated into the reagent pack for quality assurance of the test results.

STD testing: In response to increasing numbers of sexually transmitted diseases, the CDC recommends that all sexually active females between the ages of 15 and 25 be screened annually for chlamydia. To accomplish this, several tests called Nucleic Acid Amplification

Tests (NAATs) have recently been developed. These tests use urine samples to detect the presence of chlamydia or gonorrhea. By amplifying nucleic acids specific to these organisms, the test can detect the presence of very small numbers of bacteria.

Microscopic examination of urine: May show formed elements and can also determine the presence of cells, casts, crystals, bacteria, and other microorganisms. The first step is to use a centrifuge to obtain sediment for analysis. See Figures 24-14 and 24-15.

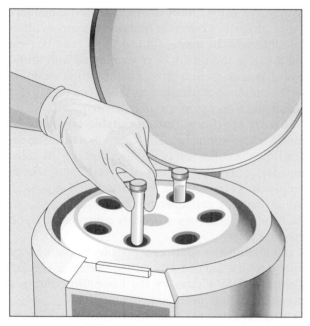

Figure 24-14 *The centrifuge must be balanced by placing test tubes on opposite sides.*

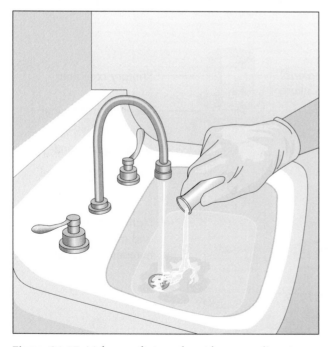

Figure 24-15 *Make sure that you do not lose any sediment when you pour off the urine.*

Crystals: Commonly found in urine specimens. They usually do not indicate a significant disorder. They are found in large numbers in patients with renal stones.

Urinary casts: Cylinder-shaped elements that form when protein accumulates in the kidney tubules and is washed down into the urine.

Mucous threads: Found in normal urine. Increased amounts usually indicate urinary tract inflammation. They are examined under low-power magnification.

Special Considerations

Pregnant patients: Pregnancy normally increases urinary frequency. Pregnant women are also prone to urinary tract infections. At each prenatal visit, they must have their urine checked for abnormal levels of glucose (indicative of diabetes) and abnormal levels of protein (preeclampsia or renal problems).

Elderly patients: Bladder muscles weaken with age, often leading to incomplete bladder emptying and chronic urine retention, which can cause urinary tract infections, nocturia, and incontinence.

Pediatric patients: Ask whether there are any problems with diaper rash (indicative of renal dysfunction), excessive thirst (possible diabetes), crying during urination (urinary tract infection), or bedwetting or enuresis (stress or urinary tract infections).

Medical Microbiology

Diagnosing infections: There are six steps in diagnosing infections: examining the patient, obtaining one or more specimens, examining the specimen, culturing the specimen, determining the culture's antibiotic sensitivity, and treating the patient. The medical assistant should work closely with the other members of the medical team.

Collecting Specimens

Guidelines for collecting specimens: Following these guidelines will make it possible to collect specimens properly:

- Try to avoid causing the patient harm, discomfort, or undue embarrassment.
- If the patient is to collect the specimen, provide clear, detailed instructions and the proper container.
- Collect the material from a site where the organism is most likely to be found and where contamination is least likely to occur.
- Obtain the specimen at a time that allows optimal chance of recovery of the microorganism.
- Use appropriate collection devices, specimen containers, transport systems, and culture media. Follow aseptic techniques.

- Obtain a sufficient quantity of the specimen.
- Obtain the specimen before antimicrobial therapy begins.
- Label the container, and include the proper requisition form.

Throat culture: A frequently performed microbiological procedure that is often performed when the patient shows signs or symptoms of an upper respiratory, throat, or sinus infection. In most cases, a throat culture is obtained to determine whether the patient has strep throat. Left untreated, strep throat can lead to rheumatic fever. To obtain sterile specimens, such as those used for throat cultures, a sterile swab is used. See Figure 24-16.

Sputum specimen: The patient should cough deeply and expectorate mucus from the lungs into a sterile container. The patient should be instructed to avoid contaminating the specimen with saliva. Follow

Universal Precautions when handling sputum specimens, and wear a face shield or mask and goggles.

Wound specimens: The procedure for obtaining specimens from infected wounds is similar to that for a throat culture. Obtain representative material from a deep area and a surface area without contaminating the swab by touching areas outside the site.

Stool culture: Ordered if the physician suspects that the patient has certain diseases such as cancer or colitis or bacterial, protozoal, or parasitic infections. Patients can collect stool specimens on a clean paper plate, in a clean waxed-paper carton, or in a collection container or collection tissue. Collection containers for stool cultures do not have to be sterile. The container must be clean, and the stool should not be contaminated with urine.

O and P specimen: A type of stool sample examined for the presence of parasites and their ova (eggs). Both a fresh and a preserved specimen are required.

Preparing specimens for an outside laboratory: If testing is to be done by an outside laboratory, be sure to follow the collection procedures and use the collection device required by the laboratory. Maintain the samples in a state as close to their original as possible. Ensure that the container has a tight-fitting lid, and place the container in a secondary container or zipper-type plastic bag.

Transporting the specimen: Specimens can be transported to an outside laboratory during a regularly scheduled daily pickup by the laboratory, during an as-needed pickup, or through the mail.

Mailing specimens: The USPS will accept microbiological specimens with a total volume of less than 50 mL that are packaged according to strict regulations of the U.S. Public Health Service. See Figure 24-17.

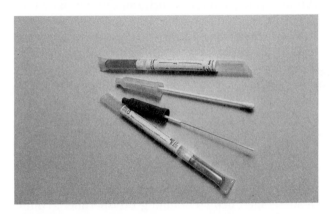

Figure 24-16 *Sterile swabs vary in size and in material.*

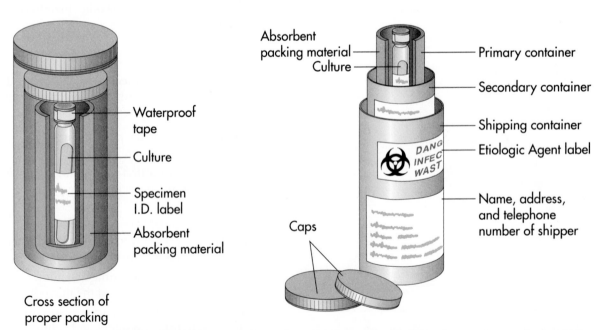

Figure 24-17 *When packaging and labeling a specimen for mail delivery, you must follow the procedures set by the CDC, based on U.S. Public Health Service regulations.*

Examining Specimens

Direct examination: Examination of the specimen under a microscope to identify the presence of microorganisms. There are two types of procedure: preparing wet mounts and preparing potassium hydroxide (KOH) mounts.

Wet mount: A type of mount that is easy to prepare and enables quick determination of many microorganisms. It requires mixing a small amount of the specimen with a drop of normal saline (0.9% sodium chloride) on a glass slide. Then a coverslip is placed over the mixture. The physician can examine the slide directly under the microscope.

Potassium hydroxide (KOH) mount: A type of mount used for identification of a fungal infection of the skin, nails, or hair. The procedure involves the following steps:

1. Suspend the specimen in a drop of 10% KOH on a glass slide.
2. Apply a coverslip.
3. Let the specimen sit for 30 minutes at room temperature.
4. Examine the slide under the microscope.

Stained specimens: Microorganisms can be seen more clearly when stained with a dye or group of dyes.

Smear: The first step in preparing a stained specimen is to prepare a smear. Apply a small amount of the specimen to a glass slide. Allow the sample to dry, then briefly heat the slide to fix the sample to the slide. Stain the smear.

Gram's stain: The stain most commonly used in examining bacteriological specimens. It involves a simple procedure, shown in Figure 24-18. If the bacteria have

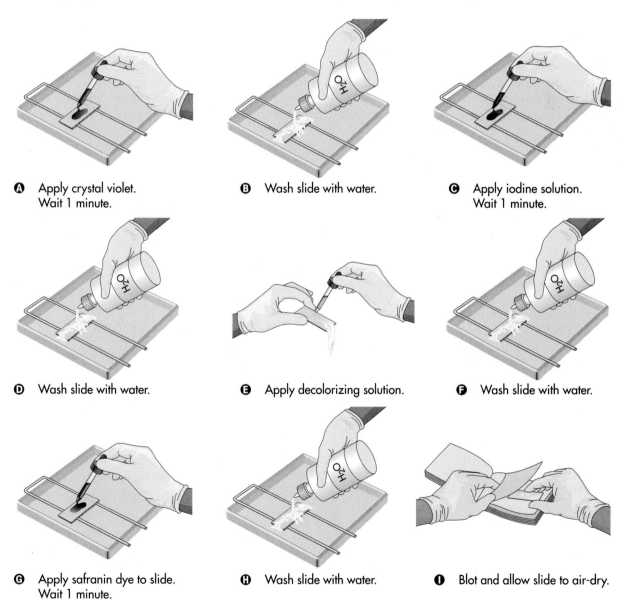

Ⓐ Apply crystal violet. Wait 1 minute.

Ⓑ Wash slide with water.

Ⓒ Apply iodine solution. Wait 1 minute.

Ⓓ Wash slide with water.

Ⓔ Apply decolorizing solution.

Ⓕ Wash slide with water.

Ⓖ Apply safranin dye to slide. Wait 1 minute.

Ⓗ Wash slide with water.

Ⓘ Blot and allow slide to air-dry.

Figure 24-18 *The procedure for performing a Gram's stain on a microbiologic specimen involves applying a series of stains, water washes, and alcohol in a specific order, for precise periods of time.*

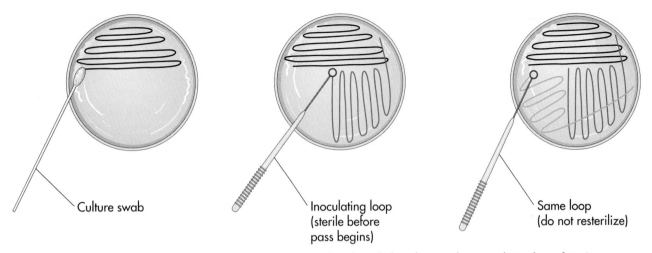

Figure 24-19 *When inoculating a plate for qualitative analysis, roll and streak the culture swab or inoculating loop of specimen material across $\frac{1}{3}$ of the surface of the culture plate. Begin the next pass with a sterile loop.*

a deep purple color, they are gram-positive. If the bacteria exhibit a pink or red color, they are gram-negative.

Acid-fast: Not readily susceptible to decolorization by acids during the staining procedure. The acid-fast nature of certain microorganisms, such as those of the genus *Mycobacterium*, allows microscopic examination and differentiation.

Culture Media

Culture media: Liquid, semisolid, and solid substances used to foster the growth of bacteria. Semisolid media are most commonly used in medical offices.

Agar: A gelatinlike substance extracted from algae that gives a semisolid culture medium its consistency.

Petri dish or **plate:** A covered glass or plastic dish that holds the culture medium. Handle Petri dishes only on the outside, so as to avoid contaminating them. Store them with the bottom (agar side) up.

Culturette® Collection and Transport System: A sterile, self-contained unit that holds a polyester swab and a small, thin-walled glass vial of transport medium in a plastic sleeve. It is used for obtaining and transporting specimens. (It is manufactured by Becton Dickinson Microbiology Systems.)

Selective culture media: Culture media that allow the growth of only certain kinds of bacteria. They are commonly used for specimens that normally contain bacteria, such as stools or vaginal samples.

Nonselective culture media: Media that support the growth of most organisms. For example, blood agar is a nonselective culture medium used to culture a throat swab specimen.

Special culture units: Commercially prepared units with specific purposes, such as performing rapid urine cultures or culturing vaginal specimens.

Preparing the plate: Before inoculating a culture plate, label it on the bottom (agar side) with the patient's name, doctor's name, source of the sample, date and time of inoculation, and your initials.

Bacitracin: An antibiotic used in cultures to give an early indication of the presence of group A streptococci.

Qualitative analysis: The determination of the type of pathogen by its appearance. Inoculate the plate as shown in Figure 24-19.

Quantitative analysis: The determination of the number of bacteria present in a sample.

Incubation: After inoculating the plate, put it in an incubator set at 35°C to 37°C, with the bottom (agar side) up, for 24 to 48 hours.

Colony: A visible growth on a culture plate, usually resulting from a single type of bacteria.

Culture isolation: One isolated, pathogenic-appearing colony is transferred from the primary culture plate. The secondary culture plate is incubated at 37°C to allow a pure culture to grow. A pure culture contains only a single type of organism.

Sensitivity testing: Determines an organism's susceptibility to specific antibiotics in order to enable the doctor to decide which one to use to treat the infection. The test involves the following steps:

1. Suspend a sample of the isolated pathogen in a small amount of liquid medium.

2. Streak the pathogen evenly on the surface of a culture plate.

3. Place small disks of filter paper containing various antimicrobial agents on top of the plate, using sterile forceps or a special dispenser.

4. Incubate the plate at 37°C for 1 day.

A clear zone around a disk indicates an effective antimicrobial agent, whereas growth next to a disk indicates an ineffective agent.

Quality control: All staining reagents should be checked frequently for effectiveness. All slides must be checked. All devices with temperature controls should be checked every day. All reagents and media must be used before the expiration date and evaluated for sterility. Equipment such as refrigerators, freezers, and incubators should be properly monitored and maintained.

Clinical Laboratory Improvement Amendments of 1988 (CLIA '88): A law enacted by Congress placing all laboratory facilities involved with human health and disease under federal regulations administered by the Health Care Financing Administration (HCFA) and the CDC. As a result, laboratories must meet complex standards, and medical assistants may perform only certain types of tests.

Instructions:

Answer the following questions. Check your answers in the *Answer Key* that follows this section.

1. Which of the following is an appropriate site for capillary blood collection?
   A. Small toe
   B. Earlobe
   C. Heel
   D. Both B and C
   E. All of the above

2. Which cells play a vital role in internal respiration?
   A. Bone marrow cells
   B. Erythrocytes
   C. Leukocytes
   D. Mast cells
   E. Basophils

3. What is the longest time a tourniquet should remain on a patient's arm?
   A. 1 minute
   B. 2 minutes
   C. 3 minutes
   D. 4 minutes
   E. 5 minutes

4. Dysuria is
   A. Inability to retain urine
   B. Painful or difficult urination
   C. Increased output of urine
   D. Decreased output of urine
   E. Micturition

5. Which of the following devices might be used to collect blood from fragile veins?
   A. A finger stick lancet
   B. A Vacutainer® system
   C. A butterfly needle
   D. An automatic puncturing device
   E. None of the above

6. A blue stopper indicates that a collection tube
   A. Is sterile
   B. Is to be used only for capillary puncture
   C. Contains the additive EDTA
   D. Contains an antiseptic
   E. Contains sodium citrate

7. To test for substances that are sporadically released into urine, a physician might order which type of urine specimen?
   A. 24-hour
   B. Clean catch
   C. Random
   D. First voided
   E. Timed

8. To follow Universal Precautions in phlebotomy, you should
   A. Wash your hands
   B. Wear examination gloves
   C. Recap the needle after blood is drawn and dispose of it in a biohazard container
   D. Both A and B
   E. All of the above

9. A medical assistant or a phlebotomist should not attempt to obtain blood from any patient more than
   A. One time
   B. Two times
   C. Three times
   D. Four times
   E. Five times

10. If a urinalysis cannot be performed within 30 minutes after collection, the urine specimen must be stored
    A. In an incubator
    B. In a freezer
    C. At room temperature
    D. In a refrigerator

11. Specific gravity may be measured by all of the following methods <u>except</u>
    A. Dipstick
    B. Urinometer
    C. Microscope
    D. Refractometer
    E. Reagent strip

12. The quality control log
    A. Lists specimens sent to another laboratory for testing
    B. Shows when the testing equipment was last calibrated
    C. Shows all the procedures completed during the workday
    D. Shows the quality testing performed on every batch of reagent product
    E. Documents maintenance done on laboratory equipment

13. Which of the following stains is specific to blood?
    A. Contrast
    B. Gram's
    C. Wright's
    D. Basic
    E. Agar

14. The color code for an evacuation tube that does <u>not</u> contain an additive is
    A. Red
    B. Lavender
    C. Gray
    D. Red and black
    E. Yellow

15. A creatine kinase test is done to help diagnose which of the following conditions?
    A. Muscular dystrophies and heart disease
    B. Infection or leukemia
    C. Cancer
    D. Kidney disorder
    E. Uterine disorder

16. Which of the following describes a centrifuge?
    A. Machine used to count blood cells
    B. Machine used to separate particles
    C. Machine used to heat cultures
    D. Machine used to analyze specimens
    E. Machine used to clean laboratory equipment

17. An erythrocyte sedimentation rate test might be used to
    A. Test for specific antibodies in the blood
    B. Determine sickle cell anemia or inflammation and infection
    C. Determine obesity and phenylketonuria
    D. Determine liver disease and hypothyroidism
    E. Determine the type and level of vitamins

18. How should the patient's arm be positioned when drawing blood in phlebotomy?
    A. Above heart level
    B. Bent at the elbow
    C. Hanging down
    D. Slightly upward
    E. Slightly downward

19. Which of the following is used in direct examination of a specimen?
    A. Wet mount
    B. Gram's stain
    C. Agar
    D. Petri dish
    E. Both B and C

20. The venipuncture site most commonly used on adults is the
    A. Basilic vein
    B. Median cubital vein
    C. Cephalic vein
    D. Brachial vein
    E. Iliac vein

21. After preparing a KOH mount,

   A. Examine the slide immediately
   B. Let the specimen sit at room temperature
   C. Refrigerate the specimen immediately
   D. Place the specimen in an incubator
   E. Either A or B

22. Before inoculating a culture plate, you should

   A. Label it on the top
   B. Label it on the bottom, agar side
   C. Label it with the patient's name and your initials only
   D. Both B and C
   E. Both A and C

23. The first step in preparing a culture plate is to

   A. Refrigerate it
   B. Warm it
   C. Add the specimen
   D. Label it
   E. Wash it

24. Albumin found in urine might indicate

   A. Renal disease
   B. Heart failure
   C. Hypertension
   D. Fever
   E. All of the above

25. Urine that is too acidic could indicate

   A. Urinary tract infection
   B. Renal failure
   C. Diabetes
   D. Gout
   E. Incontinence

26. If a drop of blood does not form after capillary puncture, which of the following should be done?

   A. Puncture the skin again
   B. Push repeatedly on the finger as if milking it
   C. Apply a tourniquet
   D. Apply steady pressure
   E. Wait until a drop does form

27. Which of the following causes would give plasma or serum a milky appearance?

   A. Hyperlipidemia
   B. Kidney disease
   C. Cancer
   D. Protein disorder
   E. Vegetarian diet

28. Which of the following is used in preparing a blood smear slide?

   A. Hemoclip
   B. Microhematocrit tube
   C. Lens paper
   D. Automatic puncturing device
   E. Spreader slide

29. Sensitivity testing is used to determine

   A. A pathogen's susceptibility to antibiotics
   B. A patient's susceptibility to antibiotics
   C. A patient's susceptibility to a pathogen
   D. A pathogen's susceptibility to antiseptic agents
   E. None of the above

30. A diaper rash on a pediatric patient may indicate which of the following?

   A. Possible diabetes
   B. Urinary tract infection
   C. Renal dysfunction
   D. Enuresis
   E. Nocturnal enuresis

31. The amylase test is used for disorders related to the

   A. Heart
   B. Brain
   C. Pancreas
   D. Lymphatic system
   E. Endocrine system

32. A physician may order a stool culture if he or she suspects
    A. Cancer
    B. Protozoal infection
    C. Bacterial infection
    D. Colitis
    E. All of the above

33. Fasting specimens are preferred for which of the following tests?
    A. Creatinine
    B. Triglycerides
    C. Thyroid function
    D. Hemoglobin
    E. Albumin

34. The anticoagulant EDTA is most appropriate for a blood specimen that has been collected for
    A. Glucose tolerance tests
    B. Complete blood cell counts
    C. Blood cultures
    D. Plasma toxicology
    E. Coagulation studies

ANSWER KEY

1.	D	18.	E
2.	B	19.	A
3.	A	20.	B
4.	B	21.	B
5.	C	22.	B
6.	E	23.	D
7.	A	24.	E
8.	D	25.	D
9.	B	26.	D
10.	D	27.	A
11.	C	28.	E
12.	B	29.	A
13.	C	30.	C
14.	A	31.	C
15.	A	32.	E
16.	B	33.	B
17.	B	34.	B

Self-Evaluation

PART

2

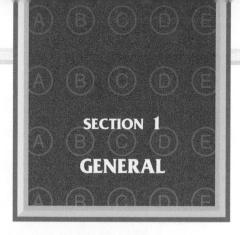

SECTION 1
GENERAL

TEST FOR MEDICAL ASSISTING KNOWLEDGE

Self-Evaluation

After you have finished reading Chapters 1 through 8, set aside some time to take this sample exam. There are 295 questions in this section. You can take them all at once or in smaller portions. Try to time yourself and answer about 60 questions in 60 minutes. Read each question carefully and circle the best answer. After you are finished, turn to Part 3, p. 540, for answers and rationales.

1. John Smith, a patient at your medical office, has been coming in for cancer treatment. After you send him a bill for the treatment, Mr. Smith's wife calls wondering what kind of treatment her husband has been receiving. What can you tell Mrs. Smith?

   A. Because you think that it is unfair that Mr. Smith has not informed his wife of his condition, you tell her about her husband's disease
   B. You don't tell Mrs. Smith on the phone, but you make sure to leave a message on the couple's answering machine detailing the test results and the reasons for Mr. Smith's visits
   C. You tell Mrs. Smith about her husband's condition, because you are legally required to do so according to public health laws because she is a family member
   D. You tell Mrs. Smith that you are not allowed to release medical information even to family members without the patient's consent and advise her to talk to Mr. Smith.
   E. You tell Mrs. Smith to call the insurance company, who would be able to inform her of all the details.

2. The word *articular* means
   A. The study of joints
   B. Pertaining to speech
   C. Pertaining to a joint
   D. Pain in the joints
   E. Difficulty with speech

3. *Trichoid* means resembling
   A. Nail
   B. Fat
   C. Skin
   D. Mole
   E. Hair

4. The sagittal plane divides the body into
   A. Front and back halves
   B. Left and right halves
   C. Upper and lower halves
   D. Four quarters: upper left, upper right, lower left, lower right
   E. Dorsal and ventral parts

5. The prefix *ambi-* means
   A. Without
   B. Both
   C. Self
   D. Good
   E. Unclear

6. Which of the following is true of DNA?

   A. Contained in the nucleus of a cell, it regulates the cell's activities
   B. It is a rod-shaped organelle that serves as the power plant of the cell
   C. It is a single chain of chemical bases
   D. It is a dense body in the nucleus composed of protein
   E. It contains water, dissolved ions, and nutrients

7. The prefix *ab-* means

   A. Without
   B. Toward
   C. Against
   D. Away from
   E. Underneath

8. The suffix *-ase* means

   A. Enzyme
   B. Noun marker
   C. Lip
   D. Condition
   E. Pain

9. Colpectomy is the excision of the

   A. Colon
   B. Rectum
   C. Vagina
   D. Uterus
   E. Testes

10. Which of the following is a type of cell division?

    A. Diffusion
    B. Osmosis
    C. Endocytosis
    D. Exocytosis
    E. Mitosis

11. Which of the following represents the highest level of Maslow's hierarchy of needs?

    A. Safety needs
    B. Survival or physiological needs
    C. Self-actualization needs
    D. Belongingness and love needs
    E. Prestige and esteem needs

12. An abnormal decrease in depth and rate of respiration is known as

    A. Dyspnea
    B. Apnea
    C. Auscultation
    D. Hypoxia
    E. Hypopnea

13. An area of necrotic tissue that has been invaded by bacteria is known as

    A. Infarction
    B. Gangrene
    C. Ischemia
    D. Atresia
    E. Inflammation

14. Privileged communication is

    A. The leading physician's conversation with a patient who has a hardship case
    B. The physician's conversation with a judge in a malpractice suit
    C. Communication between the physician and a public health agency
    D. Any conversation among patients in the reception area
    E. Information held confidential within a protected relationship such as between patient and physician or between lawyer and client

15. Which of the following cells release histamine?

    A. Lymphocytes
    B. Monocytes
    C. Basophils
    D. Erythrocytes
    E. Leukocytes

16. The prefix *retro-* means

    A. Behind
    B. Around
    C. Below
    D. Before
    E. After

17. The most common site for cancer incidence in males is the

    A. Bladder
    B. Colon
    C. Lung
    D. Prostate
    E. Brain

18. Protection against disease is called

    A. Prognosis
    B. Remission
    C. Pronation
    D. Prophylaxis
    E. Therapy

19. Which of the following types of bacteria is arranged in clusters?

    A. Streptococci
    B. Diplococci
    C. Staphylococci
    D. Protozoa
    E. Spirilla

48. In which of the following body systems are sebaceous glands located?

    A. Reproductive
    B. Integumentary
    C. Endocrine
    D. Urinary
    E. Nervous

49. The prefix *hypo-* means

    A. Excessive
    B. High
    C. Half
    D. Below
    E. Above

50. A 44-year-old woman comes to the emergency room complaining of nausea, vomiting, and pain in the upper abdomen. She also appears to have mild jaundice. These symptoms are most characteristic of

    A. Stomach cancer
    B. Diabetes insipidus
    C. Hyperinsulinism
    D. Cholelithiasis
    E. Myxedema

51. A wide-ranging prediction or explanation of everyday behavior or phenomena is

    A. Theory
    B. Hypothesis
    C. Experiment
    D. Behavior
    E. Rationale

52. Bipolar disorder is characterized by

    A. Eating disorders
    B. Euphoric and depressed moods
    C. Amnesia
    D. Autism
    E. Obsessions

53. Fread believed that personality of the ego was characterized as

    A. Basic instincts
    B. Psychic energy
    C. Reality-based thinking
    D. The pleasure principle
    E. Unconscious forces

54. According to Elisabeth Kübler-Ross, when a loved one is dying, the family may experience the same stages as the dying person. These stages are

    A. Denial, euphoria, sadness, death
    B. Trust, autonomy, guilt, inferiority, role confusion
    C. Denial, anger, bargaining, depression, acceptance
    D. Alarm, resistance, exhaustion, aftermath
    E. Repression, anger, justification, and projection

55. When is it legal to release medical information about a patient?

    A. When the person asking for it is a close relative or friend
    B. When the patient has verbally consented
    C. When an insurance company calls to request it
    D. When release of the information is ordered by a subpoena
    E. It is never legal to release information about a patient

56. In an emergency situation,

    A. Medically trained personnel can be immune from a liability suit
    B. Consent to allow touching, examination, or treatment by medically authorized personnel is waived
    C. A patient's right to confidentiality can be completely waived even if information released does not directly relate to the emergency
    D. Medically trained personnel are required to help victims according to the Good Samaritan Act
    E. Consent is necessary if the patient is a minor

57. The suffix *-penia* means

    A. Increase
    B. Enlargement
    C. Formation
    D. Abnormal reduction
    E. Pain

58. Something of value that is bargained for in a contract is called

    A. Acceptance
    B. Consideration
    C. Offer
    D. Reciprocity
    E. Registration

84. The comp...
   is called

   A. Sanit...
   B. Steril...
   C. Antis...
   D. Micro...
   E. All o...

85. The comb...

   A. cereb...
   B. ence...
   C. myel...
   D. poli...
   E. blep...

86. Prostate...
   by biops...
   ond lab...
   the initi...
   the patie...
   physicia...
   anisms i...

   A. Proj...
   B. Sub...
   C. Der...
   D. Rati...
   E. Rep...

87. As a g...
   should...

   A. No...
   B. Be...
   C. No...
   D. Bo...
   E. All...

88. A 9-yea...
   by her...
   mothe...
   to see...
   medica...

   A. N...
   B. Ye...
   C. Ye...
   D. Ye...
   E. N...

89. The so...
   the bo...

   A. F...
   B. N...
   C. A...
   D. B...
   E. L...

59. How should a medical assistant communicate with an elderly patient?

   A. Encourage the patient to write his or her questions
   B. Encourage the patient to ask questions
   C. Talk with the patient softly
   D. Avoid asking questions loudly
   E. Avoid eye contact

60. Which of the following is the role of the umbilical vein in fetal circulation?

   A. It transports oxygen from the placenta to the fetus
   B. It transports blood from the fetus to the placenta to deliver oxygen and to get rid of carbon dioxide
   C. It carries blood directly to the inferior vena cava
   D. It carries blood directly to the right atrium
   E. None of the above

61. The site of maturation for T lymphocytes is the

   A. Spleen
   B. Thymus
   C. Bone marrow
   D. Liver
   E. Blood

62. A one-sided relationship in which one member benefits and the other is unaffected is called

   A. Symbiosis
   B. Mutualism
   C. Commensalism
   D. Opportunism
   E. Parasitism

63. Costectomy means excision of a

   A. Xiphoid process
   B. Sternum body
   C. Rib
   D. Vertebra
   E. Bladder

64. Which of the following is the most common route of transmission of trichomoniasis?

   A. Saliva
   B. Urine
   C. Sputum
   C. Genital secretions
   E. Blood

65. How can you communicate to a patient that his or her main idea was understood?

   A. By allowing the patient to reflect
   B. By restating what the patient has said
   C. By being assertive and establishing rapport
   D. By folding your arms across your chest
   E. By shaking your head

66. *Bacteriostatic* means

   A. Inhibiting bacterial growth
   B. Killing bacteria
   C. Without infection
   D. Completely destroying all living organisms
   E. Maintaining a constant amount of bacteria

67. The unauthorized disclosure of client information is called

   A. Invasion of privacy
   B. Battery
   C. Breach of contract
   D. Unethical protocol
   E. None of the above

68. A 5-year-old boy has a bone deformity of the thigh. The pediatrician should order an X-ray of the patient's

   A. Tibia
   B. Humerus
   C. Femur
   D. Fibula
   E. Patella

69. Susan, the new medical assistant, reported to work on her first day and made a mistake in copying some files that her supervisor, John, asked for. When John learned of Susan's mistake, he angrily blurted out that women are always more trouble than they are worth. John was exhibiting

   A. Passive voice
   B. Sexual communication
   C. Unethical discrimination
   D. Gender bias
   E. Negligence

70. *Lithiasis* refers to

   A. A disease of the liver
   B. The formation or presence of stones
   C. A treatment for kidney failure
   D. An instrument used to examine the bladder
   E. A toxic substance found in the liver

71. Which of
of rights?
   A. The p
      the ex
   B. The p
      exper
   C. The p
      conti
   D. Both
   E. All of

72. When a p
known as
   A. Fear
   B. Deni
   C. Accep
   D. Symp
   E. Barga

73. A time wl
   A. Remi
   B. Prog
   C. Prop
   D. Mala
   E. Atres

74. Vitamin
   A. Nigh
   B. Werr
   C. Hem
   D. Pern
   E. Rick

75. Formatic
   A. Hyd
   B. Hyd
   C. Hyd
   D. Hyd
   E. Hyd

76. What is
placed t
an offic
open fr
   A. 10:0
   B. 11:0
   C. 12:(
   D. 1:0
   E. 2:0

77. Blamin;
   A. Dis
   B. Rat
   C. Pro
   D. Rep
   E. No

96. Which of the following documents explains that patients should receive respectful care?
   A. Hippocratic Oath
   B. Good Samaritan Act
   C. Patient's Bill of Rights
   D. American Medical Association Code of Ethics
   E. All of the above

97. Which of the following abbreviations means "each eye"?
   A. AU
   B. AD
   C. AS
   D. OD
   E. OU

98. A telephone inquiry about a bill should be handled
   A. By the patient's physician
   B. By the attending physician
   C. By the medical assistant who answers the phone
   D. By the attending nurse
   E. None of the above

99. Which of the following medical terms is misspelled?
   A. Abscess
   B. Homestasis
   C. Aerobic
   D. Neuron
   E. None of the above

100. As a medical assistant, what should your goals be in patient education?
   A. To promote patient health by teaching healthful habits and practices such as proper diet and exercise
   B. To help patients prevent injury
   C. To help patients visualize an upcoming procedure
   D. Both A and B, but C is the physician's responsibility
   E. A, B, and C are all responsibilities of the medical assistant

101. Which of the following structures of the eye contains the photoreceptors (rods and cones)?
   A. Choroid
   B. Sclera
   C. Vitreous humor
   D. Retina
   E. Tunic

102. Which of the following terms best describes the awareness and insight that one person has for another's feelings and emotions?
   A. Sensitivity
   B. Sympathy
   C. Empathy
   D. Emotivity
   E. Apathy

103. Carriers of pathogenic organisms are called
   A. Vectors
   B. Viruses
   C. Diseases
   D. Normal flora
   E. Bacteria

104. Which of the following hormones prepares the uterus for pregnancy?
   A. Estrogens
   B. Human chorionic gonadotropin
   C. Progesterone
   D. Androgen
   E. All of the above

105. The plural of *nucleus* is
   A. Nuclei
   B. Nucleuses
   C. Nuclea
   D. Nucleae
   E. Nucleus

106. What is the term for a group of people who are authorized by law to act as a single person?
   A. Association
   B. Group practice
   C. Corporation
   D. Partnership
   E. Sole proprietorship

107. Confidentiality may be waived
   A. When a third party such an insurance carrier requests a medical examination and pays the physician's fee
   B. When a patient sues a physician for malpractice
   C. When a waiver has been signed by the patient or legal guardian
   D. When a waiver has been signed by the patient's spouse
   E. Confidentiality may never be waived

108. The Johns Hopkins Medical Center calls to report that a patient whom your office referred there has undergone the needed surgery and is doing well. How should you handle this call?

   A. Transfer it to the physician if he or she is available
   B. Take the call yourself
   C. Take a message for the physician if the physician is out, and make sure that the physician talks to the hospital
   D. Either A or B
   E. None of the above

109. Immobility and consolidation of a joint due to disease, injury, or surgical procedure is called

   A. Scoliosis
   B. Kyphosis
   C. Lordosis
   D. Ankylosis
   E. Crepitation

110. According to Kübler-Ross, dying patients go through all of the following stages except

   A. Isolation
   B. Refusing treatment
   C. Depression
   D. Guilt and bargaining
   E. Anger

111. Who owns medical records?

   A. The patient
   B. The physician
   C. The courts
   D. The legal guardian
   E. Both A and B

112. Chronic dilation and distention of the bronchial walls is called

   A. Bronchiectasis
   B. Bronchitis
   C. Bronchiolitis
   D. Atelectasis
   E. Atelencephalia

113. Which of the following diseases can result from antidiuretic hormone deficiency?

   A. Dwarfism
   B. Diabetes mellitus
   C. Diabetes insipidus
   D. Myxedema
   E. Acromegaly

114. Which of the following is included in the SOAP approach to documentation?

   A. Applicable financial information
   B. Opinion of the medical assistant
   C. Problem
   D. System of conditions
   E. Plan of action

115. Rapid movement of the eyeball is known as

   A. Nystagmus
   B. Hyperopia
   C. Presbyopia
   D. Hordeolum
   E. Hashimoto's disease

116. Which of the following words is misspelled?

   A. Scirrhous
   B. Pneumonia
   C. Puritus
   D. Vaccine
   E. Pleurisy

117. Which of the following suffixes means "surgical repair"?

   A. -stomy
   B. -scopy
   C. -plasty
   D. -tomy
   E. -iasis

118. A patient's failure to follow the physician's instructions may result in

   A. The transfer of the patient to the care of another physician
   B. A civil case between the physician and the patient
   C. Capitation for managed care
   D. Nonmaleficence against the physician
   E. A premature termination of contract

119. Major depression and bipolar disorders are most characteristic of which of the following?

   A. Dissociative disorder
   B. Impulse-control disorder
   C. Mood disorder
   D. Personality disorder
   E. Cognitive disorder

120. What body functions does the hypothalamus control?

   A. Body temperature
   B. Water balance
   C. Sleep
   D. All of the above
   E. None of the above

121. Which endocrine gland secretes cortisol?

   A. Anterior pituitary
   B. Thyroid
   C. Adrenal cortex
   D. Ovaries
   E. None of the above

122. Which law controls the distribution and use of all drugs with abuse potential?

   A. Controlled Substance Act of 1970
   B. Drug Regulation and Reform Act of 1978
   C. Orphan Drug Act of 1983
   D. Toxic Drug Act of 1975
   E. Substance Regulation Act of 1980

123. Which of the following can be seen only with an electron microscope?

   A. Molds
   B. Bacteria
   C. Viruses
   D. Pathogens
   E. Internal organs

124. The combining form *cutane / o* means

   A. Sweat
   B. Skin
   C. Nail
   D. Tissue
   E. White

125. Which of the following blood types is considered the universal donor?

   A. Type A
   B. Type B
   C. Type AB
   D. Type O
   E. None of the above

126. Which of the following suffixes means "pain"?

   A. -ilgia
   B. -itis
   C. -olgia
   D. -otomy
   E. -algia

127. Which of the following blood types is considered to be the universal recipient?

   A. Type A
   B. Type B
   C. Type O
   D. Type AB
   E. None of the above

128. Which of the following tumors consists of multiple cysts ("a bunch of grapes")?

   A. Hydatidiform mole
   B. Adenocarcinoma of the vagina
   C. Adenocarcinoma of the breast
   D. Fibroadenoma
   E. Myeloid sarcoma

129. Bleeding between menstrual periods is called

   A. Menorrhagia
   B. Amenorrhea
   C. Metrorrhagia
   D. Amnesia
   E. Ovulation

130. The plural of *atrium* is

   A. Atrius
   B. Atrium
   C. Atriae
   D. Atriums
   E. Atria

131. Dermatitis is

   A. Inflammation of the skin
   B. Chronic itching and swelling of the skin
   C. Chronic pain under the skin
   D. Inflammation of the hair follicles
   E. Inflammation of kidneys

132. Which of the following is true about the scope of education and training for medical assistants?

   A. Medical assistants are allowed to diagnose patients when the physician is absent and the case needs urgent medical attention
   B. Medical assistants can give out diagnostic opinions when performing emergency triage
   C. In some states, medical assistants are not allowed to draw blood
   D. Medical assistants should not be responsible for keeping controlled substances secure
   E. Medical assistants should not be responsible for treating terminally ill patients, especially patients diagnosed with AIDS

133. Self-actualization, prestige, love, safety, and survival are components of the humanistic hierarchy of needs developed by which of the following psychologists?

   A. Skinner
   B. Piaget
   C. Maslow
   D. Pavlov
   E. Freud

134. In a malpractice suit that involves the accidental injury of a patient during a surgical procedure, such as the removal of a healthy body part,

A. The physician's lawyers will emphasize the concept of *respondeat superior*
B. The court has the burden of proving the physician's guilt
C. The Latin phrase *res ipsa loquitur* does not apply
D. The patient has the burden of proving the physician's guilt
E. The physician has the burden of proving innocence

135. Which of the following microbes lives only in the absence of oxygen?

A. Obligate anaerobe
B. Facultative anaerobe
C. Heterotroph
D. Facultative aerobe
E. Pathogens

136. As a medical assistant working at the receptionist desk in a medical office, you get a call from an angry individual who insists on talking to Dr. Jonezee, a physician at the office. The angry woman on the phone refuses to be identified and insists that she has a right to be heard by her own physician, and she claims that you are just some person in the front office who obviously doesn't know anything and can't help her. What should you do?

A. Tell her to calm down or you will hang up, and if she still insists on yelling at you and refuses to identify herself, hang up on her without saying anything else
B. Transfer the call to Dr. Jonezee if she is available, because the physician might be able to calm an angry patient
C. Tell the caller politely that she needs to tell you who she is in order for you to be able to help her, and that if she can't tell you, she should write a letter to the physician and mark it *Personal*
D. Trace the call to find out who the caller is, and pull her file and try to help her even if she refuses
E. Offer the caller the option of leaving a message on the physician's voice mail

137. A 6 year-old child who starts sucking his thumb when is new brother is born is exhibiting which type of defense mechanism?

A. Repression
B. Projection
C. Regression
D. Denial
E. Displacement

138. An operative report reads "fx, rt. radius." The correct meaning is

A. Flexion, right forearm
B. Fracture, right forearm
C. Fusion, right forearm
D. Fasciotomy, right forearm
E. Fixation, right forearm

139. Which part of the ear detects motion and governs balance?

A. Tympanic membrane
B. Semicircular canal
C. Cochlea
D. Cerumen
E. Auditory ossicles

140. *Intercostal* means

A. Between two coasts, in reference to the coverage area of some insurance companies
B. Pertaining to an area between the ribs
C. Between two joints
D. Pertaining to an area between the vertebrae
E. Pertaining to a disease that affects a large geographical area

141. According to the Medical Assisting Code of Ethics, members of the AAMA should

A. Render service with full respect for the dignity of humanity
B. Respect confidential information obtained through employment unless legally authorized or required to divulge such information
C. Participate in additional service activities aimed toward improving the health and well-being of the community
D. Both A and B
E. All of the above

142. Koplik's spots in the mouth are a sign of

A. Chickenpox
B. Measles
C. German measles
D. Warts
E. Diphtheria

143. Which of the following is a flat, blade like bone that forms the midanterior portion of the upper trunk?

A. Scapula
B. Sternum
C. Xphoid process
D. Clavicle
E. Pelvis

144. Thrombolysis is
    A. The surgical reconstruction of blood vessels
    B. The blockage of blood vessels
    C. The destruction of a clot
    D. The surgical removal of a clot
    E. An abnormal condition of blood

145. Which of the following receives oxygenated blood from the pulmonary veins?
    A. Right atrium
    B. Left atrium
    C. Right ventricle
    D. Left ventricle
    E. Both A and C

146. Which of the following is usually the only symptom of cancer of the larynx?
    A. Cephalalgia
    B. Aphasia
    C. Dysphonia
    D. Apnea
    E. Dyslexia

147. Which of the following is true of a living will?
    A. A living will is legal if two witnesses have signed it
    B. A living will is legal if there is a do-not-resuscitate (DNR) order
    C. A living will is legal if the patient is competent at the time of its creation
    D. A living will is legal if the patient is competent to create such a will and two witnesses sign it and attest to its accuracy
    E. Both B and D

148. When should you minimize background noise when communicating with a patient?
    A. It is not usually necessary
    B. When dealing with a fearful patient
    C. When dealing with an angry patient
    D. When dealing with a patient who has a visual impairment
    E. When dealing with a patient who has a hearing impairment

149. Retinol is another name for
    A. Vitamin A
    B. Vitamin B_9
    C. Vitamin E
    D. Vitamin B_6
    E. Vitamin B_{12}

150. Which of the following acts provides immunity from liability for any civil damages to volunteers at the scene of an accident?
    A. Self-Determination Act
    B. Good Samaritan Act
    C. Uniform Anatomical Gift Act
    D. Bill of Rights
    E. Medical Liability Emergency Act

151. Absorption of vitamin B_{12} requires
    A. Pepsin
    B. Gastrin
    C. Intrinsic factor
    D. Secretin
    E. Calcium

152. Questions that require elaboration on the part of the patient are referred to as
    A. Long answer questions
    B. Open-ended questions
    C. Direct questions
    D. Yes/no or is/do questions
    E. None of the above

153. Which of the following diseases can be caused by excessive growth hormone in an adult?
    A. Hypothyroidism
    B. Dwarfism
    C. Diabetes insipidus
    D. Acromegaly
    E. Graves' disease

154. When the eyeball is abnormally short, the condition is called
    A. Presbyopia
    B. Myopia
    C. Hyperopia
    D. Strabismus
    E. Binocular vision

155. Which of the following conditions of the eye may elevate pressure within the eye and cause blindness?
    A. Cataract
    B. Glaucoma
    C. Uveitis
    D. Entropion
    E. Myxedema

156. Which of the following cancers is most easily diagnosed in the early stages?
    A. Ovarian cancer
    B. Vaginal cancer
    C. Endometrial cancer
    D. Cervical cancer
    E. Stomach cancer

157. Which of the following muscles extends the thigh?
    A. Gluteus medius
    B. Quadriceps femoris
    C. Hamstrings
    D. Gluteus maximus
    E. Brachialis

158. The deltoid muscle may
    A. Extend the arm
    B. Raise the arm
    C. Flex the arm
    D. Adduct the arm
    E. Abduct the arm

159. The correct spelling of the plural form of *appendix* is
    A. Appandixes
    B. Appendixs
    C. Appendices
    D. Appendixces
    E. None of the above

160. Iodine deficiency may cause
    A. Hypertension
    B. Anemia
    C. Impaired growth
    D. Renal hypertrophy
    E. Goiter

161. Where does protein synthesis occur?
    A. In the nucleolus
    B. On ribosomes
    C. On lysosomes
    D. On mitochondria
    E. On the Golgi apparatus

162. A term meaning "within the vein" is
    A. Intervenous
    B. Intravenous
    C. Intravenious
    D. Intervenious
    E. None of the above

163. Which of the following procedures would require the patient's written consent?
    A. Removing a splinter from under a nail
    B. Treating a 14-year-old boy for an emergency
    C. Major surgery
    D. Giving a 25-year-old woman a Pap smear
    E. None of the above

164. A statute of limitations limits
    A. The amount of damages collected in a malpractice suit
    B. The amount a physician can charge for a service
    C. The amount of time or deadline for filing a lawsuit or legal action
    D. The type of work medical assistants can perform within the scope of their training
    E. None of the above

165. The term *malleolus* refers to a type of bone that is
    A. Straight
    B. Broken
    C. Rounded
    D. Long
    E. Fractured

166. The second cervical vertebra is called
    A. Atlas
    B. Coccyx
    C. Basilar
    D. Hyoid
    E. Axis

167. The combining form *pulmon / o* means
    A. Artery
    B. Heart
    C. Breathing
    D. Veins
    E. Lung

168. Which of the following muscles is located in the torso?
    A. Soleus
    B. Pectoralis major
    C. External oblique
    D. Biceps
    E. Masseter

169. A substance that inhibits the growth of bacteria is called
    A. Protozoa
    B. Bactericidal
    C. Bacteriostatic
    D. Aflatoxin
    E. Chemotroph

170. An abnormal lateral curvature of the spine is called
    A. Scoliosis
    B. Spondylitis
    C. Lordosis
    D. Spondylosis
    E. Kyphosis

171. What is meant by *ectopic*?
    A. Otocleisis
    B. Misplaced
    C. Dilation
    D. Surplus
    E. Maternal

172. *Dorsal* means
    A. Horizontal
    B. Anterior
    C. Frontal
    D. Posterior
    E. Vertical

173. Giardiasis is
    A. Inflammation of the appendix
    B. Infection of the small intestine, also called traveler's diarrhea
    C. Infectious inflammation of the liver
    D. Food poisoning
    E. Hereditary disease that leads to mental and physical retardation

174. Which of the following is a myelocele?
    A. Herniation of a muscle
    B. Herniation of a nerve
    C. Herniation of an umbilicus
    D. Herniation of the spinal cord
    E. Herniation of the diaphragm

175. Biofeedback is a process that can help a person learn to control
    A. Internal physiological systems
    B. External physiological systems
    C. Environmental systems
    D. Other people
    E. Emotional trauma

176. Which of the following might make you liable for invasion of privacy and breaking patient-physician confidentiality?
    A. Releasing medical records in response to a subpoena
    B. Releasing medical records to an insurance company with the patient's written consent
    C. Refusing to disclose any information to the patient's employer even though you believe that the employer should have this information
    D. Leaving a patient's medical chart as well as the patient sign-in sheet in plain view at the office
    E. Releasing information to the appropriate public health agency about a patient who has been diagnosed with AIDS

177. Touching someone to show sensitivity and empathy is
    A. Discouraged for most medical assistants
    B. Usually acceptable on the shoulder, back, or hand
    C. Acceptable, so long as you are aware of cultural and personal differences and adjust your style accordingly
    D. Both B and C
    E. None of the above

178. The suffix that means "flow" or "discharge" is
    A. -ra
    B. -rrhexis
    C. -rrho
    D. -rrhaphy
    E. -rrhea

179. Joe, a 5-year-old patient at your pediatric practice, has recently been coming in consistently bruised, looking malnourished, and too frightened to talk about what has been happening to him. You suspect child abuse; however, when you question the mother of the boy, she claims that Joe is just very accident prone and has never been a big eater, but there is really nothing else wrong. What should you do?
    A. Report it as suspected child abuse to the physician, and together report it to the authorities
    B. Do not report it, because the parents of the child might later sue you for slander
    C. Make a note of it in Joe's medical records, but acknowledge that you are powerless until Joe comes to you for help
    D. Call the police immediately
    E. None of the above

180. The energy that is necessary to keep the body functioning at a minimal level is known as
    A. Thermogenesis
    B. Catabolism
    C. Basal reaction
    D. Metabolic reaction
    E. Basal metabolism

181. A 50-year-old man has been advised by the doctor to stop smoking. He continues to smoke in spite of the advice. He knows it is unhealthy to smoke but likes to smoke. We might say that he is suffering from
    A. Development disorder
    B. Cognitive development
    C. Cognitive learning theory
    D. Cognitive dissonance
    E. Panic anxiety disorder

182. German measles is also known as

  A. Shingles
  B. Rubella
  C. Pyoderma
  D. Rubeola
  E. Pertussis

183. Which of the following is the plural of *septum*?

  A. Sepsis
  B. Septae
  C. Septa
  D. Septic
  E. Septums

184. Which of the following tissues provides insulation for the human body?

  A. Muscle tissue
  B. Nerve tissue
  C. Serous membranes
  D. Adipose tissue
  E. Epithelial tissue

185. Transportation of substances out of a cell by means of vesicles is called

  A. Endocytosis
  B. Phagocytosis
  C. Exocytosis
  D. Pinocytosis
  E. Osmosis

186. When on the telephone in the medical office, you should

  A. Speak clearly, use terms that you can pronounce correctly and that are appropriate to the situation, and not overwhelm patients with technical words they might not understand
  B. Be aware of who is in hearing range of your conversation and use discretion in the type of information you discuss
  C. Hold the telephone receiver about an inch away from your mouth and be courteous
  D. Keep any personal conversations to a minimum
  E. All of the above

187. Type A blood has

  A. Type A and type B antigens
  B. Type A antigens
  C. Type B antigens
  D. Neither type A nor type B antigens
  E. Type A antibodies

188. An irresistible urge to engage in behaviors such as repeatedly touching a spot on the nose is called

  A. Obsessive disorder
  B. Panic anxiety disorder
  C. Somatoform disorder
  D. Compulsion disorder
  E. Conversion disorder

189. Which of the following is the act of intentionally misleading?

  A. Tort
  B. Fraud
  C. Felony
  D. Burglary
  E. Misdemeanor

190. Performing a physical examination of the patient without the patient's consent would be considered

  A. Rape
  B. Assault
  C. Abuse
  D. Battery
  E. Violation

191. While on the phone with a patient discussing an appointment, you get interrupted by a second call, which you think might be an important business associate of the physician. How should you handle this situation?

  A. Finish your initial conversation with the patient and let the voice mail get the second call; after you hang up with the patient, check the voice mail and return any messages
  B. Excuse yourself to the first caller and answer the second call, then return to the first call as soon as possible; minimize waiting for all callers
  C. Tell the patient that there is a second call, that it might be an important call you've been expecting, and that you will call back after taking the call
  D. Any of the above
  E. None of the above

192. Which of the following components moves substances across the surface of the cell?

  A. Cilia
  B. Centrioles
  C. Flagella
  D. Cytoskeleton
  E. Leukocytes

193. When answering the phone, which of the following greetings is appropriate?
  A. "Hello, this is Dr. Jones-Smith's office. My name is George. How may I help you?"
  B. "Hello, this is George. How may I help you?"
  C. "Hello."
  D. "This is 555–5555. How may I help you?"
  E. All of the above

194. The contractual relationship between a patient and a physician binds the physician
  A. To cure the patient
  B. To advise the patient against needless surgery and to provide reasonable care
  C. To diagnose all conditions and prescribe treatment
  D. Both B and C
  E. All of the above

195. When you are a victim of sexual harassment at your workplace, what actions should you take?
  A. Report the harassment to your supervisor
  B. Tell the harasser to stop
  C. Quit immediately
  D. Ignore the situation
  E. Both A and B

196. A 4-year-old boy fell on a kitchen floor. After the accident, his mother saw his right leg swell and brought him to the emergency room. An X-ray showed that the bone is partially bent and partially broken. What type of fracture is this?
  A. Comminuted
  B. Impacted
  C. Greenstick
  D. Oblique
  E. Incomplete

197. According to Maslow's hierarchy of needs, which of the following can be considered one of the most basic human needs?
  A. Shelter
  B. Human contact
  C. Safety and security
  D. Both A and C
  E. All of the above

198. The combining form *gon / o* means
  A. Genitals
  B. Vagina
  C. Sexually transmitted disease
  D. Uterus
  E. Testis

199. Which of the following would be considered a positive form of body language?
  A. Looking down and nodding
  B. Facing the patient and nodding
  C. Folding your arms
  D. Both B and C
  E. All of the above

200. A 19-year-old soccer player is unable to extend his knee after a sports injury. Which of the following tendons may be injured?
  A. Extensor digitorium
  B. Patellar
  C. Biceps femoris
  D. Achilles
  E. None of the above

201. A suffix is
  A. The main part of a word
  B. The last part of a word
  C. A word ending that modifies the root
  D. A word part at the beginning that modifies the root
  E. The first part of a word

202. Which of the following foods is high in fiber?
  A. Green beans
  B. Red meat
  C. Yogurt
  D. Rice
  E. Bread

203. Quadriplegia results in the paralysis of
  A. The lower extremities
  B. The right side of the body
  C. The upper extremities and the trunk
  D. The left side of the body
  E. All four extremities and usually the trunk

204. A license to practice medicine is
  A. Required by local law
  B. Required by the local medical society
  C. Required by law in each state
  D. A right of every graduate physician
  E. Required by federal law

205. Which of the following systems is the body's first line of defense against infection?
  A. Endocrine
  B. Urinary
  C. Respiratory
  D. Integumentory
  E. Nervous

206. Which of the following terms is spelled correctly?

A. Micturation
B. Tonsilectomy
C. Dispharesis
D. Keratosis
E. Hydrocephalas

207. A physician is required to report

A. Births
B. Deaths
C. Food poisoning
D. Both A and B
E. All of the above

208. At which of the following annual state conventions was the AAMA founded in 1955?

A. Florida
B. Washington
C. Texas
D. Kansas
E. Oregon

209. Parts of the ear include all of the following except the

A. Incus
B. Iris
C. Stapes
D. Auricle
E. Malleus

210. What type of fracture is involved when the bone is broken and one of the broken ends is wedged into the interior of the other?

A. Comminuted
B. Open or compound
C. Impacted
D. Oblique
E. Incomplete

211. Which of the following bones is located in the arm?

A. Patella
B. Scapula
C. Ulna
D. Fibula
E. Femur

212. Which of the following is a malignant tumor of the connective tissues?

A. Hyperplasia
B. Carcinoma
C. Sarcoma
D. Cretinism
E. Neoplasm

213. The elbow is an example of which of the following types of joints?

A. Pivot
B. Hinge
C. Ball and socket
D. Saddle
E. Condyloid

214. A collapse of the cardiovascular system resulting in a dangerous reduction of blood flow throughout the body is called

A. Acute endocarditis
B. Rheumatic fever
C. Cardiac tamponade
D. Shock
E. Aneurysm

215. Which of the following results from the administration of a vaccine with killed or weakened organisms?

A. Natural active immunity
B. Artificial active immunity
C. Artificial passive immunity
D. Natural passive immunity
E. Both C and D

216. Keratinization

A. Is a process by which epithelial cells lose their moisture, which is replaced by protein
B. Is a process that leads to cretinism
C. Forms a translucent band that is found only in thick-skinned individuals
D. Is found at the bottom layer of the cutaneous membrane, beneath the dermis
E. None of the above

217. Which of the following body cavities is divided into the thoracic and the abdominopelvic cavities?

A. Dorsal
B. Transverse
C. Ventral
D. Frontal
E. Sagittal

218. Hay fever, anaphylaxis, asthma, and eczema are examples of which of the following types of hypersensitivities?

A. Type I
B. Type II
C. Type III
D. Type IV
E. Type V

219. Susan Johnson's insurance company calls to request that her medical records be transferred to her new physician. What should you do?
    A. Call the other physician to verify the request
    B. Tell the insurance company that you need Ms. Johnson's signed consent to release and transfer her medical records
    C. Call Ms. Johnson to verify the transfer
    D. Transfer the medical records at the request of the insurance company
    E. Instruct the insurance company to arrange the transfer with Ms. Johnson, not you

220. In which part or parts of the body are there no sweat glands?
    A. Lips
    B. Nipples
    C. Ears
    D. Palms
    E. Both A and B

221. When something is without legal force or effect, it is called
    A. Void
    B. Implied
    C. Breached
    D. Offered
    E. Tort

222. An increase in the number of cells of a body part that results from an increased rate of cellular division is called
    A. Mitosis
    B. Malignancy
    C. Atrophy
    D. Hypertrophy
    E. Hyperplasia

223. Hashimoto's disease is an abnormal, chronic condition of the
    A. Pancreas
    B. Adrenal cortex
    C. Thymus gland
    D. Thyroid gland
    E. Heart

224. The fight-or-flight response is
    A. Controlled by the cranial and spinal nerves that connect the central nervous system with the skin and skeletal muscles
    B. Communication between neurons of the somatic nervous system and the autonomic nervous system
    C. The sympathetic part of the autonomic nervous system that acts as an accelerator for organs needed to meet a stressful situation
    D. Both A and C
    E. All of the above

225. The abbreviation meaning "right eye" is
    A. OS
    B. OD
    C. AD
    D. AU
    E. RE

226. The abbreviation meaning "nothing by mouth" is
    A. Rx
    B. n.o.
    C. p.o.
    D. m.n.o.
    E. n.p.o.

227. What is the main muscle involved in the act of inspiration?
    A. Larynx
    B. Lung
    C. Diaphragm
    D. Trachea
    E. Stomach

228. Which of the following is an example of an open-ended question?
    A. "Are you in pain now?"
    B. "Have you been exercising?"
    C. "How would you describe your diet?"
    D. "Do you drink alcohol?"
    E. "Are you married?"

229. The best way to receive a positive evaluation during your externship is by
    A. Showing integrity and practicing high ethical standards
    B. Showing the office manager that you are very skillful and knowledgeable
    C. Offering the physician a cup of coffee
    D. Impressing patients that you are able to cure diseases
    E. Impressing the physician by being on time

230. Which of the following statements is true about medical law?

 A. Because of the doctrine of *respondeat superior*, the physician becomes responsible for all negligent acts of his or her employees even when he or she is not giving them direct orders
 B. A case in which a patient negligently refuses to follow a physician's instructions comes under the umbrella of the *res ipsa loquitur* doctrine
 C. The physician is contractually bound to cure a patient
 D. A physician dispensing controlled substances must be registered with the Drug Enforcement Agency
 E. All of the above

231. Which of the following is the study of hereditary improvement through the control of genetic characteristics?

 A. Genetic screening
 B. Gene therapy
 C. Eugenics
 D. Artificial insemination
 E. None of the above

232. A solution that has a higher concentration (e.g., of salt) than the fluids within a cell is called

 A. Hypertonic
 B. Hypotonic
 C. Isotonic
 D. Exotonic
 E. Endotonic

233. In which part of the lung does the exchange of gases take place?

 A. Ventricles
 B. Alveoli
 C. Trachea
 D. Bronchioles
 E. Larynx

234. Where does the chemical breakdown of carbohydrates begin within the digestive system?

 A. Esophagus
 B. Saliva in the mouth
 C. Stomach
 D. Small intestine
 E. Large intestine

235. Which of the following is a difference between the nervous and endocrine systems?

 A. The nervous system controls only conscious activities, whereas the endocrine system controls unconscious activities
 B. The nervous system is usually quicker to respond than the endocrine system
 C. Although the effects of the endocrine system are slower, they are also more prolonged
 D. Both B and C
 E. All of the above

236. Cushing's syndrome is

 A. An inflammatory autoimmune disease that attacks the thyroid gland
 B. A tickborne disease characterized by skin lesions, malaise, fatigue, and facial palsy
 C. Hyperactivity of the adrenal cortical gland that develops from an excess of the glucocorticoid hormone
 D. Inflammation of the pericardium
 E. A reduction in the quantity of either red blood cells or hemoglobin in a measured volume of blood

237. In order to comply with the Health Insurance Portability and Accountability Act (HIPAA), which of the following must be provided by the physician when requested by patients?

 A. Credentials of staff members
 B. Office policy and procedure manual
 C. Job description of medical assistants
 D. Notice of privacy practices
 E. Current fee schedule

238. Which of the following systems removes waste products, salts, and excess water from the blood and eliminates them from the body?

 A. Digestive system
 B. Cardiovascular system
 C. Endocrine system
 D. Respiratory system
 E. Urinary system

239. Which of the following is the longest part of the digestive system?

 A. Small intestine
 B. Large intestine
 C. Esophagus
 D. Anal canal
 E. Rectum

240. Which of the following interview topics is it illegal to discuss with a prospective employee?

    A. Work ethic
    B. Greatest weakness
    C. Marital status
    D. Educational background
    E. Previous employer

241. Professional medical liability insurance is used to

    A. Prevent fraud and abuse
    B. Comply with federal law
    C. Provide for legal expenses in medical liability cases
    D. Comply with state law
    E. Both B and D

242. Bitter tastes are perceived

    A. At the back of the tongue
    B. A the very tip of the tongue
    C. At the sides of the tongue
    D. In the middle of the tongue
    E. Everywhere on the tongue

243. A major concern when sending medical reports via e-mail is

    A. Ability to read the document clearly
    B. Speed of transmission
    C. Software compatibility
    D. Confidentiality
    E. Cost

244. The suffix -emesis means

    A. Pertaining to
    B. Binding
    C. Record
    D. Condition
    E. Vomiting

245. The unauthorized disclosure of client information is an example of

    A. Nonfeasance
    B. Defamation
    C. Fraud
    D. Malfeasance
    E. Invasion of privacy

246. In which of the following instances do you usually have to use a combining vowel?

    A. When connecting a prefix to a root that begins with a consonant
    B. When connecting two word roots
    C. When connecting a word root and a suffix that starts with a consonant
    D. Both B and C
    E. All of the above

247. The RMA examination may be scheduled

    A. Almost any day of the year
    B. Once a year
    C. Once a month
    D. Every two months
    E. Every six months

248. Which of the following vitamins is necessary for formation of prothrombin in the liver and is essential to blood clotting?

    A. Vitamin E
    B. Vitamin C
    C. Vitamin K
    D. Vitamin A
    E. Vitamin B_{12}

249. A person or group bringing charges in a lawsuit is called a(n)

    A. Arbitrator
    B. Defendant
    C. Lawyer
    D. Plaintiff
    E. Both A and C

250. The habit of nail-biting is called

    A. Onychomalacia
    B. Onychectomy
    C. Onychopathy
    D. Onychotrophy
    E. Onychophagia

251. Every language contains the essential element(s) of

    A. Symbols, grammar, and sounds
    B. Symbols and grammar
    C. Symbols only
    D. Grammar only
    E. Sounds only

252. Sometimes people choose a career because they want to please their parents and family. This is an example of a(n) _____ factor as a motivational source.

    A. Innate
    B. Biological
    C. Social
    D. Cognitive
    E. Traditional

253. The study of how behavior is affected by genes is known as

    A. Structuralism
    B. Functionalism
    C. Behavioral genetics
    D. Humanistic psychology
    E. Naturalism

254. The <u>best</u> way to define a stressor is as
    A. The emotional and physical process of adjusting to change
    B. An individual's response to a stressful situation
    C. An event that causes an individual to change or adapt
    D. A factor that dampens the impact of a stressful event
    E. An individual's emotional state that causes them to change

255. Kim has worked at a stressful job for 10 years. She has developed high blood pressure and an ulcer. In which stage of the GAS would Selye place Kim?
    A. Alarm reaction
    B. Attack
    C. Resistance
    D. Exhaustion
    E. Surrender

256. Dianne has an active set of defense mechanisms that constantly affect her behavior and thoughts. The defense mechanisms are her
    A. Id's attempt to promote life instincts
    B. Superego's attempt to promote morality
    C. Ego's attempt to control anxiety and guilt
    D. Death instincts coming to the surface
    E. Rationalizations of moral conflict

257. Ed always feels angry. However, instead of recognizing his anger, Ed believes that everyone around him is angry. Ed is using the defense mechanism of
    A. Projection
    B. Rationalization
    C. Sublimation
    D. Displacement
    E. Repression

258. Paul got very angry at his dog because it urinated all over his new carpet. He had an urge to hit the dog, but, instead, he punched his wall. The defense mechanism that Paul displayed is
    A. Projection
    B. Displacement
    C. Reaction formation
    D. Rationalization
    E. Compensation

259. Sally is a 4-year-old who prefers sleeping with her parents to sleeping in her own bed. However, she gets upset when she sees her father kissing her mother. In which of Freud's psychosexual stages of development is Sally likely to be?
    A. Oral
    B. Anal
    C. Phallic
    D. Genital
    E. Latency

260. Which personality approach assumes that personality is determined by the unique ways in which each individual views the world?
    A. Humanistic
    B. Social-cognitive
    C. Trait
    D. Psychodynamic
    E. Object relations

261. One of humanistic personality theories' most important concepts is
    A. Learned behavior
    B. Factor analysis
    C. Self-actulization
    D. Object relations
    E. Congruence

262. Some of the humanistic approach's best-known applications are
    A. In crisis intervention
    B. Psychotherapy methods
    C. Curriculum materials
    D. Assessment tools
    E. Interdependent

263. For the past 3 months, Tammy has been worried that something bad is going to happen. She can't pinpoint the source of this feeling, but she can't sleep or concentrate, and is irritable and jumpy. Her symptoms suggest that she may be suffering from _____ disorder.
    A. Dissociative
    B. Panic
    C. Generalized anxiety
    D. Conversion
    E. Obsessive-compulsive

264. George was in class when, suddenly, his heart began to pound, his chest felt tight, and he became very dizzy. When this type of episode happened a few more times, George decided to see his doctor. His doctor did not find anything physically wrong with him. George was most likely suffering from

   A. Generalized anxiety disorder
   B. Obsessive-compulsive disorder
   C. Panic disorder
   D. Specific phobia
   E. Dissociative disorder

265. Lynette was depressed for six months. Now, however, she feels so confident, energetic, and good that she decides to take all of her bank saving out and invest in gerbil cages and equipment. She states that she has discovered a way to make gerbils "live forever." She speaks so excitedly and rapidly to her friends about her idea that they can barely understand her. Lynette most likely suffers from _____ disorder.

   A. Bipolar
   B. Dysthymic
   C. Conversion
   D. Panic
   E. Dissociative

266. Major depressive disorder is most likely to occur in which types of twins?

   A. Identical male
   B. Nonidentical male
   C. Identical female
   D. Nonidentical female
   E. Conjoined

267. All of the following are symptoms of schizophrenia <u>except</u>

   A. Multiple personalities
   B. Disorganized thoughts
   C. Delusions
   D. Hallucinations
   E. Constantly angry demeanor

268. Six-year-old Bobby has shown no attachment to his mother or anyone else. He does not smile, and has not learned how to speak. Bobby suffers from

   A. Depression
   B. Attention deficit disorder
   C. Anxiety disorder
   D. Autistic disorder
   E. Separation anxiety disorder

269. According to Maslow's five level hierarchy of human needs, which of the following is the primary need?

   A. Safety
   B. Self-actualization
   C. Survival
   D. Esteem
   E. Love

270. An empathetic person has the ability to

   A. Engage in the process of self-enhancement
   B. Perceive and understand another person's situation
   C. Avoid intrusion of one's own emotions and feelings
   D. Remain cool and calm during a confrontation
   E. Divert another person's attention from a problem in a joking manner

271. Tom Samuel becomes a religious zealot because he fears his own violent streak. This is an example of which defense mechanism?

   A. Denial
   B. Reaction formation
   C. Repression
   D. Displacement
   E. Projection

272. According to Freud, the state of development marked by disinterest in sexual concerns is known as the

   A. Latency state
   B. Genital stage
   C. Phallic stage
   D. Oral stage
   E. Anal stage

273. Based on the Humanist theory a person has an internal force that pushes them to grow and improve. The force is known as

   A. Motive for affiliation
   B. Fear of success
   C. Unconditional regard
   D. Inner-directedness
   E. Self-actualization

274. A person with a preoccupation toward inner thoughts and a lack of responsiveness to others, is defined as having

   A. Dyslexia
   B. Dysphoria
   C. Autism
   D. Mania
   E. Paranoia

275. A 74-year-old man has severe gangrene of the right foot and right lower leg. His physician recommends above-the-knee amputation to prevent further problems. The patient refuses to consider this recommendation and states that he will stop smoking to control the condition, so that amputation will not be necessary. Which of the following defense mechanisms is this patient demonstrating?

A. Rationalization
B. Repression
C. Denial
D. Compensation
E. Sublimation

276. A patient states that she just got fired from her job. You recognize this stressor as

A. Posttraumatic syndrome
B. Cataclysmic stressor
C. Personal stressor
D. Background stressor
E. Impersonal stressor

277. When a dying patient appears less depressed and there is a quiet sense that he realizes that death happens to all living things, what stage do you think is happening (according to Kübler-Ross's stages)?

A. Denial
B. Anger
C. Bargaining
D. Acceptance
E. Depression

278. You talk with a patient, and listen to him describe how he feels. You gain some understanding of how it is to be 30 years old and dying because he explains what it is like to walk in his shoes. Your emotional experience is known as:

A. Fear
B. Anxiety
C. Sympathy
D. Empathy
E. None of the above

279. Threatening or challenging events are known as

A. Stressors
B. Stress reducers
C. Minor events
D. Events that make you feel good
E. Major events

280. A subfield of psychology whose main focus of study consists of mental processes is:

A. Health psychology
B. Social psychology
C. School psychology
D. Cognitive psychology
E. Environmental psychology

281. Which statement is true about stress?

A. Stress can be from positive and negative sources
B. Background stressors are events that happen suddenly
C. Stress does not affect the body's ability to fight off illness
D. All stress causes severe physiological disorders
E. None of the above

282. A patient is always telling the staff in the office how irritable they are and how they do not listen to her. The patient is under a lot of stress and is irritable. The office staff has been observed on multiple occasions to politely listen to this patient and try to help her. This patient may be using a defense mechanism known as

A. Repression
B. Regression
C. Denial
D. Projection
E. Sublimation

283. Humanistic theorists believe that behavior is

A. Motivated by inner unconscious forces
B. Controlled by a person naturally trying to reach his or her potential
C. Made up of biological factors
D. Controlled by reinforcers and consequences
E. Exclusively copied from others

284. A 50-year-old man has arrived at a clinic because of low weight and a skin infection. You, the medical assistant, are assigned to take his medical history. You find out that he is malnourished because he is homeless at times. According to Maslow's hierarchy of needs, you can expect this patient to

A. Be interested in joining a self-help club
B. Be focused on just meeting his biological needs
C. Feel good about himself
D. Be worried about his safety
E. Be concerned about a change in career direction

285. A 30-year-old man has been diagnosed with late stage cancer. He will probably live only 6 to 9 months. You are the medical assistant at the primary care doctor's office. Two weeks after receiving his diagnosis, you see this patient, and he tells you about how he is sending large sums of money for a "miracle cure" from Mexico. According to Kübler-Ross's stages, what stage do you think he is in?

A. Depression
B. Denial
C. Acceptance
D. Anger
E. Bargaining

286. Which of the following is an example of the fight-or-flight syndrome?

A. Fear
B. Emotion
C. Empathy
D. Projection
E. Reaction formation

287. Uplifts are designed as

A. Stressors
B. Stress reducers
C. Minor positive events
D. Events that make you feel good
E. B, C, and D

288. According to the general adaptation syndrome, if stress is not reduced, a patient will probably

A. Increase the intensity of her symptoms to the point of exhaustion
B. Become increasingly more irritable
C. Continue to have a depressed immune system
D. All of the above
E. None of the above

289. Mrs. S. shares with you that her father is very ill and likely to die soon. You recognize this stressor as a

A. Posttraumatic syndrome
B. Cataclysmic stressor
C. Personal stressor
D. Background stressor
E. Eustress

290. According to Erikson's stages of development, an adolescent who excels at athletics, trains and makes the team is showing

A. A positive outcome to his identity vs. role confusion conflict
B. A negative outcome to his identity vs. role confusion conflict
C. A positive outcome to his generativity vs. stagnation conflict
D. A negative outcome to his generativity vs. stagnation conflict
E. Positive outcome to his industry vs. inferiority

291. Maslow theorized that

A. Self-esteem was not important
B. Self actualization was the first step
C. Biological needs must be met before self actualization
D. Love and belonging never occur together
E. Shelter is less important than love

292. Identifying a problem, formulating a rationale, and performing research to support or nullify the rationale are part of the

A. Academic theory
B. Scientific method
C. Wellness method
D. Theory of personality

293. Mental processes are

A. Private thoughts, emotions, and feelings
B. Not directly observable, deducible only through inference
C. Directly observable
D. Both A and B
E. Both A and C

294. Schizophrenia is

A. Severe distortion of reality
B. Severe distortion of affect
C. Severe distortion of judgment
D. All of the above
E. None of the above

295. According to behaviorists, Mr. H. would have the best chance of changing behaviors if

A. Reinforcers were removed
B. Some consequences were present
C. If his unconscious was explored
D. Both A and B
E. All of the above

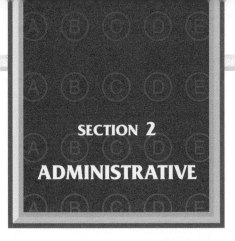

TEST FOR MEDICAL ASSISTING KNOWLEDGE

Self-Evaluation

After you have finished reading Chapters 9 through 14, set aside some time to take this sample exam. There are 250 questions in this section. You can take them all at once or in smaller portions. Try to time yourself and answer about 60 questions in 60 minutes. Read each question carefully and circle the best answer. After you are finished, turn to p. 556 in Part 3 for answers and rationales.

1. Which of the following pieces of office equipment is necessary for electronic data interchange?
   A. Scanner
   B. Transcriber
   C. Modem
   D. Photocopier
   E. Postage meter

2. A supplier offers a 10% discount when ordering 12 or more items. Each item costs $40. How much will 12 items cost?
   A. $108
   B. $480
   C. $396
   D. $432

3. The primary purpose of a patient record-filing system is to
   A. Protect patient privacy
   B. Make documents available to authorized personnel
   C. Facilitate efficient document retrieval
   D. Separate active and inactive files
   E. Arrange chart files for the physician's review

4. In a facility that has several procedure rooms and adequate personnel to staff them, which type of scheduling can be used to build in flexibility?
   A. Wave
   B. Open hours
   C. Grouping
   D. Advance
   E. Computerized

5. Which of the following explanations is a reason to keep medical records?
   A. They are used in malpractice suits
   B. They are used to provide continuity of care
   C. They are used for audits
   D. They are used to evaluate the quality of treatment in a physician's office
   E. All of the above

6. Medical assistants are expected to answer the phone
   A. Only if the answering service doesn't answer it first
   B. By the second or third ring
   C. Rarely, because it is not within their scope of training
   D. To answer diagnostic questions
   E. Only if the call pertains to an administrative matter

7. Which of the following terms is one of the six Cs of charting?
   A. Client's words
   B. Chronicle
   C. Calculation
   D. Computation
   E. Conclusive

8. A deceased patient's chart should be transferred to which of the following files?
   A. Subject
   B. Closed
   C. Follow-up
   D. Inactive
   E. Alphabetical

9. Bob Johnson goes to his participating HMO provider for a check-up and a flu shot. The allowed charge for a check-up is $80, and the physician's usual fee is $85. The allowed charge for the flu shot is $50, and the physician's usual fee is $40. How much is Mr. Johnson charged for the visit?
   A. Nothing
   B. $5
   C. $15
   D. $40
   E. $130

10. Which accounting system uses the equation *Assets = Liabilities + Owner Equity*?
   A. Pegboard
   B. Single-entry
   C. Double-entry
   D. Daily log
   E. Accounts receivable

11. The balance
   A. Equals debits plus credits
   B. Equals the difference between debits and credits
   C. Is the amount recorded on the left
   D. Is the amount recorded on the right
   E. Both A and C

12. In order to ensure the continuous accuracy of accounts, a medical assistant can
   A. Transfer the amounts in each account from the journals to the ledgers
   B. Keep track of write-offs
   C. Bank electronically
   D. Write only certified checks
   E. Take a trial balance

13. Bills and statements of account should be sent as
   A. Standard Mail (B)
   B. Standard Mail (A)
   C. Express Mail
   D. Priority Mail
   E. First-Class Mail

14. All of the following calls will require the physician's personal attention <u>except</u>
   A. Requests for prescription renewals that have not been preauthorized
   B. Reports from patients concerning unsatisfactory progress or abnormal test results
   C. Calls from insurance companies
   D. Calls from other doctors
   E. Personal calls

15. The fee an individual physician most frequently charges for a service is called the
   A. Usual fee
   B. Customary fee
   C. Reasonable fee
   D. Standard fee
   E. Prevailing charge

16. When you have 300 flyers and circulars to mail out, which mail category should you use?
   A. Standard Mail (A)
   B. Standard Mail (B)
   C. First-Class Mail
   D. Periodicals
   E. Bound Printed Matter

17. Medicare Part B covers
   A. Hospital care
   B. Outpatient services
   C. Hospice care
   D. Nursing facility care
   E. All of the above

18. Michelle Columbus is a patient at your medical facility. She has both Medicare and a type of Medigap insurance. When you file her insurance claim, where should you send the claim?

A. The claim must be filed with the Medigap insurance carrier first

B. The claim is not filed at all, because payments from both policies are automatic on a month-to-month basis

C. The claim must be filed with Medicare first

D. The charges must be filed with both insurance carriers at once

E. None of the above

19. Medicaid is

A. A secondary carrier when the patient has Medicare

B. Always the primary carrier

C. A type of Medigap insurance policy

D. A governmental insurance plan with which all physicians must comply

E. Both A and C

20. How can you protect your computerized medical office records against both fires and computer viruses?

A. Do not open attachments from people you don't know

B. Do not open e-mail messages from people you don't know

C. Make backup copies of all files nightly

D. Store backup files off the premises

E. Both C and D

21. Which of the following types of information is often stored on a medical database?

A. Provider data

B. Patient data

C. Diagnosis codes

D. Transactions

E. All of the above

22. What should you do when a bill is 30 days overdue?

A. Send a letter or a reminder statement to the patient

B. Call the patient at work to remind him or her of this oversight

C. Threaten the patient

D. Ignore the situation, and call or write only when the account is 60 days overdue

E. Pay a personal visit to the patient to offer help

23. When filing patient records, which of the following should be filed first?

A. Paul Edward Jr.

B. Paul Edward Sr.

C. Paul J. Edward Sr.

D. P. Travis Edward Jr.

E. P. Travis Edward Sr.

24. Physicians are required to keep payroll data for how many years?

A. 1

B. 2

C. 3

D. 4

E. 5

25. Employers must submit a report of all taxes owed by a business at least

A. Every week

B. Every 2 weeks

C. Monthly

D. Quarterly

E. Annually

26. HCPCS is the abbreviation for the Health Care Procedural Coding System, mandated by Congress for

A. Medicare

B. Medicaid

C. Blue Cross

D. CHAMPVA

E. TRICARE

27. When you have to file an insurance claim for a procedure that is not listed in the *Physicians' Current Procedural Terminology*, what should you do?

A. File a claim for the procedure that is closest to the unlisted one

B. Look for a code in the ICD-9-CM

C. Read the guidelines for such procedures in each section, and file a special report that describes and explains the extent and reasons for service

D. You cannot file a claim for an unlisted procedure

E. Consult the Health Care Financing Administration

28. Voucher checks are commonly used for

A. Insurance payments

B. Purchasing items that cost less than $100

C. Purchasing items that cost more than $100

D. Cash in foreign countries

E. Payroll

29. FUTA taxes are
    A. Deducted from an employee's wages based on gross income
    B. Authorized under the Federal Unemployment Tax Act
    C. Paid half by employers and half by employees
    D. Calculated annually
    E. Both A and B

30. Which of the following statements is true of non-participating Medicare providers?
    A. The patient pays the provider
    B. The patient pays Medicare
    C. Medicare pays the provider
    D. The provider pays Medicare
    E. Either A or C

31. Which of the following statements is true of medical transcription?
    A. You should listen all the way through a tape before starting to transcribe
    B. You can adjust the transcribing equipment's speed and volume
    C. You should write down the time on the digital counter for any problems so that you can find them when you request clarification
    D. You should have any needed materials at hand
    E. All of the above

32. A method of identifying and separating items to be filed into smaller subunits is called
    A. Indexing
    B. Creating tickler files
    C. Numerical filing
    D. Coding
    E. Subject filing

33. When using a computer, a list of commands or options that can be selected is called a
    A. Protocol
    B. Menu
    C. Window
    D. Link
    E. Character

34. The medical assistant responsible for coding should attend at least
    A. One CPT class each year
    B. One ICD-9 class each year
    C. One ICD-9 and one CPT class each year
    D. One CPT and one ICD-9 class every two years
    E. One CPT and one ICD-9 class every three years

35. A Form W-2 lists
    A. Gross income
    B. Taxes withheld
    C. FUTA taxes separately
    D. Both A and B
    E. All of the above

36. What is the maximum size of an item you can mail through the U.S. Postal Service?
    A. Letters should not weigh more than 13 ounces, and parcels should not weigh more than 25 pounds
    B. There are size limits only on envelopes, not on Parcel Post
    C. There are no size limits on items mailed
    D. A combined length and girth of 130 inches and weight of no more than 108 pounds
    E. A combined length and girth of 108 inches and weight of no more than 70 pounds

37. Which of the following terms is used to describe the medical records of patients who have not been in the office for several years?
    A. Reserved
    B. Restricted
    C. Purged
    D. Closed
    E. Inactive

38. Which of the following statements was true of Special Delivery?
    A. When something was marked Special Delivery, it got delivered as soon as it reached the recipient's post office
    B. It could not be used for items sent to a post office box or to a military address
    C. Special Delivery mail got a unique tracking number, and the sender was notified when the mail was received
    D. It alerted postal workers that a package or letter contained unusual contents
    E. Both A and B

39. Which of the following is considered the best type of filing system because it is designed to reduce the misfiling of patient files?
    A. Numerical
    B. Subject based
    C. Geographical
    D. Color coded
    E. Cross referenced

40. Which of the following is a federation of nonprofit organizations offering private insurance plans?
    A. CHAMPVA
    B. Blue Cross and Blue Shield Association
    C. TRICARE
    D. DEERS
    E. Medicare

41. A regular referral from a primary care physician often takes
    A. No time at all, because it is handled over the phone
    B. 24 hours
    C. From 3 to 10 days
    D. About a month
    E. None of the above

42. The CMS-1500 is
    A. A nonprofit insurance carrier
    B. An agency under Medicare
    C. An agency under Medicaid
    D. A commonly used insurance claim form
    E. A private provider of health care

43. The Blue Cross part of BCBS covers
    A. Physician services
    B. Hospital services
    C. Dental services
    D. Vision services
    E. None of the above

44. A certain patient often comes to your office for cancer treatment. When this patient comes in with a sore throat caused by the flu, what is the primary diagnosis according to the ICD-9-CM?
    A. Cancer
    B. Flu
    C. Sore throat
    D. Coughing
    E. Fever

45. Placing area rugs in the reception area of a medical office is an example of
    A. Quality assurance
    B. Quality improvement
    C. A safety hazard
    D. Universal precautions
    E. Receptionist duties

46. FICA taxes are paid
    A. Half by the employer and half by the employee
    B. Completely by the employer
    C. Completely by the employee
    D. By the employee if the employer has fewer than 4 workers
    E. Only in special circumstances

47. The place where transactions are first recorded is called the
    A. General journal
    B. Charge journal
    C. Daysheet
    D. Daily log
    E. All of the above

48. The amount charged for a medical insurance policy is the
    A. Customary fee
    B. Usual fee
    C. Copayment
    D. Coinsurance
    E. Premium

49. Preventing duplicate payment for the same service is known as
    A. Cost-share
    B. Insurance fraud prevention
    C. Co-payment
    D. Group policies
    E. Coordination of benefits

50. The process of checking transcribed materials for accuracy and clarity is called
    A. Formatting
    B. Proofreading
    C. Word processing
    D. Transcription
    E. Dictation

51. Which of the following plans covers spouses of veterans with permanent, service-related disabilities?
    A. Medigap
    B. Medicare
    C. Medicaid
    D. CHAMPUS
    E. CHAMPVA

52. The endorsement Special Handling
    A. Should be used especially on fragile items
    B. Is not required for those parcels sent as First Class, Express, or Priority Mail
    C. Should be printed in capital letters two lines below the postage
    D. Is the same as Special Delivery
    E. Both B and C

53. Which of the following types of insurance cover medical expenses for patients who are injured on the physician's property?
    A. Special risk
    B. Overhead
    C. Liability
    D. Workers' compensation
    E. Disability

54. Blue Shield makes direct payments to
    A. The hospital
    B. Physician members
    C. The patient
    D. Insurance companies
    E. Medicare recipients

55. To maximize communication with children, all of the following guidelines are good practices except
    A. To take their feelings seriously
    B. To work directly with their parents
    C. Explain all procedures, even basic ones, in simple terms
    D. To let them examine instruments
    E. To be truthful

56. Groups of procedures related directly to diagnosis are referred to as
    A. DRGs
    B. MFS
    C. RBRVS
    D. HCFA
    E. HCPCS

57. Amounts of money owed to a medical practice for professional services rendered are
    A. Usual fees
    B. Actual charges
    C. Major medical expenses
    D. Accounts receivable
    E. Accounts payable

58. What is the postal abbreviation for *Circle*?
    A. Cr
    B. C
    C. CIR
    D. Crl
    E. Cre

59. A system of payment used by managed care plans in which physicians and hospitals are paid a fixed, per capita amount for each patient enrolled over a stated period of time, regardless of the type and number of services provided, is called
    A. Premium
    B. Capitation
    C. Medigap
    D. Control plan
    E. Fee management

60. In proofreading, the ∧ mark means
    A. Insert
    B. Delete
    C. Make lowercase
    D. Capitalize
    E. None of the above

61. Medical assistants should
    A. Not have any visible tattoos or wear body-piercing jewelry other than earrings in the ears
    B. Wear perfume and cologne conservatively or not at all
    C. Polish their nails only with natural colors and cut them to an appropriate length
    D. Have clean, neat, and fresh attire
    E. All of the above

62. Under the old mail classification system, manuscript copies and circulars were sent as
    A. First Class Mail
    B. Second Class Mail
    C. Third Class Mail
    D. Fourth Class Mail
    E. None of the above

63. After opening the mail, a medical assistant should
    A. Date-stamp the letter
    B. Check for enclosures
    C. Annotate mail if necessary by highlighting key information and making notes in the margins
    D. Organize the mail so that the most important letters are on top
    E. All of the above

64. Guidelines that dictate the day-to-day workings of an office are called
    A. Procedures
    B. Planning
    C. Outlines
    D. Policies
    E. Protocols

65. Speaking clearly and articulating carefully is known as
    A. Pronunciation
    B. Enunciation
    C. Volume
    D. Intonation
    E. Salutation

66. When using a postage meter,
    A. Remember to change the date daily
    B. You can save money by printing the exact postage on envelopes
    C. You still have to hand-stamp most envelopes
    D. Both A and B
    E. All of the above

67. When writing a memo, you should
    A. Not use salutations or complimentary closings
    B. Use letterhead
    C. Always use the modified-block letter style
    D. Always indent paragraphs
    E. All of the above

68. In which letter style are all lines flush left except for the dateline, complimentary closing, and signature?
    A. Full-block
    B. Modified-block
    C. Simplified
    D. Center-block
    E. Left-block

69. The term used for the authorization to an insurance company to make payment directly to the physician is
    A. Reasonable fee
    B. Fee schedule
    C. Assignment of benefits
    D. Fee compliance
    E. Accepting fees

70. In postal addresses, *Junction* is abbreviated as
    A. J
    B. JT
    C. JCT
    D. JUNC
    E. JN

71. If you want an envelope to be processed electronically, how should you print the address?
    A. Use single spacing
    B. Use all capital letters
    C. Do not use punctuation
    D. Put the company name first, followed by the *Attention* line
    E. All of the above

72. Which of the following is the correct way to write Mary Jack's title?
    A. Dr. Mary Jack, M.D.
    B. Mary Jack, M.D.
    C. Ms. Dr. Mary Jack
    D. Both B and C
    E. All of the above

73. When dealing with an angry patient, you must learn how to
    A. Return to your work
    B. Stop the patient from talking
    C. Break off communication
    D. Remain calm
    E. Both A and D

74. *Telephone triage* means
    A. Requesting referrals to other doctors
    B. Checking with the insurance company
    C. Determining whether the caller is a new patient
    D. Documenting outgoing calls
    E. Screening and sorting emergency situations

75. Which of the following is a correct form for an inside street address of a business letter?
    A. Fourth Street
    B. 5th Street
    C. One Twelfth Street
    D. 3 Seventh St
    E. Nine Eleventh Dr

76. An independent practice association (IPA) is a type of
    A. Blue Cross and Blue Shield provider
    B. Medicare
    C. Medicaid
    D. HMO
    E. PPO

77. Which of the following is a correct signature block?
    A. Brian Knight, Group Health Physician
    B. Brian Knight
       Group Health Physician
    C. Brian Knight
    D. Group Health Physician
       Brian Knight
    E. Brian
       Group Health Physician

78. Which of the following checks is available in foreign currency?
    A. Money order
    B. Certified check
    C. Traveler's check
    D. Voucher check
    E. Cashier's check

102. A check written by a bank against its funds in another bank is called a

A. Voucher check
B. Money order
C. Certified check
D. Third-party check
E. Bank draft

103. Hospice programs were developed to provide care for patients who are

A. Postoperative
B. Rehabilitative
C. Terminally ill
D. Chronically ill
E. Acutely ill

104. A patient's medical fees come to a total of $90 from a participating provider. What can you bill the patient if the EOB lists the following itemization?

Charges: $90
Not Eligible for Payment: $12
Allowed Charge: $78
Applied to Deductible: $30
Copayment: $10
Amount Due from Carrier: $38

A. $38
B. $10
C. $40
D. $30
E. $42

105. Which of the following is the most secure way to mail something through the U.S. Postal Service?

A. Certified Mail
B. Insured Mail
C. Registered Mail
D. First Class Mail
E. Priority Mail

106. Which act funds Social Security?

A. Federal Insurance Contribution Act
B. Federal Unemployment Tax Act
C. Employer Tax Identification Number Act
D. Health Care Financing Administration Act
E. General Accounting Office Act

107. Which special service assures that mail is delivered only to a specific addressee or to someone authorized in writing to receive mail for the addressee?

A. Registered mail
B. Restricted delivery
C. Address service
D. Insured mail
E. COD

108. What action can you take when you realize that you have mailed something you did not intend to?

A. Nothing; once an item is mailed, it will be delivered
B. Ask the carrier to give you the item back
C. Fill out a written application at the post office to recall the mail, and attach an identically addressed envelope
D. Intercept it before it gets delivered to the addressee
E. Present a receipt of mailing or Certificate of Mailing at the addressee's post office

109. What information should be included in a patient's medical records?

A. Patient registration form
B. Laboratory test results
C. Copies of prescriptions
D. Informed consent forms
E. All of the above

110. Which of the following proofreaders' symbols means "move text to the right"?

A. ?
B. ^
C. lc
D.]
E. [

111. On January 1, the petty cash account balance was $150. On January 18, the balance of the petty cash account is $85. How much should the petty cash vouchers total on January 18?

A. $35
B. $65
C. $75
D. $95
E. $135

112. Which of the following is a scheduling method in which patients sign in and are seen on a first-come, first-served basis?

A. Numerical
B. Subject
C. Alphabetical
D. Chronological
E. Geographical

113. According to the American Medical Association, how long should you keep patient records after the patient's final visit?

A. 5 years
B. 10 years
C. 3 years
D. 7 years
E. Permanently

114. Which of the following acts provides federal income tax advantages to individuals who buy certain long-term care insurance policies?

   A. The Patient Self-Determination Act
   B. The Health Insurance Portability and Accountability Act
   C. The Clinical Laboratory Improvement Act
   D. The Health Maintenance Organization Act
   E. The Uniform Anatomical Gift Act

115. Which of the following notations indicates a V code that can only be used as a secondary diagnosis?

   A. MSP
   B. PDX
   C. NOS
   D. SDx
   E. DEF

116. TRICARE was formerly known as

   A. CHAMPVA
   B. CHAMPUS
   C. BCBS
   D. RBRVS
   E. Medicaid

117. Which of the following checks can be accepted without risk?

   A. A third-party check
   B. A check drawn on an out-of-town bank
   C. A check postdated 5 days
   D. A check predated 20 days
   E. None of the above

118. Which of the following steps should you take when you receive new supplies?

   A. Inventory all supplies
   B. Send back old supplies to the supplier
   C. Throw out all old supplies
   D. Place them in the front of the supply area
   E. Place them in the back of the supply area

119. What type of software is often used for accounting procedures?

   A. Word processing
   B. Mathematical
   C. Spreadsheet
   D. Graphical
   E. Calculator

120. Which of the following is a slow type of memory that uses the hard disk?

   A. Virtual
   B. ROM
   C. RAM
   D. Cache
   E. None of the above

121. Which of the following features of a transcription machine is most useful when the physician speaks quickly?

   A. Tone control
   B. Speed of the typist
   C. Indicator strip
   D. Volume control
   E. Stop-and-start control

122. When should you collate patient records?

   A. Once a month
   B. The day before a patient is seen
   C. The day a patient is seen, while the patient is in the waiting room
   D. Once a week
   E. Once a day

123. Which of the following is used for recording the difference between the debit and credit columns?

   A. Balance column
   B. Adjustment column
   C. Trial balance
   D. Credit balance
   E. Journal column

124. In each journal entry in a double-entry accounting system, the dollar amount of a debit must be equal to the dollar amount of a

   A. Receivable
   B. Credit
   C. Balance
   D. Equity
   E. None of the above

125. Overdue accounts are identified by

   A. Skip tracing
   B. Cycle billing
   C. Account aging
   D. Cost accounting
   E. Utilization review

126. Which of the following extensions is used in the website address for the American Association of Medical Assistants?

    A. .net
    B. .org
    C. .edu
    D. .com
    E. .gov

127. For which of the following reasons might a claim be denied?

    A. No preauthorization has been obtained
    B. The claim is not for a covered benefit
    C. The patient has a preexisting condition that is not covered
    D. Services were provided before the waiting period was up
    E. All of the above

128. An unpredictable small cash expenditure, such as buying a cup of coffee for a visiting physician, can be covered by a(n)

    A. Superbill
    B. Emergency bill
    C. Petty cash fund
    D. Bank draft
    E. Money order

129. If an insurance company has rejected a claim because no preauthorization was obtained, what should your medical office do?

    A. Write a letter of appeal, and review the patient's contract
    B. Bill the patient
    C. Resubmit the claim with proper preauthorization
    D. Call the carrier, and take the company to court if necessary
    E. Write off the claim as a loss

130. Which of the following statements is true about Medicare claims processing?

    A. Providers are encouraged but not required to use the CMS-1500 form
    B. Medicare forms are signed only by the patient
    C. Nonparticipating providers are required to accept assignment
    D. The allowable payment to nonparticipating providers is less than the allowable payment to participating providers
    E. None of the above

131. When a patient has both Medicare and Medicaid,

    A. You need to prepare two forms and file with Medicare first
    B. Claims are automatically forwarded from Medicare to Medicaid
    C. Claims no longer need to be filed on a CMS-1500
    D. You need to file with Medicaid and Medicare at the same time, dividing the claim amounts equally
    E. You need to file the claim with Medicaid first and then with Medicare

132. Which of the following statements is true of TRICARE claims processing?

    A. The patient may be billed for the entire deductible and the coinsurance portion of the allowed charge
    B. If the office does not accept assignment from TRICARE, the patient has to submit the claim forms
    C. The claim forms are always filed by the office, using the CMS-1500
    D. Both A and C
    E. Both A and B

133. Which of the following types of information is included in office policy manuals?

    A. Specifications for personal appearance
    B. Employer insurance contributions
    C. Employee health records
    D. Employee salaries
    E. Employee progress reports

134. Which of the following mail types will guarantee overnight delivery?

    A. Special Delivery First-Class
    B. Registered First-Class
    C. Certified First-Class
    D. Priority
    E. Express

135. According to the Truth in Lending Act, a written agreement is required if a patient agrees to pay his or her debt in a minimum of how many installments?

    A. Two
    B. Three
    C. Four
    D. Five
    E. Six

136. Rubber bands and staples are
    A. Incidental supplies
    B. Vital supplies
    C. Capital equipment
    D. Clinical supplies
    E. General supplies

137. Open-ended questions
    A. Should never be asked of patients
    B. Should be asked of all patients
    C. Should be asked of adults, but not of children
    D. Should be asked of children, but not of adults
    E. Should be asked of difficult patients only

138. Medicare claims must be filed by which of the following dates for services rendered during the previous year?
    A. February 28
    B. March 31
    C. June 15
    D. September 30
    E. December 31

139. What percentage of a practice's gross income should be devoted to purchasing supplies?
    A. Not more than 3%
    B. Not more than 20%
    C. Not more than 6%
    D. Not more than 15%
    E. Not more than 50%

140. Which of the following items serves as a reminder to the patient?
    A. A legal record
    B. An appointment book
    C. An appointment card
    D. An encounter form
    E. Any of the above

141. The most common scheduling system used in urgent care centers is
    A. Open booking
    B. Wave
    C. Modified wave
    D. Stream
    E. Cluster

142. Scheduling two or more patients in the same time slot is called
    A. Wave scheduling
    B. Advance scheduling
    C. Double booking
    D. Modified wave scheduling
    E. Doubled open hours

143. Which of the following statements is true of workers' compensation claims processing?
    A. Records of a workers' compensation case should be kept with the patient's regular medical records
    B. The medical office bills the patient, who then is responsible for submitting claims to the insurance carrier
    C. The injured person's records must be personally signed by the physician
    D. The insurance carrier gets only a claim but no other records
    E. The injured person pays the medical bills and can file claims with the insurance company later

144. When you receive a monthly statement from the practice's bank, you should first
    A. Initial and file the statement with other financial records
    B. Reconcile the bank statement with the practice's own checkbook balances and contact the bank if you notice any discrepancies
    C. Note when the account was opened and compare this date to the date listed in your records
    D. Review the caption for the total value of checks processed, the total amount of deposits made, the account's beginning and ending balance, and that month's closing date
    E. Both B and D

145. A patient whose 65th birthday was yesterday arrives at your medical office. Under the guidelines of the Social Security Act, she is now entitled to receive benefits under which of the following programs?
    A. Workers' compensation
    B. CHAMPUS
    C. Medicaid
    D. Medicare Part A
    E. Medicare Part B

146. Which of the following types of filing systems is most appropriate for the research materials maintained by a physician
    A. Tickler
    B. Numerical
    C. Subject
    D. Alphabetical
    E. Geographical

147. Computer memory is usually measured in

    A. Inches
    B. Cubic centimeters
    C. Processor time
    D. Megahertz
    E. Bytes

148. A nonnegotiable check issued for the payment of debts by an insurance company is called a

    A. Warrant
    B. Voucher check
    C. Bank draft
    D. Limited check
    E. Money order

149. When you receive a check as payment from a patient, you should

    A. Endorse it immediately and write "For deposit only" on its back
    B. Endorse it and deposit it as soon as possible
    C. Use a qualified endorsement by writing *Without recourse* above the signature
    D. Write *for deposit only* on the back and deposit it with your bank
    E. None of the above

150. What should a medical office do when its collection efforts have failed?

    A. Collect through the court system
    B. Collect through a collection agency
    C. Keep sending bills to the patient and also allow a collection agency to follow up with the account
    D. Write off the debt
    E. Either A or B

151. An addition to an insurance policy is called a(n)

    A. Addendum
    B. Rider
    C. Expansion
    D. Premium
    E. Appendix

152. Which of the following acts requires that creditors provide applicants with accurate and complete credit costs and terms, clearly and obviously?

    A. Truth in Lending Act
    B. Fair Credit Reporting Act
    C. Fair Debt Collection Practices Act
    D. Equal Credit Opportunity Act
    E. Reasonable Collection and Credit Act

153. Which of the following accounts is the most typical for patients of a medical practice?

    A. Written-contract account
    B. Single-entry account
    C. Open-book account
    D. Standard payment account
    E. Double-entry account

154. When a mistake has been made in billing, you should

    A. Rebill, noting the changes on the copy of the original form and writing Second Billing at the top
    B. Hope that the insurance provider will not notice any mistakes
    C. Wait until the insurance provider asks for corrections
    D. Trace the original claim
    E. Both C and D

155. Educational charts, sound recordings, and films are often sent as

    A. Special Standard Mail
    B. Standard Mail (C)
    C. Library Mail
    D. Standard Mail (A)
    E. Parcel Post

156. Payroll tax deductions are also called

    A. Net pay
    B. Gross pay
    C. Withholding
    D. Unused vacation pay
    E. Holiday pay

157. The nonremovable magnetic medium inside a computer where information is stored is called a

    A. Hard drive
    B. Keyboard
    C. Modem
    D. Mouse
    E. CD-ROM

158. The amounts a physician owes to others for equipment and services are called

    A. Payrolls
    B. Accounts payable
    C. Accounts receivable
    D. Delinquent accounts
    E. Payments

159. Which of the following tools is useful in showing the status of each account at a glance?

A. Single-entry account list
B. Collection ratio
C. Accounts receivable ratio
D. Aging accounts receivable
E. Open-book account list

160. All of the following are advantages of electronic banking over traditional banking except

A. Increased productivity
B. Increased accuracy
C. Greater control of cash flow
D. Ease of depositing checks
E. Computerized check access

161. According to the CPT, when coding an insurance claim for a tonsillectomy, the code should be listed under which of the following body systems?

A. Integumentary
B. Respiratory
C. Reproductive
D. Endocrine
E. Cardiovascular

162. The postal abbreviation for Minnesota is

A. MT
B. MN
C. MI
D. MA
E. MS

163. Which of the following systems is the least structured of all the scheduling systems?

A. Open hours
B. Wave scheduling
C. Advance scheduling
D. Modified wave scheduling
E. Double booking

164. Which act requires credit bureaus to supply correct and complete information to businesses to use in evaluating a person's application for credit?

A. Equal Credit Opportunity Act
B. Fair Credit Reporting Act
C. Fair Debt Collection Practices Act
D. Truth in Lending Act
E. All of the above

165. Being firm and standing up for oneself while showing respect for others is called

A. Rapport
B. Prejudice
C. Communication
D. Argumentativeness
E. Assertiveness

166. The most appropriate filing system for organizing and storing medical research material is

A. Tickler
B. Alphabetical
C. Subject
D. Numerical
E. Chronological

167. Balance billing refers to

A. A practice that all participating providers of an HMO engage in
B. Billing a third-party provider for all delinquent accounts
C. Billing the patient for the difference between the usual fee and the allowed charge
D. Auditing the office's billing practices
E. Comparing the bank statements to the practice's own financial records

168. Which of the following abbreviations refers to a procedural code book using a numerical system updated annually by the American Medical Association?

A. HCPCS
B. HCFA
C. ICD-9-CM
D. CPT
E. UCR

169. Which of the following types of file cabinet is the least efficient?

A. Movable
B. Open-shelf
C. Vertical
D. Office
E. Upright

170. What will happen when a physician in contract with an HMO plan exceeds the utilization norms set by the HMO?

A. The physician will not receive a withheld portion of the capitation payment
B. The physician will lose the contract with the HMO
C. The physician will have to switch to a fee-for-service payment option
D. All of the above
E. None of the above

171. In a network, a common connection point for the devices containing ports is called a

A. Microprocessor
B. Touch pad
C. Mouse
D. Control unit
E. Hub

172. Which of the following is determined by comparing the actual fee charged by physicians in the same specialty?

   A. Fee schedule
   B. Accepting assignment
   C. Usual fee
   D. Usual, customary, and reasonable (UCR) fee
   E. Resource-Based Relative Value Scale

173. The term *point-of-service* refers to

   A. A type of HMO
   B. An option added to some HMO plans that allows patients to choose physicians outside the HMO network
   C. The geographic place where a medical service is performed
   D. The reasons given by a physician for performing a medical service
   E. The preauthorization some HMOs require

174. Encouraging patients to think through and answer their own questions and concerns is called

   A. Focusing
   B. Restating
   C. Reflecting
   D. Stressing
   E. Completing

175. When using ICD-9-CM codes, which of the following will occur when the fourth and fifth digits are omitted?

   A. Third-party downcoding
   B. Third-party upcoding
   C. Faster payments
   D. Increased payments
   E. Claim denials

176. Which type of filing cabinet requires the least amount of room?

   A. Vertical
   B. Movable
   C. Four-drawer
   D. Open-shelf
   E. None of the above

177. Unconsciously returning to more infantile thoughts or behaviors is referred to as

   A. Repression
   B. Regression
   C. Substitution
   D. Rationalization
   E. Introjection

178. A single computer that can be accessed by other computers over a network is called a(n)

   A. Server
   B. Software-driven computer
   C. Operating system
   D. Modem computer
   E. Application computer

179. Which of the following files is used as a reminder?

   A. Subject
   B. Numerical
   C. Inactive
   D. Cue
   E. Tickler

180. On the outside of an envelope, the postal abbreviation for *Plaza* is

   A. Plaz
   B. P
   C. PL
   D. Pla
   E. PLZ

181. An example of negative communication is

   A. Verbalizing
   B. Smiling naturally
   C. Mumbling
   D. Speaking slowly
   E. Speaking clearly

182. When someone calls inquiring about a bill,

   A. You should transfer the caller to the nurse on duty
   B. You should transfer the caller to the physician
   C. Handle the call yourself
   D. Transfer the caller to the answering service
   E. Transfer the caller to the appropriate insurance provider

183. The worldwide database of people covered by CHAMPUS or TRICARE is called

   A. CHAMPVA
   B. DEERS
   C. BCBS
   D. HCPCS
   E. EOB

184. How long should copies of all bills and order forms for supplies be kept on file, in case the practice is audited by the IRS?

   A. 1 year
   B. 3 years
   C. 5 years
   D. 10 years
   E. Indefinitely

185. When a patient has both Medicaid and CHAMPVA,
    A. You should file the claim with Medicaid
    B. You should file the claim with Medicaid first, then with CHAMPVA
    C. You should file the claim with CHAMPVA first, then with Medicaid
    D. You should file the claim with both Medicaid and CHAMPVA at the same time
    E. The patient is responsible for filing these claims

186. Which of the following programs may offer the highest level of benefits to enrollees when they obtain services from a designated physician, hospital, or other health provider?
    A. Health maintenance organization
    B. Preferred provider organization
    C. Kaiser Foundation Health Plan
    D. Independent practice association
    E. Indemnity policy

187. Which portion of the CMS-1500 form contains physician or supplier information?
    A. The first part
    B. The middle part
    C. The last part
    D. Both A and B
    E. The form does not include physician or supplier information

188. After opening the mail, one of your duties as a medical assistant might be to
    A. Enunciate
    B. Proofread
    C. Edit
    D. Rewrite
    E. Annotate

189. When performing diagnostic coding, you use the
    A. *Physicians' Current Procedural Terminology*
    B. Health Care Procedural Coding System
    C. *International Classification of Diseases, 9th Revision, Clinical Modification* (ICD–9–CM)
    D. National Standard Format
    E. Health Care Financing Administration

190. Anesthesiology is a section of which type of coding?
    A. CPT
    B. ICD
    C. DRG
    D. RBRVS
    E. MFS

191. Each new employee must complete which of the following federal income tax forms at the time of hiring?
    A. W-2
    B. W-4
    C. 941
    D. 1099
    E. 1094

192. What is the time limit on refiling a denied Medicare charge?
    A. 7 days
    B. 30 days
    C. 3 months
    D. 6 months
    E. 12 months

193. Whose telephone calls require the immediate attention of the physician?
    A. Pharmacists
    B. Consulting physicians
    C. Hospital staff nurses
    D. The physician's family
    E. Important patients

194. Which of the following types of correspondence can be signed by the medical assistant?
    A. Consultation reports
    B. Referral letters
    C. Termination letters
    D. Letters to other physicians
    E. Insurance paperwork

195. Which of the following forms must be filed as the employer's quarterly federal tax return?
    A. W-2
    B. W-4
    C. 941
    D. 1099
    E. 1094

196. The annual deductible for recipients of Medicare Part B benefits is
    A. $20
    B. $50
    C. $80
    D. $100
    E. $115

197. Which of the following groups present the most common collection problem?
    A. Patients with hardship cases
    B. Younger adults
    C. Partially insured individuals
    D. Male patients
    E. Foreign patients

ADMINISTRATIVE

198. The "brain" of the computer is called the
    A. Central processing unit (CPU)
    B. Read-only memory (ROM)
    C. Random-access memory (RAM)
    D. Video display terminal (VDT)
    E. Cathode ray tube (CRT)

199. The body of a business letter begins
    A. Two lines below the salutation or subject line
    B. On the line immediately below the salutation or subject line
    C. Three lines below the salutation or subject line
    D. Two lines below the letterhead
    E. One line below the inside address

200. Notations on a business letter are placed
    A. Below the letterhead
    B. Two lines below the signature block or identification line
    C. Anywhere at the end of the letter
    D. Below the complimentary closing
    E. At the very bottom of the last page

201. In an accounting system, how should a debit balance on a patient ledger card be entered?
    A. Income
    B. Accounts receivable
    C. Payment
    D. Charge
    E. Debit

202. Which of the following persons is the principal in an insurance contract?
    A. Subscriber
    B. Beneficiary
    C. Insurer
    D. Coordinator
    E. None of the above

203. When a patient away from home on vacation consults a physician, the patient most likely is given
    A. An open account
    B. A single-entry account
    C. A one-time account
    D. A vacation account
    E. A holiday account

204. The numerals appearing in the lower left corner of a check, which are printed in magnetic ink, represent which of the following codes or numbers?
    A. NSF
    B. ABA number
    C. MICR code
    D. Dollars
    E. Bank code name

205. All of the following insurance programs are sponsored by the federal government except:
    A. TRICARE
    B. CHAMPVA
    C. Medicaid
    D. Workers' compensation
    E. Medicare

206. The abbreviation *NS* indicates
    A. New surgery
    B. Nasal cavity
    C. No-show patient
    D. Not submitted
    E. Not sanitized

207. Which of the following ratios measures how fast outstanding accounts are being paid?
    A. Collection ratio
    B. Payment ratio
    C. Accounts receivable ratio
    D. Delinquency ratio
    E. Percentage

208. Before submitting a claim for rebilling, you should
    A. Call the staff of the insurance carrier to alert them to a second billing
    B. Write the words *Second Billing* in red letters at the top of a copy of the original claim form
    C. Review procedures and then write off the debt, because the insurance company will automatically reject a rebilled claim
    D. Make a photocopy of the original claim and send it to the insurance carrier
    E. None of the above

209. In the color-coded filing system, purple includes which part of the alphabet?
    A. E through H
    B. I through N
    C. O through Q
    D. R through Z
    E. A through L

210. Which of the following devices can convert printed matter and images into information that can be interpreted by the computer?
    A. Touch screen
    B. Modem
    C. Keyboard
    D. Hard drive
    E. Scanner

211. On letters and packages, handling instructions such as *Personal* or *Confidential* are printed
    A. Two lines above the address
    B. Three lines below the postage
    C. Three lines below the return address
    D. Across from the address, on the same line
    E. Anywhere on the envelope where there might be room

212. Which of the following is a correct way to write the date on a letter?
    A. December 5, '02
    B. Dec. 5, 2002
    C. 12/5/02
    D. 12/05/2002
    E. December 5, 2002

213. Where does the dateline go on a letter?
    A. Two or three lines below the letterhead, about 15 lines ($2\frac{1}{2}$ inches) down the page
    B. Right below the letterhead, about 12 lines (2 inches) down the page
    C. To the right of the letterhead, at the same level with the last line on the letterhead
    D. One line above the letterhead
    E. None of the above

214 The postal abbreviation for *Expressway* is
    A. EX
    B. EP
    C. EXPY
    D. EW
    E. E

215. Which of the following information is most important to give to a new patient?
    A. Policy on prescription refills
    B. Office hours and payment requirements
    C. List of local specialists
    D. List of local pharmacies
    E. List of local hospitals

216. When you need to divide a word in a business letter, which of the following rules can you apply?
    A. You can divide after a prefix
    B. You can divide according to pronunciation
    C. You can divide between two consonants that appear between vowels
    D. All of the above
    E. None of the above

217. Which of the following terms refers to computer software operations that obtain a saved file?
    A. Retrieving
    B. Formatting
    C. Editing
    D. Creating
    E. Merging

218. A letter in which all the lines are flush left is
    A. In modified-block style
    B. In full-block style
    C. In simplified style
    D. A standard letter
    E. A left-flush letter

219. Which type of check endorsement is "For deposit only"?
    A. Restricted
    B. Limited
    C. Open
    D. Qualified
    E. Certified

220. What type of HMO employs its own physicians?
    A. Group model HMO
    B. Cost containment HMO
    C. Fee-for-service HMO
    D. Staff model HMO
    E. Point-of-service HMO

221. Which of the following guidelines applies to writing business letters in a medical office?
    A. The text in the body of the letter should always be double-spaced
    B. Insert an extra line between paragraphs
    C. On the second page, use letterhead and put the name of the addressee, the page number, the date, and the subject in a header
    D. Both A and C
    E. All of the above

222. The most common insurance claim form is the
    A. CPT form
    B. Charge sheet
    C. Superbill
    D. HCPCS
    E. CMS-1500

223. Which of the following keys are used to activate the calculator function on a computer keyboard?
    A. Shift/F1
    B. Shift/F4
    C. Num Lock
    D. Ctrl/Tab
    E. Ctrl/Alt/Delete

224. Bill Joentis went to a participating provider to receive a single treatment for which the provider usually charges $300. The allowed charge for such a service as prescribed by Bill's insurance carrier is $280, and Bill's copayment is $10 for each visit. How much is the provider allowed to charge Bill?

A. $10
B. $30
C. $20
D. $28
E. $38

225. According to the Labor Standards Act, employee health records should be kept for

A. 1 year
B. 2 years
C. 3 years
D. 5 years
E. 7 years

226. The process of removing outdated data from computer disks or drives is called

A. Retrieving
B. Word processing
C. Transcribing
D. Booting
E. Purging

227. Mimicking the behavior of another person in order to cope with feelings of inadequacy is called

A. Introjection
B. Identification
C. Projection
D. Compensation
E. Regression

228. Which of the following proofreaders' marks means "to center"?

A.]
B. [
C. —
D.][
E. n

229. In patient charting, which of the following abbreviations is used to note a prescription?

A. RS
B. Pt
C. Rx
D. P&P
E. CBC

230. Which of the following types of U.S. Postal Service mail guarantees overnight delivery?

A. Priority
B. Registered
C. First class
D. Express
E. Certified

231. The diseases within the Tabular List of the ICD-9-CM are organized

A. Alphabetically
B. By symptoms
C. Chronologically
D. By the external cause of injury
E. By body system

232. Which of the following is the most common pointing device for a computer?

A. Keyboard
B. Trackball
C. Mouse
D. Motherboard
E. Hard drive

233. Which of the following postal abbreviations is used to represent North Carolina?

A. NA
B. NB
C. NC
D. ND
E. NH

234. According to OSHA, how often must an exposure control plan be reviewed and updated?

A. Every month
B. Every 6 months
C. Every 9 months
D. Every 12 months
E. Every 18 months

235. Which of the following computer keys moves the cursor to a preset position?

A. Tab
B. Shift
C. Insert
D. Enter
E. Spacebar

236. In the CPT, which of the following codes refers to *Evaluation and Management*?

A. 00100
B. 10040
C. 70010
D. 90281
E. 99201

ADMINISTRATIVE

237. A detailed outline prepared for the physician that includes the trip location, date of arrival, and confirmation of hotel reservations is known as a(n)

   A. Written confirmation
   B. Reservation
   C. Itinerary
   D. Agenda
   E. Statement

238. Which of the following business letter closures is considered the most appropriate for a medical office?

   A. Sincerely yours
   B. Respectfully
   C. Yours truly
   D. Best wishes
   E. Regards

239. A list of the specific items to be discussed at a meeting is known as the

   A. Minutes
   B. Meeting schedule
   C. Agenda
   D. Meeting announcement
   E. Itinerary

240. If a medical record has been temporarily removed, it should be replaced by a(n)

   A. Out guide
   B. Index card
   C. Post-it note
   D. Cross-referenced card
   E. Divider guide

241. CPT codes are organized into how many sections?

   A. Two
   B. Three
   C. Five
   D. Six
   E. Nine

242. Which of the following patient information is essential to organizing and filing patient records in all types of filing systems?

   A. Social Security number
   B. Name
   C. Address
   D. Signs and symptoms
   E. Date of birth

243. Narcotics should be inventoried

   A. Daily
   B. Weekly
   C. Bi-weekly
   D. Monthly
   E. Yearly

244. The term *assets* refers to

   A. Notes payable
   B. Vendor inventory
   C. Bank debts
   D. Accounts receivable
   E. Accounts payable

245. Which of the following terms refers to turning on a computer?

   A. File
   B. Tab
   C. Boot
   D. Backup
   E. Byte

246. If you are processing payroll, which of the following should be calculated first?

   A. Net pay
   B. Federal income tax
   C. Social Security taxes
   D. Gross wages
   E. 401K

247. Which of the following postal abbreviations should be used for an envelope that is being sent to Phoenix?

   A. AK
   B. AR
   C. AZ
   D. AL
   E. NM

248. Which of the following forms is filed with an employee's state income tax return?

   A. W-2
   B. W-4
   C. W-9
   D. 940
   E. 940A

249. Which of the following federal statutes protects debtors from harassment?

   A. Federal Wage Garnishment Law
   B. Equal Credit Opportunity Act
   C. Fair Credit Reporting Act
   D. Fair Debt Collection Practices Act
   E. Americans With Disabilities Act

250. Which of the following patient information must be recorded when you are scheduling an appointment for a patient?

   A. Social Security number
   B. Age
   C. Telephone number
   D. Mailing address
   E. Date of birth

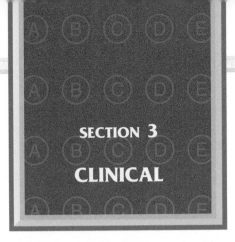

TEST FOR MEDICAL ASSISTING KNOWLEDGE

Self-Evaluation

After you have finished reading Chapters 15 through 24, set aside some time to take this sample exam. There are 250 questions in this section. You can take them all at once or in smaller portions. Try to time yourself and answer about 60 questions in 60 minutes. Read each question carefully and circle the best answer. After you are finished, turn to p. 570 in Part 3 for answers and rationales.

1. If a needlestick injury occurs, you should take all of the following actions except

   A. Washing your hands
   B. Documenting and reporting the injury
   C. Sending the report to the local health department
   D. Covering the injury
   E. Notifying your supervisor

2. Failure to comply with OSHA standards could result in penalties; the maximum penalty for the first violation is

   A. $700
   B. $1,700
   C. $7,000
   D. $10,000
   E. $15,000

3. Tetracyclines are

   A. Bactericidal antibiotics
   B. Bacteriostatic antibiotics
   C. Antiviral agents
   D. Norepinephrine
   E. Antiepileptic drugs

4. Which of the following microorganisms is the main blood-borne hazard for health-care workers?

   A. Hepatitis B virus
   B. Human immunodeficiency virus
   C. *Treponema pallidum*
   D. Cytomegalovirus
   E. Hepatitis E virus

5. Infected pregnant women can pass all of the following microorganisms to their babies during pregnancy or delivery except

   A. Syphilis
   B. Malaria
   C. HIV
   D. AIDS
   E. Hepatitis B virus

6. The early detection and treatment of a patient with Shigellosis prevents the spread of infectious disease by interrupting the chain of transmission at which of the following levels?

   A. Susceptible host
   B. Reservoir host
   C. Mode of transmission
   D. Means of entry
   E. Means of exit

7. Which of the following positions is also called the recumbent position?

   A. Fowler's
   B. Sims'
   C. Lithotomy
   D. Supine
   E. Prone

8. What does an antihypertensive drug do?

   A. It regulates the heartbeat
   B. It prevents and controls high blood pressure
   C. It prevents and relieves convulsions
   D. It prevents and decreases perspiration
   E. It controls cholesterol levels in the blood

9. The medical assistant's most effective means of preventing the spread of infection from one patient to another is to

   A. Wear a gown and mask
   B. Wear sterile gloves
   C. Disinfect the examination table
   D. Wash one's hands after each patient
   E. Disinfect the instruments

10. Which of the following is the most appropriate method of sterilizing hemostat forceps?

    A. Ultrasound
    B. Steam under pressure
    C. Gas sterilization
    D. Alcohol
    E. Dry heat

11. A measurement of the actual absorbed dose of radiation is called

    A. Rad
    B. Scan
    C. X-ray
    D. Radioactivity
    E. Radioisotope

12. Which of the following crutch gaits can be used by patients who can bear full weight on one leg and no weight on the other?

    A. Swing-to
    B. Four-point
    C. Three-point
    D. Two-point
    E. Both A and D

13. Which of the following radiological studies requires the patient to fast for 12 hours prior to the procedure?

    A. Magnetic resonance imaging of the spinal cord
    B. Angiography
    C. Nuclear medicine scan of the liver
    D. Computed tomography of the skull
    E. Upper gastrointestinal X-ray series

14. The drug of choice for Lyme disease is

    A. Penicillin
    B. Fluconazole
    C. Tetracycline
    D. Metronidazole
    E. Cephalosporin

15. Mr. Brown, who is 39 years old, received second- and third-degree burns on his chest, abdomen, upper back, and genital area. Which of the following is an estimation of the extent of his burn?

    A. 20%
    B. 28%
    C. 48%
    D. 53%
    E. 68%

16. A cut with jagged edges is called a(n)

    A. Incision
    B. Abrasion
    C. Laceration
    D. Puncture
    E. Contusion

17. The majority of accidental poisonings occur at home to children under the age of

    A. 7 years
    B. 10 years
    C. 5 years
    D. 6 years
    E. 8 years

18. A prescription reads: Ibuprofen 200 mg tabs 2 q 4–6 hr prn fever. Which of the following is indicated by the abbreviation *prn*?

    A. Every day
    B. Twice a day
    C. As needed
    D. At bedtime
    E. After meals

19. Each of the following is part of the AIDS virus infection cycle <u>except</u>
    A. Acute HIV infection
    B. AIDS-non-related complex
    C. AIDS-related complex
    D. Asymptomatic latency period
    E. Full-blown AIDS

20. The study of drugs and their actions in the body is called
    A. Pharmacognosy
    B. Pharmacy
    C. Pharmacology
    D. Posology
    E. Pharmacodynamics

21. Which of the following positions is similar to the jackknife position in that the patient's hips are flexed at a 90-degree angle?
    A. Trendelenburg's
    B. Proctological
    C. Knee-chest
    D. Prone
    E. Supine

22. Which of the following is a sign of shock?
    A. Bradycardia
    B. Tachycardia
    C. Bradypnea
    D. Hypertension
    E. Hot flash

23. A barium swallow is also called
    A. Barium enema
    B. Lower GI series
    C. Upper GI series
    D. Gastric lavage
    E. Gastric substance

24. Yeast infections may be caused by which of the following organisms?
    A. *Trichomonas vaginalis*
    B. *Clostridium perfringens*
    C. *Yersinia pestis*
    D. *Candida albicans*
    E. *Gardnerella vaginalis*

25. Destroying abnormal cells by the use of freezing temperatures is called
    A. Electrosurgery
    B. Electrocautery
    C. Laser surgery
    D. Cryosurgery
    E. Heat therapy

26. An example of an emulsion is
    A. Cod liver oil
    B. Tylenol elixir®
    C. Nutraderm lotion®
    D. Aromatic spirits of ammonia
    E. None of the above

27. In the metric system, 1000 micrograms equal
    A. 1 milligram
    B. 1 gram
    C. 1 kilogram
    D. 1 grain
    E. 1 wheat

28. Which of the following ECG curves represents recovery of the ventricles?
    A. P wave
    B. QRS complex
    C. T wave
    D. U wave
    E. QRS

29. A drug that has no pharmacological activity because it contains no active ingredients is known as
    A. Placebo
    B. Teratogen
    C. Synergistic
    D. Melanin
    E. Fluconazole

30. If you are performing a 3-hour glucose tolerance test, you should instruct an adult patient to drink a liquid that contains how many grams of glucose?
    A. 15
    B. 30
    C. 50
    D. 75
    E. 100

31. Thyroxine is classified as which of the following types of drugs?
    A. Therapeutic
    B. Replacement
    C. Diagnostic
    D. Prophylactic
    E. Palliative

32. Which of the following agents are used to relieve itching?

    A. Antipyretics
    B. Antihypertensives
    C. Antidiuretics
    D. Antitussives
    E. Antipruritics

33. Which of the following medical instruments is used to examine the pressure of the eyes?

    A. Penlight
    B. Ophthalmoscope
    C. Tonometer
    D. Otoscope
    E. Goniometer

34. Which of the following foods is an excellent source of potassium?

    A. Rice
    B. Eggs
    C. Yogurt
    D. Bananas
    E. Cheese

35. Which of the following drugs is an example of a Schedule V drug?

    A. Diazepam
    B. Lomotil®
    C. Amphetamine
    D. Heroin
    E. Talwin®

36. Microscopic structures in urine that are composed of protein are called

    A. Squamous epithelial cells
    B. Calcium oxalate crystals
    C. White blood cells
    D. Red blood cells
    E. Casts

37. All of the following waves on the ECG curve upward except

    A. Q
    B. T
    C. R
    D. P
    E. U

38. All of the following waves are part of one heartbeat on an ECG tracing except

    A. P
    B. V
    C. Q
    D. R
    E. T

39. Which of the following statements is not true regarding the preparation of a patient for MRI?

    A. The patient should avoid caffeine for 4 hours before the examination
    B. The patient should not wear eye makeup
    C. The patient should avoid alcohol for 4 hours before the procedure
    D. The patient should be asked whether any internal metallic materials are present
    E. The patient should not have a pacemaker

40. Which of the following studies does not use radiation to produce images?

    A. MRI
    B. CT scan
    C. PET scan
    D. Fluoroscopy
    E. Flat plate X-ray study

41. The flat surface of a microscope that holds the slide for viewing is called the

    A. Nosepiece
    B. Objective
    C. Stage
    D. Illuminator
    E. Condenser

42. Renal function is assessed by measuring which of the following serum levels?

    A. Leukocytes
    B. Blood amylase
    C. Blood glucose tolerance
    D. Blood urea nitrogen
    E. Aspartate aminotransferase

43. The angle of insertion of a needle for intradermal injections is

    A. 5 degrees
    B. 15 degrees
    C. 30 degrees
    D. 45 degrees
    E. 90 degrees

44. Spirometry tests measure the function of which of the following body systems?

    A. Reproductive
    B. Respiratory
    C. Integumentary
    D. Cardiovascular
    E. Urinary

45. Which of the following terms describes an agent that relieves symptoms without curing the disease?

   A. Palliative
   B. Prophylactic
   C. Diagnostic
   D. Replacement
   E. Therapeutic

46. Which of the following terms indicates increased appetite?

   A. Polyclonia
   B. Polycythemia
   C. Polydipsia
   D. Polyphagia
   E. Polyuria

47. Which of the following statements is <u>not</u> true of echocardiography?

   A. It evaluates the inner structures of the heart
   B. Echoes are obtained and heard by a stethoscope
   C. Echoes are obtained by ultrasound
   D. Echoes are recorded on paper
   E. Echoes can be used to detect the buildup of fluid

48. Which of the following techniques can show a detailed cross-section of tissue structure?

   A. MRI
   B. Myelogram
   C. EEG
   D. CT
   E. Mammogram

49. Which of the following is included in a patient's vital signs?

   A. Visual acuity
   B. Respiration rate
   C. Height and weight
   D. Head circumference
   E. Reflexes

50. Which of the following measures is equivalent to 500 mg?

   A. 0.5 g
   B. 1.0 g
   C. 2.5 g
   D. 5.0 g
   E. 10.0 g

51. Total surgical scrub (hand washing) time should be approximately

   A. 2 minutes
   B. 3 minutes
   C. 5 minutes
   D. 10 minutes
   E. 15 minutes

52. Which of the following malignancies is the most common HIV-related cancer?

   A. Osteosarcoma
   B. Kaposi's sarcoma
   C. Melanoma
   D. Leukemia
   E. Bronchogenic carcinoma

53. Destruction of all living microorganisms by specific means is called

   A. Sterilization
   B. Disinfection
   C. Sanitization
   D. Ultrasonic cleaning
   E. Both B and D

54. Which of the following terms is used by OSHA to describe the use of physical or chemical means to remove, inactivate, or destroy blood-borne pathogens?

   A. Decontamination
   B. Disinfection
   C. Sterilization
   D. Sanitization
   E. Distraction

55. When performing a venipuncture, it is necessary to

   A. Use sterile gloves
   B. Perform a surgical scrub at the venipuncture site
   C. Immediately recap the needle when finished
   D. Place the patient in the Trendelenburg position
   E. Use a tourniquet

56. Radiation exposure badges are also called

   A. Radiopaques
   B. Dosimeters
   C. Nuclear energy
   D. Scan meters
   E. Radiometers

57. When sending a specimen for a throat culture to an outside laboratory, which of the following substances should be used?
   A. Transport medium
   B. Agar medium
   C. Saline solution
   D. Fixative solution
   E. Hydrogen peroxide

58. *Atrial kick* is a term used for the surge of blood that is
   A. Pushed into the aorta as a result of ventricle contraction
   B. Pushed into the ventricle as a result of atrial contraction
   C. Pushed back into the arteries as a result of ventricle contraction
   D. Pushed back into the superior and inferior vena cava as a result of atrial contraction
   E. Leaving the ventricle

59. Which of the following is also called a bipolar lead?
   A. Precordial lead
   B. Augmented lead
   C. Standard lead
   D. Unconventional lead
   E. Conventional lead

60. The degree to which a joint is able to move is called
   A. Luxation
   B. Range of extension
   C. Range of flexion
   D. Range of motion
   E. Range of limitation

61. The style of walking is called
   A. Gag reflex
   B. Gait
   C. Gap phenomenon
   D. Gaze
   E. Hyperextension

62. When a patient lies on his or her back with lower legs supported by the extended foot rest, which position is he or she in?
   A. Radial
   B. Lithotomy
   C. Supine
   D. Prone
   E. Sims'

63. Which of the following substances in urine may indicate hyperglycemia?
   A. Bilirubin
   B. Protein
   C. Urea
   D. Glucose
   E. Ketone

64. Variation in the shape of erythrocytes is called
   A. Polychromasia
   B. Poikilocytosis
   C. Anisocytosis
   D. Polycythemia
   E. Microcytosis

65. A special container made of gelatin that is sized for a single dose is called a
   A. Tablet
   B. Troche
   C. Suppository
   D. Caplet
   E. Capsule

66. Which of the following federal agencies requires controlled substances to be stored in a locked cabinet?
   A. Food and Drug Administration
   B. Occupational Safety and Health Administration
   C. Drug Enforcement Administration
   D. Federal Department of Health and Human Services
   E. None of the above

67. How many limb leads are used in recording electrocardiograms?
   A. 3
   B. 6
   C. 10
   D. 12
   E. 13

68. In which of the following ranges is the normal specific gravity of urine?
   A. 1.010 and 1.030
   B. 1.015 and 1.035
   C. 1.020 and 1.040
   D. 1.025 and 1.045
   E. 1.025 and 1.050

69. Pneumococcal polysaccharide vaccine is administered to children or adolescents in one dose of 0.5 mL by which of the following routes?

    A. Intramuscular
    B. Intradermal
    C. Subcutaneous
    D. Sublingual
    E. Either A or C

70. Fasting specimens are preferred for which of the following tests?

    A. Creatinine
    B. Hemoglobin
    C. Globulin
    D. Albumin
    E. Triglycerides

71. The procedure for obtaining specimens from infected wounds is similar to which of the following?

    A. Pap smear
    B. Urine culture
    C. Sputum culture
    D. Stool culture
    E. Throat culture

72. Which of the following sphygmomanometers used to measure blood pressure is the most accurate?

    A. Electronic
    B. Aneroid
    C. Mercury
    D. Digital
    E. Both A and C

73. In which of the following positions does the patient lie face up with the knees flexed and the feet flat on the table?

    A. Dorsal recumbent
    B. Fowler's
    C. Prone
    D. Sims'
    E. Jackknife

74. The difference between systolic and diastolic blood pressure is called

    A. Pulse deficit
    B. Pulse pressure
    C. Unequal pressure
    D. Equal pressure
    E. Bounding pulse

75. The abbreviation *Tx* means

    A. Prescription
    B. Take
    C. Physical examination
    D. Treatment
    E. Contract

76. Which of the following arteries of the body is seldom used to take the pulse?

    A. Temporal
    B. Carotid
    C. Radial
    D. Femoral
    E. Brachial

77. Which of the following types of gloves are the most commonly used in the medical office?

    A. Nitrile
    B. Vinyl
    C. Sterol
    D. Cotton
    E. Latex

78. Lack of circulation due to a stoppage of blood flow is called

    A. Hypotension
    B. Blood stasis
    C. Myocardial infarction
    D. Stroke
    E. Phlebitis

79. A laboratory test for which of the following requires the use of serum or plasma?

    A. Bleeding time
    B. Hemoglobin
    C. Platelets
    D. Erythrocytes
    E. Cholesterol

80. A patient who has tuberculosis should use which of the following types of personal protective equipment?

    A. Gown
    B. Goggles
    C. Gloves
    D. Mask
    E. Drape

81. Sterilized instruments are considered to have a shelf life for
    A. 7 to 14 days
    B. 14 to 21 days
    C. 1 month
    D. 2 to 3 months
    E. 4 to 6 months

82. Which of the following forceps have sharp points that are useful in removing foreign objects?
    A. Dressing
    B. Towel
    C. Splinter
    D. Hemostatic
    E. Thumb

83. The following medication is prescribed for a patient: Erythromycin 500 mg bid × 7 days. The pharmacist has only the 250-mg dose in stock. How many 250-mg capsules will the pharmacist dispense to the patient?
    A. 7
    B. 14
    C. 21
    D. 28
    E. 42

84. In pregnancy testing, which of the following substances may be found in the patient's urine?
    A. Fluorescent treponemal antibody
    B. Human chorionic gonadotropin
    C. Follicle stimulating hormone
    D. Luteinizing hormone
    E. Thyroid stimulating hormone

85. Which of the following types of fractures means that the bone is crushed or splintered?
    A. Spiral
    B. Impacted
    C. Greenstick
    D. Comminuted
    E. Oblique

86. Which of the following procedures requires surgical asepsis?
    A. Digital-rectal examination
    B. Delivering a baby
    C. Aspiration of a bursa sac
    D. Flexible proctosigmoidoscopy
    E. Otoscopy

87. Which of the following ECG waves may indicate slow recovery of Purkinje fibers?
    A. P
    B. QRS
    C. T
    D. U
    E. V

88. In which of the following types of anemia may you find hemoglobin S?
    A. Iron-deficiency
    B. Aplastic
    C. Hemolytic
    D. Sickle cell
    E. Megaloblastic

89. Which of the following abbreviations should appear on a written prescription?
    A. Tx
    B. Rx
    C. Hx
    D. Fx
    E. Dx

90. The first step in responding to an emergency is to
    A. Survey the situation
    B. Shout at the patient
    C. Give oxygen
    D. Call 911
    E. Remain calm

91. Which of the following microorganisms is the most common cause of urinary tract infections?
    A. *Bacteroides fragilis*
    B. *Escherichia coli*
    C. *Proteus vulgaris*
    D. *Streptococcus pneumoniae*
    E. *Staphylococcus epidermidis*

92. A dispensing record must be kept on file for 2 years for which of the following scheduled drugs?
    A. I
    B. II
    C. III
    D. IV
    E. V

93. Which of the following instruments is used to examine the vagina?

    A. Laparoscope
    B. Otoscope
    C. Speculum
    D. Cystoscope
    E. Laryngoscope

94. Emergency pharmaceutical supplies should include which of the following basic drugs?

    A. Tylenol®
    B. Antitussives
    C. Vaseline®
    D. Epinephrine
    E. Antibiotics

95. Which of the following types of injections is used to administer antibiotics in a patient with streptococcoal pharyngitis?

    A. Subcutaneous
    B. Intradermal
    C. Intra-articular
    D. Intramuscular
    E. Intravenous

96. Abnormal black tarry stools that have a distinctive odor and contain digested blood are called

    A. Melanoma
    B. Melena
    C. Melatonin
    D. Melanin
    E. Megoloblastoma

97. Which of the following is the most appropriate type of specimen for detecting the presence of *Giardia lamblia*?

    A. Blood
    B. Urine
    C. Stool
    D. Saliva
    E. Sputum

98. Beginning at what age should children have annual checkups?

    A. 1 year
    B. 2 years
    C. 3 years
    D. 5 years
    E. 12 years

99. Alpha-fetoprotein testing from amniotic fluid is used for early diagnosis of which of the following?

    A. Fetal neural tube defects
    B. Fetal alcoholism
    C. Anencephaly
    D. Fetal drug addiction
    E. Both A and C

100. When using the high-power objective (45×), which of the following parts of the compound microscope is used to focus the image?

    A. Fine adjustment
    B. Revolving nosepiece
    C. Stage
    D. Coarse adjustment
    E. Eyepiece

101. Which of the following methods of collecting urine is the most common?

    A. Clean-catch midstream
    B. First-voided morning
    C. 24-hour
    D. Timed
    E. Random

102. The DEA requires

    A. That physicians register every 2 years
    B. That records be kept when drugs are dispensed
    C. That drugs be disposed of in the presence of a witness
    D. Both B and C
    E. All of the above

103. The best time to perform a breast self-examination is

    A. Immediately after the menstrual period is completed
    B. While showering in cold water
    C. While you are in bed
    D. After intercourse
    E. Before you sleep

104. All of the following statements about preparation for mammography are true except

    A. The patient should not use perfume on the underarm area or breasts before the examination
    B. The patient should avoid caffeine for a week
    C. The patient should avoid drinking water 2 hours prior to the procedure
    D. The patient should not use deodorant or powder on the underarm area or breasts before the examination
    E. Both A and D

105. Which of the following types of agents do physicians use to prevent cell growth in a malignant tumor?

    A. Beta-adrenergic blockers
    B. Anticoagulants
    C. Antineoplastics
    D. Antiseptics
    E. Antimicrobials

106. Annual vaccination may be indicated in some adolescents for which of the following diseases?

    A. Rabies
    B. Chickenpox
    C. Hepatitis A
    D. Influenza
    E. Hepatitis B

107. Which of the following is a slow crutch gait used by patients who can bear weight on both legs?

    A. Swing-to gait
    B. Two-point gait
    C. Three-point gait
    D. Four-point gait
    E. Five-point gait

108. In phlebotomy, at approximately what angle is the needle inserted into the vein?

    A. 10 degrees
    B. 15 degrees
    C. 30 degrees
    D. 45 degrees
    E. 90 degrees

109. The part of the prescription that contains the names and quantities of the ingredients is the

    A. Superscription
    B. Subscription
    C. Inscription
    D. Signature
    E. Drug label

110. Which of the following tests for color blindness may be administered by medical assistants?

    A. Snellen
    B. Weber's
    C. Rinne
    D. Ishihara
    E. Pap smear

111. Cocaine is a

    A. Schedule I drug
    B. Schedule II drug
    C. Schedule III drug
    D. Schedule IV drug
    E. Schedule V drug

112. Which of the following indicates a positive result of a tuberculin test?

    A. Papules
    B. Pustules
    C. Infection
    D. Infraction
    E. Induration

113. Serological tests are performed on samples collected in evacuation tubes with which stopper color?

    A. Blue
    B. Red
    C. Yellow
    D. Lavender
    E. Black

114. The position used to treat patients in shock is

    A. Jackknife
    B. Sims'
    C. Trendelenburg's
    D. Supine
    E. Standing

115. Which of the following terms means the displacement of bones at a joint?

    A. Sprain
    B. Strain
    C. Dislocation
    D. Fracture
    E. Inflammation

116. Which of the following techniques may prevent the extreme skin irritation and occasional discoloration caused by iron preparations?

    A. The Z-track method
    B. Deep IM injection
    C. IV injection
    D. Intradermal injection
    E. None of the above

117. In which of the following conditions may HCG levels be lower?

    A. First trimester of pregnancy
    B. Ectopic (tubal) pregnancy
    C. Hydatidiform mole
    D. Twin pregnancy
    E. Both A and D

118. Which of the following positions is suitable for the examination of the rectum for both male and female patients?

    A. Sims'
    B. Fowler's
    C. Jackknife
    D. Knee-chest
    E. Standing

119. Organisms that cause disease are called

    A. Fulminate
    B. Pathogens
    C. Acute
    D. Chronic
    E. Inflammation

120. The destruction of pathogens by physical or chemical means is called

    A. Sterilization
    B. Disinfection
    C. Asepsis
    D. Auscultation
    E. Pathogenesis

121. Hematemesis should be recorded under which of the following body systems?

    A. Integumentary
    B. Circulatory
    C. Respiratory
    D. Lymphatic
    E. Gastrointestinal

122. Which of the following types of drugs decreases appetite?

    A. Antiemetics
    B. Antacids
    C. Analgesics
    D. Anorectics
    E. Analeptics

123. The process of listening for sounds within the body is called

    A. Palpation
    B. Percussion
    C. Auscultation
    D. Menstruation
    E. Inspection

124. For injection of the vastus lateralis site, the patient may be in which of the following positions?

    A. Recumbent
    B. Knee-chest
    C. Standing
    D. Prone
    E. Trendelenburg's

125. Which of the following tests requires fasting specimens (that is, specimens taken after the patient has fasted)?

    A. Pregnancy
    B. Creatinine
    C. Hematocrit
    D. Triglyceride level
    E. Hemoglobin

126. A colposcopy is used for which of the following systems?

    A. Reproductive
    B. Respiratory
    C. Digestive
    D. Urinary
    E. Nervous

127. Which of the following instruments is used in measuring pressure of the intraocular region?

    A. Tuning fork
    B. Tonometer
    C. Ophthalmoscope
    D. Snellen chart
    E. Goniometer

128. Which of the following positions is the best for musculoskeletal and neurological examinations?

    A. Knee-chest
    B. Prone
    C. Sims'
    D. Standing
    E. Fowler's

129. Flushing of the ear canal to remove impacted cerumen is called

    A. Ear instillation
    B. Ear irrigation
    C. Tympanectomy
    D. Weber's test
    E. Rinne test

130. What gauge of needle is used for the Mantoux test?

    A. 18 to 19
    B. 20 to 21
    C. 23 to 24
    D. 26 to 27
    E. 28 to 29

131. A score on a color vision acuity test may indicate color vision deficiency only if it is

    A. Less than 7
    B. Less than 10
    C. Greater than 10
    D. Less than 5
    E. Less than 1

132. Which procedure is performed to view an organ in cross-section?

    A. Ultrasonography
    B. Venography
    C. Tomography
    D. Angiography
    E. Pyelography

133. Electrocardiograms are most commonly recorded at which of the following speeds?

    A. 5 mm per second
    B. 15 mm per second
    C. 25 mm per second
    D. 30 mm per second
    E. 60 mm per second

134. Which of the following instruments is used to drain an abscess?

    A. Probe
    B. Cannula
    C. Scalpel
    D. Specula
    E. Bandage scissors

135. Which type of drug may be refilled five times in 6 months when authorized by the physician?

    A. Schedule I drug
    B. Schedule II drug
    C. Schedule III drug
    D. Schedule IV drug
    E. Schedule V drug

136. A needle has all of the following parts <u>except</u>

    A. Hub
    B. Shaft
    C. Flange
    D. Bevel
    E. Lumen

137. Which of the following medications is most appropriate for a patient with depression?

    A. Pioglitazone (Actos)®
    B. Sertraline (Zoloft)®
    C. Orlistat (Xenical)®
    D. Simvastatin (Zocor)®
    E. Streptokinase (Streptase)®

138. The two most important components of hand washing are

    A. Surgical soap and cold water
    B. Surgical soap and warm water
    C. Alcohol and surgical soap
    D. Betadine and warm water
    E. Running water and friction

139. Which of the following terms means *surgical removal of the gallbladder*?

    A. Colostomy
    B. Cholelithotomy
    C. Cholangiostomy
    D. Cholectomy
    E. Cholecystectomy

140. In a normal adult, the ratio of respirations to pulse rate is

    A. 1:2
    B. 1:4
    C. 1:6
    D. 1:8
    E. 1:10

141. When a tuberculin test is performed, at which of the following angles is the needle inserted?

    A. 5 degrees
    B. 15 degrees
    C. 30 degrees
    D. 45 degrees
    E. 90 degrees

142. Wrapped items must be autoclaved for 20 minutes and unwrapped items for

    A. 30 minutes
    B. 25 minutes
    C. 20 minutes
    D. 15 minutes
    E. 10 minutes

143. Which of the following procedures requires a general anesthetic?

    A. Pap smear
    B. Colposcopy
    C. Barium enema
    D. Gastric lavage
    E. Laparoscopy

144. In testing for candidiasis, which of the following substances should be mixed with the vaginal specimen?

    A. Sterile water
    B. Tap water
    C. Iodine solution
    D. Sodium hydroxide
    E. Potassium hydroxide

145. Which of the following arteries is most commonly used to monitor lower limb circulation?

    A. Dorsalis pedis
    B. Posterior tibial
    C. Popliteal
    D. Femoral
    E. Internal iliac

146. Which of the following is described as a contrast bath?

A. Two baths, one filled with hot water and the other with cold milk
B. Two baths, one agitated by jets of air under pressure and the other not
C. Two baths, one filled with cold water and the other with hot water
D. Two baths, one dry and the other wet
E. None of the above

147. The distance between the patient and the Snellen eye chart for visual acuity should be

A. 3 meters
B. 5 meters
C. 10 feet
D. 20 feet
E. 25 feet

148. The instrument used to measure blood pressure is called a(n)

A. Manometer
B. Tonometer
C. Sphygmomanometer
D. Spirometer
E. Echogram

149. Which of the following abbreviations means "every 2 hours"?

A. q2h
B. q2
C. qid
D. qod
E. qh2

150. Which of the following information is considered demographic data?

A. Drug allergies
B. Occupation
C. Date of birth
D. Family medical history
E. Past medical history

151. Treatment using dry-cold or wet-cold applications is called

A. Diathermy
B. Cryotherapy
C. Hydrotherapy
D. Exercise therapy
E. Manipulation

152. Which of the following ECG curves represents the time between contraction of the ventricles and recovery?

A. Q-T interval
B. P-R interval
C. S-T segment
D. QRS complex
E. U wave

153. A sweet, fruity odor in urine may indicate the presence of

A. Phosphates
B. Uric acid
C. Albumin
D. Bilirubin
E. Ketones

154. The suture materials carried by surgical suture needles are also called

A. Ligation
B. Ligatures
C. Litigation
D. Needle holders
E. Suture forceps

155. When measuring the temperature of uncooperative patients of any age, which of the following thermometers should be used?

A. Oral mercury glass
B. Oral electronic
C. Tympanic
D. Axillary
E. Disposable

156. Which of the following is a treatment in which the patient places the hand or foot in a container of glass beads that are heated and agitated with hot air?

A. Ultraviolet therapy
B. Infrared therapy
C. Hot soak therapy
D. Fluidotherapy
E. Cryotherapy

157. Which of the following statements about nonabsorbable sutures is <u>incorrect</u>?

A. Sizes 2-0 through 6-0 are the most commonly used
B. They range in thickness from size 16-0 to 0-0
C. Size 0 is the thickest
D. They are made of polyester, steel, silk, or nylon
E. Generally they are used for outer tissues of the body

158. Nicotine and nitroglycerin patches are examples of which of the following methods of drug administration?

A. Subcutaneous
B. Intramuscular
C. Transdermal
D. Intravenous
E. Intracapillary

159. Death rates from HIV infection have been declining in the United States mostly as a result of

A. Immunization
B. Condom use
C. Increased research
D. Antiretroviral therapy
E. Changes in attitudes about sex among young individuals

160. Which of the following positions is not suitable for patients who are pregnant (late stage), elderly, or obese?

A. Standing
B. Trendelenburg's
C. Sims'
D. Lithotomy
E. Prone

161. Wounds in which the outer layers of the skin are rubbed off are called

A. Lacerations
B. Abrasions
C. Incisions
D. Contusions
E. Punctures

162. Which of the following drug types controls nausea, vomiting, and motion sickness?

A. Antihidrotic
B. Anticonvulsant
C. Vasodilator
D. Antiemetic
E. Sedative

163. Which of the following muscles of the body is the preferred injection site for infants?

A. Gluteus medius
B. Deltoid
C. Vastus lateralis
D. Ventrogluteal
E. Gluteus maximus

164. Which of the following antibiotics is used in cultures to give an early indication of the presence of group A streptococcus?

A. Penicillin
B. Tetracycline
C. Erythromycin
D. Amoxicillin
E. Bacitracin

165. Which of the following conditions may give plasma or serum a milky, or turbid, appearance?

A. Hyperglycemia
B. Hyperlipidemia
C. Hypercalcemia
D. Hypolipidemia
E. Hypoglycemia

166. Acetone breath can be smelled in which of the following conditions?

A. Septic shock
B. Insulin shock
C. Diabetic coma
D. Hyperlipidemia
E. Hypercalcemia

167. Which of the following conditions may cause plasma outside the body to be pink or red in color?

A. Hemotomes
B. Hemoptysis
C. Hemolysis
D. Hematoma
E. Icterus

168. A mucous membrane represents which of the following in the chain of infection transmission?

A. Infectious agent
B. Means of exit
C. Means of entry
D. Reservoir
E. Susceptible host

169. Which of the following drugs is most commonly used for local anesthesia that is injected?

A. Tetracaine (Pontocaine®) 2%
B. Mepivacaine (Carbocaine®) 0.5%
C. Lidocaine (Xylocaine®) 1%
D. Lidocaine (Xylocaine®) 5%
E. Lidocaine (Xylocaine®) 10%

195. Which of the following procedures or techniques involves injecting isotopes combined with glucose?
    A. CT
    B. MRI
    C. Ultrasound
    D. PET
    E. Arthrography

196. Which of the following arteries is the best location to take a pulse during an emergency?
    A. Radial
    B. Femoral
    C. Brachial
    D. Carotid
    E. Popliteal

197. Which diagnostic X-ray technique, used primarily for mammography, produces images electrically rather than chemically and permits shorter exposure times and lower radiation levels than ordinary X-rays?
    A. Xeroradiography
    B. Thermography
    C. Xerography
    D. Fluoroscopy
    E. Both A and C

198. Hypodermic syringes are commonly used to administer medication by which of the following routes?
    A. Intravenous
    B. Intramuscular
    C. Intradermal
    D. Subcutaneous
    E. Transdermal

199. Proctology is
    A. The study of disorders of the colon
    B. The study of disorders of the female reproductive system
    C. The study of disorders of the internal body cavities
    D. Concerned with treating disorders of the colon, rectum, and anus
    E. Both A and D

200. Which of the following is used to detect alcohol levels in blood samples?
    A. Betadine®
    B. Zephiran®
    C. Isopropyl alcohol
    D. Povidone-iodine
    E. Pure iodine

201. Which of the following statements about a Pap smear is false?
    A. The patient should not douche within 48 hours before the test
    B. The patient should not use vaginal medications within 48 hours before the test
    C. The patient should not have intercourse within 8 hours after the test
    D. The test should not be done during a patient's menstrual period
    E. The patient should not have intercourse within 48 hours before the test

202. The first MMR vaccination should be given to a child by which of the following ages?
    A. At birth
    B. 2 to 4 months
    C. 6 to 7 months
    D. 12 to 15 months
    E. 4 to 6 years

203. Your physician has ordered 120 mg of a drug that comes only in 15 mg tablets. How many tablets constitute a dose?
    A. 4
    B. 6
    C. 8
    D. 10
    E. 12

204. What is meant by a patient's gait?
    A. Style of walking
    B. Vital signs
    C. Muscle tone
    D. Weight
    E. Sharpness and awareness of the patient

205. Which of the following terms means an increased number of white blood cells?
    A. Leukoplakia
    B. Leukopenia
    C. Leukoblast
    D. Leukopoiesis
    E. Leukocytosis

206. Which of the following is the best specimen on which to conduct an occult blood test?
    A. Whole blood
    B. Serum
    C. Plasma
    D. Feces
    E. Sputum

207. Which of the following color codes indicates a blood collection tube containing EDTA?

A. Purple
B. Green
C. Black
D. Yellow
E. Red

208. Forearm crutches are also called

A. Lofstrand crutches
B. Axillary crutches
C. Walkers
D. Canadian crutches
E. Both A and D

209. All of the following statements about preparing a patient for intravenous pyelography are true except

A. The patient should be asked about possible allergies to iodine
B. The patient should take a prescribed amount of electrolyte solution or other laxative
C. The patient may eat no solid food starting the morning before the procedure
D. The patient may have one cup of coffee on the morning of the test
E. The patient should be asked about possible allergies to shellfish

210. Albuterol aerosol inhalants are a type of

A. Vasodilator
B. Antitussive
C. Antihistamine
D. Expectorant
E. Bronchodilator

211. Autoclave indicator tape turns which color after autoclaving?

A. Red
B. Yellow
C. Green
D. Blue
E. Black

212. Which of the following types of urine specimen is helpful in diagnosing dehydration and pheochromocytoma?

A. Random
B. Clean-catch midstream
C. Timed
D. 24-hour
E. First-voided morning

213. The temperature of an autoclave is commonly set for

A. 150°F to 180°F
B. 180°F to 210°F
C. 210°F to 245°F
D. 250°F to 270°F
E. 270°F to 295°F

214. Abnormal, temporary low blood pressure, especially when a patient moves rapidly, is called

A. Anemic hypotension
B. Orthostatic hypotension
C. Very mild hypertension
D. Very mild hypotension
E. Hypovolemic shock

215. Which of the following types of shock may occur following allergic reactions?

A. Cardiogenic
B. Hypovolemic
C. Neurogenic
D. Anaphylactic
E. Septic

216. Which of the following color codes indicates a tube that does not contain any additive?

A. Lavender
B. Green
C. Red
D. Blue
E. Yellow

217. Which of the following instruments is used to separate particles of different densities within a liquid?

A. Seralyzer
B. Autoclave
C. Ultrasound generator
D. Spectrophotometer
E. Centrifuge

218. Which of the following groups of microorganisms can be seen only with an electron microscope?

A. Fungi
B. Rickettsiae
C. Protozoa
D. Bacteria
E. Viruses

219. Drugs with a low abuse potential that have an accepted medical use are classified as

  A. Schedule I drugs
  B. Schedule II drugs
  C. Schedule III drugs
  D. Schedule IV drugs
  E. Schedule V drugs

220. Treatment for which of the following diseases requires a series of six injections over a 4-week period?

  A. Rabies
  B. Viral meningitis
  C. Hepatitis B
  D. Influenza
  E. AIDS

221. Which of the following items should be used to clean the lenses of a microscope?

  A. Soft facial tissue
  B. Cotton cloth
  C. Paper towel
  D. Lens paper
  E. Either A or B

222. OSHA regulations require all health-care workers who may be at risk to be vaccinated against which of the following diseases?

  A. Tuberculosis
  B. AIDS
  C. Hepatitis A
  D. Hepatitis B
  E. Hepatitis C

223. The most commonly used site for measuring the pulse rate is the

  A. Carotid artery
  B. Radial artery
  C. Brachial artery
  D. Femoral artery
  E. Temporal artery

224. A dilute solution of formaldehyde used to preserve biological specimens is

  A. Formalin
  B. Selective culture medium
  C. Fixative
  D. Lactated Ringer's solution
  E. EDTA

225. Which of the following drugs prevents or inhibits sleep?

  A. Antianxiety
  B. Antihypnotic
  C. Analgesic
  D. Antipruritic
  E. Antitussive

226. What structure separates each atrium and its respective ventricle?

  A. Septum
  B. Valve
  C. Base of the heart
  D. Apex
  E. Sinus

227. Valproic acid may be used to treat

  A. Petit mal epilepsy
  B. Grand mal epilepsy
  C. Parkinson's disease
  D. Viral infections
  E. Heart disease

228. The Ishihara test is used for which of the following organs of the body?

  A. Gallbladder
  B. Ear
  C. Urinary bladder
  D. Eye
  E. Uterus

229. Which of the following leads is also called unipolar?

  A. Standard
  B. Limb
  C. Precordial
  D. Augmented
  E. Chest

230. Which of the following agents is used in the treatment of inflammatory conditions?

  A. Prednisone
  B. Penicillin
  C. Acetaminophen (Tylenol®)
  D. Axid®
  E. Zolpidem

231. Which of the following color codes indicates tubes used for blood cultures?
    A. Red
    B. Yellow
    C. Green
    D. Blue
    E. Black

232. Which of the following antibiotics can soften contact lenses and discolor the urine, saliva, and sweat, causing each to become reddish-orange in color?
    A. Nystatin
    B. Ampicillin
    C. Metronidazole
    D. Rifampin
    E. Vancomycin

233. The administration of a drug by placing it under the tongue until it dissolves is called
    A. Transdermal
    B. Sublingual
    C. Buccal
    D. Oral
    E. Topical

234. The coughing up of blood from the respiratory tract is called
    A. Hemolysis
    B. Hemostasis
    C. Hemothorax
    D. Hemopneumothorax
    E. Hemoptysis

235. Which of the following vaccines can be administered at birth?
    A. BCG
    B. Polio
    C. Hepatitis A
    D. Hepatitis B
    E. Measles

236. Most drugs are eliminated by the
    A. Liver
    B. Lungs
    C. Kidneys
    D. Colon
    E. Skin

237. According to Good Samaritan laws,
    A. Emergency care is permitted when it is within the scope of competence of the person administering first aid
    B. Emergency care is permitted only with the explicit (e.g., verbal) consent of the patient
    C. All medical personnel are required to provide care in all emergency situations
    D. When providing emergency care, medical personnel are protected against possible claims of negligence
    E. The permission of the patient (or the person holding power of attorney) is required in any situation, emergency or otherwise

238. Which of the following colors indicates specific hazards such as radioactivity?
    A. White
    B. Red
    C. Yellow
    D. Blue
    E. Green

239. Administration of a drug by placing it in the mouth between the gums and the cheek is called
    A. Oral
    B. Topical
    C. Sublingual
    D. Transdermal
    E. Buccal

240. Which of the following colors is most frequently used to designate a biohazardous sharps container?
    A. Green
    B. Yellow
    C. Blue
    D. Red
    E. Black

241. Pentazocine is used as a(n)
    A. Opioid analgesic to relieve severe acute or chronic pain
    B. Nonopioid analgesic to relieve mild to moderate pain
    C. Anticoagulant used to prevent venous thrombosis
    D. Antiarrhythmic drug to slow the heart rate
    E. A barbiturate used to promote sleep and treat convulsions

242. In the erythrocyte sedimentation rate test, the normal rate at which cells fall is 1 mm every
  A. Minute
  B. 5 minutes
  C. 30 minutes
  D. Hour
  E. 2 hours

243. Which of the following classes of drugs is used to constrict the pupils?
  A. Mydriatics
  B. Miotics
  C. Anticholinergics
  D. Styptics
  E. Cardiotonics

244. The increasing resistance to the usual effects of an established dosage of a drug is called
  A. Adverse effect
  B. Dependence
  C. Antagonism
  D. Synergism
  E. Tolerance

245. Excessive EDTA causes erythrocytes to
  A. Shrink
  B. Rupture
  C. Swell
  D. Reproduce
  E. Be destroyed

246. A device used to measure the degree of joint movement is called a
  A. Tonometer
  B. Torsiometer
  C. Glucometer
  D. Goniometer
  E. Gonioscope

247. Which of the following statements is true of centrally acting muscle relaxants?
  A. Examples include baclofen (Lioresal®), carisoprodol (Soma®), and tizandine (Zanaflex®)
  B. They are used for therapy of muscle strain and multiple sclerosis
  C. They are used for surgical procedures to relax abdominal muscles, and examples include dantrolene
  D. Both A and B
  E. All of the above

248. Which of the following classes of drugs is most appropriate for a patient with a persistent cough?
  A. Antiemetics
  B. Antipruritics
  C. Antitussives
  D. Antibiotics
  E. Antidotes

249. The needle gauge range most commonly used for venipuncture is
  A. 17–19
  B. 19–20
  C. 21–23
  D. 24–25
  E. 17–25

250. A corticosteroid is used to treat
  A. Asthma
  B. Epilepsy
  C. Pain
  D. Obesity
  E. Hypertension

Self-Evaluation Answers and Rationales

PART

3

General	Medical Assisting Knowledge

Administrative	Medical Assisting Knowledge

Clinical	Medical Assisting Knowledge

28. **(C)** *Dactyl/o* means "finger" or "toe." Polydactyly is the presence of extra fingers or toes. Polydipsia is excessive thirst. Polyphagia is excessive, uncontrolled eating. Polysomy is the presence of a chromosome in at least triplicate form in an otherwise diploid somatic cell. Polychoria is the condition of having more than one pupil in one eye.

29. **(D)** The scapula is one of the pair of large, flat, triangular bones that form the dorsal part of the pectoral girdle. It is also known as the shoulder blade. The pectoral girdle includes the clavicles (collarbones) and scapulae. The olecranon process is the bony point of the elbow. The sternum forms the anterior portion of the thoracic cavity. The styloid process is a projection on the temporal bone.

30. **(E)** In a bench trial, a judge serves without a jury and rules on the law as well as on the facts.

31. **(A)** The specific immune response is required if the nonspecific immune response cannot cope with invasion or injury. It is directed and controlled by T and B cells. These cells can remember pathogens and respond more quickly in subsequent invasions.

32. **(A)** Angioplasty is the reconstitution of a blood vessel. Venectomy (or phlebectomy) is the excision of a vein. Arterectomy or arteriectomy is the excision of an artery. Angiorrhaphy is the repair by suture of any blood vessel. Cardiotomy is surgical incision of the heart.

33. **(D)** The heart is located in the anterior thorax region. The pulse of infants can generally be measured by auscultating this region.

34. **(E)** *Opt / o* refers to vision, and *phot / o* refers to light. *Ocul / o* and *ophthalm / o* both mean "eye."

35. **(C)** Life events, whether positive (such as marriage) or negative, can cause a great deal of stress.

36. **(A)** *Res ipsa loquitur* is a Latin phrase that means "the matter speaks for itself." It is also known as the doctrine of common law. This doctrine is usually applied when the physician clearly could have prevented a negligent act, such as leaving foreign bodies (e.g., instruments) inside a patient's body during surgery, damaging healthy tissue during an operation, burning or otherwise unnecessarily injuring the patient while the patient is under anesthesia, or causing an infection by the use of unsterilized instruments.

37. **(C)** Proteins such as albumin help maintain water balance that affects osmotic pressure, which prevents the accumulation of fluids in body tissues, which would cause edema.

38. **(C)** *Bacteria* is the plural form of *bacterium*.

39. **(B)** The tibia is another name for the shin bone.

40. **(E)** Parathyroid hormone is able to increase the absorption of calcium from the wall of the small intestine. The blood calcium level is therefore regulated by the parathyroid glands.

41. **(A)** Vitamin C deficiency may result in scurvy.

42. **(A)** "After meals" is abbreviated as *pc*, from the Latin phrase *post cibum*. The abbreviation *pm (post meridiem)* means "after noon," *po (per os)* means "by mouth," and *prn (pro re nata)* means "as needed." PS is not an abbreviation.

43. **(A)** Professional negligence is the proximate cause of injury or harm to a patient, resulting from a lack of professional knowledge, experience, or skill. It is also known as malpractice.

44. **(A)** Erikson believed that at ages 3 to 6 years, the conflict is initiative *vs.* guilt.

45. **(E)** Wernicke's area is responsible for language comprehension. Broca's area is responsible for motor speech and for controlling the mouth, tongue, and larynx. The occipital lobe is responsible for visual recognition. The parietal lobe is responsible for the interpretation of sensory input, such as taste. The insular lobe is responsible for visceral or primitive emotions, drives, and reactions.

46. **(E)** The duodenum is the first portion of the small intestine and is followed by the jejunum and ileum.

47. **(B)** Meningitis is inflammation of the meninges, the membranes covering the brain and spinal cord. Diphtheria affects the mucous membranes of the respiratory tract. Parotitis is mumps, the inflammation of one or both parotid glands. Infectious mononucleosis is an acute infectious disease that changes leukocytes. Myocarditis is an inflammation of the myocardium commonly caused by viruses, bacteria, fungi, or protozoa.

48. **(B)** Sebaceous glands are small organs found in the dermis; therefore, they are found in the integumentary system. Sebum secreted by the glands lubricates the hair and the surrounding skin. It helps prevent the evaporation of sweat and aids in the retention of body heat.

49. **(D)** *Hypo-* means "below" or "under." Hypoglycemia is low blood sugar.

50. **(D)** These symptoms are characteristic of cholelithiais, which is the presence of gallstones in the gallbladder. It is more common in women over 40 years of age.

51. **(A)** A wide-ranging prediction or explanation of everyday behavior or phenomena is called theory.

52. **(B)** Bipolar disorder is a condition in which a person alternates between periods of euphoric feelings and mania and periods of depression.

53. **(C)** The ego is one of Freud's personality components, and is based in reality.

54. **(C)** Elisabeth Kübler-Ross thought that a person passes through five distinct stages, when a loved one is dying. These stages include denial, anger, bargaining, depression, and acceptance.

55. **(D)** When giving out confidential information, you should always get the patient's written consent. Other legally required disclosures include those ordered by subpoena, those dictated by statute to protect public welfare, and those considered necessary to protect the welfare of the patient or a third party.

56. **(B)** Consent to allow touching, examination, or treatment by medically authorized personnel is unnecessary in an emergency situation.

57. **(D)** The suffix *-penia* means "abnormal reduction" (leukopenia), *-osis* means "increase" (leukocytosis), *-megaly* means "enlargement" (cardiomegaly), and *-plasia* means "formation" (dysplasia). The suffix *-algia* means "pain" (neuralgia).

58. **(B)** Contracts have three parts: offer, acceptance, and consideration. The offer sets the stage, and it must be communicated effectively and in good faith. Acceptance involves agreeing to take the offer. The consideration is something of value bargained for as part of the contract.

59. **(B)** A medical assistant should communicate with an elderly patient by encouraging the patient to ask questions.

60. **(A)** The umbilical vein in fetal circulation transports oxygen from the placenta to the fetus. The umbilical artery transports blood from the fetus to the placenta to get oxygen and to get rid of carbon dioxide.

61. **(B)** The thymus is the primary, central gland of the lymphatic system and is the site of maturation for T cells. The T cells of the cell-mediated specific immune response develop in this gland before migrating to the lymph nodes and spleen.

62. **(C)** Commensalism is a one-sided relationship in which one member benefits and the other is unaffected. Mutualism is a relationship in which both organisms benefit. Symbiosis is the living together of two species. Opportunism is a relationship in which an organism that was previously harmless becomes pathogenic when the host's defenses are weakened. In parasitism, one organism lives at the expense of another organism.

63. **(C)** Costectomy is the surgical removal of a rib.

64. **(D)** Trichomoniasis is a vaginal infection caused by the protozoan *Trichomonas vaginalis*. This infection can be transmitted by genital secretions.

65. **(B)** By restating or repeating what you believe is the main thought or idea expressed in a conversation, you can make sure that you understand what is being communicated. Allowing patients to reflect will not tell them that you understood what they said; it will, however, allow them to think through and answer their own questions. Being assertive involves standing up for yourself while showing respect to others; it has little to do with whether you understood the patient or not. A rapport can develop between you and a patient through good communication skills, but rapport itself does not mean that you specifically understood what the patient has communicated to you. Crossing your arms over your chest or shaking your head is displaying negative body language, which conveys anger, disagreement, or lack of caring.

66. **(A)** *Bacteriostatic* means "inhibiting bacterial growth." Bactericidal substances destroy or kill bacteria. *Aseptic* means "free of infective material." *Sterile* means "free of living microorganisms."

67. **(A)** Invasion of privacy is the intrusion into a person's seclusion or into his or her private affairs. The unauthorized disclosure of medical records or financial or personal information of the patient is considered an invasion of privacy. For example, if you tell a patient's employer without the patient's written consent that the patient has AIDS, you are violating the patient's right to privacy.

68. **(C)** The thigh bone, which extends from the pelvis to the knee, is called the femur.

69. **(D)** John was exhibiting gender bias. Gender bias is any type of action or language that unjustly favors one gender over another. Discrimination involves acting unfairly on the basis of bias or prejudice against a certain group or class. For example, if Susan does not get a promotion because John tends to view women unfavorably, then John could be sued for discriminating against her.

70. **(B)** *Lith / o* is a combining form that means "stone," and the suffix *-iasis* means "condition or formation of."

71. **(E)** The patient has the right to all of the choices listed in this question. For all patient rights, review Table 8-3 in Chapter 8, "Medical Law and Ethics."

72. **(D)** When a person feels sad for another person, the emotion is called sympathy.

73. **(A)** Remission is the partial or complete disappearance of the clinical and subjective characteristics of a chronic or malignant disease. Prognosis is a prediction of the probable outcome of a disease. Prophylaxis is prevention or protection against disease. Malaise is a vague, uneasy feeling of body weakness, distress, or discomfort, often marking the onset of and persisting throughout a disease. Atresia is the absence or closure of a normal body opening, duct, or canal such as the external ear canal or anus.

74. **(E)** Night blindness is caused by a deficiency in vitamin A. Vitamin B_1 deficiency may lead to Wernicke-Korsakoff syndrome. Hemorrhage can be a symptom of vitamin K deficiency. Pernicious anemia may be caused by vitamin B_{12} deficiency.

75. **(B)** Hidrosis is the production and secretion of sweat. Hydrops is an abnormal accumulation of clear, watery fluid in a body tissue or cavity. Hydrolase is an enzyme. Hydropenia is a lack of water in the body tissues. Hydrolysis is a chemical process of decomposition that involves splitting a bond and adding a hydrogen ion.

76. **(E)** The time difference between Miami, Florida, and Honolulu, Hawaii, is 5 hours. If the time in Hawaii is 9:00 a.m., then it is 2:00 p.m. in Florida.

77. **(C)** Projection is a defense mechanism that involves the attribution of one's own difficulties to external causes. Rationalization is the justification of problems or unacceptable behavior by giving acceptable reasons rather than real ones (i.e., by making up plausible excuses). Repression involves pushing unpleasant thoughts or problems into the unconscious to avoid dealing with them. You should be aware of these defense mechanisms and avoid using them, because they do not lead to effective communication.

78. **(B)** Herpes zoster is an acute viral infection that is also called shingles.

79. **(E)** When you talk to patients who have a visual impairment, you should use larger print materials, make sure that there is adequate lighting in the room, and as always talk directly and honestly.

80. **(E)** Geriatrics is the treatment of elderly individuals, not necessarily the treatment of individuals with terminal illnesses. Palliative care is care given to make someone, such as a dying person, more comfortable. Patients should never be abandoned. They should have emotional support, pain control, respect for their autonomy, and effective communication.

81. **(E)** *Disphagia* is misspelled. The correct spelling is *dysphagia,* meaning difficulty swallowing.

82. **(C)** Afferent neurons conduct nerve impulses toward the spinal cord and brain.

83. **(D)** When dealing with children, you should work directly with the children rather than communicating through the parents, take their feelings seriously, explain all the procedures in simple terms, let them examine the instruments, use praise, be truthful, and do not talk down to them.

84. **(B)** Sanitization reduces the number of microorganisms, and antisepsis inhibits the growth and multiplication of microorganisms.

85. **(B)** *Encephal / o* refers to the brain, as in the word *encephalitis,* meaning "inflammation of the brain." *Cerebr / o* refers to the cerebrum, not to the brain as a whole. *Myel / o* means "spinal cord." *Poli / o* means "gray matter." *Blephar / o* means "eyelid."

86. **(C)** Denial is an unconscious defense mechanism in which a person avoids emotional conflict and anxiety by refusing to acknowledge thoughts, feelings, desires, or facts that are consciously unacceptable.

87. **(E)** As part of a medical team, medical assistants should be ready to compromise and admit if they are wrong, treat others with respect, listen to everyone equally, avoid putting others on the defensive, refrain from reinforcing or adopting negative attitudes, work to solve problems, learn from others, and remember the common goal of providing excellent health care to patients.

88. **(A)** The girl's legal guardian, her mother, must give written consent before the girl's medical records are released.

89. **(E)** The soleus muscle is located in the leg.

90 **(C)** The most appropriate initial response to an incoming telephone call is "Dr. Brown's office, Melinda speaking."

91. **(A)** Privilege is the authority granted to a physician by a hospital to provide patient care in the hospital.

92. **(D)** Digestion is the conversion of food into absorbable substances within the gastrointestinal tract. Digestion occurs through the mechanical and chemical breakdown of food; therefore, the process of digestion begins in the mouth.

93. **(E)** The liver and gallbladder are located in the right upper quadrant of the abdomen.

94. **(E)** Calls that require the attention of the physician include emergency calls, calls from other doctors and physicians, calls from patients who want to discuss test results (particularly abnormal results), calls from patients who want to discuss symptoms with the physician, reports from patients concerning unsatisfactory progress, requests for prescription renewals when they have not been previously authorized by the physician, and personal calls. In general, all emergencies should be routed to the physician immediately. Calls from other physicians should also be routed to the doctor immediately if possible.

95. **(B)** Anosmia is the loss or impairment of the sense of smell. Aphonia is a condition characterized by loss of the ability to produce normal speech sounds. Amnesia is a loss of memory caused by brain damage or by severe emotional trauma. Anorexia is a lack or loss of appetite. Something lacking new development or pertaining to the failure of a tissue to produce normal cell division is referred to as aplastic.

96. **(C)** The Patient's Bill of Rights is a document that explains that patients should receive respectful care.

97. **(E)** The abbreviation that indicates each eye is *OU*.

98. **(C)** An inquiry about a bill is an administrative call that can be handled by the medical assistant who answers the phone. Other calls that the medical assistant can handle include appointment scheduling, rescheduling, and canceling; insurance questions; X-ray and laboratory reports; routine reports from hospitals regarding a patient's progress; satisfactory progress reports from patients; requests for referrals to other doctors; questions concerning office policies, fees, and hours; complaints about administrative matters; and prescription refills when they have been previously authorized by the physician.

99. **(B)** *Homestasis* should be spelled *homeostasis*.

100. **(E)** As a medical assistant, you might be required to give patients instructions prior to surgery, a test, or a procedure. It may be easier for patients to visualize the conditions or procedures if you use an anatomical model or a video tape. Other instructional materials include brochures, booklets, fact sheets, educational newsletters, and community directories. Another one of your goals as a medical assistant should be to promote good health behaviors and to teach patients how to prevent common injuries. Encourage patients to eat well, exercise regularly, get adequate rest, limit alcohol consumption, stop smoking, and balance work and leisure to avoid stress.

101. **(D)** The retina is the innermost layer of the eye, composed of delicate nervous tissue that receives images of external objects and transmits visual impulses through the optic nerve to the brain.

102. **(C)** Empathy involves a person's experiencing another person's emotional state by viewing the situation through that person's eyes.

103. **(A)** Vectors are carriers of pathogenic organisms. For example, mosquitoes can be vectors for malaria and encephalitis.

104. **(C)** Progesterone is a natural progestational hormone. It prepares the uterus for pregnancy.

105. **(A)** When a word ends in -*us*, you can usually (not always) form the plural by dropping the -*us* and adding -*i*.

106. **(C)** A corporation is a body formed by a group of people who are authorized by law to act as a single person.

107. **(C)** Confidentiality should not be waived in a malpractice suit, nor for an insurance carrier, nor for the patient's spouse. Confidentiality should be waived only when the patient or his or her legal guardian gives written consent, the medical records are subpoenaed, or there is a statute requiring a waiver to protect the public.

108. **(B)** Routine reports from hospitals regarding a patient's progress can be handled by the medical assistant. Only calls regarding a patient's unsatisfactory progress need to be handled by a physician.

109. **(D)** Ankylosis is the fixation of a joint, often in an abnormal position, resulting from the destruction of articular cartilage and subchondral bone. It is common in rheumatoid arthritis.

110. **(B)** Elisabeth Kübler-Ross defines five stages or responses of dying patients: denial and isolation, anger, bargaining and guilt, depression, and acceptance.

111. **(B)** Physicians are considered the owners of the medical records they have written.

112. **(A)** Bronchiectasis is an abnormal condition of the bronchial tree characterized by irreversible dilation and destruction of the bronchial walls.

113. **(C)** Diabetes insipidus is a metabolic disorder caused by injury of the neurohypophyseal system. It is caused by deficient production or secretion of the antidiuretic hormone (ADH) or the inability of the kidney tubules to respond to ADH.

114. **(E)** SOAP provides a series of steps for dealing with a medical case: the patient's symptoms (*s*ubjective data), the diagnosis (*o*bjective data), *a*ssessment, and *p*lan of action.

115. **(A)** Nystagmus is the involuntary, rhythmic movement of the eyes, in which the oscillations may be horizontal, vertical, rotary, or mixed.

116. **(C)** *Puritus* should be spelled *pruritus*, which means "severe itching."

117 **(C)** The suffix -*stomy* means "the (surgical) creation of a new opening," -*tomy* means "cutting" or "incision," and -*scopy* means "the process of viewing (something) with a scope." The suffix -*iasis* refers to a condition or the formation of something, such as the formation of stones, lithiasis.

118. **(E)** A contract may be prematurely terminated as a result of failing to pay for services, missing appointments, failing to follow the physician's instructions, or obtaining the services of another physician.

119. **(C)** Mood disorders involves all aspects of a person's behavior or perception of external events. Major depression and bipolar disorders are example of the mood disorders.

120. **(D)** The hypothalamus assists in controlling body temperature, water balance, sleep, appetite, emotions of fear and pleasure, and involuntary functions.

121. **(C)** The adrenal cortex secretes aldosterone, cortisol, and androgens. Cortisol increases blood glucose levels and contributes to stress adaptation.

122. **(A)** The Controlled Substance Act of 1970 controls the distribution and use of all drugs of abuse potential as designated by the DEA. It divides narcotics, stimulants, and some sedatives into five classes, called schedules.

123. **(C)** Viruses are infectious agents that are even simpler in nature than prokaryotes. They are composed of a small amount of DNA or RNA wrapped in a protein covering, and they are usually not considered cellular. Only an electron microscope is powerful enough to magnify them sufficiently to be seen.

124. **(B)** *Cutane* / *o* means "skin," *hidr* / *o* means "sweat," *onych* / *o* means "nail," *hist* / *o* means "tissue," and *albin* / *o* means "white."

125. **(D)** Type O Rh− blood is the universal donor because it has neither A nor B antigens and has both A and B antibodies.

126. **(E)** The suffixes *-algia* and *-algy* mean "pain" or "painful condition."

127. **(D)** Type AB Rh⁺ blood is the universal recipient because it has both A and B antigens on red blood cells but neither A nor B antibodies in plasma.

128. **(A)** A hydatidiform mole is an intrauterine tumor mass of grapelike enlarged cysts.

129. **(C)** Metrorrhagia is uterine bleeding other than that caused by menstruation. It may be caused by uterine lesions and may be a sign of a urogenital malignancy, especially cervical cancer. Menorrhagia is abnormally heavy or long menstrual periods. Amenorrhea is the absence of menstruation.

130. **(E)** When a word ends in *-um*, you can usually form the plural by dropping the *-um* and adding *-a*.

131. **(A)** *Dermat / o* means "skin," and the suffix *-itis* means "inflammation." The term *dermatitis* refers to the inflammation of skin.

132. **(C)** Often, laws dictate what medical assistants may or may not do. For example, in some states it is illegal for medical assistants to draw blood. It is illegal in all states for a medical assistant to diagnose a condition, prescribe treatment, and engage in deception about certification, title, and level of education.

133. **(C)** Abraham Maslow believed that the basic needs of humans are safety, love, survival, prestige and self-actualization.

134. **(E)** In cases involving negligence, the doctrine of *res ipsa loquitur* applies, and the physician has the burden of proving innocence and nonnegligence. This doctrine implies that injury would not have occurred unless someone had been clearly negligent.

135. **(A)** An obligate anaerobe lives only in the absence of oxygen. The majority of microbes are aerobes, meaning that they live and grow in the presence of oxygen.

136. **(C)** Before you can properly transfer a call, the person calling needs to identify himself or herself and give you a brief description of the nature of the call. If the person refuses to be identified, you should not put the call through to the physician; instead, ask the person to write a letter to the physician and to mark it *Personal*. Even if the patient is angry, you should remain calm and professional and offer to help solve the caller's problem. Genuinely listen to complaints, and help the patient express his or her anger in a constructive manner.

137. **(C)** According to Freud, regression is a defense mechanism whereby a person seeks to relieve stress by seeking an earlier developmental period.

138. **(B)** The abbreviation *fx* means "fracture" and the abbreviation *rt.* means "right."

139. **(B)** The semicircular canal is one of three curved passages in the inner ear that detect motion and govern balance. The tympanic membrane transmits sound vibrations. The cochlea is the receptor for hearing. Cerumen is ear wax. The auditory ossicles are three tiny bones in the middle ear: the malleus (hammer), the incus (anvil), and the stapes (stirrup). These bones transmit and amplify vibrations.

140. **(B)** The prefix *inter-* means "between," and *cost / o* means "rib."

141. **(E)** The AAMA publishes a code of ethics for all of its certified medical assistants. According to the AAMA, all its members should be dedicated to the conscientious pursuit of their profession in order to deserve the high regard of the entire medical profession. The AMT holds its certified medical assistants to similarly high standards. Whether you are seeking RMA or CMA certification, you should familiarize yourself with the AAMA Code of Ethics.

142. **(B)** Koplik's spots are small red spots with bluish-white centers on the buccal mucosa, characteristic of measles.

143. **(B)** The sternum is a flat, bladelike bone that is located in the front of chest.

144. **(C)** *Thromb / o* means "clot," and the suffix *-lysis* means "destruction." Thrombolysis is the destruction or dissolving of a clot.

145. **(B)** The atria are the upper chambers of the heart. The right atrium receives deoxygenated blood through the superior and inferior venae cavae, and the left atrium receives oxygenated blood from the lungs through the pulmonary veins. Blood then passes through the atria to the ventricles. As the ventricles contract, they pump blood through the arteries. The right ventricle pumps blood into the pulmonary artery to the lungs, and the left ventricle pumps blood into the aorta to the rest of the body.

146. **(C)** Dysphonia is any abnormality in the speaking voice. In cancer of the larynx, dysphonia is usually the only symptom.

147. **(D)** In a living will, the individual expresses his or her wishes regarding medical treatment. It may detail circumstances under which treatment should be discontinued, which treatments to suspend, and which to maintain. A living will is legal if the patient is competent to create such a will and two witnesses sign it and attest to its accuracy.

148. **(E)** Minimizing background noise, positioning yourself close to and facing the patient, using body language to supplement your voice, speaking slowly, and using written materials all help you communicate more effectively with an individual who has a hearing impairment.

149. **(A)** Retinol is another name for vitamin A. Carotene is a precursor that is converted to vitamin A in the liver.

150. **(B)** The Good Samaritan Act provides immunity from liability to a volunteer at the scene of an accident for any civil damages in rendering emergency care, so long as the volunteer acts within his or her scope of education and training.

151. **(C)** Intrinsic factor is a substance secreted by the gastric mucosa that is essential for the intestinal absorption of Vitamin B_{12} (cyanocobalamin).

152. **(B)** Open-ended questions usually ask "how" and "why." They allow the patient to describe in detail the symptoms and any related thoughts and feelings he or she may have. Such questions are usually used in a patient interview to obtain more complete information by allowing patients to elaborate on responses they may have previously given to simple yes/no or is/do questions.

153. **(D)** Acromegaly is a chronic metabolic condition characterized by a gradual, marked enlargement and elongation of the bones of the face, jaw, and extremities. This condition mostly affects middle-aged and older persons and is caused by the overproduction of growth hormone.

154. **(C)** Hyperopia is farsightedness, or an inability of the eye to focus on nearby objects. It results from an error of refraction, brought on by the abnormal shortness of the eyeball, which causes rays of light entering the eye to be brought into focus behind the retina.

155. **(B)** Glaucoma is an abnormal condition of elevated pressure within an eye caused by obstruction in the outflow of aqueous humor. The most serious complication of glaucoma is blindness.

156. **(D)** Cervical cancer is a neoplasm of the uterine cervix that can be detected in the early, curable stage by the Papanicolaou test (Pap test or Pap smear).

157. **(D)** The gluteus maximus is a large muscle, originating in the iliac and the sacrum, that acts to extend the thigh. The gluteus medius abducts and rotates the thigh. The quadriceps femoris extends the leg. The hamstrings flex the leg. The brachialis flexes the forearm.

158. **(E)** The deltoid muscle is a large, thick, triangular muscle that covers the shoulder joint. It is the prime mover of the arm for abduction.

159. **(C)** The plural form of *appendix* is *appendices*.

160. **(E)** Iodine deficiency may cause goiter or cretinism. Goiter is more common among women.

161. **(B)** A ribosome is a cytoplasmic organelle composed of RNA and protein that functions in the synthesis of protein.

162. **(B)** *Intravenous* means "pertaining to the inside of a vein," as of a thrombus or an injection, infusion, or catheter.

163. **(C)** Only major surgery, an invasive procedure, the prescription of experimental drugs, admittance to a hospital, and procedures with high risk would require written expressed consent. Routine procedures such as Pap smears, minor surgical procedures such as removing splinters or broken glass, and emergency situations, even when they involve a minor, do not require written consent.

164. **(C)** A statute of limitations prescribes a fixed amount of time in which a lawsuit can be filed for an alleged wrongdoing.

165. **(C)** The malleolus is a rounded bony process, such as the rounded bone on each side of the ankle.

166. **(E)** The axis is the second cervical vertebra, about which the atlas rotates, allowing the head to be turned, extended, and flexed.

167. **(E)** *Pulmon / o* means "lung." The word *pulmonary* means "relating to the lungs."

168. **(C)** The external oblique muscle is located in the lower eight ribs of the torso or trunk.

169. **(C)** A bactericidal substance destroys or kills bacteria. A bacteriostatic substance inhibits the growth of bacteria.

170. **(A)** Abnormal lateral curvature of the spine is called scoliosis.

171. **(B)** *Ectopic* means "away from the normal location" (i.e., situated in an unusual place). For example, in an ectopic pregnancy, the fertilized egg is implanted somewhere other than in the uterus.

172. **(D)** *Dorsal* means "pertaining to the back" or "posterior."

173. **(B)** Giardiasis is a protozoan infection of the small intestine caused by *Giardia lamblia*, usually acquired from contaminated and untreated water.

174. **(D)** Myelocele is a saclike protrusion of the spinal cord through a congenital defect in the vertebral column.

175. **(A)** A process that can help a person learn to control internal physiological systems is called biofeedback.

176. **(D)** In order to guard the privacy of patients, you should not leave medical charts, insurance reports, or patient sign-in sheets where patients or office visitors can see them. Imagine a friend or an employer of your patient walking in and finding out that the patient has had multiple appointments for cancer treatment or multiple appointments with an OB/GYN.

177. **(D)** Touching someone on the shoulder, back, or hand can show sensitivity and empathy, but not everyone will be accepting. Be aware of cultural and personal differences, and adjust your style to the preferences of others.

178. **(E)** The suffix *-rrhea* means "flow" or "discharge."

179. **(A)** Child abuse commonly affects children younger than 3 years of age, but it can happen at any age. You should not expect children to come to you for help, because they may be unaware that what is happening to them is wrong and that it can and should be stopped, they may not realize that you would be able to help, and they may also be frightened of their abusers. The Child Abuse Prevention and Treatment Act of 1974 mandates the reporting of cases of child abuse. Child abuse should be reported by teachers, physicians, and other licensed health-care practitioners. A report should immediately be made to the proper authorities, and a written report is usually required within a specific time frame, such as 72 hours. Depending on state law, failure to report suspected cases of child abuse may be considered a misdemeanor. Those who report child abuse are granted absolute immunity from criminal and civil liability resulting from the reported incident. Even if you turn out to be wrong about Joe's symptoms, the parents will not be able to sue the practice because you had just cause in reporting a suspected case.

180. **(E)** Basal metabolism is the amount of energy needed for the body when it is at digestive, physical, and emotional rest.

181. **(D)** Cognitive dissonance occurs when a person holds two conflicting attitudes about the same event.

182. **(B)** German measles is also known as rubella. It is a contagious viral disease.

GENERAL

183. **(C)** When a word such as *septum* ends in *-um*, you can usually form the plural by dropping the *-um* and adding *-a*. A septum is a wall dividing two cavities.

184. **(D)** Adipose tissue is a collection of fat cells or loose connective tissue with many cells that contain fat vacuoles. It provides insulation for the human body.

185. **(C)** Exocytosis is the formation of vesicles to transfer substances from inside the cell to the outside of the cell.

186. **(E)** To handle incoming calls, follow these guidelines: Answer the telephone by the second or third ring, hold the mouthpiece about an inch away from your mouth and leave one hand free to write with, greet the caller with the name of the office and then with your name, identify the caller, be courteous, pay attention to the caller, use appropriate terminology and enunciate and pronounce correctly, avoid unnecessarily long conversations, and keep personal calls to a minimum.

187. **(B)** Type A blood has type A antigens and type B antibodies. The type A antigens sit on red blood cells, and the antibodies are found in the serum. Type A blood has type B antibodies, type B blood has type A antibodies, type AB has no antibodies, and type O has both types of antibodies. A handy rule to remember is that each blood group has the same type antigen as its name and the opposite antibody.

188. **(D)** An irresistible urge to engage in behaviors such as repeatedly touching a spot on arm is called compulsion disorder.

189. **(B)** Fraud is the act of intentionally misleading or deceiving another person by any means so as to cause him or her legal injury. Fraud usually leads to the loss of something valuable or the surrender of a legal right.

190. **(D)** Assault is the threat of bodily harm to another. Battery is an action that causes bodily harm to another. Battery is often broadly defined as the illegal touching of another person. In health care, battery may be charged for unauthorized touching of a patient, including such actions as suturing a wound, administering an injection, performing surgery, or performing a physical examination without consent.

191. **(B)** If you are interrupted by a second call, excuse yourself to the first caller and answer the second call. Determine the identity of the second caller and the nature of the call. Return to the first call as soon as possible and minimize waiting for all callers. In fact, if you have callers on hold, return to them occasionally to reassure them that you have not forgotten about them and to update them on what is going on. For example, if someone is waiting to talk to the physician but the physician is still busy, offer the caller an opportunity to leave a message or have the physician return the call as soon as possible.

192. **(A)** Cilia are membrane-enclosed bundles of microtubules that extend outward from cell membranes. They are short and numerous. Cilia move substances across the surface of the cell.

193. **(A)** Greet callers with the name of the office and then with your name. Do not answer the phone by simply giving the telephone number of your office or by saying "hello."

194. **(B)** The physician must advise patients against needless surgery, and the physician must advise patients of any risks associated with major surgery or a difficult procedure, but the physician is not bound to fully cure a patient or to restore a patient to a previous condition. The physician should not be negligent, but no physician is infallible. The physician is obligated only to treat the patient to the scope of the physician's training and education and to provide reasonable care according to his or her capabilities. For example, an ophthalmologist, trained in the disorders of the eye, might not recognize a disorder of the ear.

195. **(E)** Sexual harassment is persistent, unwanted sexual advances, attention, or communication, and it is prohibited in the workplace. Sexual harassment can be physical or verbal, expressed in gestures, in images, or in written and spoken words. It can occur at any level of the hierarchy within a workplace. It can result in personal distress for the recipient and legal trouble for the medical facility. When faced with sexual harassment, you may find that the easiest way to stop this behavior is to tell the harasser that the behavior has made you uncomfortable and that you wish it to stop. If this approach does not work, you should go to your supervisor or even seek help outside of your employment, either in support groups or with legal counsel.

196. **(C)** In a greenstick fracture, the bone is partially broken and partially bent. This type of fracture commonly occurs in children.

197. **(A)** According to Abraham Maslow's systematized theory of human behavior, all human needs can be organized into five successive categories or levels. The first level includes basic needs, such as for food, water, shelter, and clothing. The second level includes needs for safety and security. The third level includes needs for human companionship and a sense of belonging to a group. The fourth level includes needs for respect and self-esteem. The fifth level includes the need to achieve one's highest level of potential, a concept referred to as self-actualization.

198. **(A)** *Gon / o* means "genitals" or "semen." Gonorrhea is a contagious inflammation of the genital mucous membrane.

199. **(B)** Your body language complements your verbal messages, and it's important that your body language reflect what you are trying to say. Maintain eye contact with the patient when talking to him or her. Eye contact shows interest, attention, and sensitivity. Looking away might imply disinterest, boredom, or anger. Similarly, crossing or folding your arms creates a closed position that implies anger, distrust, and lack of caring. On the other hand, turning and leaning your body toward a person usually shows interest and focuses your attention.

200. **(B)** If a soccer player is unable to extend his knee after a sports injury, he may have injured the patellar tendon of the rectus femoris muscle.

201. **(C)** A suffix is word ending that modifies the meaning of the root. Not all words have a suffix. An example of a suffix can be found in the word *ganglionectomy*. *Ganglion* is the root, and *-ectomy* is the suffix.

202. **(A)** Green beans contain a high amount of fiber.

203. **(E)** Quadriplegia is the paralysis of the lower and upper extremities (the legs and arms) and the trunk, which results from spinal cord injury in the region of the fifth to seventh cervical vertebrae.

204. **(C)** A license to practice medicine is required by law in each state.

205. **(D)** Intact skin is the first line of defense against infection. The integumentary system protects the body from invading pathogens.

206. **(D)** *Keratosis* is the correctly spelled term.

207. **(E)** Physicians are required to submit statutory reports on a regular basis to various governmental agencies. Certain reports are required from all practicing physicians, including reports of births, deaths, and cases of food poisoning and communicable diseases (AIDS, hepatitis, neonatal herpes, Lyme disease, rabies, and sexually transmitted diseases). Physicians also need to report known or suspected abuse of any individual (e.g., child, elderly adult, or battered woman), drug abuse, and evidence of criminal acts (e.g., injuries resulting from violence, such as gunshot or stab wounds).

208. **(D)** The AAMA was founded at the 1955 annual state convention in Kansas.

209. **(B)** The iris is the anterior division of the vascular tunic of the eye.

210. **(C)** A comminuted fracture describes a bone that has broken into pieces. In an open or compound fracture, the broken bone creates an external wound that leads to the site of fracture; fragments of the bone commonly pierce through the skin. An oblique fracture is a slanted fracture of the shaft of the bone on its long axis. An incomplete fracture does not continue along the whole bone.

211. **(C)** The ulna and radius are bones located in the arm.

212. **(C)** Sarcoma is a malignant neoplasm or tumor of connective tissues such as bone or muscle. This type of cancer might affect the bones, bladder, kidneys, liver, lungs, and spleen.

213. **(A)** A pivot joint is a synovial joint in which movement is limited to rotation. The elbow is a type of pivot joint.

214. **(D)** Shock is the collapse of the cardiovascular system resulting in a dangerous reduction of blood flow throughout body tissues. Shock can be caused by sepsis, hemorrhage, heart failure, respiratory distress, or anaphylaxis.

215. **(B)** Active immunity is a long-term immunity in which the body produces its own antibodies. Active immunity can be natural or artificial. Natural active immunity results from the exposure to disease-causing organisms. Artificial active immunity results from the administration of a vaccine with killed or weakened organisms. Passive immunity results from the introduction into the body of antibodies that were produced outside the body. Natural passive immunity results when antibodies from the mother cross the placenta to the fetus. Artificial passive immunity results from immunization with antibodies to a disease-causing organism.

216. **(A)** Keratinization is the process by which epithelial cells lose their moisture and are replaced by keratin (protein). The stratum lucidum is the translucent band that is found only in thick-skinned individuals. The subcutaneous layer is the bottom layer of the cutaneous membrane, beneath the dermis, or true skin. The dermis contains hairs, nails, glands, fibers, sense receptors, and blood vessels. Cretinism is a congenital condition characterized by severe hypothyroidism and often associated with other endocrine abnormalities. Typical signs of cretinism include dwarfism, mental deficiency, puffy facial features, dry skin, and a large tongue.

217. **(C)** There are two main body cavities: dorsal and ventral. The dorsal cavity is divided into two separate cavities: the cranial cavity, which contains the brain, and the spinal cavity, which contains the spinal cord. The ventral cavity comprises the thoracic and the abdominopelvic cavities.

218. **(A)** Hypersensitivity is an abnormal condition characterized by an exaggerated response of the immune system to an antigen. High fever, anaphylaxis, asthma, and eczema are examples of type I hypersensitivities.

219. **(B)** You need to have such a request in writing from the patient authorizing the transfer.

220. **(E)** Sweat glands, also called sudoriferous glands, are widely distributed over the body, except for the lips, nipples, and parts of the external genitalia. Sweat glands are abundant on the palms of the hands and on the soles of the feet.

221. **(A)** Void is the correct description for something that is without legal force or effect. An implied contract is an unwritten or unspoken agreement, the terms of which result from the actions of the parties involved.

222. **(E)** Hyperplasia is an increase in the number of cells of a body part that results from an increased rate of cellular division.

223. **(D)** Hashimoto's disease is an autoimmune thyroid disorder. It is characterized by the production of antibodies in response to thyroid antigens.

224. **(C)** The fight-or-flight response is controlled by the sympathetic part of the autonomic nervous system, which acts as an accelerator for organs, especially the adrenal gland, whose functions are needed to meet a stressful situation. Heart rate, respiratory rate, blood pressure, and blood flow increase in response to an emergency situation. In addition, the pupils dilate, sweat glands are stimulated, the liver increases the release of glucose, and there is a reduction in the secretion of enzymes in the digestive system.

225. **(B)** *OD (oculus dexter)* is the abbreviation meaning "right eye."

226. **(E)** The abbreviation for "nothing by mouth" is *NPO* or *n.p.o.*, which stands for the Latin phrase *non per os*, "not by mouth." *PO* or *p.o.* stands for *per os*, "by mouth."

227. **(C)** Inspiration is the process of bringing air into the lungs. The major muscle of inspiration or inhalation is the diaphragm, the contraction of which creates negative pressure in the chest, allowing air to fill the lung along a pressure gradient.

228. **(C)** An open-ended question is one that is answered by more than a simple yes or no. "How would you describe your diet?" is an example of an open-ended question.

229. **(A)** Showing integrity and practicing high ethical standards is the best way to receive a positive evaluation during your externship.

230. **(D)** Even with the doctrine of *respondeat superior,* as a medical assistant you can be sued for your own negligent actions unless you were directly ordered to perform a certain task. The *respondeat superior* doctrine makes physicians responsible for the employee's actions; however, supervising someone is not the same as giving an order. You should not act negligently, and you should not go beyond the scope of your education and training. The doctrine of *res ipsa loquitur* applies to cases in which the physician clearly demonstrated negligence, such as by leaving surgical instruments in patients or by injuring a healthy body part during surgery. A physician is not contractually bound to cure every patient and every disease, because to do so would be an impossible task. The physician is contractually bound to perform to the best of his or her capabilities and to provide reasonable care to patients.

231. **(C)** Eugenics is the study of improving a population by selective breeding. This process is considered unethical in humans.

232. **(A)** *Hyper-* means "high," and *-tonic* means "pertaining to tension or contraction." *Hypertonic* applies to solutions that are of higher osmotic pressure than the fluid in cells as well as to muscles that are tense.

233. **(B)** The alveoli are clusters of air sacs at the end of the bronchioles in the lungs. The exchange of gases occurs in the alveoli.

234. **(B)** Food is chewed in the mouth and mixed with saliva to form a moist, soft lump called the bolus. The saliva moistens food and begins the chemical breakdown of carbohydrates.

235. **(D)** The endocrine system coordinates many body functions. Its response to change is slower and more prolonged than that of the nervous system. It would be incorrect to say that the nervous system controls only conscious activities. For example, the autonomic nervous system controls unconscious activities such as reflexes.

236. **(C)** Cushing's syndrome is the hyperactivity of the adrenal cortical gland. The patient experiences fatigue, weakness, fat deposits in the scapular area, a protruding abdomen, hypertension, edema, and hyperlipidemia.

237. **(D)** In order to comply with HIPAA, the physician must provide a notice of privacy practices to patients.

238. **(E)** The urinary system removes waste products, salts, and excess water from the blood and eliminates them from the body. The organs of the urinary system include the kidneys, ureters, urinary bladder, and the urethra.

239. **(A)** The small intestine is the longest part of the digestive tract, where the chemical digestion of fats and the final breakdown of carbohydrates and proteins take place. Most of the nutrients in food are absorbed in the small intestine.

240. **(C)** It is illegal to ask a prospective employee about his or her marital status.

241. **(C)** Liability insurance provides legal expenses in the event of a medical liability case, but it is not required by federal or state law.

242. **(A)** There are four basic taste sensations: salty, sweet, sour, and bitter. The very tip of the tongue contains sweet and salty receptors, the sides of the tongue contain sour receptors, and the back of the tongue contains bitter receptors.

243. **(D)** Confidentiality is one of the major concerns when sending medical reports via e-mail.

244. **(E)** Hyperemesis is excessive vomiting.

245. **(E)** The unauthorized disclosure of client information is an example of an invasion of privacy.

246. **(D)** Most prefixes can be connected to other word parts without a combining vowel. When two word roots are connected, a combining vowel is usually used even if vowels are present at the junction. Connecting a word root and a suffix that starts with a consonant usually requires a combining vowel. When a word root and a suffix are connected, a combining vowel is usually not used if the suffix begins with a vowel.

247. **(A)** The RMA examination may be scheduled almost any day of the year.

248. **(C)** Vitamin K represents a group of fat-soluble vitamins, known as quinones, that are essential for the synthesis of prothrombin in the liver.

249. **(D)** A plaintiff is a person who files a lawsuit, thereby initiating a legal action.

250. **(E)** Onychophagia is the habit of excessively biting and chewing one's fingernails and periungual skin, sometimes leading to cutaneous injury.

251. **(B)** Language is a symbolic code structured in a specific way, used to communicate ideas.

252. **(C)** A person's parents and family are part of his or her social network.

253. **(C)** Behavioral genetics is the study of how behavior is affected by genes.

254. **(C)** A stressor is an event, good or bad, that causes an individual to change or adapt.

255. **(D)** The exhaustion phase of GAS occurs when the patient is unable to adapt to the stressors.

256. **(C)** The ego works on the reality principle to help bring impulses into the norms of society.

257. **(A)** Projection is a defense mechanism attributing unwanted feelings onto someone else.

258. **(B)** Shifting feelings towards an unacceptable object onto a more acceptable one is known as displacement.

259. **(C)** The phallic stage of personality development is the stage when a child is coming to terms with identification with the same-sex parent.

260. **(A)** The humanistic theory of personality asserts that humans are striving to reach their full potential.

261. **(C)** The humanistic theory of personality asserts that humans are striving to reach their full potential and can do so with encouragement and unconditional positive regard.

262. **(B)** Humanists believe that humans possess an internal force that pushes them to grow, improve, and become the best individuals that they are capable of being.

263. **(C)** The experience of long-term, persistent anxiety and worry is known as generalized anxiety disorder.

264. **(C)** Panic disorder is a pattern of anxiety in which long periods of calm are broken by intensely uncomfortable attacks of anxiety.

265. **(A)** Bipolar disorder is characterized by periods of depression followed by periods of mania.

266. **(C)** Identical female twins are more likely to have a major depressive disorder.

267. **(A)** Schizophrenia is a psychological disorder involving cognitive disturbances, disorganization, and reduced enjoyment and interests.

268. **(D)** Autism is a mental disorder characterized by extreme withdrawal and an abnormal absorption in fantasy, accompanied by delusions, hallucinations, and the inability to communicate verbally or otherwise relate to people.

269. **(C)** According to Maslow the biological needs are primary. These include air, food, water, clothing, and shelter.

270. **(B)** Empathy involves a person experiencing another person's emotional state by viewing the situation through that person's eyes.

271. **(B)** A person who changes an unacceptable motive to its exact opposite is using a defense mechanism known as reaction formation.

272. **(A)** Freud describes the latency stage as the stage that occurs between the ages of 5 and adolescence. During this stage a child puts his sexual concerns aside.

273. **(D)** According to Humanists, humans possess an internal force, an inner-directedness, that pushes them to grow, to improve, and to become the best individuals that they are capable of being.

274. **(C)** Autism is a mental disorder characterized by extreme withdrawal and an abnormal absorption in fantasy, accompanied by delusions, hallucinations, and the inability to communicate verbally or otherwise relate to people.

275. **(C)** Denial is a refusal to accept an anxiety-producing event as reality.

276. **(C)** A personal stressor is caused by life events.

277. **(D)** The acceptance stage of death is characterized by a sense of peace that death will happen and a quiet state of recognition that all livings things die.

278. **(D)** Empathy involves a person experiencing another person's emotional state by viewing the situation through that person's eyes.

279. **(A)** Anything that threatens or challenges a person is known as a stressor.

280. **(D)** Cognitive psychology is the study of intellectual processes and how these processes affect development.

281. **(A)** Stress can result from positive or negative events.

282. **(D)** Attributing unwanted feelings to someone else is known as projection.

283. **(B)** The humanistic theory of personality states that humans are striving to reach their full potential and can do so with encouragement and unconditional positive reward.

284. **(B)** According to Maslow's hierarchy of needs, a person must first fulfill his primary or biological needs.

285. **(B)** Ross describes denial as a person's attempt to deny a terminal diagnosis.

286. **(A)** Fight-or-flight syndrome is invoked by fear.

287. **(E)** An uplift is a stress-reducing, minor event that can make a person feel good.

288. **(D)** GAS theory suggests that persons under stress experience the same set of psychological reactions, including alarm and mobilization, resistance, and exhaustion.

289. **(C)** A personal stressor is caused by life events.

290. **(A)** According to Erikson, conflict in adolescence is identity *vs.* role confusion. A positive outcome in this stage of development is awareness of one's own uniqueness.

291. **(C)** According to Maslow's hierarchy of needs, a person must first fulfill his primary or biological needs.

292. **(B)** Scientific method uses a systematic approach to gain knowledge. There are three steps used in this method. These steps include identifying the problem, formulating a rationale, and performing supportive research.

293. **(D)** Mental processes are private thoughts, emotions, and feelings and cannot be directly observed.

294. **(D)** Schizophrenia is a psychological disorder involving cognitive disturbances, disorganization, and reduced enjoyment and interests.

295. **(D)** Behaviorists believe that behaviors are changed by removing reinforcers and imposing consequences for the actions.

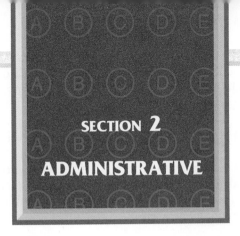

MEDICAL ASSISTING KNOWLEDGE

Self-Evaluation Answers and Rationales

Here you'll find the answers to the test on General Medical Assisting Knowledge on p. 497 in Part 2. Check your answers and note which questions you missed. Study the rationales for any questions you feel you had difficulty with, and if you need more review, go back to the appropriate section in the chapters.

1. **(C)** A modem is necessary for electronic data interchange. Modem-to-modem connections provide secure and reliable high-speed, continuous transmissions.

2. **(D)** $40 \times 12 = $480. You then need to deduct 10% of $480 to find the discounted price. 10% of $480 = $48. Subtract $48 from $480 to find the discounted price of $432, which is the cost of the 12 items.

3. **(C)** The primary purpose of a patient record-filing system is to facilitate efficient document retrieval. All files should be able to be accessed quickly and economically, whether on paper or in an electronic format.

4. **(A)** Wave scheduling can provide flexibility to accommodate unforeseen situations, such as a patient who requires more time or a patient who arrives late. For wave scheduling to work, the medical facility should have multiple procedure rooms and adequate personnel.

5. **(E)** Good medical records help a physician provide continuity in a patient's medical care. They also supply statistical information which can be used to revise techniques and treatments. Medical records can also be used in lawsuits and malpractice cases either to support a patient's claim or to support the physician's defense against such a claim. They can also help to evaluate the quality of treatment a doctor's office provides. Medical records also provide documentation for insurance billing and the basis for defending audits by managed care and government (Medicare and Medicaid) regulatory agencies.

6. **(B)** Medical assistants should answer the phone promptly by the second or third ring. Hold the phone's mouthpiece about an inch away from your mouth and leave at least one hand free to write with. Greet callers first with the name of the office and then with your name. Do not answer the phone by simply repeating the number of your office or by saying "hello." Although the type of calls you usually handle as a medical assistant will be administrative, you will still be expected to answer the phone and transfer the patient to the physician when it is necessary. You should never give a diagnostic opinion to a patient either on the phone or in person.

7. **(A)** In order to maintain accurate patient records, you should keep these six concepts in mind: client's words, clarity, completeness, conciseness, chronological order, and confidentiality.

8. **(B)** Closed files are records of patients who have died, moved away, or otherwise terminated their relationship with the physician.

9. **(A)** In managed care, a participating provider agrees to accept allowed charges in return for various incentives, such as fast payment. If a participating provider charges more for a service than the allowed charge, the physician must write off the difference. The patient, like Mr. Johnson, may not be billed for this amount.

10. **(C)** The double-entry system is based on the accounting equation: *Assets = Liability + Owner Equity*. This system requires more extensive knowledge of accounting procedures than the simpler single-entry or pegboard systems.

11. **(B)** The balance equals the difference between the debit and credit totals. The balance column is usually on the far right side of a ledger. A debit is recorded on the left side of an account and is also called a charge. A credit is recorded on the right side of an account and is also referred to as revenue or net worth.

12. **(E)** Taking a trial balance is a method of checking the accuracy of accounts. It should be done once a month after all posting has been completed and before preparing the monthly statements. The purpose of a trial balance is to disclose any discrepancies between the journal and the ledger.

13. **(E)** Items that weigh 13 oz or less may be sent as First Class Mail. First Class Mail that weighs over 13 oz becomes Priority Mail. Anything the post office accepts for mailing can be mailed as First Class Mail; however, some things *must* be mailed as First Class Mail (or Priority Mail). Handwritten or typewritten material, bills, statements of account or invoices, and credit cards should be mailed First Class.

14. **(C)** Generally, calls from insurance companies will not require the physician's personal attention.

15. **(A)** The usual fee is what an individual physician most frequently charges for a service to private patients. The customary fee is a range of fees charged by most physicians in the community for a particular service. For example, the range of fees for a check-up could be from $40 to $50 in a community. The prevailing charges are fees most frequently charged in an area. For example, for a check-up, fees could range from $40 to $50; however, upon closer investigation an insurance company could learn that 10 physicians in the community charge $45, three charge $40, one charges $42, and four charge $50. In this case, the prevailing fee would be $45.

16. **(A)** Standard Mail (A) is designed for printed matter, flyers, circulars, advertising, newsletters, bulletins, catalogs, and small parcels. All Standard Mail (A) must be mailed in bulk. There must be at least 200 pieces of mail or 50 pounds of mail to get this low rate. The periodicals classification is designed for newspapers, magazines, and other periodical publications whose primary purpose is transmitting information to an established list of subscribers or requesters. Periodicals must be published at regular intervals at least four times a year from a known office of publication and be formed of printed sheets. There are specific standards for, among other things, circulation, record keeping, and advertising limits. There is a nonrefundable application fee to become authorized for Periodicals mailing privileges.

17. **(B)** Medicare Part B covers outpatient services, services by physicians, durable medical equipment, and other services and supplies. This coverage is optional. Medicare Part A covers hospital, nursing, facility, home health, hospice, and inpatient care.

18. **(C)** Medigap policies are private insurance contracts that supplement regular Medicare coverage. They often pay for the beneficiary's deductibles, coinsurance, and in some cases for services not covered by Medicare. If the subscriber has Medigap insurance, Medicare is still the primary payer, which means claims must be filed with Medicare first.

19. **(A)** Medicaid is a health cost assistance program for needy individuals. Coverage may vary from month to month based on the recipient's income. Physicians are not obligated to treat Medicaid patients, but if they do accept Medicaid patients, they also accept Medicaid reimbursement for covered services and they cannot bill the patients for any differences in cost. Medicaid is always a secondary carrier to Medicare.

20. **(E)** In order to protect essential computerized information, it is important to make regular back ups of files onto disks, CD-ROMs, or zip drives. It's also important to store these back-up files off premises. While not opening an email attachment from someone you don't know or an attachment you did not expect to receive provides good protection against certain computer viruses, it will definitely not protect your computer from a fire. Opening an email is usually harmless, since viruses are usually programs sent as an attachment to emails. Another good way to protect your computers from viruses is by purchasing an up-to-date virus detection and protection program.

21. **(E)** Provider data, patient data, insurance carriers, diagnosis codes, procedure codes, and transactions are usually stored on large medical databases. A database is a collection of related data organized within a specific structure. For example, the procedures code database would contain data needed to create charges such as the *Physician's Current Procedural Terminology*, as well as place of service. The source of these codes is often the patient superbill.

22. **(A)** You should send out the first collection letter or statement when an account is 30 days overdue, and follow up at 60, 90, and 120 days. You should not call the patient at work nor pay the patient a personal visit. Write a letter that reminds the patient of a possible oversight of debt and call the patient at home only during reasonable hours.

23. **(A)** Out of the given list of names, Paul Edward Jr. would be the first patient record filed.

24. **(D)** The physician is required by law to keep payroll data for 4 years. The records should include the employee's Social Security number, the number of withholding allowances claimed, gross salary, and deductions for Social Security tax; Medicare tax; federal; state and other tax; state disability insurance; and state unemployment tax.

25. **(D)** An employer must file and submit a quarterly federal tax return.

26. **(A)** HCPCS, pronounced "hic-pics," is mandated by Congress for Medicare claims and updated annually. It is a five-digit alphanumerical coding system that can accommodate the addition of modifiers.

27. **(C)** If a procedure is unlisted, the insurance form has guidelines at the beginning of each section on what codes to use. In these cases, a special report must be attached to the claim to describe and explain the extent of and reasons for service. ICD-9-CM refers to the *International Classification of Diseases, 9th revision, Clinical Modification*, which is used to list what is wrong with the patient and what initially brought the patient to see the doctor.

28. **(E)** A voucher check is frequently used for payroll checks since it allows additional information such as deductions to be supplied to the payee.

29. **(B)** FUTA is the Federal Unemployment Tax Act, which requires employers to pay a percentage of each employee's gross income. This amount should not be deducted from the employee's wages.

30. **(A)** When a patient goes to a nonparticipating provider of Medicare, the patient pays the practice, and then the patient receives reimbursement from Medicare.

31. **(E)** To ensure accurate transcription, you should have needed materials at hand; adjust the transcribing equipment's speed, tone, and volume; listen all the way through before starting to transcribe; write down the time on the digital counter for any problems so that you can find them quickly when requesting clarification; and listen carefully.

32. **(A)** Indexing refers to a method of deciding where to file a letter or paper. Indexing is an organized method of identifying and separating items to be filed into small subunits. Each unit is identified according to unit number. The key individual's unit, unit 1, is the individual's last name. Unit 2 is the individual's first name. Unit 3 is the middle initial. Unit 4 is a title or special name such as Mrs. or Dr.

33. **(B)** A menu is a list of commands or options that can be selected when using a computer. For example, the File menu of most word processing programs includes the commands New File, Open File, Close File, and Save File.

34. **(C)** The medical assistant responsible for coding should attend at least one CPT and one ICD-9 class each year.

35. **(D)** The W-2 form lists the total gross income; total federal, state, and local taxes that were withheld; and taxable fringe benefits such as tips. The amount of wages that were taxable under Social Security and Medicare are listed separately.

36. **(E)** The maximum size for mail pieces is 108 inches in combined length and girth. The maximum mailable weight of any mail piece is 70 pounds. Items mailed as Parcel Post can have a maximum combined length and girth of 130 inches.

37. **(E)** *Inactive* is the term used to describe the medical records of patients who have not been in the office for several years.

38. **(E)** Special Delivery allowed mail to be delivered as soon as it reached the recipient's post office. Special Delivery stamps could be purchased at the post office. Special Delivery was used for regular First Class, Second Class, and insured mail. Special Delivery could not be used for mail addressed to a post office box or military installation. Please note that this is an outdated service that might still appear on the certification exams.

39. **(D)** A color-coded filing system is the best type of filing system because it is designed to reduce the misfiling of patient folders. An out-of-place file folder is easily seen because the color tab attached to it breaks the color sequence of the surrounding files.

40. **(B)** The Blue Cross and Blue Shield Association is a nationwide federation of local nonprofit service organizations that offer prepaid health-care services to subscribers.

41. **(C)** A regular referral usually takes 3 to 10 days, an urgent referral takes 24 hours, and STAT referrals are done over the phone and take place immediately.

42. **(D)** The Health Care Financing Administration designed a form called the CMS-1500 to handle Medicare and Medicaid claims. It is the most commonly accepted insurance form by private insurance providers as well.

43. **(B)** The Blue Cross part of the BCBS covers hospital services, home care services, and other institutional care. Blue Shield covers physician services, dental, vision, and other outpatient benefits.

44. **(B)** The primary diagnosis refers to the main condition for which a patient is treated. When a cancer patient comes in with the flu, the primary diagnosis will be the flu, not cancer.

45. **(C)** Placing area rugs in the reception area of a medical office is an example of a safety hazard. Area rugs may be tripping hazards because of turned-up corners and the potential of patients to slip when walking on them.

46. **(A)** FICA stands for the Federal Insurance Contribution Act, which funds Social Security. The employee pays half and the employer pays the other half of these taxes. Taxes are based on the level of taxable earnings, the length of the payroll period, marital status, and the number of withholding allowances claimed.

47. **(E)** The general journal is known also as the daily log, daybook, daysheet, daily journal, and charge journal. This journal is where all transactions are first recorded.

48. **(E)** The amount charged for a medical insurance policy, in which the insurer agrees to provide certain benefits, is called the premium.

49. **(E)** Coordination of benefits can prevent duplicate payment for the same service.

50. **(B)** The process of checking transcribed materials for accuracy and clarity is referred to as proofreading. Proofreading business letters and transcribed documents helps to reduce the possibility of medication, legal, or information errors that could result in medical malpractice charges or problems with patient care.

51. **(E)** CHAMPVA covers spouses of veterans with permanent, service-related disabilities. Survivors of veterans who died from service-related injuries or in the line of duty are also covered.

52. **(E)** A *Special Handling* endorsement is required for parcels whose unusual contents require additional care in transit and handling. Special handling is not required for those parcels sent by First Class, Express, or Priority Mail. Special handling is available for Standard Mail only, including insured and COD mail. Special handling service is not necessary for sending ordinary parcels even when they contain fragile items. Breakable items will receive adequate protection if they are packed with sufficient cushioning and clearly marked *FRAGILE*. If special handling is required, the words *SPECIAL HANDLING*, (similar to other mailing notations such as *CERTIFIED*, *HAND CANCEL*, or *REGISTERED*) should be printed in capital letters two lines below the postage.

53. **(C)** Liability insurance covers medical expenses for patients who are injured on the physician's property. For example, in Florida, the law limits a doctor's liability for injuries occurring to patients in the medical facility to $750,000 in most cases.

54. **(B)** Blue Cross makes direct payment to physician members.

55. **(B)** To maximize communication with children, you must work directly with them, rather than communicating through parents.

56. **(A)** Diagnostic-related groups, or DRGs, are groups of procedures or tests related directly to diagnosis. The fixed fees paid by Medicare Part A are based on DRGs.

57. **(D)** Accounts receivable are the amounts owed to a business for services or goods supplied.

58. **(C)** The postal abbreviation for *Circle* is *CIR*.

59. **(B)** Capitation is a reimbursement type often used in group-model HMOs. A fixed fee is paid to the physician monthly regardless of the number of times the patient visits the physician.

60. **(A)** ∧ is a proofreader's mark meaning *insert*. This mark is usually followed by some text to be inserted or # indicating that a space should be inserted.

61. **(E)** In the medical assisting profession, appearance is very important. Every medical facility will have its own dress code, but these general rules will apply in most places.

62. **(C)** Under the old classification system, Third Class Mail included books and catalogues of 24 or fewer bound pages, manuscript copies, identification cards, circulars, and other printed materials, as well as all other matter weighing less than 16 ounces that was not sent First or Second Class.

63. **(E)** In general, mail processing involves sorting, opening, recording, annotating, and distributing. Some physicians prefer to open letters from attorneys or accountants. Mail such as routine office expense bills, insurance forms, and checks for deposit may not need to be opened by the physician. In general, when you transmit letters to the physician, place the most important letters on the top and the least important ones on the bottom. Usually something marked *Special Delivery* is considered important mail. After opening the mail, medical assistants usually need to date stamp the letters, check for enclosures, and in some cases annotate the letter. You should not open mail marked *Personal* or *Confidential* unless you have the addressee's explicit permission.

64. **(D)** Guidelines that dictate the day-to-day workings of an office are policies.

65. **(B)** The term *enunciation* means "to speak clearly and to articulate carefully."

66. **(D)** Most medical offices use a postage meter that automatically stamps large mailings. The postage can be printed directly onto an envelope with a meter. The advantages of using a postage meter include saving trips to the post office and saving money by providing exact postage without having to have every denomination of stamps at hand.

67. **(A)** Memos are usually intended for interoffice correspondence. The purpose is to expedite the communication of a message in a manner that provides a record without becoming cumbersome. They are used to inform personnel about meetings and general changes that affect everyone. You should not use salutations and complimentary closes in memos. The standard format for a memorandum contains a to, from, date, and subject line before the body of the memo. The body of the memo starts two blank lines after the subject line and has no paragraph indentations.

68. **(B)** When using a modified-block letter style, begin all lines at the left margin, with the exception of the date line, complimentary closure, and keyed signature, which usually begin at the center position.

69. **(C)** Assignment of benefits is the authorization to the insurance company to make payments directly to the physician.

70. **(C)** *Junction* should be abbreviated as *JCT*.

71. **(E)** The address must be typed on the envelope using single spacing and all capital letters with no punctuation. Put the addressee's name on the first line, the department on the second line, and the company name on the third line. If the letter is being sent to someone's attention at the company, put the company name first and *ATTENTION: [NAME]* on the second line. The last line in the address must include the city, the two-digit state code, and the zip code.

72. **(B)** For a doctor, the title should read as either *Dr. Mary Jack* or *Mary Jack, M.D.* The form *Dr. Mary Jack, M.D.*, is incorrect. It is also preferable to use a professional degree such as *M.D.* instead of an academic title such as *Dr.* The degree designations should be abbreviated.

73 **(D)** As a medical assistant, you must learn how to remain calm when you deal with an angry patient.

74. **(E)** *Triage* refers to the screening and sorting of emergency situations.

75. **(C)** On the inside address of a business letter, spell out numerical names of streets but use numerals for the street address except for single numbers one through nine, which should be spelled out. Also spell out the words *Street, Drive, Boulevard, Place,* and so on.

76. **(D)** An Independent Practice Association is a type of HMO in which a program administrator contracts with a number of physicians who agree to provide treatment to subscribers in their own office for a fixed capitation payment per month.

77. **(B)** The signature block contains the sender's name on the first line and title on the second line. The block should be aligned with the closing and be typed four lines below it to allow for the signature.

78. **(C)** Travelers' checks are available in foreign currencies. Travelers' checks are designed for people who are traveling where personal checks may not be accepted and for people who don't want to carry large amounts of cash.

79. **(A)** Things of a routine business nature such as ordering supplies are often signed by the medical assistant; however, medical reports, letters to insurance companies, consultation or referral letters, and letters clinical in nature should be signed by the physician.

80. **(E)** The most common types of envelopes used in the medical office are the Number $6\frac{3}{4}$ and Number 10.

81. **(A)** A return address for the sender should always be placed in the upper lefthand corner.

82. **(B)** There are three types of file cabinets used in the medical office: vertical, lateral, and movable file cabinets.

83. **(A)** Modems may be used to transfer information from one computer to another by means of telephone lines and servers.

84. **(C)** Established diagnoses are coded on insurance claim forms.

85. **(B)** Vital supplies are absolutely essential to ensure the smooth running of the practice. An example of these supplies is prescription pads.

86. **(B)** Minutes are the official record of the proceedings of a meeting. An agenda is the order of business for a meeting. When keeping minutes, you should note the date, location, time, and purpose of the meeting, the presiding officer, names of people in attendance, the agenda, motions made, and summaries of discussions.

87. **(E)** The collection ratio measures the effectiveness of the billing system.

88. **(C)** *Reschedule* is abbreviated as *RS*.

89. **(D)** An encounter form is referred to as a fee schedule. Claims that are filed for a prepaid service are called encounter claims.

90. **(D)** According to the National Childhood Vaccine Injury Act of 1986, all immunization records must be kept permanently.

91. **(A)** Advanced scheduling refers to when appointments are made weeks or months in advance.

92. **(E)** The Resource-Based Relative Value Scale (RBRVS) is a system used by Medicare since 1992 to determine uniform payments for medical services that take geographical differences into account. A relative value unit is determined for each medical service on the basis of the physician's work, which requires time and skill, and the provider's expenses, such as running the office and having malpractice insurance. The MFS is developed using the RBRVS. The participating physician may bill the patient for coinsurance and deductibles but may not collect excess charges.

93. **(B)** Carol Jones can be billed for only 10% of the set fee, which is $140. Therefore, her bill would be for $14. The physician, by accepting Medicare patients, accepts the Medicare fee schedule, and the medical office may not bill the patient for any difference between usual fees and the Medicare assigned fee.

94. **(A)** An 80:20 plan means that the insurance carrier will pay for 80% of all medical fees, making the subscriber, Mark, responsible for coinsurance, 20% of all medical fees. Twenty percent of 200 equals $40. An easy way to calculate this without a calculator is to first determine 10% by moving the decimal point one space to the left (10% of $200 is $20). Then multiply the 10% figure by 2.

95. **(A)** Forwarding is offered free of charge to Priority, First Class, and Standard Mail (A). Standard Mail (B) is forwarded locally at no charge, but if it is going out of town, extra postage will be due. First Class and Priority mail are returned at no charge; Standard Mail (A) is returned for a charge based on weight; and Standard Mail (B) return is charged at the appropriate single-piece rate. Return service is free for First Class and Priority Mail, but Standard Mail (A) is charged First Class or Priority Mail rates for the return. Certificates of mailing are not free. They can be purchased at the time of mailing.

96. **(B)** According to the ICD-9-CM, V codes are used to classify factors that influence the patient's health status and contact with health services. These codes are updated frequently and become more specific to new diseases every year.

97. **(B)** Steps toward having a positive attitude include using positive statements instead of negative statements, smiling instead of frowning, and saying something pleasant instead of complaining.

98. **(D)** Some physicians prefer to open letters from attorneys or accountants. Mail such as routine office expense bills, insurance forms, and checks for deposit may not need to be opened by the physician. Personal letter or letters marked *Confidential* also should not be opened unless you have the expressed permission of the addressee. It's always good to check with the physician to find out what mail falls under your responsibility and what mail he or she prefers to open.

99. **(D)** The explanation of benefits is a document that the medical practice receives from the insurance carrier, and it shows how the amount of the benefit was determined. The insurance carrier keeps a running account of the deductible, and this deductible will be listed on the explanation of benefits. Until the deductible has been met, the physician may bill the patient for the amount listed as the deductible on the explanation of benefits.

100. **(B)** When a patient goes to a nonparticipating provider, the patient is responsible for any difference between the allowed charge and the physician's usual fee as well as any deductible, co-payment, or coinsurance. If the patient had gone to a participating provider, the physician would not be able to bill the patient for any difference between the physician's usual fee and the allowed charge. Any difference would have to become a write-off for the physician.

101. **(B)** Filing business and organizational records is based on subject and topic.

102. **(E)** Bank drafts are checks written by a bank against its funds in another bank.

103. **(C)** Hospice programs were developed to provide care for patients who are terminally ill. Most hospices service all patients, regardless of their ability to pay.

104. **(C)** The patient cannot be charged the difference between the allowed charge and the physician's usual fees. So the $12 difference will be a write-off for the practice. However, the patient is responsible for the deductible and the co-payment. The allowed charge is $78 and the carrier will pay $38 of that. The difference is $40, which is the total of the copayment and the deductible.

105. **(C)** Registered Mail is the most secure service offered by the post office. Registered Mail provides insurance coverage for valuable items and is controlled from the point of mailing to the point of delivery. This service should be reserved for mailing items of tangible value, such as gifts or items that cannot be replaced in case of loss or damage. Both First Class Mail and Priority Mail can be registered.

106. **(A)** Federal Insurance Contribution Act (FICA) funds Social Security.

107. **(B)** Restricted delivery means that the mail is delivered only to a specific addressee or someone authorized in writing to receive mail for the addressee. Restricted delivery is available only for Registered Mail, Certified Mail, COD mail, and mail insured for more than $50.

108. **(C)** You can recall mail by filling out a written application at the post office and by giving it to the post office along with an envelope that is addressed identically to the one you want to recall. A mail carrier is not permitted to simply give mail back to you.

109. **(E)** For adequate legal protection, a patient's medical record should include the following items: patient registration form, patient medical history, physical examination results, results of laboratory tests, copies of prescription notes on refill authorizations, diagnosis and treatment plan, patient progress reports, follow-up visits, and telephone calls, informed consent forms, discharge summary, and correspondence with and about the patient.

110. **(D)** In proofreading, the direction to "move text to the right" is symbolized by the following character:].

111. **(B)** The easiest way to determine what the petty cash vouchers should total on January 18 is to subtract the $85 balance from the balance on January 1, which was $150; the difference between these two is $65. Therefore, the vouchers should show that $65 was taken out of petty cash.

112. **(D)** Patients seen on a first-come, first-served basis are scheduled chronologically. *Chronological* means "in order of date or time."

113. **(B)** According to the American Medical Association and the American Hospital Association, patient records should be kept for 10 years after the patient's final visit.

114. **(B)** The Health Insurance Portability and Accountability Act (HIPAA) gives some federal income tax advantages to individuals who buy certain long-term care insurance policies. As a result of HIPAA, qualifying persons who purchase long-term care policies can deduct the premiums when medical expenses exceed 7.5% of their adjusted gross income.

115. **(D)** *SDx* is a notation that indicates a V code that can only be used as a secondary diagnosis. *S* stands for *secondary* and *Dx* stands for *diagnosis*.

116. **(B)** TRICARE was formerly known as CHAMPUS, a health-care benefit for families of uniformed personal and retirees from the uniformed services.

117. **(D)** Accepting a predated check is not a risk unless the check is predated more than 6 months.

118. **(E)** When new supplies are received, you should place them in the back of the supply area.

119. **(C)** A spreadsheet is a computer program that simulates a business or scientific worksheet and performs the necessary calculations when data is changed. It is used most often in accounting procedures.

120. **(A)** Virtual memory is the slowest type of memory that uses the hard disk to store programs and data when all the RAM has been used.

121. **(E)** The stop-and-start control on a transcription machine is useful when the physician speaks quickly.

122. **(B)** Collating records involves collecting all records, test results, and information pertaining to the patient who is scheduled to be seen by the physician. This is usually done the day before the patient is seen.

123. **(A)** A balance column is used for recording the difference between the debit and credit columns.

124. **(B)** In a journal entry, the dollar amount of debit must be equal to the dollar amount of the credit. For example, an amount owed by a patient to the medical facility is a debit for the patient and a credit to the facility.

125. **(C)** Overdue accounts are identified by account aging.

126. **(B)** The AAMA's website address is www.aama.org.

127. **(E)** Claims might be denied because a claim is not for a covered benefit, the patient has a preexisting condition that is not covered, the patient's coverage has been cancelled, the physician's procedure was experimental, no preauthorization was obtained, and the physician provided services before the patient's health insurance contract went into effect.

128. **(C)** The petty cash fund is maintained to pay small, unpredictable cash expenditures.

129. **(A)** Your best course of action is to write a claim appeal, a written request to the insurance carrier to review the reimbursement. Perhaps the patient's condition was an emergency and there was no time to obtain preauthorization. It is best to review the patient's contract with the insurance carrier. You should bill the patient when a claim is rejected for the reasons that the patient's coverage has been canceled or the physician provided services before the patient's health insurance went into effect. If the claim is rejected because the insurance company considers the physician's procedure experimental, your office might request a peer review or call the carrier to discuss options.

130. **(D)** Claims for Medicare must be filed by December 31 of the year following that in which the services were rendered. Medicare forms must be signed by both the patient and the physician. Nonparticipating providers are not required to accept assignment of benefits, and the allowable payment to nonparticipating providers is less than the payments to participating providers. Providers are required by law to file the CMS-1500 for all eligible patients.

131. **(B)** When a patient has both Medicare and Medicaid, the claim form is first processed through Medicare, the primary provider, and then the claim is automatically forwarded to Medicaid, the secondary provider. This is sometimes referred to as a crossover claim.

132. **(E)** When processing TRICARE claims, if the provider accepts assignment, the patient will be billed for the deductible and any coinsurance. If the provider does not accept assignment, the patient is responsible for filing claims with TRICARE.

133. **(A)** Specifications for personal appearance are included in office policy manuals. Generally, these specifications indicate conservative, professional clothing, hairstyles, makeup, and jewelry.

134. **(E)** Express mail is available seven days a week and it guarantees overnight delivery of an item. Federal Express and the United Parcel Service also offer next-day delivery.

135. **(D)** For installment payments (such as for prenatal care), administrative medical assistants need to know the conditions of the Truth in Lending Act. Patients who pay their bill in more than 4 installments must have a written contract with their physician.

136. **(A)** Incidental supplies can be clinical, administrative, or general in nature. They do not threaten the efficiency of the office if the supplies run low. Incidental supplies include rubber bands and staples.

137. **(B)** Open-ended questions should be asked of all patients. They allow the patient to elaborate on feelings and symptoms, and they help you understand the patient better. Children should be treated with the same respect and attention as adults.

138. **(E)** Claims for Medicare must be filed by December 31 of the year following that in which the services were rendered.

139. **(C)** The average medical practice spends 4% to 6% of its annual gross income on supplies. If costs exceed 6%, reevaluate the office's spending practices and impose some cost-saving measures.

140. **(C)** An appointment card often serves as a reminder to the patient about an appointment scheduled with the medical office.

141. **(A)** Open booking is the most common scheduling system used in urgent care centers. Some types of treatment provided in urgent care facilities cover work-related injuries, sprains, fractures, and lacerations.

142. **(C)** Double booking means two or more patients are scheduled into the same time slot.

143. **(C)** The records of the workers' compensation case should be kept separate from the patient's regular history. The insurance carrier is entitled to receive copies of all records pertaining to the industrial injury. The injured person's records must be personally signed by the physician. The insurance carrier may provide its own billing forms. The patient is not billed.

144. **(E)** The bank statement's caption provides a summary of account activity that has taken place during the month up to the closing date. It includes the beginning balance, total value of checks processed, total amount of deposits made, service charges, and an ending balance. You should reconcile this statement with the practice's own records.

145. **(D)** Under the guidelines of the Social Security Act, a patient who has had his or her 65th birthday is entitled to receive benefits under Medicare Part A.

ADMINISTRATIVE

146. **(C)** There are many reasons why material would be filed using a system of subjects in a medical office. If physicians are doing research, they might wish to index research according to disease.

147. **(E)** Memory is usually measured in bytes.

148. **(A)** A warrant is a nonnegotiable check, issued to indicate that a debt should be paid, for example, by an insurance company.

149. **(A)** When you accept a check, immediately endorse it and write the words *For deposit only* on the back.

150. **(E)** Before writing off the amount, you can try to collect through the court system or through a collection agency. After an account has been released to a collection agency, your medical office should make no further attempts to collect the debt.

151. **(B)** A rider constitutes an addition to an insurance policy, often attached on a separate piece of paper. The premium is the amount charged for a medical insurance policy.

152. **(A)** The Truth in Lending Act requires creditors to provide applicants with accurate and complete credit costs and terms, clearly and obviously.

153. **(C)** Open-book accounts are the most typical accounts for patients of a medical practice.

154. **(A)** You should never ignore mistakes made in billing. You should rebill the claim. Waiting for the insurance provider to notice the mistake might take too long, and they might not notice the mistake. It is best to correct any mistakes as soon as you catch them.

155. **(A)** Special Standard Mail is generally used for books (at least 8 pages long), film (16mm or narrower), printed music, printed test materials, sound recordings, play scripts, educational charts, loose-leaf pages, binders consisting of medical information, and computer-readable material.

156. **(C)** Payroll deductions are the amounts withheld. *Withholding* means that a certain amount of money is set aside from each paycheck and is put toward the employee's taxes for the approaching tax period.

157. **(A)** The magnetic medium inside the computer where information is permanently stored for later retrieval is known as the hard drive.

158. **(B)** Accounts payable refers to the accounts a physician owes to others for equipment and services.

159. **(D)** Aging accounts receivable is a procedure that classifies accounts by age from the first date of billing. It should list all patient account balances, when charges were incurred, the most recent payment date, and any notes regarding the account. The age analysis is a good tool to show the status of each account at a glance.

160. **(D)** Productivity, accuracy, and cash flow are advantages of electronic banking over traditional banking. A medical assistant is still responsible for recording and depositing checks.

161. **(B)** According to the CPT, when coding an insurance claim for a tonsillectomy, the code should be listed under the respiratory system.

162. **(B)** The postal abbreviation for Minnesota is *MN*. The other choices stand for the following states: *MT* is the abbreviation for Montana, *MI* for Michigan, *MA* for Massachusetts, and *MS* for Mississippi.

163. **(A)** Some providers do not schedule appointments; they prefer to conduct their practices with open office hours. This system is the least structured.

164. **(B)** The Fair Credit Reporting Act (FCRA) requires credit bureaus to supply correct and complete information to businesses to use in evaluating a person's application for credit, insurance, or a job. If an applicant sues the practice in federal court for violating the FCRA, the practice may have to pay damages, punitive damages, court costs, and lawyers' fees.

165. **(E)** Assertiveness means someone being firm and standing up for oneself while showing respect for others.

166. **(C)** The subject system is the most appropriate filing system for organizing and storing medical research material. In this system, documents are grouped and filed alphabetically by related subjects. Information retrieval is very fast because all related information is stored together.

167. **(C)** Balance billing refers to billing the patient for the difference between the usual and the allowed charges. Whether balance billing is acceptable depends on the physician's contract with the insurance company. Most participating providers of an HMO are not allowed to do any balance billing.

168. **(D)** *Physicians' Current Procedural Terminology* (CPT) is a procedural code book using a numerical system updated annually by the American Medical Association.

169. **(C)** Vertical file cabinets are the least efficient type of cabinet because half of the filing time goes into opening and closing drawers.

170. **(A)** The "withhold" is the portion of the monthly capitation payment to physicians retained by an HMO until the end of the year to create an incentive for efficient care. If the physician exceeds the utilization norms, he or she will not receive this portion.

171. **(E)** In a network, a common connection point for the devices containing ports is called a hub. Hubs are often used to connect segments of a local-area network (LAN) and contain multiple ports. They allow information to be shared among LAN users.

172. **(D)** The usual, customary, and reasonable fee is determined by comparing the actual fee charge by physicians in the same geographical area and specialty.

173. **(B)** With increased deductibles and coinsurance, the point-of-service option was added to some HMO plans to allow patients to choose physicians outside of the regular HMO network.

174. **(C)** *Reflecting* means encouraging patients to think through and answer their own questions and concerns.

175. **(E)** When using ICD-9-CM codes, claim denials will occur when the fourth and fifth digits are omitted. It is essential to make sure that the complete set of digits is used so that claims are processed efficiently.

176. **(B)** Movable file units allow easy access to large record systems and require less space than either the vertical or lateral (open-shelf) files.

177. **(B)** *Regression* is the term used when a patient unconsciously returns to more infantile thoughts or behaviors.

178. **(A)** A server is a single computer that can be accessed by other computers over a network.

179. **(E)** Tickler files are chronological files used as reminders that something needs to be done on a certain date.

180. **(E)** The postal abbreviation for *Plaza* is *PLZ*.

181. **(C)** Mumbling is a type of negative communication. Other examples of negative communication include smiling artificially, speaking too quickly, and exhibiting a less-than-friendly attitude.

182. **(C)** An inquiry about a bill is an administrative-type call a medical assistant should handle.

183. **(B)** DEERS stands for the Department of Defense's Defense Enrollment Eligibility Reporting System.

184. **(D)** Copies of all bills and order forms for supplies should be kept on file for 10 years in case the practice is audited by the IRS.

185. **(C)** CHAMPVA or TRICARE are primary providers. Medicaid is always a secondary provider. Therefore, claims must be filed with CHAMPVA first, and only then with Medicaid.

186. **(B)** Preferred provider organizations can offer the highest level of benefits to enrollees when they obtain services from a physician, hospital, or other health provider.

187. **(C)** The CMS-1500 is divided into two main sections. Blanks 1 through 13 are used for patient and insured information. Blanks 14 through 33 are used for the physician or supplier information.

188. **(E)** *Annotate* means you must highlight key points of the letter and write comments in the margins.

189. **(C)** The *International Classification of Diseases, 9th Revision, Clinical Modification* (ICD-9-CM) is a three-volume system for classifying diseases and surgical procedures.

190. **(A)** CPT codes are five-digit numbers, organized into six sections: Evaluation and Management, Anesthesiology, Surgery, Radiology, Pathology and Laboratory, and Medicine. To find the correct procedure codes using the CPT, look for the service in the index.

191. **(B)** A W-4 form must be completed at the time of hiring.

192. **(D)** A denied Medicare charge can be reconsidered only within 6 months after denial.

193. **(B)** Consulting physicians should always be transferred to the physician.

194. **(E)** The medical assistant may sign claim forms to insurance carriers and other vendors.

195. **(C)** Form 941 must be filed to report employers' quarterly federal tax returns.

196. **(D)** The annual deductible for recipients of Medicare Part B benefits is $100. This means that a patient covered by this plan has to pay $100 per calendar year for medical services that are covered under Medicare Part B. Once the patient pays the deductible, all other costs are paid by the plan.

197. **(A)** Patients who are poor, uninsured, underinsured, or elderly and on a limited income are known as hardship cases. Collecting on these types of accounts is one of the most common collection problems in health care. Physicians sometimes decide to treat hardship cases for a reduced fee or for free.

198. **(A)** The "brain" of the computer is also called the central processing unit, or CPU.

199. **(A)** The body of a letter begins two lines below the salutation or subject line. It is single spaced with double spaces between paragraphs. Leave an extra line above and below a list and indent each item on the list five spaces from the margin.

200. **(B)** Notations include such information as the number and type of enclosures and the names of other people who receive copies of the letter. The notation is typed two lines below the signature or identification line.

201. **(B)** The accounts receivable balance represents the debit balance.

202. **(A)** The subscriber is the principal. A beneficiary is the person who receives the benefits. The terms *insurer* and *coordinator* are not used.

203. **(B)** A single-entry account is an account with only one charge, as, for example, when a vacationer consults a physician for illness.

204. **(C)** The magnetic ink character recognition code (MICR code) appears on the bottom of a check and consists of numbers and characters printed in magnetic ink.

205. **(D)** Government-sponsored insurance coverage for eligible individuals includes Medicare, Medicaid, TRICARE, and CHAMPVA.

206. **(C)** The abbreviation of *NS* indicates "no-show patient."

207. **(C)** An accounts receivable measures how fast outstanding accounts are being paid. The formula for figuring out the accounts receivable ratio is to divide the current accounts receivable balance by the average gross monthly charges.

208. **(B)** When rebilling is necessary, make a copy of the original claim form submitted and write *SECOND BILLING* in red letters at the top. Reasons to rebill include to correct a mistake in billing, to detail charges to receive maximum reimbursement, to respond to a carrier's request and supply missing information, or to correct any wrong diagnosis or procedure codes.

209. **(D)** Color coding filing breaks the alphabet up into five different colors: red, yellow, green, blue, and purple. The last color, purple, covers the letters from R through Z.

210. **(E)** A scanner is a device that can convert printed matter and images to information that can be interpreted by the computer.

211. **(C)** Handling instructions should be placed three lines below the return address.

212. **(E)** You should always completely write out the date.

213. **(A)** The date is usually keyed on line 15, or two or three lines below the letterhead.

214. **(C)** *Expressway* is abbreviated as *EXPY*.

215. **(B)** A new patient must be familiar with office hours and payment requirements.

216. **(D)** You can divide according to pronunciation, compound words between the two words, hyphenated compound words at the hyphen, after a prefix, before a suffix, between two consonants that appear between vowels, and being -*ing* unless the last consonant id doubled, in which case divide before the second consonant. Do not divide such suffixes as -*sion*, -*tial*, and -*gion*. Also do not divide a word so that only one letter is left on a line.

217. **(A)** *Retrieving* is the term used when computer software obtains a saved file. This process is also sometimes referred to as *accessing*.

218. **(B)** A full-block letter is typed with all the lines flush left. It is quick and easy to write. It is often used in medical practices.

219. **(A)** A restrictive endorsement includes the words *For deposit only*, making it impossible for anyone other than the bank to cash the check.

220. **(D)** Under a staff model HMO, the physicians are employees of the HMO and work full time seeing member patients. In this type of HMO, a primary care physician is assigned as the gatekeeper for patients.

221. **(B)** The body of the letter should be single-spaced. Between paragraphs, use double spacing. For multipage letters, use letterhead only for the first page and blank quality bond paper for the second page. The second page should contains the name of the addressee, page number, date, and subject in the header.

222. **(E)** The most common insurance claim form is the CMS-1500.

223. **(C)** The Num Lock key must be pressed to activate the calculator function on a computer keyboard. When that key is not pressed, the calculator pad key area functions to move the cursor around the screen and cannot perform any calculations.

224. **(A)** A participating provider is not allowed to charge the patient for any differences between the actual charges and allowed charge. The patient is responsible for the copayment, coinsurance, and deductible.

225. **(C)** The Labor Standards Act requires that you should keep employee health records on file for 3 years.

226. **(E)** *Purging* is the process of removing outdated data from computer disks or drives. Purging essentially erases data, completely removing outdated files from the disk or drive.

227. **(B)** Mimicking the behavior of another person in order to cope with feelings of inadequacy is referred to as identification. Identification is a common defense mechanism.

228. **(D)** The following proofreaders' mark means "to center:"][.

229. **(C)** In patient charting, *Rx* is the abbreviation used to note a prescription.

230. **(D)** Express Mail, which is offered by the United States Postal Service, guarantees overnight delivery. It is always a good idea to verify when your package will arrive by asking the postal clerk.

231. **(E)** Diseases within the Tabular List of the ICD-9-CM are organized by body system.

232. **(C)** The most common pointing device for a computer is the mouse. It is favored by the majority of computer users worldwide.

233. **(C)** The postal abbreviation for North Carolina is *NC*. The other choices stand for the following states: *ND* is the abbreviation for North Dakota and *NH* for New Hampshire. *NA* and *NB* are not USPS state abbreviations.

234. **(D)** According to OSHA, an exposure control plan must be reviewed and updated every 12 months.

235. **(A)** The Tab key is used to move the cursor to a preset position. The user can instruct the computer to set tab stops at any point across the page that is being created.

236. **(E)** In the CPT, 99201 is the code that refers to *Evaluation and Management.*

237. **(C)** An itinerary is a detailed trip outline that includes the trip location, date of arrival, and a confirmation of hotel reservations.

238. **(A)** The most appropriate business letter closure for a medical office is "Sincerely yours." The other choices may be acceptable in some offices, but "Sincerely yours" is considered the most appropriate business letter closure overall.

239. **(C)** An agenda is a list of the specific items to be discussed at a meeting.

240. **(A)** An out guide should replace a medical record if it has been temporarily removed. When all or part of a file is removed, an out guide is put in its place.

241. **(D)** CPT codes are organized into six sections: (1) physician services, (2) physical and occupational therapy services, (3) radiological procedures, (4) clinical laboratory tests, (5) other medical diagnostic procedures, and (6) hearing and vision services.

242. **(B)** The patient's name is essential to organizing and filing charts in all types of filing systems.

243. **(A)** Narcotics should be inventoried daily to ensure that they are not removed by any person who is not authorized to do so.

244. **(D)** The term *assets* refers to accounts receivable. *Current assets* refers to cash and other assets that can be sold or otherwise converted to cash within a 12-month period.

245. **(C)** The term *boot* refers to turning on a computer. The booting sequence of start-up commands is stored inside the computer.

246. **(D)** If you are processing payroll, gross wages should be calculated first. Gross wages is the amount earned by each employee before taxes (withholding) are deducted.

247. **(C)** The city of Phoenix is located in Arizona. Therefore, the correct postal abbreviation is *AZ*. The other choices stand for the following states: *AK* is the abbreviation for Alaska, *AR* for Arkansas, *AL* for Alabama, and *NM* for New Mexico.

248. **(A)** A W-2 form is filed with an employee's state income tax return.

249. **(D)** The Fair Debt Collection Practices Act protects debtors from harassment.

250. **(C)** The most important information that you must record when scheduling an appointment for a patient is the patient's telephone number.

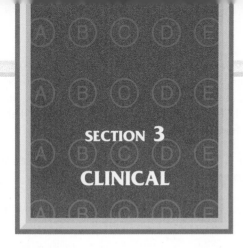

MEDICAL ASSISTING KNOWLEDGE

Self-Evaluation Answers and Rationales

Here you'll find the answers to the test on General Medical Assisting Knowledge in Part 2 on p. 518. Check your answers and note which questions you missed. Study the rationales for any questions you feel you had difficulty with and if you need more review, go back to the appropriate section in the chapters.

1. **(C)** If an injury occurs, you must take the following actions: Wash your hands, cover the injury, report and document the injury, and get the injury treated. It is not necessary to send the report to the local health department.

2. **(C)** Failure to comply with OSHA standards could result in a maximum penalty of $7,000 for the first violation.

3. **(B)** Tetracyclines are a group of broad-spectrum bacteriostatic antibiotics that are effective against both gram-negative and gram-positive micro-organisms. Tetracyclines inhibit protein synthesis in bacterial cells. Examples are Aureomycin®, Vibramycin®, and Achromycin®. Tetracyclines are commonly used in the treatment of urethritis, cholera, lower respiratory tract infections, meningitis, rickettsiae, and Lyme disease.

4. **(A)** Hepatitis B virus is the main blood-borne hazard for health-care workers.

5. **(B)** Infected pregnant women can pass the spirochete of syphilis, HIV, and HBV to their babies during pregnancy or delivery.

6. **(B)** The chain of infection begins with the infectious agent. To prevent the spread of any infectious disease, the chain must be interrupted at any level, especially in transmission to the reservoir host.

7. **(D)** The supine position is also called the recumbent position.

8. **(B)** Antihypertensive drugs treat high blood pressure or hypertension. Vasodilators, calcium antagonists (e.g., diltiazem and varapamil), sympathetic blocking drugs (e.g., clonidine), and thiazides are a few types of antihypertensive drugs.

9. **(D)** Before and after each patient is examined or treated, the medical assistant should use the correct technique to wash his/her hands. Hand washing is the most effective method to prevent the spread of infection from one person to another.

10. **(B)** Steam under pressure in the autoclave is the best method of sterilization because it kills all pathogens. Pressurized steam is fast, convenient, and dependable.

11. **(A)** A rad is a measurement of the actual absorbed dose of radiation.

12. **(C)** A three-point gait is used by patients who can bear full weight on one leg and no weight on the other.

13. **(E)** An upper gastrointestinal (GI) series uses the oral administration of a barium sulfate suspension to diagnose ulcers, tumors, and other abnormalities of the esophagus, stomach, and duodenum. Therefore, the upper part of the GI tract must be emptied, which requires that the patient fast for 12 hours prior to the test.

14. **(C)** Treatment for Lyme disease includes tetracycline or amozicillin/probenecid for early symptoms. The drug of choice for candidiasis is fluconazole and for trichomoniasis it is metronidazole. Urinary and respiratory infections are treated with cephalosporin.

15. **(B)** To calculate the amount of skin surface burned on an adult, you should use the rule of nines. Mr. Brown's chest, abdomen, and upper back each accounts for approximately 9% of the skin surface; 9% × 3 = 27%. His genital area counts as 1%. The total comes to 28%.

16. **(C)** Lacerations are cuts with jagged edges.

17. **(C)** The majority of accidental poisonings occur at home to children under the age of 5 years.

18. **(C)** The abbreviation *prn* means *as needed*.

19. **(B)** The AIDS virus infection cycle has four stages: acute HIV infection, asymptomatic latency period, AIDS-related complex, and full-blown AIDS.

20. **(C)** Pharmacology is the study of the origin, nature, chemistry, effects, and uses of drugs. Pharmacy is the art of compounding, preparing, dispensing, and properly using drugs. Pharmacognosy is the branch of pharmacology dealing with natural drugs. Posology is the study of the amount of a drug that is required to produce therapeutic effects. Pharmacodynamics is the study of the mechanisms of actions of drugs on living organisms.

21. **(B)** In both the proctologic and the jackknife position, the hips of the patient are flexed at a 90-degree angle. In the proctologic position, the patient lies face down with both the torso and the legs lowered. In the jackknife position, the patient lies face up with both the torso and the legs raised.

22. **(B)** Tachycardia, a condition in which the heart contracts at a rate greater than 100 times per minute, is a sign of shock. This condition acts to increase the amount of oxygen delivered to the cells by increasing the blood circulation rate through the vessels.

23. **(C)** A barium swallow is also called an upper GI series.

24. **(D)** Yeast infections may be caused by the organism *Candida albicans*, which is normally present in the mucous membranes of the vagina.

25. **(D)** Cryosurgery can destroy abnormal cells by freezing.

26. **(A)** An example of an emulsion is cod liver oil, which is a mixture of oils in water.

27. **(A)** In the metric system, 1000 micrograms equal one milligram.

28. **(C)** The T wave represents the recovery of the ventricles.

29. **(A)** A placebo has no pharmacological activity. A teratogen is any agent that interferes with normal prenatal development, causing the formation of one or more developmental abnormalities in the fetus. Synergism is the joint action of agents in which their combined effect is greater than the sum of their individual effects.

30. **(E)** In administering a 3-hour glucose test to an adult, 100 grams of glucose is included in the liquid mixture given to the patient. After fasting the night before the test, the patient drinks the liquid. The patient's blood and urine are then collected periodically for up to 6 hours. This test is most often used to assist in the diagnosis of diabetes or other disorders that affect carbohydrate metabolism.

31. **(B)** Thyroxine is classified as a replacement drug because it is used when the thyroid gland does not properly manufacture the correct amounts of this substance.

32. **(E)** Antipruritics are used to relieve itching. Antipruritic agents include topical anesthetics, corticosteroids, and antihistamines.

33. **(C)** A tonometer is used to examine the pressure of the eyes. By applying force, it determines the resistance of the eyeball to indentation.

34. **(D)** Bananas are an excellent source of potassium, a nutrient that is important in glycogen formation, protein synthesis, and correcting imbalances of acid-base metabolism.

35. **(B)** Lomotil® is a trademark for an antidiarrheal drug, classified as a Schedule V drug with low abuse potential and accepted medical use. Diazepam and Talwin® are examples of Schedule IV drugs, amphetamine is listed in Schedule II, and heroin is classified as a Schedule I drug. Talwin® is a schedule IV drug.

36. **(E)** Casts are microscopic structures in urine that are composed of protein. These tiny structures are formed by deposits of minerals or other substances on the walls of renal tubules, bronchioles, or other organs.

37. **(A)** On the ECG, the P, R, T, and U waves curve upward. The Q and S waves curve downward.

38. **(B)** One heartbeat produces a pattern of waves designated P, Q, R, S, T, and sometimes U.

39. **(C)** The preparation for an MRI includes asking the patient about possible allergies to contrast media, iodine, or shellfish. You should also ask whether any internal metallic materials are present, and the patient should avoid caffeine for 4 hours before the examination.

40. **(A)** An MRI does not use radiation to produce images. Magnetic resonance imaging is based on the resonance of atomic nuclei in a strong magnetic field, which means that this type of study uses radiofrequencies instead of ionizing radiation to produce images.

41. **(C)** The stage is the flat surface of a microscope that holds the slide for viewing. In order to aid viewing, light is projected through the slide when it is positioned on the stage.

42. **(D)** Renal function is assessed by measuring the serum levels of urea nitrogen in the blood. These levels are directly related to the metabolic function of the liver and the excretory function of the kidneys.

43. **(B)** The angle of insertion of a needle for intradermal injections is 15 degrees.

44. **(B)** Spirometry tests measure the function of the respiratory system. A spirometer measures and records the volume of air that is inhaled and exhaled.

45. **(A)** An agent that relieves symptoms without curing the disease is referred to as being palliative. Types of palliative treatment include narcotics to dull pain, a colostomy to bypass further bowel problems, and removing dead tissue in a patient whose cancer is progressing to multiple locations in the body.

46. **(D)** Polyphagia indicates increased appetite as well as excessive uncontrolled eating. It is also called hyperphagia.

47. **(B)** Echocardiography is recorded on paper. It is obtained by ultrasound (not by stethoscope). It is used to evaluate the inner structures of the heart and can indicate such conditions as fluid accumulation.

48. **(D)** CT is a radiographic technique that produces a film representing a detailed cross-section of tissue structure.

49. **(B)** The respiration rate is included in a patient's vital signs. The normal rate of respirations for adults is between 12 and 24 breaths per minute.

50. **(A)** 0.5 g is equivalent to 500 mg. This calculation is based on the fact that 1 g = 1000 mg.

51. **(D)** Total hand washing time should be approximately 10 minutes.

52. **(B)** Kaposi's sarcoma is a malignancy of the skin and lymph nodes that often occurs in AIDS patients. It is the most common HIV-related cancer.

53. **(A)** Destruction of all living microorganisms by specific means is called sterilization.

54. **(A)** *Decontamination* is a term used by OSHA to describe the use of physical or chemical means to remove, inactivate, or destroy blood-borne pathogens on a surface or item to the point where they are no longer capable of transmitting infection.

55. **(E)** When performing a venipuncture, it is necessary to use a tourniquet. The tourniquet is wrapped around the arm proximal to the intended site of the puncture—usually on the outside of the forearm.

56. **(B)** Radiation exposure badges are also called dosimeters.

57. **(A)** When sending a specimen for a throat culture to an outside laboratory, a transport medium should be used. The fragile nature of many pathogens means that they are vulnerable to drying as well as to temperature changes. These specimens are usually placed in a liquid transport medium immediately after sampling them from the patient so that they will be unharmed and ready for laboratory testing.

58. **(B)** Atrial kick occurs when blood is pushed into the ventricles as a result of atrial contraction.

59. **(C)** Standard leads are also called bipolar leads because they monitor two electrodes. Leads I, II, and III are standard or bipolar leads.

60. **(D)** Range of motion is the degree to which a joint is able to move.

61. **(B)** Gait is the style of walking.

62. **(C)** A patient lying on his or her back with lower legs supported by the extended foot rest is in the supine position. It is also called the dorsal decubitus or dorsal recumbent position.

63. **(D)** Glucose in the urine may represent hyperglycemia. This condition is most frequently associated with diabetes mellitus.

64. **(B)** Variation in the shape of erythrocytes is called poikilocytosis.

65. **(E)** A special container made of gelatin that is sized for a single dose is called a capsule. Capsules are intended to be swallowed, usually with a glass of water.

66. **(C)** The Drug Enforcement Administration is the part of the federal government that enforces regulations that control the import or export of narcotic drugs and certain other substances. It also controls the trafficking of these substances across state lines.

67. **(B)** Electrocardiography requires six limb leads, three of which are standard (bipolar) and three of which are augmented.

68. **(A)** The normal range of the specific gravity of urine is between 1.010 and 1.030.

69. **(E)** Pneumococcal polysaccharide vaccine may be administered intramuscularly or subcutaneously to children who are at risk for and to adolescents who have chronic illnesses with increased risk for pneumococcal disease.

70. **(E)** Fasting specimens are preferred for a triglycerides test. This test detects the levels of fats within the bloodstream.

71. **(E)** The procedure for obtaining specimens from infected wounds is similar to that of a throat culture.

72. **(C)** There are three types of sphygmomanometers: mercury, aneroid, and electronic. The mercury type is the most accurate.

73. **(A)** In the dorsal recumbent position, the patient lies face up with the knees flexed and the feet flat on the table.

74. **(B)** The difference between systolic and diastolic blood pressure is called the pulse pressure. The range is normally between 30 mm Hg and 50 mm Hg.

75. **(D)** Treatment is abbreviated as *Tx* or *Tr. Rx* is commonly used to mean "prescription"; it is an abbreviation of the Latin verb *recipe*, which means "take."

76. **(A)** The temporal artery is located in the temple area of the skull. It is seldom used to detect a pulse.

77. **(E)** Latex gloves are the most commonly used in the medical office.

78. **(B)** Blood stasis is lack of circulation due to a stoppage of blood flow.

79. **(E)** Tests to measure cholesterol in the blood are done with serum or plasma.

80. **(D)** A patient who has tuberculosis should use a mask. This condition is generally transmitted by the inhalation or ingestion of infected droplets.

81. **(C)** Instruments are considered sterile for 21 to 30 days.

82. **(C)** Splinter forceps have sharp points that are useful in removing foreign objects.

83. **(D)** In this example, 28 capsules of a 250-mg dose of erythromycin should be dispensed to the patient. The formula is the following: 28 × 250 mg = 7000 mg, which is the same total amount as the original prescription (500 mg twice a day for 7 days: 500 × 2 × 7 = 7000 mg total).

84. **(B)** When testing for pregnancy, human chorionic gonadotropin may appear in the urine. This hormone is secreted by placental trophoblastic cells and indicates pregnancy.

85. **(D)** Comminuted bone fractures consist of crushed or splintered bones. Comminuted fractures often consist of bones that are broken in several places or shattered into numerous fragments.

86. **(C)** The aspiration of a bursa sac requires surgical asepsis. A bursa sac is a fibrous sac between certain tendons and the bones beneath them; this sac is lined with a membrane that secretes synovial fluid. Surgical asepsis is required because of the possible spread of pathogens via the synovial fluid.

87. **(D)** The presence of a U wave that appears after the T wave may be due to slow recovery of the Purkinje fibers.

88. **(D)** Hemoglobin S is found in sickle cell anemia and also in sickle cell trait.

89. **(B)** The abbreviation *Rx* should appear on a written prescription.

90. **(E)** The first step in responding to an emergency is to remain calm. Remaining calm will allow you to be able to competently perform all other emergency procedures.

91. **(B)** The microorganism *Escherichia coli*, commonly abbreviated as *E. coli*, is the most common cause of urinary tract infections. It is normally present in the intestines and is a serious gram-negative pathogen. Septicemia (blood poisoning) from this microorganism may rapidly result in shock or death.

92. **(B)** A dispensing record for Schedule II drugs must be kept on file for 2 years because of the strong potential for abuse of or addiction to these drugs. Schedule II drugs include morphine, cocaine, pentobarbital, oxycodone, alphaprodine, and methadone.

93. **(C)** A speculum is used to examine the vagina. This instrument is a retractor used to separate the vaginal walls in order to allow for examination of internal structures.

94. **(D)** Emergency pharmaceutical supplies should include epinephrine. This drug is used to treat anaphylaxis, acute bronchial spasm, and nasal congestion and to increase the effectiveness of a local anesthetic.

95. **(D)** An intramuscular injection of antibiotics is the most appropriate type of injection for streptococcal pharyngitis. Penicillin G benzanthine or erythromycin are commonly injected intramuscularly.

96. **(B)** Melena is an abnormal black tarry stool that contains digested blood.

97. **(C)** Stool specimens are most appropriate for detecting *Giardia lamblia*. This protozoan causes giardiasis, which results in diarrhea.

98. **(B)** Children 2 years of age and older should have annual checkups.

99. **(E)** Alpha-fetoprotein testing from amniotic fluid is used for early diagnosis of fetal neural tube defects and anencephaly.

100. **(D)** The coarse adjustment on a compound microscope is used to focus the image when using the high-power objective (45×).

101. **(E)** The random specimen is the most common method of urine collection.

102. **(D)** The DEA requires physicians to renew their registration every 3 years; to keep records for 2 years about who was given what drug, what dosage, on what date, and for what reason; to keep inventory; and to log the disposal of drugs with a witness present.

103. **(A)** The best time to perform a breast self-examination is immediately after the menstrual period is completed. At this time, the breasts are less tender and less swollen. Early diagnosis greatly improves the cure rate in cancer of the breast.

104. **(C)** In preparation for mammography, patients should avoid caffeine for a week and also avoid the use of powder, deodorant, or perfume on the underarm area or breast before the examination.

105. **(C)** To prevent cell growth in a malignant tumor, a physician must use antineoplastic agents. These agents control or kill cancer cells and are generally more damaging to dividing cells than to resting cells.

106. **(D)** Adolescents who are at increased risk for complications caused by influenza or who have contact with persons at increased risk for these complications can receive an annual influenza vaccine (in the period from September through December).

107. **(D)** A four-point crutch gait is a slow gait used by patients who can bear weight on both legs.

108. **(B)** In phlebotomy, the needle is inserted into the vein at approximately a 15-degree angle.

109. **(C)** The inscription lists the names and quantities of the ingredients. The superscription includes the patient's name, address, date, and the symbol *Rx*. The subscription gives directions to patients. The drug label is not part of the prescription.

110. **(D)** The medical assistant may be responsible for administering the Ishihara color vision acuity test.

111. **(B)** Schedule II drugs have high abuse potential, but have some accepted medical use. Cocaine is such a drug. Prescriptions for Schedule II drugs cannot be refilled without a new prescription from the physician.

112. **(E)** Induration, which is the hardening of the skin caused by inflammation (a reaction to the tuberculin protein derivative), indicates a positive result of a tuberculin test.

113. **(B)** Serological tests are performed on samples that do not contain additives, the color code for which is red.

114. **(C)** Trendelenburg's position is the "shock position."

115. **(C)** Dislocation is the displacement of bones at a joint.

116. **(A)** The use of the Z-track method prevents the deposited iron from seeping back into the skin layers.

117. **(B)** HCG levels will be lower in an ectopic pregnancy.

118. **(D)** The rectum is examined in the knee-chest (genupectoral) position for both males and females.

119. **(B)** Pathogens are organisms that cause disease.

120. **(B)** The destruction of pathogens by physical or chemical means is called disinfection. This process causes pathogens to become inactive.

121. **(C)** Hematemesis should be recorded under the respiratory system. Patients with this condition vomit bright red blood, which indicates rapid upper GI bleeding (commonly associated with esophageal dilation of the veins, arteries, or lymphatic vessels) or a peptic ulcer.

122. **(D)** Anorectic drugs decrease appetite. Some amphetamines have anorectic effects.

123. **(C)** The process of listening for sounds within the body is called auscultation. It is done to evaluate the condition of the heart, blood vessels, lungs, pleura, intestines, or other organs, or to detect fetal heart sounds.

124. **(A)** For injection of the vastus lateralis site, the patient may be in the recumbent position.

125. **(D)** Triglycerides are simple fat compounds consisting of three molecules of fatty acid. Measuring triglyceride levels in the blood requires fasting specimens.

126. **(A)** Colposcopy is the examination of the vagina and cervix with an optical magnifying instrument. It is commonly performed after a Pap smear to obtain biopsy specimens of the cervix.

127. **(B)** Tonometers are instruments for measuring tension or pressure of the intraocular region. They are used for the detection of glaucoma.

128. **(D)** The standing position is used for musculoskeletal, neurological, and peripheral vascular system examinations.

129. **(B)** Ear irrigation is the flushing of the ear canal to remove impacted cerumen, to relieve inflammation, or to remove a foreign body.

130. **(D)** The Mantoux tuberculin test requires the use of a short needle with a gauge of 26 to 27.

131. **(A)** A score of 10 or above indicates average color vision. A score of less than 7 may indicate color vision deficiency.

132. **(C)** Tomography is the procedure performed to view a cross-section of an organ.

133. **(B)** Electrocardiograms are most commonly recorded at 15 mm per second. They depict a graphic (paper) record of the heart's electrical conduction.

134. **(C)** A scalpel is used to drain an abscess. An abscess, which is a cavity containing pus and surrounded by inflamed tissue, may form as a result of localized infection.

135. **(D)** Schedule IV drugs have low abuse potential and an accepted medical use. They may be refilled five times in 6 months when authorized by a physician. Examples of Schedule IV drugs include chloral, hydrate, diazepam, and alprazolam.

136. **(C)** The hub, shaft, lumen, point, and bevel are parts of a needle. The flange (rim) is a part of the syringe.

137. **(B)** Sertraline (Zoloft®) is most appropriate for a patient with depression. This drug is an SSRI, a type of antidepressant that helps correct the chemical imbalance of serotonin in the brain.

138. **(E)** The two most important components of hand washing are running water and friction. The ideal method involves warm water and more than 2 minutes of vigorous scrubbing. The combination of friction and warm water is important in removing bacteria.

139. **(E)** Cholecystectomy means surgical removal of the gallbladder.

140. **(C)** In a normal adult, the ratio of respirations to pulse rate is 1:6. The average rate of adult respiration is 12 to 24 per minute, and the average pulse rate of adults is 60 to 80 per minute.

141. **(B)** The angle of insertion for performing tuberculin tests is 15 degrees, almost parallel to the skin surface.

142. **(E)** Wrapped items autoclaved with steam require 30 pounds of pressure at 132°C (270°F) for 20 minutes. Unwrapped items require only 10 minutes of autoclaving, which is known as flashing.

143. **(E)** Laparoscopy is the examination of the abdominal cavity with a laparoscope through one or more small incisions in the abdominal wall. A general anesthetic is used.

144. **(E)** In testing for candidiasis, vaginal specimens should be mixed with potassium hydroxide. Potassium hydroxide has many uses as an alkalinizing agent, including preparing clinical specimens for examination.

145. **(D)** The femoral artery is most commonly used to monitor lower limb circulation. It is palpated in the groin.

146. **(C)** A contrast bath is actually two baths, one filled with hot water and the other with cold water. The patient quickly moves the affected body part from one to the other.

147. **(D)** In the distance vision acuity test, which is usually given with the Snellen chart, the distance between the patient and the chart should be 20 feet.

148. **(C)** Sphygmomanometers are the instruments used to measure blood pressure. A manometer is an instrument used to measure the pressure of a liquid or a gas.

149. **(A)** The abbreviation *q2h* is short for *quaque secunda hora*, meaning "every second hour." The abbreviation *qid* (for *quater in die*) means "four times a day." The abbreviation *qod* stands for "every other day."

150. **(C)** Date of birth is considered demographic data. Demographics are used to arrive at standards on which many different business functions are based, including insurance packages.

151. **(B)** Cryotherapy is treatment using dry cold or wet cold applications to prevent swelling, to control bleeding, and to reduce inflammation.

152. **(C)** The S-T segment, which connects the end of the QRS complex with the beginning of the T wave, represents the time between contraction of the ventricles and recovery.

153. **(E)** A sweet and fruity odor in urine may indicate the presence of ketones. This can signify an extensive breakdown of fats caused by faulty carbohydrate metabolism, which occurs primarily as a complication of diabetes mellitus.

154. **(B)** Suture material is also called ligature.

155. **(C)** Tympanic thermometers can be used with uncooperative patients of any age. They measure the temperature of the tympanic membrane of the ear by detecting infrared radiation from the tissue.

156. **(D)** Fluidotherapy is a relatively new technique in which the patient places the hand or foot in a container of glass beads that are heated and agitated with hot air.

157. **(B)** Nonabsorbable sutures range in thickness from size 11-0 to size 7-0.

158. **(C)** Nicotine and nitroglycerin patches deliver medication by the transdermal route. The drug is absorbed continuously through the skin and enters the bloodstream directly.

159. **(D)** Death rates from HIV infections have been declining in the United States, mostly as a result of antiretroviral therapy.

160. **(E)** In the prone position, the patient lies face down. This position is used for examination of the back and feet. It is not appropriate for patients who are obese, pregnant (late stage), or elderly or who have difficulties of the respiratory system.

161. **(B)** Abrasions are wounds in which the outer layers of the skin are rubbed off, resulting in an oozing of blood from ruptured capillaries.

162. **(D)** Antiemetics control nausea, vomiting, and motion sickness. Antihidrotics prevent or decrease perspiration. Anticonvulsants prevent or relieve convulsions. Vasodilators relax and dilate blood vessels. Sedatives have a soothing, relaxing effect.

163. **(C)** The vastus lateralis muscle in the thigh is the preferred injection site for infants and children younger than 3 years of age.

164. **(E)** Bacitracin is used in cultures to give an early indication of the presence of group A streptococci.

165. **(B)** Hyperlipidemia may give plasma or serum a milky, or turbid, appearance.

166. **(C)** The end result of severe hyperglycemia is the development of diabetic coma. Symptoms are rapid breathing, dry skin, acetone breath, and confusion.

167. **(C)** Hemolysis is the breakdown of red blood cells and the accompanying release of hemoglobin that occurs normally at the end of the life span of the cells. In the laboratory, hemolysis sometimes causes plasma to become pink or red in color.

168. **(B)** A mucous membrane represents the means of exit in the chain of infection transmission. Mucous membranes line cavities or canals of the body that are open to the outside, such as the linings of the mouth, respiratory passages, and the GI tract.

169. **(C)** Lidocaine (Xylocaine®) 1% is most commonly used for local anesthesia that is injected. The advantages of using local anesthesia include low cost, ease of administration, low toxicity, and rapid recovery.

170. **(C)** Cardiomalacia is the softening of the heart.

171. **(A)** BCG vaccination is not recommended for children infected with HIV.

172. **(D)** Cystoscopy is the examination of the bladder by visualization and inspection with a special instrument called a cystoscope.

173. **(C)** OSHA regulations mandate training within 90 days of the effective date of assignment and annually thereafter.

174. **(C)** The appropriate medium for throat cultures (to detect streptococcus) is blood agar.

175. **(A)** Heme (part of hemoglobin) can be responsible for changing the color of serum to green.

176. **(D)** A loss of 25% to 40% of a patient's total blood volume can be life-threatening or fatal.

177. **(C)** In sensitivity testing, a clear zone around the disk indicates that the antimicrobial agent is effective.

178. **(D)** Stroking is the most common massage modality used in the medical office.

179. **(A)** In preparation for cholecystography, the oral contrast medium should be taken about 2 hours after dinner.

180. **(E)** According to the USDA's Food Guide Pyramid, 6 to 11 servings of bread, rice, and pasta should be consumed daily. This chart was developed in 1992 by the U.S. Department of Agriculture and replaced the chart of the four food groups that had been in use since the 1950s.

181. **(E)** Prefilled syringes are known as cartridges.

182. **(C)** Glucagon is stored on the crash cart to treat patients with insulin shock. Glucagon may be administered orally or parenterally, or as an intramuscular or intravenous injection.

183. **(C)** Specific gravity can be measured with urinometers, reagent strips (dipsticks), and refractometers.

184. **(A)** The patient's skin is the most likely source of contamination during a lumbar puncture. The normal flora of the skin can enter the lumbar puncture site, allowing pathogens to be transferred to the site by errors in aseptic technique.

185. **(E)** Blood-borne pathogens in the office can be destroyed by sodium hypochlorite, the active ingredient in household bleach.

186. **(B)** Tilting the patient's head backward is the most appropriate position during an episode of epistaxis. Epistaxis is bleeding from the nose caused by local irritation of mucous membranes, violent sneezing, fragility of the mucous membrane or of the arterial walls, chronic infection, trauma, hypertension, leukemia, vitamin K deficiency, or scratching the inside of the nose.

187. **(C)** Aspirin impairs the ability of platelets to form aggregates.

188. **(D)** Leads aVR, aVL, and aVF are augmented limb leads.

189. **(C)** Needles used for administering medication commonly range in gauge from 18 to 27.

190. **(A)** Needle biopsy of the breast requires surgical asepsis.

191. **(E)** In Trendelenburg's position, the patient lies on the back with the head lower than the legs. This position is used for abdominal surgery and for patients who are in shock.

192. **(C)** Surgical asepsis must be performed during a lumbar puncture. Strict aseptic technique is used to avoid the possibility of infection, which can result in pain, a change in alertness, leakage of CSF from the puncture site, fever, and urinary retention.

193. **(E)** Autoclaves should be cleaned after each load.

194. **(C)** A prognosis is the likely outcome of a disorder, that is, a prediction of the probable course of a disease in an individual and the chances of recovery.

195. **(D)** PET involves injecting isotopes combined with other substances, such as glucose. The positrons that are emitted are processed by a computer and displayed on a screen. This technique is useful for diagnosis of brain-related conditions, such as epilepsy and Parkinson's disease.

196. **(D)** The carotid artery is the best location to take a pulse during an emergency. It is easily accessible and seldom causes any discomfort to the patient.

197. **(E)** Xeroradiography, also called xerography, produces images electrically, permits shorter exposure times, and requires less radiation than standard X-rays.

198. **(B)** Hypodermic syringes are available in 2-, 2.5-, 3-, and 5-cc sizes. They are commonly used to administer intramuscular injections.

199. **(D)** Proctology is a branch of medicine concerned with treating disorders of the colon, rectum, and anus.

200. **(B)** Zephiran® (benzalkonium chloride) is used to detect alcohol levels in blood.

201. **(C)** The Pap smear is used to determine the presence of abnormal or precancerous cells in the cervix and vagina. The patient is instructed not to have intercourse within 48 hours before the test.

202. **(D)** According to recommended childhood immunization schedules, the first MMR vaccination should be given at between 12 and 15 months, and the second should be given at 4 to 6 years of age.

203. **(C)** A drug dose of 120 mg administered in 15 mg tablets would require that 8 tablets be taken.

204. **(A)** The patient's gait means the style of walking.

205. **(E)** Leukocytosis is an abnormal increase in the number of circulating white blood cells.

206. **(D)** An occult blood test is a chemical test or microscopic examination for the presence of blood, especially in the feces.

207. **(A)** A blood collection tube containing EDTA is colored purple.

208. **(E)** Forearm crutches are also called Lofstrand or Canadian crutches.

209. **(D)** In preparation for intravenous pyelography, the patient should have no food or liquids after the preceding midnight. Patients who are to be given a barium enema may have one cup of coffee, tea, or water on the morning of the procedure.

210. **(E)** Albuterol aerosol inhalants are a type of bronchodilator. These substances relax the contractions of the smooth muscle of the bronchioles in order to improve ventilation to the lungs.

211. **(E)** Autoclave indicator tape turns black after autoclaving.

212. **(D)** Measuring the amount of urine output in a 24-hour period is helpful in diagnosing renal disease, dehydration, urinary tract obstructions, and pheochromocytoma.

213. **(D)** The autoclave temperature is most commonly set between 250°F and 270°F.

214. **(B)** Orthostatic hypotension is abnormal, temporary low blood pressure. It occurs when a patient moves rapidly from a lying to a standing position. It is also called postural hypotension.

215. **(D)** Anaphylactic shock, or anaphylaxis, may occur following allergic reactions.

216. **(C)** Tubes coded red contain no additive. They are used for blood chemistries, AIDS antibody tests, viral studies, serological tests, and blood typing.

217. **(E)** A centrifuge is a laboratory machine used to separate particles of different densities within a liquid by spinning them at very high speeds.

218. **(E)** Viruses can be seen only with an electron microscope. They are the smallest microorganisms.

219. **(D)** Drugs with low abuse potential that have an accepted medical use are classified as Schedule IV drugs.

220. **(A)** Studies have shown that a regimen of one dose of HRIG and five doses of HDCV over a 28-day period is safe and effective against rabies.

221. **(D)** Lens paper may be used to clean microscope lenses.

222. **(D)** OSHA regulations require hepatitis B vaccination for all health-care employees who are at risk.

223. **(B)** The radial artery is the most commonly used site for measuring the pulse rate.

224. **(A)** Formalin is a diluted solution of formaldehyde used to preserve biological specimens.

225. **(B)** Antianxiety drugs depress the central nervous system, analgesics relieve pain, antipruritics relieve itching, and antitussives relieve coughing.

226. **(B)** The tricuspid valve separates the right atrium and the right ventricle, and the mitral valve separates the left atrium and the left ventricle. The septum separates the left and right halves of the heart (each containing one atrium and one ventricle).

227. **(A)** Valproic acid (Depakenel®) is used to treat petit mal epilepsy. Its side effects include nausea, vomiting, tremors, and liver toxicity in young patients.

228. **(D)** The Ishihara test is used to measure color vision acuity.

229. **(D)** Augmented leads are also called unipolar leads.

230. **(A)** Prednisone is prescribed in the treatment of severe inflammation and immunosuppression.

231. **(B)** For blood cultures, tubes coded yellow are used.

232. **(D)** Rifampin is an antibacterial drug prescribed in the treatment of tuberculosis, in meningococcal prophylaxis, and as an antileprotic. Among the more serious adverse reactions to rifampin is liver toxicity. Discoloration of urine, saliva, and sweat and softening of the contact lenses commonly occur.

233. **(B)** Sublingual administration is the placement of a medication under the tongue until it dissolves.

234. **(E)** Hemoptysis is the coughing up of blood from the respiratory tract.

235. **(D)** A baby born to a woman who carries the hepatitis B virus must receive the first vaccination at birth.

236. **(C)** A drug must pass through four basic stages: absorption, distribution, metabolism, and excretion. Absorption is the process by which a drug is brought into circulation. Distribution is the process by which the circulatory system transports drugs to the affected areas. Metabolism is the process by which drugs are broken down into useful by-products by enzymes in the liver. The liver is the main body part involved in metabolism. The kidney is responsible for filtering out the drugs from the blood. Drugs are also excreted by the lungs, the sweat glands, and the intestines.

237. **(A)** Good Samaritan laws permit emergency care on the condition that it is within the scope of competence of the person administering first aid.

238. **(A)** OSHA regulations require that hazard warning labels display a color code. White indicates specific hazards such as radioactivity.

239. **(E)** Buccal administration is the placement of a drug in the mouth between the cheek and gum.

240. **(D)** The color red is most frequently used to designate a biohazardous sharps container. Biohazards include anything that is a potential health risk due to the presence of ionizing radiation or harmful bacteria or viruses.

241. **(A)** Pentazocine (Talwin®) is an opioid analgesic used to relieve severe acute and chronic pain, pain associated with myocardial infarction, posttrauma, cancer, and chronic inflammatory conditions. Other opioid analgesics include codeine, meperidine, morphine, and propoxyphene. Codeine is also an antitussive drug.

242. **(B)** The normal rate (in ESR tests) at which red blood cells fall, often referred to as the sed rate, is 1 mm every 5 minutes.

243. **(B)** Miotic drugs are used to constrict the pupils. These agents are used to treat glaucoma. A commonly used miotic drug is pilocarpine.

244. **(E)** Tolerance is the increasing resistance to the usual effects of an established dosage of a drug as a result of continued use. Dependence is a state of reliance on a drug, either psychological or physiological, that may result in withdrawal symptoms if drug use is discontinued.

245. **(A)** Excessive EDTA may shrink erythrocytes.

246. **(D)** Goniometers are devices used to measure the degree of joint movement.

247. **(D)** Centrally acting skeletal muscle relaxants inhibit skeletal contraction by blocking conduction within the spinal cord.

248. **(C)** Antitussives are most appropriate for a patient with a persistent cough. These drugs act on the central and peripheral nervous systems to suppress the cough reflex.

249. **(B)** The most common gauge range of needles used for venipuncture is 19–20.

250. **(A)** Corticosteroid is the drug of choice for chronic asthma. Other drugs used to treat asthma include metaproterenol (Alussent®) and theophylline.

Credits

Chapter 1

Figures 1.1, 1.2: © Total Care Programming.

Chapter 9

Figures 9.1, 9.7, 9.8: © Terry Wild.

Chapter 10

Figure 10.2: © Cliff Moore.

Chapter 15

Figures 15.2, 15.3: © The McGraw-Hill Companies, Inc./Jill Braaten, photographer; **Figure 15.7:** © David Kelly Crow.

Chapter 16

Figure 16.3: Courtesy of Richmond Products; **Figures 16.4, 16.5:** © Terry Wild; **Figure 16.8:** © David Kelly Crow; **Figures 16.9, 16.10, 16.11, 16.12:** © Cliff Moore.

Chapter 17

Figure 17.1: © David Kelly Crow; **Figure 17.5:** Courtesy of Shirley Zeiberg.

Chapter 21

Figures 21.1a–d: © Martin Rotker.

Chapter 24

Figure 24.4: © Total Care Programming; **Figure 24.16:** © Cliff Moore.

Index

Note: "b" indicates boxed material; "f" indicates a figure; "t" indicates a table.

Frontal plane, 57, 58f
Frostbite, 419
Full-block letter style, 184f
Fungi, 117

G

Gait, 405, 405f
Gallbladder, 75f
Gastritis, 103
Gastroenteritis, 97
Gastrointestinal system. *See* Digestive system
General adaptation syndrome (GAS), 135
General medical assisting knowledge sample
    exam, 472–496
General supplies, 233t
Genital herpes, 105
GERD (gastroesophageal reflux disease), 103
    medication, 337t
GI series, 395t
Glands, 77f, 77t–79t
Glandular secretion, 57t
Golgi apparatus, 54
Goniometry, 406, 406t, 407f
Gonorrhea, 105
Good Samaritan Act, 160
Gram's stain, 114, 463–464
    procedure, 463f
Gram-negative bacteria, 114, 116t
Gram-positive bacteria, 114, 116t
Grief, stages of, 169
Gynecologic/obstetric examination, 303–313

H

Hand washing, aseptic, 124, 292f, 292–293
Hard disk drive, 225
Hardware, computer, 222, 223f
Harvard Healthy Eating Pyramid, 151f
HCPCS (Health-Care Procedure Coding
    System), 277
HDL (high-density lipoprotein), 143
Head injuries, 424
Health and wellness, promotion, 135–136
Health care proxy, 168f, 169
Health insurance plans, 257–258
    government, 258–260
    managed care, 261–262
    private, 260–261
Health-Care Financing Administration
    (HCFA), 277
Heart, 71–72, 72f, 383f
    anatomy and physiology, 383
    conditions and procedures, 388
    ECG, 383–387
    monitoring, 387–388
Heart attack, 425
Heatstroke, 419
Height measurement, 329
Hematology, 439–440
    tests, 449–451
Hemispheres, brain, 64
Hemocytometer, 454, 461f
Hemostats, 317f
Hepatitis, 287–288
Hepatitis A vaccine, 376
Hereditary diseases, 94

Hernia types, 103t
HIPAA (Health Insurance Portability
    and Accountability Act), 164, 165,
    262, 304
    claims processing, 262
HIPPA Privacy Rule, 164, 227, 262
Histology, 56
HIV (human immunodeficiency virus)
    infection, 105–106, 288–289
    antiretroviral drugs, 290t–291t, 346
HMO (Health Maintenance
    Organization), 261
Holter monitor, 387
Honesty, 7–8
Hormone replacement therapy (HRT),
    357–358
Hormones, 77t–79t, 80t
Household measurement system, 365, 368t
Human body
    abdominal regions and quadrants, 57, 59f
    blood, 69–72
    blood vessels, 73
    bone distribution, 60t
    brain, 65f
    cavities, 57, 58t
    cells, 53–55
    chemistry, 53
    digestive system, 75–77
    division planes, 57, 58t
    endocrine system, 77–79
    heart, 72f
    joints, 61f
    lymphatic system, 73–74
    membranes, 57
    microbes in, 118–124
    muscles, 62f, 63t
    nervous system, 63–67
    organization, 53f
    reproductive system, 81–84
    respiratory system, 74–75
    sensory system, 67–69
    skeleton, 60f
    tissues, 56–56
    urinary system, 79–81
Humanistic theory of personality, 131
Hydrotherapy, 408–409
Hypersensitivity, types, 93t
Hypertension, 328
Hyperthermia, 419
Hypertonic solution, 54
Hypodermic syringes, 373
Hypoglycemia, 424
Hypolipidemic drugs, 353
Hypothalamus, 65, 77f, 77t
Hypothermia, 419
Hypotonic solution, 54

I

ICD-9-CM (International Classification
    of Diseases, 9th revision, Clinical
    Modification) codes, 272–275, 272f,
    273t, 274t
Immune system, 92
    microbial disease, 122t
    organs, 94
Immunity, acquisition, 93t

Immunization, 375
    schedule, 375t–376t
Immunodeficiency disorders, 92
Immunohematology, 452
Immunology, 92–94, 440
Impotence, 82, 107
    medication, 358
Incoming calls, 190
Incontinence, 105
Induced vomiting, poisons, 428
Infarction, 92
Infection
    control, 293–294
    cycle of, 123f
    nosocomial, 92, 291
    vectors, 124t
Infectious diseases, 96–97, 116t, 117t
    specimen collection, 461–462
Infectious waste disposal, OSHA
    violations, 295t
Influenza, 97
Inhaled poisons, 429
Injectible drug forms, 340
Injury prevention, 194t
Insect stings, 422
Inspiration, 74
Instruments, physical examination, 306f
Insulin, 357
Insulin shock, 424
Insulin syringe, 373
Insurance
    government health plans, 258–260
    medical terminology, 256–257
    types, 257
Integrity, 7–8
Integumentary system, 58–59. *See also* Skin
    abbreviations, 24t
    burns, 419–421
    combining forms, 23t
    disease and disorders, 97–98
    medications, 338t, 346
    microbial disease, 119t
    terms, 23t–24t
Interpersonal skills, 212
Interviewing, patient, 304
Intestines, 75f, 76
    normal flora, 123t
Intradermal injection, 370, 371f
Intramuscular (IM) injection, 371,
    372f, 374
Ischemia, 92
Isotonic solution, 54
IVP (intravenous pyelography), 397

J

Jock itch (*tinea cruris*), 98
Joints, 60, 61f
Jung, Carl, theories, 131

K

Kaiser Foundation Health Plan, 260
Kidney, 79, 81f, 456f
Kübler-Ross, Elizabeth, stages of death,
    134–135